mjf

Books by Corinne T. Netzer

THE CORINNE T. NETZER ANNUAL CALORIE COUNTER

THE BRAND-NAME CALORIE COUNTER

THE BRAND-NAME CARBOHYDRATE GRAM COUNTER

THE CHOLESTEROL CONTENT OF FOOD

THE COMPLETE BOOK OF FOOD COUNTS

THE CORINNE T. NETZER CALORIE COUNTER

THE CORINNE T. NETZER CARBOHYDRATE GRAM COUNTER

THE CORINNE T. NETZER DIETER'S DIARY

THE CORINNE T. NETZER ENCYCLOPEDIA OF FOOD VALUES

THE CORINNE T. NETZER FAT GRAM COUNTER

THE CORINNE T. NETZER FIBER COUNTER

THE CORINNE T. NETZER LOW-FAT DIARY

THE DIETER'S CALORIE COUNTER

THE COMPLETE BOOK OF VITAMIN & MINERAL COUNTS

THE COMPLETE BOOK OF FOOD COUNTS COOKBOOK SERIES:

100 LOW FAT SMALL MEAL AND SALAD RECIPES

100 LOW FAT VEGETABLE AND LEGUME RECIPES

100 LOW FAT SOUP AND STEW RECIPES

100 LOW FAT PASTA AND GRAIN RECIPES

100 LOW FAT FISH AND SHELLFISH RECIPES

100 LOW FAT CHICKEN AND TURKEY RECIPES

THE COMPLETE BOOK OF
FOOD COUNTS

Fourth Edition

CORINNE T. NETZER

MJF BOOKS

NEW YORK

Published by MJF Books
Fine Communications
Two Lincoln Square
60 West 66th Street
New York, NY 10023

The Complete Book of Food Counts
ISBN 1-56731-213-6

Manufactured in the United States of America on acid-free paper

MJF Books and the MJF colophon are trademarks of Fine Creative Media, Inc.

10   9   8   7   6   5   4   3   2   1

Introduction

The fourth edition of *The Complete Book of Food Counts* is the largest compilation of essential food data in this format. It contains data (calories, protein, carbohydrates, fat, cholesterol, sodium, and fiber) for basic generic foods, brand-name foods, and restaurant chains. Whether you are interested in dieting or nutrition—or both—you will find this book unique and invaluable as a reference. Should you need even more data, you may wish to consult *The Corinne T. Netzer Encyclopedia of Food Values.*

Since this book is alphabetized, you should have no difficulty finding whatever you wish to look up. There are, however, times when you may have to look in more than one place. If you are searching for a particular food and cannot find it immediately, look for it under a category, such as cakes, puddings, cookies, soups. Wherever sensible, I have cross-referenced listings, but the pressure of space has made it impossible to do that for every item.

Compare only foods listed in similar measures. This rule particularly applies to the confusion between measures by capacity and measures by weight. Eight ounces is not necessarily equivalent to eight fluid ounces or one cup. Eight ounces is a measure of how much something weighs; one cup is a measure of how much space it occupies. For instance, a cup of lightweight food, such as puffed rice or popcorn, weighs about one ounce, and eight ounces of the same product would fill many cups. Naturally, you can convert a similar unit of measure into a smaller or larger amount. The following table may be useful in making such conversions.

Equivalents by Capacity
(all measures level)
1 quart	=	4 cups
1 cup	=	8 fluid ounces
	=	½ pint
	=	16 tablespoons
2 tablespoons	=	1 fluid ounce
1 tablespoon	=	3 teaspoons

Equivalents by Weight

1 pound = 16 ounces
3.57 ounces = 100 grams
1 ounce = 28.35 grams

All the material contained in *The Complete Book of Food Counts* is based on information from the United States government, from producers and processors of brand-name foods, and from food chains. The data contained herein is the most complete and accurate information available as this book goes to press. Please bear in mind that seasonal and regional differences can affect the nutritional value of foods. Also, the food industry often changes recipes and sizes and may discontinue products or add new ones. In the future I will revise and update this book to keep you completely informed.

Good luck and good dieting.

CORINNE T. NETZER

Abbreviations and Symbols

cal.	calories
carbo.	carbohydrates
chol.	cholesterol
cont.	container
diam.	diameter
fl.	fluid
gms	grams
"	inch
<	less than
(o)	may contain trace amounts
mgs	milligrams
lb(s).	pound(s)
n.a.	not available
oz.	ounces
pc(s).	piece(s)
pkg.	package
pkt.	packet
prot.	protein
sod.	sodium
sq.	square(s)
tbsp.	tablespoon
tsp.	teaspoon
tr.	trace
w/	with
*	prepared according to basic package directions, except as noted

---

Note: Brand-name foods and restaurants listed in italics denote registered trademarks.

A

Food and Measure	cal.	prot. (gms)	carbo. (gms)	fat (gms)	chol. (mgs)	sod. (mgs)	fiber (gms)
A la king sauce mix							
(*Durkee*), 1 cup*	60	1.0	8.0	4.0	0	800	0
Abalone, meat only,							
raw, 4 oz.	119	19.4	6.8	.9	96	341	0
Abruzzese sausage							
(*Boar's Head Cinghi-*							
ale), 1 oz.	100	8.0	<1.0	8.0	15	540	0
Acerola, fresh:							
trimmed, ½ cup . . .	16	.2	3.8	.1	0	4	<1.0
juice, 6 fl. oz.	36	.7	8.7	.5	0	6	<1.0
Acorn squash, ½ cup:							
baked, cubed	57	1.1	14.9	.1	0	4	2.9
boiled, mashed . . .	41	.8	10.7	.1	0	3	3.4
Adobo (*Durkee*),							
¼ tsp.	0	0	0	0	0	320	0
Adzuki beans:							
dry (*Arrowhead Mills*),							
¼ cup	160	11.0	29.0	.5	0	0	6.0
boiled, ½ cup	147	8.7	28.5	.1	0	9	n.a.
canned, ½ cup:							
(*Eden*)	100	7.0	18.0	0	0	10	5.0
(*Eden* Jars)	90	6.0	16.0	0	0	35	4.0
sweetened	351	5.6	81.4	<.1	0	323	n.a.
Agar, see "Seaweed"							
Alcapurrias, frozen							
(*Goya*), 1 piece . .	170	4.0	26.0	6.0	10	450	1.0
Alfalfa sprouts,							
1 cup:							
(*Arrowhead Mills*) . .	30	4.0	4.0	.5	0	5	2.0
(*Jonathan's*)	25	3.0	3.0	.5	0	5	2.0

Food and Measure	cal.	prot. (gms)	carbo. (gms)	fat (gms)	chol. (mgs)	sod. (mgs)	fiber (gms)
Alfalfa sprouts *(cont.)*							
w/dill or radish							
sprouts *(Jonathan's)*	30	3.0	4.0	.5	0	15	2.0
w/garlic *(Jonathan's)*	27	3.0	4.0	.5	0	5	2.0
w/onion *(Jonathan's)*	25	3.0	3.0	.5	0	5	2.0
Alfredo sauce:							
(Ragu), ¼ cup	110	2.0	3.0	10.0	40	430	0
(Progresso), ½ cup	300	8.0	5.0	28.0	70	810	2.0
cheese, three							
(Lawry's), 3 tbsp.	70	2.0	0	3.0	5	830	0
refrigerated, ½ cup:							
(Contadina)	400	7.0	8.0	38.0	80	510	0
(Contadina Light)	190	8.0	10.0	13.0	40	560	0
Alfredo sauce mix:							
(Knorr), ⅓ pkg. . . .	60	3.0	7.0	2.5	5	670	0
(Spice Islands),							
½ pkg.	45	3.0	3.0	2.5	10	610	0
Alfredo seasoning							
mix *(Lawry's)*,							
1½ tbsp.	35	<1.0	4.0	1.5	<5	420	0
All-purpose season-							
ing *(Aromat)*,							
¼ tsp.	0	0	0	0	0	240	0
Allspice:							
1 tsp.	5	.1	1.4	.2	0	1	.4
(McCormick), ¼ tsp.	2	0	.3	0	0	<1	.2
Almond, shelled,							
1 oz., except as							
noted:							
(Dole)	170	6.0	5.0	14.0	0	4	n.a.
(Planters)	170	6.0	5.0	15.0	0	0	3.0
dried:							
1 oz.	167	5.7	5.8	14.8	0	3	3.1
slivered, 1 cup . . .	795	26.9	27.5	70.5	0	15	14.7
dry-roasted, salted	167	4.6	6.9	14.7	0	221	3.9
honey-roasted:							
1 oz.	168	5.2	7.9	14.2	0	37	n.a.
(Planters)	160	5.0	7.0	14.0	0	190	2.0
oil-roasted, salted . .	176	5.8	4.5	16.4	0	221	3.2

Food and Measure	cal.	prot. (gms)	carbo. (gms)	fat (gms)	chol. (mgs)	sod. (mgs)	fiber (gms)
slivered:							
(*Paradise/White Swan*), ¼ cup, 1.1 oz.	200	8.0	3.0	17.0	0	0	2.0
(*Planters Gold Measure*), 2-oz. pkg.	340	12.0	11.0	31.0	0	390	6.0
tamari-roasted (*Eden*)	170	8.0	8.0	12.0	0	35	4.0
toasted	167	5.8	6.5	14.4	0	3	3.2
Almond butter:							
crunchy or creamy:							
(*Roaster Fresh*), 1 oz.	184	5.0	6.0	16.0	0	56	0
(*Roaster Fresh* Unsalted), 1 oz. . .	184	5.0	6.0	16.0	0	4	0
salted, 1 tbsp.	101	2.4	3.4	9.5	0	72	.5
Almond meal, partially defatted, 1 oz.	116	11.2	8.2	5.2	0	2	n.a.
Almond paste:							
1 oz.	127	3.4	12.4	7.2	0	3	4.2
(*Solo*), 2 tbsp.	180	4.0	19.0	11.0	0	0	1.0
Alum (*Durkee*), ¼ tsp.	0	0	0	0	0	0	0
Amaranth, ½ cup:							
raw, trimmed	4	.3	.6	<.1	0	3	n.a.
boiled, drained	14	1.4	2.7	.1	0	14	n.a.
Amaranth, whole-grain, 1 oz.	106	4.1	18.8	1.8	0	6	4.3
Amaranth entree, canned (*Health Valley* Fast Menu), 1 cup	160	8.0	31.0	0	0	290	9.0
Amaranth flour (*Arrowhead Mills*), ¼ cup	110	4.0	25.0	2.0	0	0	3.0
Amaranth seeds (*Arrowhead Mills*), ¼ cup	170	7.0	29.0	2.0	0	0	3.0
Anasazi beans (*Arrowhead Mills*), ¼ cup	150	10.0	27.0	.5	0	0	9.0

Food and Measure	cal.	prot. (gms)	carbo. (gms)	fat (gms)	chol. (mgs)	sod. (mgs)	fiber (gms)
Anchovy, meat only:							
fresh, European, raw,							
1 oz.	37	5.8	0	1.4	n.a.	29	0
canned, in olive oil:							
drained, 1 oz. . . .	60	8.2	0	2.8	n.a.	1040	0
5 medium, .7 oz.	42	5.8	0	1.9	n.a.	734	0
Anchovy paste							
(*Reese*), 1 tbsp. . .	30	2.0	0	2.5	55	940	0
Angel hair pasta:							
dry, see "Pasta"							
refrigerated (*Con-*							
tadina), 1¼ cup . .	240	10.0	43.0	3.0	90	30	2.0
Angel hair pasta en-							
tree, frozen, 1 pkg.:							
(*Lean Cuisine*)	210	9.0	35.0	4.0	0	420	4.0
(*Smart Ones*)	170	8.0	29.0	2.0	0	520	4.0
w/sausage (*Marie Cal-*							
lender's)	370	14.0	43.0	15.0	10	630	4.0
Angel hair pasta mix:							
chicken (*Golden*							
Saute), ½ pkg. dry	210	8.0	44.0	1.5	0	850	2.0
w/herbs (*Noodle-*							
Roni), 1 cup* . . .	320	9.0	42.0	13.0	5	850	2.0
Parmesan:							
(*Golden Saute*),							
½ pkg. dry . . .	240	8.0	42.0	5.0	10	890	2.0
(*Noodle-Roni*							
Parmesano),							
1 cup*	320	9.0	40.0	15.0	5	890	2.0
Anise:							
(*McCormick*), ¼ tsp.	4	.2	.4	0	0	<1	.3
seeds, 1 tsp.	7	.4	1.1	.3	0	<1	.3
Apple, ½ cup, except							
as noted:							
fresh:							
w/peel, 2¾" apple	81	.3	21.1	.5	0	1	3.7
w/peel, sliced . . .	32	.1	8.4	.2	0	<1	3.0
peeled, 2¾" apple	72	.2	19.0	.4	0	<1	2.4
peeled, sliced . . .	31	.1	8.2	.2	0	<1	1.0

Food and Measure	cal.	prot. (gms)	carbo. (gms)	fat (gms)	chol. (mgs)	sod. (mgs)	fiber (gms)
fresh, cooked, peeled:							
sliced, boiled . . .	46	.2	11.7	.3	0	1	2.1
sliced, microwaved	48	.2	12.3	.4	0	1	2.4
canned:							
baked, Dutch (*Lucky Leaf/Musselman's*)	170	0	41.0	0	0	90	3.0
escalloped (*White House*)	160	0	35.0	0	0	25	0
fried (*Apple Time/ Lucky Leaf*) . . .	170	0	43.0	0	0	20	2.0
sliced (*Lucky Leaf/ Musselman's*) . .	50	0	12.0	0	0	20	2.0
sliced (*Musselman's* Home Style) . . .	170	0	43.0	0	0	20	2.0
sliced (*White House*)	100	0	22.0	0	0	15	2.0
spiced rings (*Lucky Leaf/Mus- selman's*), 1.1-oz. ring	35	0	9.0	0	0	5	0
spiced rings (*S&W*), 2 rings	25	7.0	7.0	0	0	20	1.0
spiced rings (*White House*), 1/2-oz. ring	30	0	5.0	0	0	5	0
dried:							
(*Sonoma*), 1.4 oz.	110	0	29.0	0	0	0	4.0
chips (*Smart Snack- ers*), .75 oz. . . .	70	0	19.0	0	0	125	3.0
sliced (*Del Monte*), 1/3 cup, 1.4 oz.	80	0	23.0	0	0	310	5.0
Apple, escalloped:							
canned, see "Apple"							
frozen (*Stouffer's*), 6 oz.	180	0	37.0	3.0	0	70	3.0
Apple-almond crisp,							
freeze-dried (*Alpine- Aire*), 1 1/2 cups . .	275	6.0	44.0	10.0	0	2	n.a.

Food and Measure	cal.	prot. (gms)	carbo. (gms)	fat (gms)	chol. (mgs)	sod. (mgs)	fiber (gms)
Apple butter, 1 tbsp.:							
(*Apple Time/Lucky Leaf/Musselman's*)	30	0	8.0	0	0	0	0
(*Dutch Girl/Mary Ellen*)	35	0	9.0	0	0	0	0
(*Eden*)	25	0	3.0	0	0	0	0
(*R. W. Knudsen*) . .	35	0	9.0	0	0	0	0
(*Smucker's/Simply Fruit*)	45	0	11.0	0	0	10	0
(*White House*)	35	0	9.0	0	0	5	0
spread (*Apple Time*)	25	0	6.0	0	0	0	0
spread (*New Morning*)	25	0	6.0	0	0	0	0
Apple cider, see "Apple juice"							
Apple drink:							
(*Hi-C Jammin'*), 8.45 oz.	120	0	33.0	0	0	30	0
(*Lincoln*), 8 fl. oz. . .	130	0	31.0	0	0	10	0
Apple drink blends, 8 fl. oz., except as noted:							
berry, frozen* (*Dole Burst*)	120	0	31.0	0	0	20	0
black cherry–white grape (*Veryfine Quenchers*)	120	0	30.0	0	0	10	0
cranberry:							
(*Dole*), 10 fl. oz. . .	160	0	40.0	0	0	25	0
(*Tree Top*), 10 fl. oz.	200	0	51.0	0	0	30	0
(*Tree Top*), 11.5 fl. oz.	230	0	58.0	0	0	35	0
cranberry-tangerine (*Veryfine Quenchers*)	120	0	31.0	0	0	10	0
peach-kiwi (*Veryfine Quenchers*)	130	0	33.0	0	0	25	0
peach-plum (*Veryfine Quenchers*)	130	0	32.0	0	0	25	0

Food and Measure	cal.	prot. (gms)	carbo. (gms)	fat (gms)	chol. (mgs)	sod. (mgs)	fiber (gms)
pear–passion fruit (*Veryfine Quenchers*)	120	0	31.0	0	0	25	0
punch (*Minute Maid*)	120	0	33.0	0	0	30	0
raspberry:							
(*Tree Top*), 10 fl. oz.	190	0	47.0	0	0	30	0
(*Tree Top*), 11.5 fl. oz.	220	0	54.0	0	0	35	0
raspberry-blackberry:							
(*Tropicana Twister*)	130	0	32.0	0	0	20	0
(*Tropicana Twister*), 11.5 fl. oz.	180	0	44.0	0	0	25	0
raspberry-cherry (*Veryfine Quenchers*)	120	0	31.0	0	0	25	0
raspberry-lime (*Veryfine Quenchers*) . .	120	0	30.0	0	0	25	0
strawberry-banana (*Veryfine Quenchers*)	120	0	30.0	0	0	20	0
Apple fritters, frozen (*Mrs. Paul's*), 2 pcs.	260	3.5	36.0	11.0	5	570	2.0
Apple juice, 8 fl. oz., except as noted:							
(*After the Fall*)	90	0	22.0	0	0	20	0
(*Apple & Eve*)	110	1.0	26.0	0	0	10	0
(*Apple Time/Lincoln/ Lucky Leaf/Speas Farm* Regular/Cider)	120	0	31.0	0	0	25	0
(*Apple Time/Lucky Leaf/Musselman's*), 5.5 fl. oz.	80	0	20.0	0	0	10	0
(*Dole*), 10 fl. oz. . . .	160	0	39.0	0	0	25	0
(*Goya*)	120	0	30.0	0	0	25	0
(*Heinke's* Organic/ Gravenstein)	120	0	30.0	0	0	25	0
(*Minute Maid*)	120	0	29.0	0	0	30	0
(*Mott's* Natural) . . .	120	0	29.0	0	0	20	0

Food and Measure	cal.	prot. (gms)	carbo. (gms)	fat (gms)	chol. (mgs)	sod. (mgs)	fiber (gms)
Apple juice *(cont.)*							
(*Musselman's* Regular/Natural/Cider)	120	0	31.0	0	0	25	0
(*Musselman's* Premium Natural) . . .	130	0	33.0	0	0	15	0
(*R.W. Knudsen* Clear)	110	0	28.0	0	0	5	0
(*R.W. Knudsen* Organic/Gravenstein)	120	0	30.0	0	0	25	0
(*Red Cheek*)	120	0	29.0	0	0	20	0
(*S&W*)	120	0	30.0	0	0	0	0
(*Santa Cruz* Organic)	120	0	30.0	0	0	25	0
(*Season's Best*), 11.5 fl. oz.	160	0	40.0	0	0	25	0
(*Snapple*), 10 fl. oz.	140	0	36.0	0	0	30	0
(*Tree Top*)	120	0	29.0	0	0	25	0
(*Tree Top*), 11.5 fl. oz.	170	0	38.0	0	0	35	0
(*Tree Top* Fiber Rich)	150	0	36.0	0	0	45	5.0
(*Veryfine*)	120	0	35.0	0	0	35	0
(*Veryfine*), 11.5 fl. oz.	170	0	43.0	0	0	50	0
(*White House*)	120	0	30.0	0	0	25	0
sparkling cider (*Apple Time/Lucky Leaf/ Musselman's*) . . .	150	0	36.0	0	0	20	0
spiced (*Apple & Eve* Cider & Spice) . . .	110	1.0	26.0	0	0	5	0
frozen*:							
(*Minute Maid*) . . .	110	0	28.0	0	0	5	0
(*R.W. Knudsen*) . .	120	0	30.0	0	0	25	0
(*Tree Top*)	120	0	29.0	0	0	15	0
Apple juice blends, 8 fl. oz., except as noted:							
all blends, except apricot and cherry cider (*R.W. Knudsen*)	120	0	30.0	0	0	25	0
apricot:							
(*After the Fall*) . . .	100	-1.0	22.0	0	0	20	0
(*R.W. Knudsen*) . .	120	0	30.0	0	0	35	0

Food and Measure	cal.	prot. (gms)	carbo. (gms)	fat (gms)	chol. (mgs)	sod. (mgs)	fiber (gms)
(*Tree Top* Fiber Rich)	160	0	40.0	0	0	40	5.0
boysenberry or rasp- berry (*Heinke's*) . .	120	0	30.0	0	0	25	0
cherry:							
(*After the Fall*) . . .	100	1.0	24.0	0	0	20	0
cider (*R.W. Knud- sen*)	130	0	33.0	0	0	35	0
cranberry:							
(*Apple & Eve*) . . .	120	1.0	30.0	0	0	20	0
frozen* (*Tree Top*)	130	0	32.0	0	0	15	0
grape:							
(*Apple & Eve*), 8.45 fl. oz.	130	0	32.0	0	0	15	0
(*Juicy Juice*)	130	1.0	30.0	0	0	10	0
(*Minute Maid*) . . .	130	0	32.0	0	0	30	0
(*Tree Top*)	130	0	32.0	0	0	30	0
(*Tree Top*), 11.5 fl. oz.	190	0	46.0	0	0	45	0
frozen* (*Tree Top*)	130	0	32.0	0	0	20	0
orange (*Tree Top* Fi- ber Rich)	170	0	41.0	0	0	30	5.0
pear (*Tree Top*) . . .	120	0	29.0	0	0	25	0
raspberry:							
(*After the Fall*) . . .	90	0	23.0	0	0	20	0
(*Tree Top*), 5.5 fl. oz.	80	0	19.0	0	0	15	0
(*Tree Top*), 11.5 fl. oz.	160	0	40.0	0	0	35	0
frozen* (*Tree Top*)	110	0	28.0	0	0	15	0
strawberry (*After the Fall*)	100	1.0	24.0	0	0	20	0
Apple pastry (see also specific list- ings), 1 pc.:							
dumpling, frozen (*Pepperidge Farm*)	290	3.0	44.0	11.0	0	160	3.0
pocket (*Tastykake*) . .	380	3.0	40.0	23.0	5	170	2.0
puffs (*Entenmann's*)	260	2.0	36.0	12.0	0	220	1.0

Food and Measure	cal.	prot. (gms)	carbo. (gms)	fat (gms)	chol. (mgs)	sod. (mgs)	fiber (gms)
Apple pastry *(cont.)*							
squares, frozen (*Pep-*							
peridge Farm) . . .	210	2.0	27.0	10.0	0	210	2.0
Apple syrup (*R.W.*							
Knudsen), ¼ cup	150	0	38.0	0	0	0	0
Applesauce, ½ cup,							
except as noted:							
(*Apple Time* Regular/							
Granny Smith/Red							
Delicious/McIntosh)	90	0	22.0	0	0	10	2.0
(*Apple Time/Lucky*							
Leaf/Musselman's							
Lite)	50	0	13.0	0	0	10	2.0
(*Eden*)	50	0	15.0	0	0	15	0
(*Lincoln*)	90	0	22.0	0	0	10	2.0
(*Lucky Leaf*), 4-oz. jar	80	0	21.0	0	0	10	2.0
(*Lucky Leaf* Regular/							
Chunky/Delicious)	90	0	22.0	0	0	10	2.0
(*Lucky Leaf* Regular/							
Cinnamon), 6-oz. jar	120	0	30.0	0	0	10	3.0
(*Lucky Leaf* Cinna-							
mon)	100	0	25.0	0	0	10	2.0
(*Mott's*)	110	0	28.0	0	0	0	0
(*Mott's* Chunky) . . .	110	0	26.0	0	0	0	0
(*Mott's* Cinnamon)	120	0	29.0	0	0	0	0
(*Musselman's* Chunky/							
Cinnamon)	100	0	25.0	0	0	10	2.0
(*Musselman's* Regu-							
lar/Cinnamon), 4 oz.	80	0	21.0	0	0	10	2.0
(*Musselman's*), 6 oz.	120	0	30.0	0	0	10	3.0
(*Musselman's* Cinna-							
mon), 6 oz.	130	0	31.0	0	0	10	3.0
(*Musselman's* Regu-							
lar/Delicious/McIn-							
tosh/Premium) . . .	90	0	22.0	0	0	10	2.0
(*S&W* Gravenstein)	90	0	21.0	0	0	5	1.0
(*Tree Top* Original/Cin-							
namon)	100	0	25.0	0	0	0	1.0

Food and Measure	cal.	prot. (gms)	carbo. (gms)	fat (gms)	chol. (mgs)	sod. (mgs)	fiber (gms)
(*Tree Top* Original/Cinnamon), 4 oz. . . .	90	0	21.0	0	0	0	1.0
(*White House*)	90	0	23.0	0	0	15	2.0
(*White House* Cinnamon)	100	0	25.0	0	0	15	2.0
unsweetened/natural:							
(*Apple Time*), 4 oz.	50	0	12.0	0	0	10	2.0
(*Apple Time/Lincoln*)	50	0	13.0	0	0	10	2.0
(*Lucky Leaf*), 6 oz.	70	0	18.0	0	0	10	3.0
(*Lucky Leaf* Regular/ Cinnamon)	50	0	13.0	0	0	20	2.0
(*Lucky Leaf* Regular/ Cinnamon), 4 oz.	50	0	12.0	0	0	10	2.0
(*Musselman's* Regular/Cinnamon) . .	50	0	13.0	0	0	20	2.0
(*Musselman's* Regular/Cinnamon), 4 oz.	50	0	12.0	0	0	20	2.0
(*Musselman's*), 6 oz.	70	0	18.0	0	0	25	3.0
(*S&W* Gravenstein)	50	0	13.0	0	0	5	2.0
(*Santa Cruz* Regular/ Gravenstein) . . .	45	0	15.0	0	0	5	n.a.
(*Tree Top*)	70	0	18.0	0	0	0	1.0
(*Tree Top*), 4 oz. . .	70	0	16.0	0	0	0	1.0
(*White House*) . . .	70	0	15.0	0	0	15	2.0
Applesauce blends, ½ cup or 4 oz.:							
all blends (*Santa Cruz*)	45	0	15.0	0	0	5	n.a.
w/apricot or cherry (*Musselman's Fruit 'N Sauce*)	100	0	24.0	0	0	5	2.0
w/cherry (*Musselman's Fruit 'N Sauce*)	90	0	20.0	0	0	10	1.0
w/peach (*Musselman's Fruit 'N Sauce*)	90	0	22.0	0	0	5	1.0

Food and Measure	cal.	prot. (gms)	carbo. (gms)	fat (gms)	chol. (mgs)	sod. (mgs)	fiber (gms)
Apricot:							
fresh:							
3 medium, 12 per							
lb.	51	1.5	11.8	.4	0	1	2.5
pitted, halves,							
½ cup	37	1.1	8.6	.3	0	1	1.9
canned, ½ cup:							
(*Del Monte* Lite) . .	60	0	16.0	0	0	10	1.0
in juice (*Libby's*							
Lite)	60	1.0	13.0	0	0	10	1.0
in heavy syrup (*Del*							
Monte)	100	0	26.0	0	0	10	1.0
in heavy syrup							
(*S&W*)	110	1.0	26.0	0	0	15	1.0
dried:							
(*Dole Sun Giant*),							
1.4 oz.	90	1.0	22.0	0	0	0	2.0
(*Sonoma*), 1.4 oz.	120	2.0	31.0	0	0	0	1.0
sulfured, 2 oz. . . .	135	2.1	35.0	.3	0	6	5.1
sun-dried (*Del*							
Monte), ⅓ cup,							
1.4 oz.	80	2.0	25.0	0	0	5	6.0
frozen, sweetened,							
½ cup	119	.9	30.4	.1	0	5	2.1
Apricot nectar,							
8 fl. oz., except as							
noted:							
(*Goya*)	160	1.0	38.0	0	0	10	4.0
(*Libby's/Kern's*) . . .	150	<1.0	36.0	0	0	5	0
(*Libby's/Kern's*),							
11.5 fl. oz.	220	1.0	52.0	0	0	10	0
(*R.W. Knudsen*) . . .	120	0	30.0	0	0	35	0
(*S&W*)	140	1.0	35.0	0	0	15	1.0
(*S&W*), 12-oz. can	210	2.0	53.0	0	0	20	1.0
(*Santa Cruz*)	120	0	30.0	0	0	35	0
pineapple (*Kern's*),							
11.5 fl. oz.	220	<1.0	53.0	0	0	5	0

Food and Measure	cal.	prot. (gms)	carbo. (gms)	fat (gms)	chol. (mgs)	sod. (mgs)	fiber (gms)
Arby's, 1 serving:							
breakfast items:							
bacon, 2 strips . .	90	5.0	0	7.0	15	220	0
biscuit, plain	280	6.0	34.0	15.0	0	730	1.0
blueberry muffin . .	230	2.0	35.0	9.0	25	290	0
cinnamon-nut dan-							
ish	360	6.0	60.0	11.0	0	105	1.0
croissant, plain . .	220	4.0	25.0	12.0	25	230	0
egg portion	95	.5	.5	8.0	180	54	0
French-Toastix, 6	430	10.0	52.0	21.0	0	550	3.0
ham	45	7.0	0	1.0	20	405	0
sausage	163	7.0	0	15.0	25	321	0
Swiss cheese, ½ oz.	45	4.0	.5	3.0	12	175	0
table syrup	100	0	25.0	0	0	30	0
chicken fingers, 2 . .	290	16.0	20.0	16.0	32	677	.5
sandwich, chicken:							
breaded fillet	536	28.0	46.0	28.0	45	1016	5.0
Cordon Bleu	623	38.0	46.0	33.0	77	1594	5.0
grilled, deluxe . . .	430	23.0	41.0	20.0	61	848	3.0
grilled, BBQ	388	23.0	47.0	13.0	43	1002	2.0
roast, club	546	31.0	37.0	31.0	58	1103	2.0
roast, deluxe, light	276	20.0	33.0	6.0	33	777	4.0
roast, deluxe, ses-							
ame seed bun . .	433	24.0	36.0	22.0	34	763	2.0
roast, Santa Fe . .	436	29.0	35.0	22.0	54	818	1.0
sandwich, ham 'n							
cheese	359	24.0	34.0	14.0	53	1283	2.0
sandwich, ham 'n							
cheese melt	329	20.0	34.0	13.0	40	1013	2.0
sandwich, fish fillet	529	23.0	50.0	27.0	43	864	2.0
sandwich, roast beef:							
Arby's Melt w/ched-							
dar	368	18.0	36.0	18.0	31	937	2.0
Arby-Q	431	22.0	48.0	18.0	37	1321	3.0
Bac'n Cheddar							
deluxe	539	22.0	38.0	34.0	44	1140	3.0
Beef'n Cheddar . .	487	25.0	40.0	28.0	50	1216	2.0
deluxe, light	296	18.0	33.0	10.0	42	826	6.0
giant	555	35.0	43.0	28.0	71	1561	5.0

Food and Measure	cal.	prot. (gms)	carbo. (gms)	fat (gms)	chol. (mgs)	sod. (mgs)	fiber (gms)
Arby's, sandwich, roast beef *(cont.)*							
junior	324	17.0	35.0	14.0	30	779	2.0
regular	388	23.0	33.0	19.0	43	1009	3.0
super	523	25.0	50.0	27.0	43	1189	5.0
sandwich, roast turkey							
deluxe, light	260	20.0	33.0	7.0	33	1262	4.0
sandwich, sub roll:							
French dip	475	30.0	40.0	22.0	55	1411	3.0
hot Ham'n Swiss	500	30.0	43.0	23.0	68	1664	2.0
Italian sub	675	30.0	46.0	36.0	83	2089	2.0
Philly Beef 'n Swiss	755	39.0	48.0	47.0	91	2025	3.0
roast beef sub . . .	700	38.0	44.0	42.0	84	2034	4.0
triple cheese melt	720	37.0	46.0	45.0	91	1797	2.0
turkey sub	550	31.0	47.0	27.0	65	2084	2.0
salads:							
garden	61	3.0	12.0	.5	0	40	5.0
roast chicken . . .	149	20.0	12.0	2.0	29	418	5.0
side salad	23	1.0	4.0	.3	0	15	2.0
soups:							
Boston clam chow-							
der	190	9.0	18.0	9.0	25	965	1.0
broccoli, cream of	160	7.0	15.0	8.0	25	1005	2.0
cheese, Wisconsin	280	10.0	20.0	18.0	35	1065	2.0
chicken noodle . .	80	6.0	11.0	2.0	20	850	1.0
chili, Timberline . .	220	18.0	17.0	10.0	30	1130	7.0
potato w/bacon . .	170	6.0	23.0	7.0	20	905	2.0
vegetable, lumber-							
jack	90	2.0	10.0	4.0	5	1150	1.0
potatoes:							
baked, plain,							
11.5 oz.	355	7.0	82.0	.3	0	26	7.0
baked, w/margarine							
and sour cream	578	9.0	85.0	24.0	25	209	7.0
baked, Broccoli 'n							
Cheddar	447	14.0	89.0	20.0	12	565	9.0
baked, deluxe . . .	736	19.0	86.0	36.0	59	499	7.0
cakes, 2 pcs. . . .	204	2.0	20.0	12.0	0	397	0
fries, curly	300	4.0	38.0	15.0	0	853	0
fries, cheddar curly	333	5.0	40.0	18.0	3	1016	0

Food and Measure	cal.	prot. (gms)	carbo. (gms)	fat (gms)	chol. (mgs)	sod. (mgs)	fiber (gms)
fries, french	246	2.0	30.0	13.0	0	114	0
sauces/dressings:							
Arby's Sauce. . . .	15	.1	4.0	.2	0	113	0
barbecue sauce . .	30	0	7.0	0	0	185	0
beef stock au jus	10	0	1.0	0	0	440	0
blue cheese dressing	290	2.0	2.0	31.0	50	580	0
buttermilk ranch dressing, reduced calorie	50	0	12.0	0	0	710	0
cheddar dressing	35	1.0	1.0	3.0	4	139	0
honey French dressing	280	0	18.0	23.0	0	400	0
honey mayonnaise, reduced calorie	70	0	1.0	7.0	20	135	0
Horsey Sauce . . .	60	0	2.0	5.0	5	150	0
Italian dressing, reduced calorie . .	20	0	3.0	1.0	0	1000	0
Italian sub sauce	70	0	1.0	7.0	0	240	0
mayonnaise	110	0	0	12.0	5	80	0
mayonnaise, light	12	0	.5	1.0	0	64	.5
Parmesan sauce . .	70	1.0	2.0	7.0	5	130	0
red ranch dressing	75	0	5.0	6.0	0	115	0
tartar sauce	140	0	0	15.0	30	220	0
Thousand Island dressing	260	0	7.0	26.0	30	420	0
desserts:							
apple turnover . . .	330	4.0	48.0	14.0	0	180	0
cheesecake, plain	320	5.0	23.0	23.0	95	240	0
cherry turnover . .	320	4.0	46.0	13.0	0	190	0
chocolate chip cookie	125	2.0	16.0	6.0	10	85	0
Polar Swirl:							
Butterfinger . . .	457	15.0	62.0	18.0	28	318	0
Heath	543	15.0	76.0	22.0	39	346	0
Oreo	482	15.0	66.0	22.0	35	521	0
Snickers	511	15.0	73.0	19.0	33	351	1.0
peanut butter cup	517	20.0	61.0	24.0	34	385	1.0

Food and Measure	cal.	prot. (gms)	carbo. (gms)	fat (gms)	chol. (mgs)	sod. (mgs)	fiber (gms)
Arby's, desserts *(cont.)*							
shake, chocolate . .	451	15.0	76.0	12.0	36	341	0
shake, jamocha . .	384	15.0	62.0	10.0	36	281	0
shake, vanilla . . .	360	15.0	50.0	12.0	36	318	0
Arrowhead, raw,							
2⅝"-diam. corm . .	12	.6	2.4	<.1	0	3	<1.0
Arrowroot *(Durkee),*							
¼ tsp.	0	0	0	0	0	0	0
Arrowroot flour,							
1 cup	457	.4	112.8	.1	0	2	4.4
Artichoke, globe:							
fresh:							
(Dole), 1 large . . .	23	2.0	5.0	.1	0	65	3.0
boiled, 10.6-oz.							
choke	60	4.2	13.4	.2	0	114	6.5
hearts, boiled,							
drained, ½ cup	42	2.9	9.4	.1	0	80	4.5
canned or in jars (see							
also "Artichoke ap-							
petizer"):							
(Progresso), 2 pcs.	35	2.0	6.0	0	0	240	1.0
bottoms *(S&W),*							
3 pcs.	25	2.0	4.0	0	0	90	0
hearts *(S&W),*							
3 pcs.	30	2.0	5.0	0	0	200	0
frozen, hearts, 9-oz.							
pkg.	96	6.7	19.8	1.1	0	120	9.9
Artichoke, Jerusalem,							
see "Jerusalem ar-							
tichoke"							
Artichoke appetizer,							
marinated:							
(Contorno Caponata di							
Carciofi), ⅓ cup . .	130	2.0	7.0	6.0	0	460	3.0
(Progresso), ⅓ cup	160	1.0	6.0	14.0	0	290	1.0
in brine *(Goya),*							
4.5 oz.	65	2.7	13.0	4.0	0	350	1.8
in olive oil *(Goya),*							
3 oz.	210	.9	5.6	0	0	200	.8

Food and Measure	cal.	prot. (gms)	carbo. (gms)	fat (gms)	chol. (mgs)	sod. (mgs)	fiber (gms)
quarters (*S&W*), 2 pcs.	20	0	2.0	2.0	0	80	1.0
Arugula, trimmed:							
1 oz.	7	.7	1.0	.2	0	8	n.a.
(*Frieda's*), 3.5 oz. . .	23	2.2	4.0	.3	0	15	n.a.
Asparagus, ½ cup, except as noted:							
fresh:							
raw, 4 spears, 3.8 oz.	14	1.3	2.6	.1	0	1	1.2
raw (*Dole*), 5 spears	18	2.0	2.0	0	0	0	2.0
boiled, 4 spears, ½"-diam. base	14	1.6	2.5	.2	0	7	1.3
boiled, drained, cuts	22	2.3	3.8	.3	0	10	1.9
canned:							
(*S&W* Blended), 6 pcs.	15	2.0	4.0	0	0	260	1.0
(*S&W* Colossal), 3 pcs.	10	1.0	3.0	0	0	170	1.0
(*Stokely*)	25	2.0	3.0	0	0	350	1.0
(*Stokely* No Salt)	25	2.0	3.0	0	0	10	1.0
all varieties (*Del Monte*)	20	2.0	3.0	0	0	420	1.0
spears (*Green Giant*), 4.5 oz. . . .	20	2.0	3.0	0	0	450	1.0
spears, extra large (*Green Giant Le-Sueur*), 4.5 oz.	20	2.0	3.0	0	0	440	1.0
spears, extra long (*Green Giant*), 4.5 oz.	20	2.0	3.0	0	0	400	1.0
cuts (*Green Giant*)	20	2.0	3.0	0	0	420	1.0
cuts (*Green Giant* 50% Less Sodium)	20	2.0	3.0	0	0	210	1.0
frozen:							
boiled, 4 spears . .	17	1.8	2.9	.3	0	2	1.2

Food and Measure	cal.	prot. (gms)	carbo. (gms)	fat (gms)	chol. (mgs)	sod. (mgs)	fiber (gms)
Asparagus, frozen *(cont.)*							
cuts *(Green Giant Harvest Fresh)*,							
⅔ cup	25	2.0	4.0	0	0	85	1.0
Asparagus bean, see "Winged bean"							
Atemoya *(Frieda's)*,							
3½ oz.	94	1.3	24.0	.4	0	n.a.	n.a.
Au jus gravy, ¼ cup:							
(Franco-American) . .	10	1.0	2.0	.5	<5	310	0
mix*:							
(Durkee/French's)	5	0	1.0	0	0	220	0
(Knorr)	15	0	3.0	0	0	310	0
Au jus seasoning mix *(Durkee/French's* Roasting Bag),							
⅛ pkg.	10	0	2.0	0	0	340	0
Aubergine, see "Eggplant"							
Avocado, California:							
1 medium, 8 oz. . . .	306	3.6	12.0	30.0	0	21	4.7
trimmed, 1 oz.	50	.6	2.0	4.9	0	3	.8
pureed, ½ cup	204	2.4	8.0	19.9	0	14	3.1
Avocado dip, 2 tbsp.:							
(Kraft)	60	1.0	4.0	4.0	0	240	0
(Nalley)	120	0	3.0	12.0	10	200	0

B

Food and Measure	cal.	prot. (gms)	carbo. (gms)	fat (gms)	chol. (mgs)	sod. (mgs)	fiber (gms)
Bacalaitos, mix							
(*Goya*), 3 tbsp. . .	100	5.0	19.0	.5	0	490	1.0
Bacon, cooked,							
2 slices, except as							
noted:							
(*Agar Prestige*) . . .	80	4.0	0	7.0	15	260	0
(*Black Label*)	80	5.0	0	7.0	15	330	0
(*Black Label* Center							
Cut), 3 slices . . .	60	4.0	0	4.5	15	210	0
(*Black Label* Low Salt)	80	5.0	0	7.0	15	210	0
(*Black Label* Thin) . .	60	4.0	0	4.5	15	260	0
(*Black Label* Thin Low							
Salt)	60	4.0	0	4.5	15	170	0
(*Boar's Head*)	60	4.0	0	5.0	10	190	0
(*Hormel* Microwave)	70	5.0	0	5.0	15	230	0
(*Hormel Layout Pack*)	80	5.0	0	7.0	15	330	0
(*Hormel Layout Pack*							
Low Salt)	80	5.0	0	7.0	15	210	0
(*John Morrell* Hard-							
wood Smoked) . .	100	4.0	0	9.0	10	300	0
(*Jones Dairy Farm*)	90	4.0	0	8.0	15	350	0
(*Jones Dairy Farm*							
Thick), 1 slice . . .	70	3.0	0	6.0	15	290	0
(*Old Smokehouse*) . .	80	5.0	0	7.0	15	280	0
(*Oscar Mayer*)	60	4.0	0	5.0	10	250	0
(*Oscar Mayer* Thick),							
1 slice	60	4.0	0	5.0	10	250	0
(*Oscar Mayer* Center							
Cut), 3 slices . . .	90	6.0	0	7.0	20	380	0
(*Oscar Mayer* Lower							
Sodium)	60	4.0	0	4.0	10	170	0

Food and Measure	cal.	prot. (gms)	carbo. (gms)	fat (gms)	chol. (mgs)	sod. (mgs)	fiber (gms)
Bacon *(cont.)*							
(Patrick Cudahy) . . .	80	4.0	0	7.0	15	260	0
(Patrick Cudahy Rind)	100	5.0	0	9.0	15	330	0
(Red Label)	80	5.0	0	7.0	15	330	0
(Range Brand Thick)	100	7.0	0	9.0	20	460	0
(Rock River/Sinnis-							
sippi)	80	3.0	0	8.0	15	350	0
(Sweet Applewood							
Farms)	80	4.0	0	7.0	15	260	0
precooked *(Fast'N*							
Easy)	80	4.0	0	7.0	15	290	0
turkey, see "Turkey							
bacon"							
Bacon, Canadian:							
(Boar's Head), 2 oz.	70	12.0	0	2.5	30	560	0
(Hormel), 2 oz. . . .	70	10.0	0	3.0	30	610	0
(Jones Dairy Farm							
Lean Choice),							
3 slices	70	11.0	0	3.0	30	460	0
(Oscar Mayer),							
2 slices	50	9.0	0	2.0	25	600	0
Bacon, Irish, back							
2 slices, 2 oz. . . .	130	10.0	1.0	10.0	30	570	0
"Bacon," vegetarian,							
frozen, 2 strips:							
(Morningstar Farms							
Breakfast Strips) . .	60	2.0	2.0	4.5	0	220	<1.0
(Worthington Strip-							
ples)	60	2.0	2.0	4.5	0	220	<1.0
Bacon bits, 1 tbsp.							
except as noted:							
(Hormel)	30	3.0	0	1.5	5	250	0
(Hormel Pieces) . . .	25	3.0	0	1.5	10	170	0
(Oscar Mayer)	25	3.0	0	1.5	5	220	0
imitation:							
*(Bac*Os)*	30	3.0	2.0	1.0	0	130	0
(Durkee)	0	0	2.0	0	0	180	.5
(McCormick),							
1½ tbsp.	30	3.0	2.0	1.5	0	220	0

Food and Measure	cal.	prot. (gms)	carbo. (gms)	fat (gms)	chol. (mgs)	sod. (mgs)	fiber (gms)
chips (*Durkee*) . . .	0	0	2.0	0	0	190	.5
Bacon snack, see "Pork rind snack"							
Bacon dip, 2 tbsp.:							
cheese, see "Cheese dip"							
horseradish:							
(*Heluva* Good) . . .	60	1.0	2.0	5.0	20	200	0
(*Heluva* Good Free)	25	1.0	4.0	0	0	210	0
(*Kraft*)	60	1.0	3.0	5.0	0	220	0
(*Kraft* Premium) . .	50	1.0	2.0	5.0	15	200	0
onion:							
(*Breakstone's*) . . .	60	1.0	2.0	5.0	20	170	0
(*Knudsen* Premium)	60	1.0	2.0	5.0	20	170	0
(*Kraft* Premium) . .	60	1.0	2.0	5.0	15	160	0
(*Nalley*)	110	1.0	2.0	11.0	15	220	0
Bagel, 1 pc.:							
plain:							
(*Awrey's*)	200	7.0	40.0	1.0	0	340	<1.0
(*Thomas'*)	150	6.0	33.0	1.0	0	280	2.0
cinnamon raisin:							
(*Awrey's*)	200	7.0	42.0	1.0	0	250	<1.0
(*Thomas'*)	160	6.0	34.0	1.0	0	260	2.0
egg (*Thomas'*)	160	7.0	33.0	1.0	15	280	2.0
mini (*Awrey's*)	100	3.0	22.0	0	0	160	0
multigrain (*Thomas'*)	150	6.0	33.0	1.0	0	240	3.0
onion (*Thomas'*) . . .	150	6.0	33.0	1.0	0	280	2.0
Bagel, frozen, 1 pc., except as noted:							
plain:							
(*Lender's*)	160	6.0	30.0	1.0	0	320	1.0
(*Lender's* Bagel-ettes), 2 pcs. . .	140	5.0	28.0	1.0	0	260	1.0
(*Lender's* Big'N Crusty)	220	8.0	43.0	2.0	0	430	2.0
blueberry (*Lender's*)	200	6.0	38.0	2.0	0	330	2.0
cinnamon raisin:							
(*Lender's*)	200	7.0	39.0	1.5	0	290	2.0

Food and Measure	cal.	prot. (gms)	carbo. (gms)	fat (gms)	chol. (mgs)	sod. (mgs)	fiber (gms)
Bagel, frozen, cinnamon raisin *(cont.)*							
(*Lender's Big'N* Crusty)	240	8.0	47.0	2.5	0	330	2.0
(*Sara Lee*)	220	8.0	45.0	1.0	0	320	3.0
egg:							
(*Lender's*)	160	6.0	30.0	1.5	10	320	1.0
(*Lender's Big'N* Crusty)	230	8.0	44.0	2.0	15	400	2.0
garlic (*Lender's*) . . .	150	6.0	29.0	1.0	0	280	2.0
oat bran (*Lender's*)	190	7.0	36.0	1.5	0	300	4.0
onion:							
(*Lender's*)	160	5.0	30.0	1.5	0	300	2.0
(*Lender's Big'N* Crusty)	220	8.0	43.0	1.5	0	410	3.0
poppy (*Lender's*) . .	150	6.0	30.0	1.0	0	290	2.0
pumpernickel							
(*Lender's*)	150	5.0	31.0	1.0	0	340	2.0
rye (*Lender's*)	150	5.0	30.0	1.0	0	320	2.0
sesame (*Lender's*) . .	150	6.0	29.0	1.5	0	290	1.0
soft (*Lender's* Original)	210	6.0	37.0	3.5	10	330	2.0
Bagel chips (*Pepperidge Farm*), 1 oz.:							
cheese, three	140	4.0	16.0	7.0	5	240	<1.0
onion and garlic . . .	110	3.0	18.0	4.5	0	280	2.0
onion multigrain . . .	120	3.0	19.0	3.5	0	200	1.0
Bagel sandwich, see specific listings							
Baked beans, ½ cup:							
(*Allens*)	150	6.0	29.0	1.0	0	350	8.0
(*B&M* Brick Oven) . .	180	8.0	32.0	2.0	5	390	7.0
(*B&M* Extra Hearty)	190	8.0	36.0	2.0	<5	450	8.0
(*B&M* 99% Fat Free)	160	8.0	31.0	1.0	0	220	7.0
(*Bush's*)	150	7.0	29.0	1.0	<5	550	7.0
(*Bush's*)	160	6.0	28.0	1.5	5	480	8.0
(*Campbell's* New England Style)	180	5.0	32.0	3.0	5	460	6.0
(*Campbell's* Homestyle)	150	3.0	27.0	2.0	5	490	7.0

Food and Measure	cal.	prot. (gms)	carbo. (gms)	fat (gms)	chol. (mgs)	sod. (mgs)	fiber (gms)
(*Campbell's* Old Fashioned)	180	5.0	32.0	3.0	5	460	6.0
(*Friend's*)	170	8.0	32.0	1.0	<5	390	7.0
(*Grandma Brown's*)	160	8.0	28.0	1.5	0	340	8.0
(*Green Giant/Joan of Arc*)	160	6.0	31.0	1.5	<5	580	7.0
(*Heartland* Iron Kettle)	150	5.0	29.0	1.0	<5	400	5.0
(*S&W* Brick Oven) . .	160	7.0	32.0	.5	0	620	7.0
(*Van Camp's* Fat Free)	130	7.0	28.0	0	0	350	5.0
(*Van Camp's* Premium)	140	7.0	29.0	1.0	0	520	5.0
w/bacon (*Grandma Brown's* Saucepan)	150	7.0	26.0	2.5	0	300	7.0
bacon/brown sugar:							
(*Campbell's/Campbell's* Old Fashioned)	170	5.0	29.0	3.0	5	490	7.0
(*S&W*)	140	7.0	31.0	1.5	0	530	6.0
barbecue:							
(*B&M* Brick Oven)	170	7.0	32.0	.5	<5	360	6.0
(*Campbell's* Old Fashioned/Tangy)	170	4.0	29.0	2.5	5	460	6.0
(*Green Giant/Joan of Arc*)	140	6.0	28.0	.5	0	460	5.0
Texas style (*S&W*)	140	6.0	25.0	1.5	0	640	8.0
brown sugar (*Van Camp's*)	170	7.0	31.0	3.0	5	410	6.0
and franks, see "Beans and franks"							
honey:							
(*B&M*)	170	8.0	30.0	1.5	0	450	8.0
(*Health Valley*) . . .	110	7.0	24.0	0	0	135	7.0
(*Health Valley* No Salt)	110	7.0	24.0	0	0	25	7.0
bacon (*Green Giant/Joan of Arc*) . . .	160	6.0	34.0	.5	0	490	6.0
mustard (*S&W*) . .	130	7.0	31.0	0	0	500	7.0
maple sugar (*S&W*)	150	7.0	29.0	.5	0	80	6.0

Food and Measure	cal.	prot. (gms)	carbo. (gms)	fat (gms)	chol. (mgs)	sod. (mgs)	fiber (gms)
Baked beans *(cont.)*							
Mexican style, see							
"Mexican beans"							
w/onion (*Bush's*) . .	150	7.0	26.0	1.5	0	500	6.0
w/onion (*Green Giant/							
Joan of Arc*)	150	5.0	28.0	1.5	0	620	5.0
w/pork:							
(*Campbell's*)	130	3.0	24.0	2.0	5	420	6.0
(*Crest Top*)	130	7.0	21.0	1.0	0	330	6.0
(*Green Giant/Joan of							
Arc*)	120	5.0	23.0	1.0	0	490	4.0
(*Hunt's*)	130	6.0	27.5	1.0	0	515	4.0
(*Stokely* Sugar) . .	150	7.0	29.0	1.0	0	340	6.0
(*Stokely* Tomato)	140	7.0	26.0	1.0	0	530	6.0
(*Van Camp's*) . . .	110	6.0	24.0	1.5	0	490	6.0
(*Wagon Master/							
Trappey's*)	110	5.0	21.0	1.0	0	710	7.0
(*Wagon Master/							
Trappey's* 4.2 oz.)	130	7.0	23.0	1.0	0	420	9.0
w/jalapeño (*Trap-							
pey's*)	130	5.0	24.0	2.0	0	610	6.0
peas (*East Texas							
Fair* Peas 'n Pork)	110	6.0	19.0	1.5	0	540	5.0
vegetarian:							
(*Bush's*)	140	6.0	24.0	1.0	0	550	6.0
(*Campbell's*)	130	3.0	24.0	2.0	0	460	6.0
(*Stokely*)	140	7.0	26.0	.5	0	530	6.0
(*Van Camp's*) . . .	110	6.0	23.0	.5	0	360	5.0
brown sugar sauce							
(*Stokely*)	150	7.0	29.0	.5	0	340	6.0
yellow eye (*B&M*) . .	170	8.0	28.0	2.0	<5	460	7.0
Baking mix, all pur-							
pose (*Arrowhead							
Mills*), ¼ cup . . .	140	5.0	30.0	.5	0	320	2.0
Baking powder:							
(*Calumet*), ¼ tsp. . .	0	0	0	0	0	100	0
(*Davis*), 1 tsp.	8	0	2.0	0	0	330	0
Baking soda (*Tone's*),							
1 tsp.	0	0	0	0	0	821	0

Food and Measure	cal.	prot. (gms)	carbo. (gms)	fat (gms)	chol. (mgs)	sod. (mgs)	fiber (gms)
Balsam pear, ½ cup:							
leafy tips:							
raw	7	1.3	.8	.2	0	3	.6
boiled, drained . . .	10	1.0	2.0	.1	0	4	.6
pods, ½″ pcs.:							
raw	8	.5	1.7	.1	0	3	1.3
boiled, drained . . .	12	.5	2.7	.1	0	4	1.2
Bamboo shoots:							
fresh, ½ cup:							
raw, slices	21	2.0	4.0	.2	0	3	.7
boiled, drained,							
½″ slices	8	.9	1.2	.1	0	3	<1.0
canned:							
drained, ½ cup . .	13	1.1	2.1	.3	0	5	2.0
(*La Choy*), ¼ cup	5	0	1.0	0	0	0	1.0
Banana:							
fresh:							
whole, 1 lb.	271	3.1	69.1	1.4	0	3	7.1
8¾″ banana	105	1.2	26.7	.6	0	1	2.7
mashed, ½ cup . .	104	1.2	26.4	.5	0	1	2.7
dehydrated, ¼ cup	87	1.0	22.1	.5	0	1	1.9
dried (*Sonoma*),							
2 pcs.	140	2.0	33.0	0	0	0	1.0
Banana, baking, see							
"Plantain"							
Banana, manzano							
(*Frieda's*), 1 oz. . .	24	.3	6.3	.1	0	<1	n.a.
Banana, red, 7¼″ . .	118	1.6	30.7	.3	0	1	n.a.
Banana drink (*After*							
the Fall Casablanca),							
8 fl. oz.	80	1.0	19.0	0	0	10	0
Banana milk drink:							
chilled, lowfat (*Nestlé*							
Quik), 1 cup	200	7.0	30.0	5.0	20	95	0
mix (*Nestlé Quik*),							
2 tbsp.	90	0	22.0	0	0	0	0
Banana nectar,							
11.5-fl.-oz. can:							
(*Libby's/Kern's*) . . .	190	0	47.0	0	0	35	0

Food and Measure	cal.	prot. (gms)	carbo. (gms)	fat (gms)	chol. (mgs)	sod. (mgs)	fiber (gms)
Banana nectar *(cont.)*							
blends:							
(*Libby's* Quanabana)	210	0	50.0	0	0	25	0
pineapple (*Kern's*)	220	<1.0	52.0	0	0	5	0
Banana squash,							
baked (*Frieda's*),							
1 oz.	18	.5	4.4	.1	0	3	n.a.
Bananaberry shake							
(*Nestlé Killer*),							
14 oz.	450	13.0	66.0	15.0	70	240	3.0
Barbecue beans, see							
"Baked beans"							
Barbecue dip (*Heluva*							
Good), 2 tbsp. . . .	60	1.0	2.0	5.0	20	160	0
Barbecue sauce,							
2 tbsp., except as							
noted:							
(*Heinz* Thick & Rich							
Old Fashioned) . .	40	0	10.0	0	0	370	0
(*Hunt's* Light)	25	0	6.0	0	0	170	<1.0
(*Hunt's* Original) . . .	40	0	9.0	0	0	400	1.0
(*Hunt's* Original Bold)	45	0	10.0	0	0	315	1.0
(*KC Masterpiece* Orig-							
inal)	60	<1.0	11.0	1.0	0	640	0
(*Kraft* Char-Grill) . . .	60	0	12.0	1.0	0	440	0
(*Kraft* Original)	40	0	10.0	0	0	460	0
(*Kraft* Original Extra							
Rich)	50	0	12.0	0	0	360	0
(*Kraft* Thick'N Spicy							
Original)	50	0	12.0	0	0	440	0
(*Lea & Perrins* Origi-							
nal/Bold & Spicy)	50	1.0	13.0	0	0	125	0
(*Maull's*)	40	0	10.0	0	0	320	0
(*Mississippi*)	60	0	16.0	0	0	550	1.0
(*Open Pit* Original)	50	0	11.0	0	0	490	0
(*Rice Road*), 1 tsp.	5	.2	1.0	<1.0	0	270	0
(*Woody's* Cook-In')	50	<1.0	4.0	4.0	0	490	1.0
all varieties (*Healthy*							
Choice)	25	0	6.0	0	0	230	0

Food and Measure	cal.	prot. (gms)	carbo. (gms)	fat (gms)	chol. (mgs)	sod. (mgs)	fiber (gms)
Buffalo wing (*Heinz*)	15	0	4.0	0	0	750	1.0
Cajun (*Luzianne*) . . .	110	0	19.0	4.0	0	350	0
Dijon, mild (*Hunt's*)	40	0	9.0	0	0	400	0
Dijon and honey							
(*Lawry's*)	60	<1.0	12.0	1.0	0	750	0
garlic (*Kraft*)	40	0	9.0	0	0	420	0
garlic and herb (*Lea*							
& Perrins)	40	0	9.0	0	0	110	0
hickory:							
(*Hunt's* Bold) . . .	45	0	10.0	0	0	285	<1.0
(*Open Pit*)	50	0	11.0	.5	0	380	0
(*Open Pit* Thick and							
Tangy)	50	0	12.0	0	0	390	0
and brown sugar							
(*Hunt's*)	75	0	18.0	0	0	380	0
hickory or honey hick-							
ory (*Hunt's*)	40	0	9.0	0	0	410	0
hickory smoke:							
(*Kraft*)	40	0	10.0	0	0	440	0
(*Kraft Thick'N Spicy*)	50	0	12.0	0	0	440	0
(*Open Pit*)	50	0	11.0	.5	0	430	0
hot (*Kraft*)	40	0	9.0	0	0	360	0
onion bits (*Kraft*)	50	0	11.0	0	0	340	<1.0
honey:							
(*Heinz* Thick &							
Rich)	45	0	11.0	0	0	480	0
(*Kraft*)	50	0	13.0	0	0	320	0
(*Kraft Thick'N Spicy*)	60	0	13.0	0	0	350	0
mustard (*Hunt's*)	45	0	11.5	0	0	450	<1.0
and spice (*Open Pit*							
Thick and Tangy)	45	0	11.0	0	0	340	0
honey Dijon (*KC Mas-*							
terpiece)	50	0	10.0	1.0	0	570	0
hot:							
(*Kraft*)	40	0	9.0	0	0	540	0
(*Open Pit*)	50	0	11.0	0	0	380	0
and spicy (*Hunt's*)	45	0	11.5	0	0	450	<1.0
and spicy (*Master*							
Choice), 1 tbsp.	30	0	7.0	0	0	140	0

Food and Measure	cal.	prot. (gms)	carbo. (gms)	fat (gms)	chol. (mgs)	sod. (mgs)	fiber (gms)
Barbecue sauce *(cont.)*							
Italian:							
(*Porino's*)	40	0	7.0	1.5	0	310	0
seasonings (*Kraft*)	45	0	10.0	.5	0	280	0
jalapeño (*Maull's*) . .	60	0	12.0	0	0	320	0
Kansas City style:							
(*Kraft*)	45	0	11.0	0	0	280	<1.0
(*Kraft Thick'N Spicy*)	60	0	13.0	0	0	280	<1.0
(*Maull's*)	60	0	15.0	0	0	320	0
mesquite:							
(*Hunt's*)	40	<1.0	9.0	0	0	360	<1.0
(*Open Pit*)	50	0	11.0	.5	0	440	0
smoke (*Kraft*) . . .	40	0	9.0	0	0	410	0
smoke (*Kraft*							
Thick'N Spicy) . .	50	0	12.0	0	0	440	0
mild (*Hunt's*)	40	0	10.0	0	0	380	<1.0
onion:							
(*Open Pit*)	50	0	11.0	0	0	480	0
(*Open Pit* Thick and							
Tangy)	50	0	12.0	0	0	380	0
bits (*Kraft*)	50	0	11.0	0	0	340	0
bits (*Maull's*) . . .	45	0	9.0	0	0	310	0
Oriental:							
(*House of Tsang*							
Hong Kong),							
1 tsp.	10	0	2.0	0	0	150	0
pork (*House of*							
Tsang)	90	1.0	20.0	.5	0	1300	0
salsa style (*Kraft*) . .	40	0	9.0	0	0	420	0
smoky (*Maull's*) . . .	40	0	10.0	0	0	310	0
sweet:							
(*Maull's*							
Sweet-N-Mild) . .	60	0	12.0	0	0	280	0
(*Maull's* Sweet-N-							
Smokey)	60	0	13.0	0	0	300	0
(*Open Pit*)	50	0	12.0	0	0	300	0
sweet and sour:							
(*Lawry's*)	80	0	20.0	0	0	890	0
(*Open Pit*)	45	0	10.0	0	0	420	0

Food and Measure	cal.	prot. (gms)	carbo. (gms)	fat (gms)	chol. (mgs)	sod. (mgs)	fiber (gms)
teriyaki:							
(*Hunt's*)	45	1.0	11.0	0	0	350	<1.0
(*Kraft*)	60	<1.0	12.0	1.0	0	430	0
Barbecue seasoning							
(*Durkee*), ¼ tsp. . .	0	0	0	0	0	70	0
Barley, pearled:							
dry:							
1 cup	704	19.8	155.5	2.3	0	18	31.2
(*Arrowhead Mills*),							
¼ cup	170	5.0	37.0	.5	0	0	6.0
(*Goya*), ¼ cup . . .	100	3.0	24.0	0	0	0	5.0
(*Quaker* Scotch							
Quick), ⅓ cup . .	170	5.0	37.0	1.0	0	0	5.0
medium (*Quaker*							
Scotch), ¼ cup	170	5.0	37.0	1.0	0	0	5.0
cooked, 1 cup	193	3.6	44.3	.7	0	5	6.0
Barley flakes (*Arrow-*							
head Mills), ⅓ cup	110	4.0	28.0	1.0	0	0	5.0
Barley flour (*Arrow-*							
head Mills), ¼ cup	75	3.0	19.0	.5	0	0	3.0
Barley malt syrup							
(*Eden*), 1 tbsp. . .	60	1.0	14.0	0	0	0	0
Barley pilaf mix*							
(*Near East*), 1 cup	220	6.0	41.0	4.0	0	620	5.0
Basil:							
fresh:							
1 oz.	8	.7	1.2	.2	0	0	n.a.
5 medium leaves	1	.1	.1	<.1	0	0	n.a.
chopped, 2 tbsp.	1	.1	.2	<.1	0	0	n.a.
dried:							
(*McCormick*),							
¼ tsp.	<1	.1	.1	0	0	<1	.1
leaf (*Tone's*), ¼ tsp.	0	0	0	0	0	0	0
ground, 1 tbsp. . . .	11	.7	2.7	.2	0	2	.5
ground, 1 tsp.	4	.2	.9	.1	0	<1	.2
frozen (*Seabrook*),							
1 tbsp., ¼ oz.	2	.2	.3	0	0	<1	.3

Food and Measure	cal.	prot. (gms)	carbo. (gms)	fat (gms)	chol. (mgs)	sod. (mgs)	fiber (gms)
Baskin-Robbins,							
½ cup, except as							
noted:							
ice cream:							
Baby Ruth	170	2.0	18.0	10.0	30	65	0
banana nut	150	2.0	15.0	10.0	25	40	0
banana strawberry	130	2.0	17.0	7.0	25	40	0
Baseball nut	160	2.0	18.0	9.0	30	55	0
black walnut	160	3.0	13.0	11.0	30	50	0
blackberry	130	2.0	16.0	6.9	29	39	0
butter pecan	160	2.0	13.0	11.0	35	50	0
Butterfinger	160	2.0	21.0	8.0	20	65	0
caramel chocolate							
crunch	160	2.0	19.0	10.0	30	85	0
chocolate	150	2.0	18.0	9.0	30	60	0
chocolate ribbon . .	140	2.0	17.0	8.0	30	45	0
chocolate, winter							
white	150	2.0	18.0	9.0	25	50	0
chocolate, world							
class	160	2.0	18.0	9.0	30	60	0
chocolate almond	180	3.0	17.0	11.0	30	55	1.0
chocolate cake, Ger-							
man	170	3.0	21.0	11.0	25	60	1.0
chocolate chip . . .	150	2.0	15.0	10.0	35	45	0
chocolate chip							
cookie dough . .	170	2.0	20.0	9.0	35	70	0
chocolate fudge . .	160	2.0	20.0	9.0	30	75	0
chocolate mousse							
royale	170	2.0	20.0	10.0	25	60	1.0
chocolate raspberry							
truffle	160	2.0	20.0	8.0	30	55	0
Chocoholic's Reso-							
lution	170	2.0	21.0	9.0	30	65	0
Choc o' the Irish	160	2.0	17.0	9.0	30	60	0
Chunk a Cherry							
Burnin' Love . . .	140	2.0	16.0	8.0	30	45	0
cinnamon tax							
crunch	160	2.0	20.0	8.0	25	70	0
coconut	160	2.0	14.0	11.0	35	50	1.0

Food and Measure	cal.	prot. (gms)	carbo. (gms)	fat (gms)	chol. (mgs)	sod. (mgs)	fiber (gms)
coconut, nutty . . .	170	3.0	15.0	12.0	30	50	1.0
Everyone's Favorite Candy Bar	170	2.0	22.0	9.0	25	65	0
Fudge, Here Comes the	150	2.0	20.0	7.0	20	55	0
gold medal ribbon	150	2.0	20.0	8.0	30	95	0
Heath Bar	170	2.0	19.0	10.0	30	70	0
jamoca	140	2.0	14.0	9.0	35	50	0
jamoca almond fudge	160	3.0	17.0	9.0	25	40	1.0
Kahlua and choco- late cream	150	2.0	16.0	8.0	30	50	0
lemon custard . . .	150	2.0	16.0	8.0	45	55	0
mint, Martian . . .	160	2.0	19.0	9.0	25	90	0
mint chocolate chip	150	2.0	15.0	10.0	35	45	0
Mississippi mudd	160	2.0	22.0	8.0	25	80	0
Naughty New Year's Resolution	170	3.0	22.0	11.0	25	70	0
Nutty or Nice . . .	160	2.0	20.0	9.0	30	75	0
peach	130	2.0	16.0	7.0	30	40	0
peanut butter:							
'n chocolate . .	180	3.0	16.0	12.0	30	95	1.0
Reese's	180	5.0	17.0	11.0	30	70	0
peppermint	150	2.0	18.0	8.0	30	45	0
peppermint winter wondermint . . .	150	2.0	16.0	8.0	30	45	0
pink bubble gum	150	2.0	19.0	8.0	30	45	0
pistachio-almond	170	3.0	13.0	12.0	30	45	1.0
pralines 'n cream	160	2.0	19.0	9.0	30	75	0
pumpkin patch . . .	140	2.0	17.0	8.0	25	50	0
Quarterback Crunch	160	2.0	18.0	10.0	30	75	0
Red, White & Boo	150	2.0	20.0	7.0	25	45	0
rocky road	170	3.0	19.0	10.0	30	60	0
rum raisin	140	2.0	18.0	7.0	30	40	0
S'mores	170	2.0	23.0	7.5	16	55	0
Snickidy Doo Dah	170	2.0	20.0	9.0	30	90	0
strawberry short- cake	160	2.0	18.0	9.0	30	70	0

Food and Measure	cal.	prot. (gms)	carbo. (gms)	fat (gms)	chol. (mgs)	sod. (mgs)	fiber (gms)
Baskin-Robbins, ice cream *(cont.)*							
strawberry very							
berry	120	2.0	16.0	6.0	20	45	0
toffee, English . . .	160	2.0	19.0	9.0	30	70	0
vanilla	140	3.0	14.0	8.0	35	40	0
vanilla, decorating	140	2.0	14.0	9.0	35	50	0
vanilla, French . . .	160	2.0	15.0	11.0	70	45	0
ice cream, light:							
chocolate caramel							
nut	130	4.0	20.0	4.0	10	70	1.0
espresso 'n cream	110	3.0	18.0	4.0	10	55	0
praline dream . . .	120	3.0	18.0	4.0	10	65	0
raspberry, double	90	3.0	16.0	2.0	10	40	0
rocky path	130	4.0	19.0	4.0	10	55	1.0
ice cream, fat free:							
cheesecake, berry	110	3.0	24.0	0	0	100	0
chocolate marsh-							
mallow	110	4.0	26.0	0	2	75	1.0
chocolate vanilla							
twist	100	4.0	22.0	0	3	75	1.0
jamoca swirl	110	3.0	23.0	0	1	105	0
vanilla bean	100	4.0	20.0	0	0	110	0
soft serve:							
caramel praline	120	4.0	25.0	0	3	85	0
vanilla	120	5.0	25.0	0	3	85	0
ice cream, no sugar:							
berries 'n banana	80	4.0	15.0	1.0	5	55	0
Call Me Nuts	100	3.0	19.0	2.0	5	55	1.0
cherry cordial . . .	100	3.0	19.0	2.0	5	55	0
chocolate, mad							
about	100	3.0	19.0	2.0	4	40	0
jamoca Swiss al-							
mond	100	3.0	16.0	2.5	5	65	0
mint, thin	100	4.0	17.0	2.5	5	70	0
raspberry revelation	100	3.0	20.0	1.0	5	55	1.0
ices, sherbets,							
sorbets:							
daiquiri ice	110	0	27.0	0	0	10	0
grape ice	100	0	27.0	0	0	10	0

Food and Measure	cal.	prot. (gms)	carbo. (gms)	fat (gms)	chol. (mgs)	sod. (mgs)	fiber (gms)
mandarin mimosa							
sorbet	120	0	28.0	0	0	20	0
margarita ice	110	0	28.0	0	0	10	0
orange sherbet . .	120	1.0	25.0	1.5	5	25	0
peachy keen sorbet	100	0	24.0	0	0	10	0
rainbow sherbet . .	120	1.0	25.0	1.5	5	25	0
raspberry sherbet,							
blue	120	1.0	25.0	1.5	5	0	0
raspberry sorbet,							
red	120	0	30.0	0	0	10	0
raspberry lemonade							
sorbet, pink . . .	110	0	29.0	0	0	20	0
strawberry island							
delight ice	100	0	26.0	0	0	5	0
novelties, 1 pc.:							
Cappy Blast bar:							
cappuccino . . .	120	2.0	18.0	5.0	20	35	0
mocha cappuc-							
cino	120	2.0	21.0	4.0	15	35	0
chillyburger, regular							
or mint chocolate							
chip	220	4.0	27.0	11.0	25	100	1.0
sundae bar:							
jamoca almond							
fudge	280	5.0	28.0	17.0	20	60	0
peanut butter							
chocolate . .	340	7.0	22.0	27.0	20	115	2.0
pralines 'n cream	280	4.0	28.0	17.0	10	105	2.0
Tiny Toon bar:							
chocolate or mint							
chocolate chip	240	3.0	20.0	17.0	25	40	2.0
vanilla	210	3.0	18.0	16.0	25	40	0
yogurt, frozen, hard:							
brownie madness,							
Maui	140	5.0	26.0	3.0	5	80	1.0
Have Your Cake . .	110	4.0	22.0	1.0	4	100	0
Jumpin' Java Bean	120	4.0	25.0	0	0	75	0
Last Mango In Para-							
dise, nonfat . . .	130	4.0	28.0	0	0	70	1.0

Food and Measure	cal.	prot. (gms)	carbo. (gms)	fat (gms)	chol. (mgs)	sod. (mgs)	fiber (gms)
Baskin-Robbins, yogurt, frozen, hard (cont.)							
Praline, Perils of . .	130	4.0	24.0	3.0	5	95	0
raspberry cheese							
Louise	130	4.0	24.0	3.0	10	95	0
yogurt, frozen, lowfat:							
blueberry	120	4.0	24.0	1.5	5	70	0
cheesecake	120	4.0	21.0	1.5	10	75	0
chocolate	120	5.0	23.0	1.5	5	75	0
vanilla	120	4.0	22.0	2.0	10	75	0
yogurt, frozen, nonfat:							
cherry, black	110	3.0	24.0	0	0	50	0
chocolate, Dutch . .	100	4.0	23.0	0	0	60	1.0
chocolate mint . . .	100	4.0	23.0	0	0	60	1.0
Kahlua	100	3.0	21.0	0	0	55	0
key lime	100	3.0	22.0	0	0	55	0
maple walnut . . .	100	3.0	22.0	0	0	55	0
peach	100	3.0	22.0	0	0	50	0
peppermint twist . .	100	3.0	22.0	0	0	55	0
piña colada	110	3.0	22.0	0	0	50	0
raspberry	100	3.0	22.0	0	0	55	0
strawberry	100	3.0	23.0	0	0	55	0
vanilla	110	4.0	23.0	0	0	65	0
yogurt, frozen, nonfat, reduced sugar:							
apple pie	80	4.0	16.0	0	2	75	1.0
banana, whata . . .	80	4.0	15.0	0	3	75	1.0
berry, tripple delight	90	4.0	16.0	0	2	75	1.0
chocolate	80	5.0	15.0	0	0	80	1.0
mocha, cafe	80	4.0	15.0	0	2	75	1.0
vanilla	80	4.0	15.0	0	3	75	1.0
drinks,1 serving:							
blueberry strawberry smoothie	150	4.0	31.0	0	0	70	2.0
Cappy Blast:							
regular	280	6.0	42.0	10.0	50	105	0
nonfat	210	6.0	46.0	.5	4	110	0
chocolate	470	7.0	91.0	11.0	35	220	0
chocolate, lowfat	390	8.0	90.0	1.0	3	220	1.0
mocha	330	6.0	55.0	11.0	50	130	1.0

Food and Measure	cal.	prot. (gms)	carbo. (gms)	fat (gms)	chol. (mgs)	sod. (mgs)	fiber (gms)
malt shake, vanilla							
ice cream	660	15.0	84.0	31.0	145	250	1.0
Paradise Blast:							
piña colada . . .	360	3.0	55.0	9.0	40	55	0
piña colada,							
nonfat	300	3.0	67.0	0	2	60	0
strawberry luau	340	2.0	64.0	6.0	25	80	0
strawberry luau,							
lowfat	290	3.0	65.0	0	2	90	0
smoothie:							
orange banana	120	5.0	24.0	0	5	75	1.0
strawberry ba-							
nana	170	4.0	39.0	0	5	75	2.0
cones, plain, 1 pc.:							
cake cone	25	0	4.0	0	0	35	0
sugar cone	60	1.0	7.0	0	0	50	0
waffle cone, large	120	0	14.0	1.5	0	55	0
waffle cone, fresh							
baked	146	n.a.	30.0	2.0	13	5	1.0
toppings:							
butterscotch, 2 oz.	200	1.0	47.0	2.0	6	160	0
gummy bears, baby,							
75 pcs.	130	3.0	30.0	0	0	15	0
hot fudge, 1 oz. . .	100	1.0	17.0	3.0	0	45	0
hot fudge, no sugar							
added, 1 oz. . . .	90	2.0	20.0	0	2	96	1.0
praline caramel,							
1 oz.	90	0	19.0	0	0	105	0
strawberry, 1 oz.	60	0	14.0	0	0	5	0
whipped cream,							
Rod's, 2 tsp. . .	30	0	1.0	2.5	5	0	0
Bass, meat only:							
freshwater, 4 oz.:							
raw	129	21.4	0	4.2	77	79	0
baked, broiled, or							
microwaved . . .	166	27.4	0	5.4	99	102	0
sea, see "Sea bass"							
striped, 4 oz.:							
raw	110	20.1	0	2.7	91	78	0

Food and Measure	cal.	prot. (gms)	carbo. (gms)	fat (gms)	chol. (mgs)	sod. (mgs)	fiber (gms)
Bass, striped *(cont.)*							
baked, broiled, or							
microwaved . . .	141	25.8	0	3.4	117	100	0
Batter, seasoning							
(*House of Tsang*							
Cantonese), 4 tbsp.	120	0	29.0	3.0	0	1110	0
Bay leaf, dried:							
(*McCormick*), 1 leaf	<1	0	.1	0	0	0	.1
(*Tone's*), 2 leaves . .	0	0	0	0	0	0	0
crumbled, 1 tsp. . . .	5	.1	.3	.1	0	<1	<1.0
Bean dip, 2 tbsp.:							
(*Chi-Chi's* Fiesta) . .	35	1.0	4.0	1.5	0	140	1.0
(*Marie's* Fiesta) . . .	140	2.0	2.0	14.0	10	160	<1.0
(*Old Dutch*)	30	1.0	5.0	.5	0	90	1.0
black bean:							
(*Old El Paso*) . . .	20	1.0	4.0	0	0	150	1.0
(*Tostitos*)	30	2.0	5.0	0	0	190	1.0
spicy (*Guiltless*							
Gourmet) . . . . •	30	2.0	5.0	0	0	100	1.0
hot (*Frito-Lay's*) . . .	35	2.0	5.0	1.0	0	220	2.0
jalapeño (*Frito-Lay's*)	40	2.0	6.0	1.0	0	140	0
pinto, spicy (*Guiltless*							
Gourmet)	35	2.0	6.0	0	0	100	2.0
Bean dip mix, 1 tsp.:							
black (*Knorr*)	10	0	2.0	0	0	170	0
Mexican (*Knorr*) . . .	10	1.0	2.0	0	0	100	0
Bean dishes, canned,							
see specific beans							
Bean dishes, mix							
(see also specific							
beans):							
Italian (*Knorr* Cup),							
1 pkg.	230	9.0	50.0	2.0	0	920	8.0
w/pasta, ½ cup*:							
Florentine, w/bow							
ties (*Bean Cui-*							
sine)	199	9.0	27.0	7.0	6.0	450	n.a.

Food and Measure	cal.	prot. (gms)	carbo. (gms)	fat (gms)	chol. (mgs)	sod. (mgs)	fiber (gms)
French, country, w/gemelli (*Bean Cuisine*)	214	0	27.0	8.0	0	369	n.a.
red, Barcelona, w/radiatore (*Bean Cusine*)	170	6.0	27.0	4.0	0	379	n.a.
w/rice, see "Rice dishes"							
Bean entree, frozen, white, Parisian (*Weight Watchers*), 9.87 oz.	220	13.0	23.0	9.0	20	690	13.0
Bean loaf, frozen (*Natural Touch*), 1″ slice	160	8.0	13.0	8.0	<5	350	5.0
Bean salad, ½ cup, except as noted:							
deli style (*S&W*) . .	80	4.0	20.0	0	0	670	4.0
marinated (*S&W*) . .	70	3.0	16.0	0	0	1410	3.0
three:							
(*Green Giant*) . . .	70	2.0	16.0	0	0	470	3.0
(*Hanover*), ⅓ cup	100	2.0	22.0	.5	0	120	3.0
Bean sauce, brown, spicy (*House of Tsang*), 1 tsp. . . .	15	0	3.0	0	0	125	0
Bean sprouts, see "Sprouts" and specific listings							
Beans, see specific listings							
Beans, mixed, canned (*Stokely Chulent*), ½ cup . .	110	6.0	19.0	.5	0	350	3.0
Beans, snap or string, see "Green beans"							

Food and Measure	cal.	prot. (gms)	carbo. (gms)	fat (gms)	chol. (mgs)	sod. (mgs)	fiber (gms)
Beans and franks,							
1 cup, except as							
noted:							
(*Campbell's*)	330	20.0	39.0	13.0	25	1080	8.0
(*Hormel*), 7½ oz. . . .	290	11.0	32.0	13.0	45	1270	6.0
(*Kid's Kitchen*),							
7½ oz.	310	13.0	37.0	13.0	45	760	8.0
(*Libby's Diner*),							
7¾ oz.	330	13.0	36.0	16.0	40	840	9.0
(*Van Camp's Beanie*							
Weenee)	320	16.0	35.0	14.0	40	1240	8.0
baked (*Van Camp's*							
Beanee Weenee) . .	410	18.0	58.0	14.0	40	1210	10.0
barbecue (*Van Camp's*							
Beanee Weenee) . .	340	17.0	43.0	14.0	40	1150	8.0
chili (*Van Camp's*							
Beanee Weenee),							
1 can	240	14.0	27.0	12.0	35	1090	9.0
Beans and rice, see							
"Rice dishes"							
Bearnaise sauce mix							
(*Knorr*), ¹⁄₁₀ pkg. . .	10	0	2.0	0	0	100	0
Beechnuts, dried,							
shelled, 1 oz. . . .	164	1.8	9.5	14.2	0	n.a.	n.a.
Beef, choice grade,							
meat only[1], 4 oz.:							
brisket, whole:							
braised, lean w/fat	437	26.6	0	35.8	107	69	0
braised, lean only	274	33.7	0	14.5	105	79	0
chuck, arm pot roast:							
braised, lean w/fat	395	30.6	0	29.2	112	67	0
braised, lean only	255	37.4	0	10.5	115	75	0
chuck, blade roast:							
braised, lean w/fat	412	29.7	0	31.5	117	73	0
braised, lean only	298	35.2	0	16.3	120	81	0

[1] *Retail cuts trimmed to ¼″ fat, except as noted.*

Food and Measure	cal.	prot. (gms)	carbo. (gms)	fat (gms)	chol. (mgs)	sod. (mgs)	fiber (gms)
flank steak[1]:							
braised, lean only	269	31.8	0	14.7	81	82	0
broiled, lean only	256	30.0	0	14.2	77	92	0
ground, raw:							
extra lean	265	21.1	0	19.3	78	75	0
lean	298	20.0	0	23.4	85	78	0
regular	351	18.8	0	30.0	96	77	0
ground, broiled, medium:							
extra lean	290	28.8	0	18.5	95	79	0
lean	308	28.0	0	20.9	99	87	0
regular	328	27.3	0	23.5	102	94	0
porterhouse steak:							
broiled, lean w/fat	346	28.2	0	25.1	94	69	0
broiled, lean only	247	31.9	0	12.2	91	75	0
rib, whole:							
roasted, lean w/fat	426	25.1	0	35.4	96	71	0
roasted, lean only	276	30.9	0	15.9	91	82	0
rib, large end (ribs 6–9):							
roasted, lean w/fat	434	25.3	0	36.2	96	71	0
roasted, lean only	284	31.2	0	16.7	92	83	0
rib, small end (ribs 10–12):							
broiled, lean w/fat	376	26.7	0	31.3	95	70	0
broiled, lean only	264	31.8	0	14.3	91	78	0
round, bottom:							
braised, lean w/fat	322	32.5	0	20.3	109	57	0
braised, lean only	249	35.8	0	10.7	109	58	0
round, eye of:							
roasted, lean w/fat	273	30.2	0	16.0	82	67	0
roasted, lean only	198	32.9	0	6.5	78	70	0
round, full cut:							
broiled, lean w/fat	272	31.0	0	15.4	91	69	0
broiled, lean only	217	33.1	0	8.3	88	73	0
round, tip:							
roasted, lean w/fat	280	30.1	0	16.9	94	70	0

[1] *Trimmed to 0″ fat.*

Food and Measure	cal.	prot. (gms)	carbo. (gms)	fat (gms)	chol. (mgs)	sod. (mgs)	fiber (gms)
Beef, round, tip *(cont.)*							
roasted, lean only	213	32.6	0	8.3	92	74	0
round, top:							
broiled, lean w/fat	254	34.2	0	12.0	96	68	0
broiled, lean only	214	35.9	0	6.7	95	69	0
fried, lean w/fat . .	314	36.7	0	17.4	110	77	0
fried, lean only . .	257	39.8	0	9.7	110	81	0
shank, crosscuts:							
braised, lean w/fat	298	34.8	0	16.6	91	69	0
braised, lean only	228	38.2	0	7.2	88	73	0
shortribs:							
braised, lean w/fat	534	24.5	0	47.6	107	57	0
braised, lean only	335	34.9	0	20.6	105	66	0
sirloin, top:							
broiled, lean w/fat	305	31.3	0	19.0	102	70	0
broiled, lean only	229	34.4	0	9.1	101	75	0
fried, lean w/fat . .	370	31.9	0	25.9	111	79	0
fried, lean only . .	270	36.8	0	12.4	112	87	0
T-bone steak:							
broiled, lean w/fat	338	28.3	0	24.0	94	69	0
broiled, lean only	243	31.9	0	11.8	91	75	0
tenderloin:							
broiled, lean w/fat	345	28.4	0	24.8	98	67	0
broiled, lean only	252	32.0	0	12.7	95	71	0
top loin:							
broiled, lean w/fat	338	28.8	0	23.8	90	71	0
broiled, lean only	243	32.5	0	11.5	86	77	0
Beef, canned (see also "Beef entree, canned" and specific listings):							
corned, 2 oz.:							
(Goya)	120	14.0	0	7.0	n.a.	450	0
(Hormel)	120	15.0	0	7.0	50	490	0
(Libby's)	120	15.0	0	7.0	50	490	0
cubed *(Hormel)*, ½ cup	130	25.0	0	3.0	20	600	0
roast, w/gravy:							
(Libby's), ⅔ cup . .	140	26.0	2.0	3.0	80	1390	4.0

Food and Measure	cal.	prot. (gms)	carbo. (gms)	fat (gms)	chol. (mgs)	sod. (mgs)	fiber (gms)
(*Hormel*), 2 oz. . .	60	11.0	1.0	2.0	30	280	1.0
Beef, corned (see also "Beef, canned" and "Beef lunch meat"), brisket, cooked, 4 oz. . . .	285	20.6	.5	21.5	111	1286	0
Beef, dried, 1 oz.:							
cured	47	8.3	.4	1.1	n.a.	984	0
sliced (*Hormel*) . . .	50	8.0	1.0	1.5	25	1240	0
sliced (*Hormel* 2.5 oz. can)	45	8.0	1.0	1.0	20	810	0
Beef, freeze-dried (*AlpineAire*), ⅓ cup	106	15.0	n.a.	5.0	n.a.	30	0
Beef, refrigerated, rib eye, salted (*Hebrew National*), 4 oz. . .	400	16.0	0	37.0	80	260	0
"Beef," vegetarian:							
burger, see " 'Hamburger,' vegetarian"							
canned:							
(*Worthington* Savory Slices), 3 slices	150	10.0	6.0	9.0	0	540	3.0
(*Worthington Prime Stakes*), 1 pc. . .	140	9.0	4.0	9.0	0	440	4.0
(*Worthington Vegetable Steaks*), 2 slices	80	15.0	3.0	1.5	0	300	3.0
stew (*Worthington Country*), 1 cup	210	13.0	20.0	9.0	0	830	5.0
frozen:							
corned (*Worthington* Roll), ⅜" slice . .	130	9.0	4.0	9.0	0	510	2.0
corned (*Worthington* Slices), 4 slices	140	10.0	5.0	9.0	0	520	2.0
smoked (*Worthington* Roll), ⅜" slice	120	10.0	5.0	6.0	0	700	3.0
smoked (*Worthington* Sliced), 6 slices	120	11.0	6.0	6.0	0	150	3.0

Food and Measure	cal.	prot. (gms)	carbo. (gms)	fat (gms)	chol. (mgs)	sod. (mgs)	fiber (gms)
Beef dinner, frozen, 1 pkg.:							
and broccoli:							
(*Swanson*)	340	15.0	51.0	10.0	30	770	4.0
(*Swanson Hungry Man*)	500	25.0	73.0	16.0	50	1200	6.0
chicken fried steak:							
(*Banquet*)	800	29.0	73.0	44.0	55	2050	6.0
(*Marie Callender's*)	650	23.0	69.0	31.0	50	2260	7.0
w/gravy (*Swanson*)	450	35.0	44.0	23.0	50	1320	3.0
and gravy (*Swanson*)	310	11.0	37.0	7.0	40	760	5.0
and peppers Cantonese (*Healthy Choice*)	270	16.0	40.0	5.0	35	560	5.0
pot roast, Yankee:							
(*The Budget Gourmet* Light & Healthy)	270	19.0	32.0	7.0	30	430	8.0
(*Healthy Choice*) . .	280	19.0	38.0	5.0	45	460	5.0
(*Swanson*)	260	8.0	36.0	5.0	40	770	6.0
(*Swanson Hungry Man*)	400	17.0	47.0	11.0	45	910	10.0
roast beef sandwich, smothered (*Swanson*)	350	17.0	46.0	11.0	30	590	5.0
Salisbury steak:							
(*Banquet*)	740	31.0	52.0	46.0	75	1860	11.0
(*The Budget Gourmet* Light & Healthy)	260	19.0	31.0	8.0	35	430	6.0
(*Healthy Choice*) . .	320	18.0	48.0	6.0	45	470	7.0
(*Swanson*)	420	31.0	40.0	20.0	60	980	5.0
(*Swanson Hungry Man*)	590	49.0	45.0	32.0	80	1610	11.0
con queso (*Patio*)	390	18.0	33.0	20.0	40	1570	10.0
sirloin:							
(*The Budget Gourmet* Light & Healthy Special Recipe)	310	20.0	42.0	7.0	25	550	5.0

Food and Measure	cal.	prot. (gms)	carbo. (gms)	fat (gms)	chol. (mgs)	sod. (mgs)	fiber (gms)
chopped, w/gravy							
(*Swanson*)	310	14.0	34.0	9.0	30	840	5.0
meatballs and gravy							
(*The Budget*							
Gourmet Light &							
Healthy)	310	22.0	37.0	8.0	35	540	5.0
tips (*Swanson Hun-*							
gry Man)	450	25.0	49.0	16.0	120	870	9.0
tips, w/noodles							
(*Swanson*)	280	15.0	32.0	10.0	50	510	5.0
in wine sauce (*The*							
Budget Gourmet							
Light & Healthy)	270	19.0	36.0	6.0	40	460	5.0
Stroganoff (*Healthy*							
Choice)	310	21.0	44.0	6.0	60	440	3.0
teriyaki (*The Budget*							
Gourmet Light &							
Healthy)	310	19.0	46.0	6.0	45	600	7.0
tips:							
(*Healthy Choice*) . .	260	20.0	32.0	5.0	40	390	6.0
sauce (*Healthy*							
Choice)	290	19.0	40.0	6.0	40	270	5.0
Beef entree, canned:							
chow mein (*La Choy*							
Bi-Pack), 1 cup . .	110	10.0	15.0	1.5	10	760	4.0
goulash (*Hormel*),							
7½-oz. can	230	13.0	19.0	11.0	50	1040	3.0
hash, see "Beef hash"							
pepper (steak):							
(*La Choy*), ⅕ pkg.	35	2.0	7.0	0	0	940	1.0
Oriental (*La Choy*							
Bi-Pack), 1 cup	105	11.0	11.0	2.5	20	1065	3.0
Oriental, w/noodles							
(*La Choy* Bi-							
Pack), 1 cup . . .	160	18.0	18.0	2.5	15	900	4.0
pot roast (*Dinty*							
Moore American							
Classics), 10 oz. . .	210	25.0	22.0	3.0	45	730	2.0

Food and Measure	cal.	prot. (gms)	carbo. (gms)	fat (gms)	chol. (mgs)	sod. (mgs)	fiber (gms)
Beef entree, canned *(cont.)*							
roast, w/mashed potato (*Dinty Moore American Classics*), 10 oz.	240	24.0	25.0	5.0	35	860	2.0
Salisbury steak: (*Dinty Moore American Classics*), 10 oz. . . .	310	23.0	22.0	14.0	60	1090	3.0
stew, 7½ oz., except as noted:							
(*Dinty Moore*), 1 cup	230	11.0	16.0	14.0	40	950	2.0
(*Dinty Moore* Can)	190	11.0	15.0	10.0	30	840	2.0
(*Dinty Moore* Cup)	190	11.0	15.0	10.0	30	870	2.0
(*Dinty Moore American Classics*), 10 oz.	260	15.0	21.0	13.0	45	1160	3.0
(*Hormel* Micro Cup)	180	11.0	15.0	9.0	30	880	2.0
(*Hunt's* Homestyle), 1 cup	155	14.0	20.0	4.5	20	1140	5.0
(*Libby's Diner*), 7¾ oz.	290	12.0	19.0	20.0	40	850	5.0
(*Nalley*)	180	10.0	18.0	8.0	15	680	3.0
(*Nalley* Big Chunk), 1 cup	260	13.0	25.0	12.0	25	1140	4.0
burger (*Dinty Moore* Hearty Cup) . . .	240	12.0	19.0	13.0	40	930	3.0
Beef entree, freeze-dried, 1 cup:							
w/peppers, onions, rice (*Mountain House*)	230	13.0	32.0	5.0	25	890	2.0
stew (*Mountain House*)	150	10.0	24.0	2.0	20	920	3.0
Stroganoff, w/noodles (*Mountain House*)	240	10.0	28.0	10.0	15	800	1.0
teriyaki, w/rice (*Mountain House*)	250	12.0	42.0	4.0	15	850	2.0

Food and Measure	cal.	prot. (gms)	carbo. (gms)	fat (gms)	chol. (mgs)	sod. (mgs)	fiber (gms)
Beef entree, frozen, 1 pkg., except as noted:							
barbecue, mesquite (*Healthy Choice*) . .	310	23.0	45.0	4.0	45	490	6.0
broccoli Beijing (*Healthy Choice*) . .	330	20.0	55.0	3.0	20	500	5.0
Cantonese (*The Budget Gourmet*) . . .	280	16.0	36.0	8.0	30	1670	3.0
chipped: (*Banquet* Topper), 4 oz.	100	9.0	8.0	3.0	25	700	0
creamed (*Stouffer's*), 4.4 oz.	160	10.0	6.0	11.0	40	690	1.0
enchilada, see "Enchilada entree"							
ground, w/rice (*Goya*)	860	30.0	111.0	35.0	70	1000	4.0
mesquite, w/rice (*Lean Cuisine* Cafe Classics)	280	16.0	38.0	7.0	35	470	6.0
Oriental: (*The Budget Gourmet* Light & Healthy)	270	16.0	35.0	8.0	35	1070	3.0
(*Lean Cuisine*) . . .	250	14.0	30.0	8.0	30	480	4.0
(*Stouffer's Lunch Express*)	290	12.0	43.0	8.0	15	880	4.0
patty: (*Swanson Fun Feast*)	470	29.0	54.0	19.0	40	490	5.0
charbroiled, gravy and (*Morton*) . .	290	11.0	25.0	16.0	25	1210	6.0
gravy and (*Banquet*)	300	11.0	21.0	20.0	35	1060	3.0
mushroom gravy and (*Banquet*), 1 patty	180	8.0	7.0	13.0	25	640	2.0
onion gravy and (*Banquet*), 1 patty	180	8.0	7.0	14.0	20	630	2.0

Food and Measure	cal.	prot. (gms)	carbo. (gms)	fat (gms)	chol. (mgs)	sod. (mgs)	fiber (gms)
Beef entree, frozen *(cont.)*							
pepper steak:							
(*The Budget Gourmet*)	290	18.0	38.0	8.0	40	1060	4.0
(*Stouffer's*)	330	17.0	45.0	9.0	35	640	3.0
(*Weight Watchers*)	240	18.0	33.0	4.5	35	690	4.0
Oriental (*Healthy Choice*)	250	19.0	34.0	4.0	35	470	3.0
pie or pot pie:							
(*Banquet*)	330	9.0	38.0	15.0	25	1000	3.0
(*Stouffer's*)	450	19.0	36.0	26.0	65	1140	3.0
(*Swanson*)	400	35.0	39.0	23.0	30	830	3.0
(*Swanson Hungry Man*)	710	58.0	71.0	38.0	55	1440	6.0
pot pie, Yankee:							
(*Marie Callender's*)	690	16.0	57.0	44.0	25	1390	3.0
(*Marie Callender's*), 1 cup	640	19.0	53.0	39.0	10	950	3.0
pot roast, w/potatoes:							
(*Lean Cuisine*) . . .	210	16.0	21.0	7.0	40	570	3.0
(*Stouffer's* Homestyle)	270	19.0	25.0	10.0	40	640	4.0
roast:							
(*Healthy Choice* Hearty Handfuls), 6.1 oz.	310	14.0	52.0	4.5	15	550	5.0
open face (*The Budget Gourmet*) . .	340	15.0	33.0	17.0	40	890	3.0
Salisbury steak:							
(*Banquet*)	310	14.0	28.0	16.0	35	910	5.0
(*Healthy Choice*) . .	260	18.0	32.0	6.0	30	500	5.0
(*Lean Cuisine*) . . .	270	23.0	27.0	8.0	60	590	4.0
(*Stouffer's* Homestyle)	370	24.0	26.0	19.0	50	1220	0
gravy and (*Banquet*), 1 patty . .	200	12.0	7.0	14.0	25	610	2.0
gravy and (*Banquet Toppers*), 5 oz.	220	9.0	8.0	16.0	25	790	2.0
gravy and (*Morton*)	210	9.0	23.0	9.0	20.0	950	3.0

Food and Measure	cal.	prot. (gms)	carbo. (gms)	fat (gms)	chol. (mgs)	sod. (mgs)	fiber (gms)
gravy, mashed po- tato (*Swanson*)	310	26.0	23.0	17.0	30	1070	2.0
grilled (*Weight* *Watchers*)	250	19.0	24.0	9.0	40	590	3.0
sirloin (*The Budget* *Gourmet* Light & Healthy)	240	21.0	28.0	5.0	40	550	2.0
sandwich, see "Beef sandwich"							
shredded, w/rice (*Goya*)	830	38.0	118.0	24.0	55	230	5.0
sirloin:							
cheddar melt (*The* *Budget Gourmet*)	370	17.0	29.0	21.0	85	800	3.0
in herb sauce (*The* *Budget Gourmet* Light & Healthy)	260	19.0	30.0	7.0	30	850	5.0
peppercorn (*Lean* *Cuisine* Cafe Clas- sics)	210	13.0	24.0	7.0	25	480	4.0
roast supreme (*The* *Budget Gourmet*)	300	16.0	32.0	13.0	65	850	3.0
tips, and noodles (*Swanson*)	200	12.0	20.0	8.0	35	380	2.0
tips, w/vegetables (*The Budget* *Gourmet*)	250	14.0	20.0	13.0	40	1060	4.0
sliced:							
(*Banquet* Country)	240	26.0	19.0	7.0	70	660	4.0
gravy and (*Ban-* *quet*), 2 slices . .	100	13.0	7.0	3.0	40	850	<1.0
gravy and (*Banquet* Topper), 4 oz. . . .	70	8.0	5.0	2.0	25	440	<1.0
steak:							
chicken fried (*Ban-* *quet* Country) . .	400	15.0	39.0	20	30	1180	4.0
Philly (*Healthy* *Choice* Hearty Handfuls), 6.1 oz.	290	15.0	47.0	5.0	15	550	5.0

Food and Measure	cal.	prot. (gms)	carbo. (gms)	fat (gms)	chol. (mgs)	sod. (mgs)	fiber (gms)
Beef entree, frozen *(cont.)*							
stew:							
(*Banquet*), 1 cup	160	14.0	17.0	4.0	25	1120	4.0
w/rice (*Goya*) . . .	770	38.0	117.0	18.0	55	360	4.0
stir-fry (*Tyson* Kit),							
1 cup	180	11.0	30.0	2.0	20	660	2.0
Stroganoff:							
(*The Budget Gour-*							
met Light &							
Healthy)	290	20.0	32.0	7.0	35	580	3.0
(*Stouffer's*)	390	23.0	30.0	20.0	85	110	2.0
tips, Français (*Healthy*							
Choice)	280	20.0	40.0	5.0	30	520	4.0
Beef entree mix, see							
specific listings							
Beef gravy, ¼ cup:							
(*Franco-American*) . .	30	3.0	4.0	2.0	<5	300	0
hearty (*Pepperidge*							
Farm)	25	2.0	4.0	1.0	<5	360	0
Beef hash, canned,							
1 cup, except as							
noted:							
(*Broadcast Morning*							
Classics Original)	240	8.0	22.0	13.0	20	930	1.0
corned beef:							
(*Castleberry's*) . . .	430	21.0	25.0	28.0	55	1070	3.0
(*Dinty Moore* Cup),							
7½ oz.	200	19.0	19.0	22.0	60	850	2.0
(*Goya*)	410	16.0	20.0	29.0	n.a.	1000	0
(*Libby's*)	490	22.0	26.0	36.0	95	1250	4.0
(*Mary Kitchen*) . . .	390	21.0	22.0	24.0	70	930	2.0
(*Mary Kitchen*),							
7½ oz.	350	19.0	22.0	22.0	60	850	2.0
(*Nalley*)	490	22.0	26.0	34.0	65	1110	4.0
roast beef:							
(*Libby's*)	460	19.0	23.0	33.0	80	1390	3.0
(*Mary Kitchen*) . . .	390	21.0	22.0	24.0	70	790	2.0
(*Mary Kitchen*),							
7½ oz.	348	19.0	21.0	21.0	58	707	2.0

Food and Measure	cal.	prot. (gms)	carbo. (gms)	fat (gms)	chol. (mgs)	sod. (mgs)	fiber (gms)
sausage flavor (*Broadcast Morning Classics*)	240	8.0	22.0	13.0	20	1120	1.0
Beef hash, refrigerated, corned (*Jones Dairy Farm*), 2 oz.	120	5.0	7.0	8.0	30	280	n.a.
Beef jerky, see "Sausage sticks"							
Beef lunch meat (see also "Bologna," etc.), 2 oz., except as noted:							
corned, cooked:							
(*Hebrew National*)	80	15.0	0	3.0	35	450	0
brisket (*Boar's Head*)	80	12.0	0	3.0	40	460	0
round (*Healthy Deli*)	80	11.0	2.0	3.0	30	480	0
round (*Hebrew National*)	60	11.0	0	2.0	30	490	0
cut (*Boar's Head Deluxe Low Sodium*)	90	14.0	0	4.0	35	80	0
roast:							
(*Hormel*)	60	11.0	0	2.0	30	620	0
(*Hormel* Chuck) . .	110	11.0	0	9.0	35	300	0
(*Hormel* Top Round)	50	11.0	0	1.0	20	580	0
(*Hormel Light & Lean 97*)	60	10.0	0	2.0	25	600	0
(*Oscar Mayer Deli-Thin*), 4 slices, 1.8 oz.	60	11.0	1.0	1.5	25	530	0
Cajun (*Boar's Head*)	80	14.0	0	2.5	35	200	0
Italian (*Healthy Deli*)	70	11.0	1.0	1.5	30	320	0
seasoned (*Healthy Deli*)	70	12.0	0	2.0	30	320	0
top round (*Boar's Head* No Salt) . .	90	14.0	0	3.0	30	40	0

Food and Measure	cal.	prot. (gms)	carbo. (gms)	fat (gms)	chol. (mgs)	sod. (mgs)	fiber (gms)
Beef lunch meat *(cont.)*							
round:							
(*Boar's Head* No							
Salt)	90	14.0	0	4.0	35	40	0
eye, pepper sea-							
soned (*Boar's*							
Head)	90	14.0	0	3.0	40	90	0
top (*Boar's Head*							
Low Sodium) . .	90	14.0	0	3.0	30	80	0
Beef pie, see "Beef							
entree, frozen"							
Beef sandwich, fro-							
zen, 1 pc.:							
barbecue:							
(*Hormel Quick*							
Meal)	360	15.0	39.0	16.0	55	560	2.0
(*Hot Pockets*) . . .	340	13.0	45.0	12.0	25	850	<1.0
broccoli (*Lean Pock-*							
ets)	250	9.0	37.0	7.0	50	710	7.0
cheddar (*Hot Pockets*)	360	14.0	36.0	18.0	50	830	<1.0
cheeseburger:							
(*Hormel Quick*							
Meal)	400	21.0	35.0	20.0	80	580	2.0
bacon (*Hormel*							
Quick Meal) . . .	440	23.0	34.0	22.0	80	740	1.0
chili (*Hormel Quick*							
Meal)	450	23.0	39.0	23.0	85	780	3.0
fajita (*Hot Pockets*)	360	14.0	39.0	17.0	40	780	5.0
hamburger: (*Hormel*							
Quick Meal)	350	18.0	34.0	15.0	65	360	2.0
steak:							
biscuit (*Hormel*							
Quick Meal) . . .	320	13.0	36.0	14.0	50	750	2.0
mushroom (*Mrs.*							
Paterson's Aussie							
Pie)	420	11.0	39.0	24.0	40	860	2.0
Beef sauce, see							
"Steak sauce" and							
specific listings							

Food and Measure	cal.	prot. (gms)	carbo. (gms)	fat (gms)	chol. (mgs)	sod. (mgs)	fiber (gms)
Beef seasoning mix (see also specific listings):							
ground (*Durkee* Pouch), ¼ pkg. . . .	25	0	5.0	0	0	490	0
marinade:							
(*Durkee* Pouch), ¹⁄₁₀ pkg.	0	0	.5	0	0	220	0
(*Lawry's*), ¾ tsp.	0	0	1.0	0	0	590	0
Beef seasoning and coating mix:							
pot roast (*McCormick Bag 'n Season*), 1 tsp.	10	<1.0	1.0	0	0	390	0
spare ribs (*McCormick Bag 'n Season*), 1 tbsp.	30	<1.0	6.0	0	0	590	<1.0
Swiss steak (*McCormick Bag 'n Season*), 1 tsp.	15	0	3.0	0	0	430	0
Beef spread, roast (*Underwood*), ¼ cup	130	9.0	0	11.0	45	390	0
Beef stew, see "Beef entree"							
Beef stew seasoning:							
(*Durkee*), ¹⁄₉ pkg. . .	10	0	3.0	0	0	660	0
(*Durkee* Roasting Bag), ¹⁄₁₀ pkg. . . .	15	.5	3.0	0	0	310	0
(*Lawry's*), 2 tsp.	20	0	5.0	0	0	530	0
(*McCormick*),¹⁄₈ pkg.	15	<1.0	3.0	0	0	410	0
Beefalo, meat only, roasted, 4 oz. . . .	213	34.8	0	7.2	66	93	0
Beer, 12 fl. oz.:							
regular	146	.9	13.2	0	0	19	0
light	100	.7	4.8	0	0	10	0

Food and Measure	cal.	prot. (gms)	carbo. (gms)	fat (gms)	chol. (mgs)	sod. (mgs)	fiber (gms)
Beet, ½ cup, except as noted:							
fresh, raw:							
2 medium, 2″ diam.	70	2.6	15.6	.3	0	126	4.6
trimmed, sliced ..	29	1.1	6.5	.1	0	53	1.9
fresh, boiled, drained:							
2 medium, 2″ diam.	44	1.7	10.0	.2	0	77	1.7
sliced	38	1.4	8.5	.2	0	65	1.4
canned:							
w/liquid	36	1.0	8.3	.1	0	324	1.4
whole (*Stokely*), 4.5 oz.	80	1.0	8.0	0	0	300	2.0
whole, baby (*Green Giant LeSueur*)	35	1.0	8.0	0	0	260	2.0
whole or sliced (*Del Monte*).	35	1.0	8.0	0	0	290	2.0
whole or sliced (*Green Giant*) . .	35	1.0	8.0	0	0	260	2.0
whole, sliced, or julienne (*S&W*) . .	30	1.0	7.0	0	0	230	1.0
sliced (*Goya*) . . .	45	1.0	9.0	0	0	50	2.0
sliced (*Green Giant No Salt*)	35	1.0	8.0	0	0	60	2.0
sliced (*Stokely*) . .	40	1.0	2.0	0	0	60	1.0
canned, Harvard:							
w/liquid	89	1.0	22.4	.1	0	199	1.0
(*Green Giant*), ⅓ cup	60	<1.0	15.0	0	0	270	2.0
(*Stokely*), ⅓ cup . .	80	0	19.0	0	0	270	2.0
canned, pickled:							
(*S&W*), 1 oz. . . .	15	0	4.0	0	0	50	1.0
(*Stokely* Can), 1 oz.	25	0	5.0	0	0	65	1.0
(*Stokely* Jar), 1 oz.	25	0	5.0	0	0	90	1.0
crinkle (*Del Monte*)	80	1.0	19.0	0	0	380	2.0
Beet greens, ½ cup:							
raw, 1″ pcs.	4	.4	.8	<.1	0	38	.7
boiled, drained, 1″ pcs.	20	1.9	3.9	.1	0	173	2.1

Food and Measure	cal.	prot. (gms)	carbo. (gms)	fat (gms)	chol. (mgs)	sod. (mgs)	fiber (gms)
Berliner, pork and beef, 1 oz.	65	4.3	.7	4.9	13	368	0
Berries, mixed, frozen (*Big Valley Burst O' Berries*), ¾ cup	70	0	16.0	0	0	0	3.0
Berry drink, 8 fl. oz., except as noted:							
(*After the Fall* Oregon)	100	0	25.0	0	0	25	0
(*Capri Sun Yo Yogi Berry*), 6.75 fl. oz.	100	0	27.0	0	0	20	0
(*Hi-C Boppin'*)	120	0	33.0	0	0	30	0
(*Hi-C* Wild)	120	0	31.0	0	0	30	0
(*R.W. Knudsen* Razzleberry)	130	0	33.0	0	0	35	0
citrus (*Five Alive*) . .	110	0	30.0	0	0	5	0
nectar (*Santa Cruz*)	110	0	27.0	0	0	25	0
punch:							
(*Minute Maid*) . . .	120	0	32.0	0	0	25	0
(*Minute Maid* Box)	120	0	32.0	0	0	30	0
(*Tropicana*)	130	0	32.0	0	0	15	0
frozen* (*Minute Maid*)	120	0	32.0	0	0	5	0
Berry juice, 8 fl. oz.:							
(*Apple & Eve Nothin' But Juice*)	120	1.0	29.0	0	0	30	0
(*Heinke's* Berry Patch)	120	0	30.0	0	0	25	0
(*Juicy Juice*)	130	1.0	31.0	0	0	15	0
(*Veryfine* Juice-Ups)	140	0	34.0	0	0	15	0
Biryani paste (*Patak's*), 2 tbsp.	160	1.0	4.0	16.0	0	990	2.0
Biscuit, 1 pc., except as noted:							
(*Arnold* Old Fashioned), 2 pcs. . . .	130	3.0	18.0	5.0	0	250	<1.0
(*Awrey's* Country) . .	140	3.0	21.0	5.0	0	490	<1.0
(*Awrey's* Round), 1 oz.	70	2.0	10.0	3.0	0	230	0

Food and Measure	cal.	prot. (gms)	carbo. (gms)	fat (gms)	chol. (mgs)	sod. (mgs)	fiber (gms)
Biscuit *(cont.)*							
(*Awrey's* Round),							
2 oz.	150	3.0	22.0	5.0	0	480	<1.0
Biscuit, refrigerated,							
1 pc., except as							
noted:							
(*Big Country Butter*							
Tastin')	100	2.0	13.0	4.0	0	300	0
(*Grands!* Homestyle)	190	4.0	24.0	9.0	0	600	<1.0
plain or buttermilk							
(*Ballard Extra Lights*							
Ovenready), 3 pcs.	150	4.0	29.0	2.0	0	490	<1.0
baking powder or but-							
termilk (*1869*							
Brand)	100	2.0	12.0	5.0	0	300	0
butter (*Grands!*) . . .	200	4.0	23.0	10.0	0	580	<1.0
butter or country							
(*Pillsbury*), 3 pcs.	150	4.0	29.0	2.5	0	490	<1.0
buttermilk:							
(*Big Country*) . . .	100	2.0	14.0	4.0	0	300	0
(*Grands!*)	200	4.0	23.0	10.0	0	570	<1.0
(*Pillsbury*), 3 pcs.	150	4.0	29.0	2.5	0	490	<1.0
(*Pillsbury* Tender							
Layer), 3 pcs. . .	160	4.0	27.0	4.5	0	480	<1.0
cinnamon raisin							
(*Grands!*)	200	4.0	28.0	8.0	0	580	<1.0
flaky:							
(*Grands!*)	190	4.0	24.0	9.0	0	550	<1.0
(*Hungry Jack*),							
2 pcs.	170	3.0	23.0	7.0	0	600	<1.0
(*Hungry Jack Butter*							
Tastin'), 2 pcs.	170	3.0	23.0	7.0	0	580	<1.0
(*Hungry Jack Honey*							
Tastin'), 2 pcs.	180	3.0	25.0	7.0	0	580	<1.0
fluffy (*Hungry Jack*),							
2 pcs.	180	3.0	23.0	8.0	0	570	<1.0
Southern style:							
(*Big Country*) . . .	100	2.0	14.0	4.0	0	300	0
(*Grands!*)	200	4.0	23.0	10.0	0	580	<1.0

Food and Measure	cal.	prot. (gms)	carbo. (gms)	fat (gms)	chol. (mgs)	sod. (mgs)	fiber (gms)
flaky (*Hungry Jack*), 2 pcs.	170	3.0	23.0	7.0	0	600	<1.0
Biscuit, frozen, garlic and cheese (*Pepperidge Farm*), 1 pc.	170	4.0	24.0	6.0	10	510	2.0
Biscuit mix:							
(*Arrowhead Mills*), ¼ cup	120	5.0	23.0	1.0	0	200	3.0
(*Bisquick*), ⅓ cup . .	170	3.0	25.0	6.0	0	490	<1.0
Biscuit sandwich, see "Sausage biscuit"							
Bitter melon, see "Balsam pear"							
Black bean dip, see "Bean dip"							
Black bean mix:							
(*Fantastic*), ½ cup*	160	10.0	29.0	1.5	0	310	7.0
w/fusilli (*Bean Cuisine*), ½ cup* . . .	174	6.0	27.0	4.0	0	453	n.a.
Black bean garlic sauce (*Lee Kum Kee*), 1 tbsp.	25	1.0	3.0	1.0	0	1270	<1.0
Black beans:							
dried:							
(*Frieda's*), 1 oz. . .	40	2.7	6.8	.2	0	79	3.7
(*Goya*), ¼ cup . . .	70	9.0	23.0	0	0	20	15.0
boiled, ½ cup . . .	113	7.6	20.4	.5	0	1	7.5
canned:							
(*Eden* Organic) . .	100	7.0	17.0	0	0	15	6.0
(*Goya*)	90	7.0	19.0	0	0	460	6.0
(*Green Giant/Joan of Arc*)	100	6.0	18.0	0	0	520	5.0
(*Old El Paso*) . . .	100	7.0	17.0	1.0	0	400	7.0
(*Progresso*)	100	7.0	17.0	1.0	0	400	7.0
(*S&W*)	70	5.0	17.0	0	0	520	6.0
(*S&W* 50% Less Salt)	70	5.0	17.0	0	0	260	6.0
(*Stokely*)	110	6.0	19.0	.5	0	350	3.0
(*Sun-Vista*)	70	5.0	20.0	1.0	0	630	7.0

Food and Measure	cal.	prot. (gms)	carbo. (gms)	fat (gms)	chol. (mgs)	sod. (mgs)	fiber (gms)
Black beans, canned *(cont.)*							
refried, see "Refried beans"							
seasoned *(Allens/ Trappey's)*	120	7.0	20.0	1.5	0	410	7.0
turtle soup, dried:							
½ cup	312	19.6	58.2	.8	0	8	22.9
(Arrowhead Mills),							
¼ cup	150	10.0	28.0	.5	0	10	9.0
boiled, ½ cup . . .	120	7.5	22.4	.3	0	3	4.9
Blackberry:							
fresh, trimmed, ½ cup	37	.5	9.2	.3	0	tr.	3.6
canned:							
(Allens/Wolco),							
⅔ cup	60	2.0	13.0	.5	0	20	9.0
heavy syrup, ½ cup	118	1.7	29.6	.2	0	3	4.4
frozen:							
(Stilwell), 1 cup . .	100	2.0	22.0	0	0	0	7.0
unsweetened, ½ cup	49	.9	11.8	.3	0	1	3.8
Blackberry syrup							
(Knott's Berry Farm), 2 tbsp.	120	0	30.0	0	0	0	0
Black-eyed peas,							
½ cup:							
fresh or frozen, see "Cowpeas"							
canned, fresh shell:							
(Allens/East Texas Fair/Homefolks)	120	7.0	21.0	1.0	0	350	6.0
(Goya Cowpeas) . .	90	6.0	17.0	0	0	500	3.0
(Green Giant/Joan of Arc)	90	6.0	16.0	0	0	250	3.0
(Stokely)	110	6.0	19.0	.5	0	350	3.0
(Sun-Vista)	70	6.0	15.0	0	0	550	4.0
w/jalapeño *(Homefolks)* . . .	120	7.0	20.0	1.0	0	580	5.0
w/snaps *(Allens/East Texas Fair/ Homefolks)* . . .	120	8.0	20.0	1.0	0	420	5.0

Food and Measure	cal.	prot. (gms)	carbo. (gms)	fat (gms)	chol. (mgs)	sod. (mgs)	fiber (gms)
canned, dry:							
(*Allens/East Texas*							
Fair)	110	7.0	18.0	1.0	0	340	4.0
w/bacon (*Allens*) . .	105	7.0	20.0	1.5	0	390	5.0
w/bacon (*Trappey's*)	120	7.0	19.0	2.0	0	350	5.0
w/bacon and							
jalapeño (*Trap-*							
pey's)	110	6.0	19.0	1.5	0	470	5.0
frozen (*Stilwell*) . . .	110	7.0	21.0	1.0	0	10	4.0
Blintz, frozen (*Empire*							
Kosher), 2 pcs.:							
apple	220	6.0	36.0	5.5	<5	260	5.0
blueberry	190	4.0	36.0	4.0	10	260	2.0
cheese	200	11.0	29.0	6.0	20	310	3.0
cherry	200	5.0	38.0	4.0	10	280	3.0
potato	190	6.0	32.0	6.0	10	530	3.0
Blood sausage, 1 oz.	107	4.1	.4	9.8	34	n.a.	0
Bloody Mary mixer:							
(*Mr. & Mrs. "T"*),							
8 fl. oz.	40	1.0	9.0	0	0	1350	1.0
(*V-8*), 11.5 fl. oz. . .	70	0	13.0	0	0	1800	2.0
rich and spicy (*Mr. &*							
Mrs. "T"), 8 fl. oz.	50	2.0	12.0	0	0	990	2.0
Blueberry:							
fresh, ½ cup	41	.5	10.2	.3	0	5	2.0
canned, heavy syrup:							
(*Lucky Leaf/Mus-*							
selman's), ½ cup	120	0	29.0	0	0	15	3.0
(*S&W* Wild Maine),							
⅓ cup	70	0	16.0	0	0	0	6.0
dried (*Sonoma*),							
¼ cup	140	1.0	33.0	0	0	0	5.0
freeze-dried (*Alpine-*							
Aire), 1 oz.	60	.7	15.0	.5	0	1	n.a.
frozen:							
(*Cascadian Farm* Or-							
ganic), 1 cup . .	50	0	12.0	1.0	0	1	2.0
(*Stilwell*), 1 cup . .	90	0	21.0	0	0	0	6.0
sweetened, ½ cup	94	.5	25.2	.2	0	2	2.4

Food and Measure	cal.	prot. (gms)	carbo. (gms)	fat (gms)	chol. (mgs)	sod. (mgs)	fiber (gms)
Blueberry juice (*After the Fall*), 8 fl. oz.	90	0	25.0	0	0	20	0
Blueberry syrup:							
(*Knott's Berry Farm*), 2 tbsp.	120	0	30.0	0	0	0	0
(*R.W. Knudsen*), ¼ cup	150	0	38.0	0	0	0	0
(*S&W* Reduced Cal), ¼ cup	60	0	15.0	0	0	105	0
Bluefish, meat only:							
raw, 4 oz.	141	22.7	0	4.8	67	68	0
baked, broiled, or microwaved, 4 oz. . .	180	29.1	0	6.2	86	87	0
Boar, wild, meat only, roasted, 4 oz.	181	32.1	0	5.0	n.a.	n.a.	0
Bockwurst, raw, 1 oz.	87	3.8	.1	7.8	n.a.	n.a.	0
Bok choy, see "Cabbage, Chinese"							
Bologna (see also "Ham bologna," etc.), 2 oz., except as noted:							
(*Boar's Head*)	150	7.0	0	13.0	35	530	0
(*Boar's Head* 28% Lower Sodium) . .	150	8.0	0	13.0	30	410	0
(*Healthy Deli* Regular/ German 95% Fat Free)	70	8.0	3.0	2.5	15	460	0
(*John Morrell*)	180	6.0	4.0	16.0	50	600	0
(*Oscar Mayer*), 1-oz. slice	90	3.0	0	8.0	20	270	0
(*Oscar Mayer* Fat Free), 2 slices, 1.6 oz.	35	6.0	2.0	0	15	480	0
(*Oscar Mayer* Light), 1-oz. slice	50	3.0	1.0	4.0	15	310	0
(*Oscar Mayer* Wisconsin Ring)	180	6.0	2.0	16.0	35	460	0

Food and Measure	cal.	prot. (gms)	carbo. (gms)	fat (gms)	chol. (mgs)	sod. (mgs)	fiber (gms)
beef:							
(*Boar's Head*) . . .	150	7.0	0	13.0	35	520	0
(*Hebrew National*)	180	7.0	0	16.0	40	440	0
(*Hebrew National* Lean)	90	8.0	0	6.0	25	430	0
(*Hebrew National* Reduced Fat) . .	130	6.0	2.0	12.0	35	320	0
(*Oscar Mayer*), 1-oz. slice	90	3.0	1.0	8.0	15	300	0
(*Oscar Mayer* Light), 1-oz. slice	60	3.0	2.0	4.0	10	310	0
garlic:							
(*Boar's Head*) . . .	150	7.0	0	13.0	35	530	0
(*Oscar Mayer*), 1.5-oz. slice . . .	130	5.0	1.0	12.0	30	400	0
"Bologna," vegetarian, frozen:							
roll (*Worthington Bolono*), ⅜" slice	80	10.0	2.0	3.0	0	690	2.0
sliced (*Worthington Bolono*), 3 slices	80	10.0	2.0	3.5	0	720	2.0
Bonito, meat only, raw, 4 oz.	146	29.3	.5	2.3	n.a.	50	0
Borage:							
raw, 1" pcs., ½ cup	9	.8	1.4	.3	0	35	<1.0
boiled, drained, 4 oz.	28	2.4	4.0	.9	0	98	<2.0
Bouillabaisse seasoning mix (*Knorr* Recipe), 1 tbsp.	20	1.0	3.0	.5	<5	550	0
Bouillon (see also "Broth concentrate"), 1 tsp. or cube, except as noted:							
beef:							
(*Herb-Ox*)	10	0	1.0	0	0	700	0
(*Herb-Ox* Instant)	10	0	1.0	0	0	840	0
(*Knorr*)	20	1.0	<1.0	1.5	0	1290	0

Food and Measure	cal.	prot. (gms)	carbo. (gms)	fat (gms)	chol. (mgs)	sod. (mgs)	fiber (gms)
Bouillon, beef *(cont.)*							
(*MBT/Wyler's* Instant), 1 pkt. . .	15	1.0	2.0	0	0	810	0
(*MBT/Wyler's* Low Sodium), 1 pkt.	15	<1.0	3.0	0	0	5	0
beef or chicken:							
(*Wyler's/Steero*) . .	5	0	1.0	0	0	900	0
(*Wyler's/Steero* Reduced Sodium)	5	0	1.0	0	0	600	0
chicken:							
(*Herb-Ox*)	10	0	1.0	0	0	1040	0
(*Herb-Ox* Instant)	10	0	0	0	0	1040	0
(*Knorr*)	20	<1.0	<1.0	1.5	0	1200	0
(*MBT/Wyler's* Instant), 1 pkt. . .	15	<1.0	2.0	0	0	930	0
(*MBT/Wyler's* Low Sodium), 1 pkt.	15	<1.0	3.0	0	0	0	0
fish (*Knorr*), ½ cube	10	1.0	0	1.0	0	960	0
onion (*MBT* Instant), 1 pkt.	15	0	3.0	0	0	800	0
vegetable:							
(*Herb-Ox*)	10	0	0	0	0	1000	0
(*MBT* Instant), 1 pkt.	10	0	2.0	0	0	860	0
(*Wyler's*)	5	0	1.0	0	0	870	0
vegetarian (*Knorr*), ½ cube	15	1.0	1.0	1.0	0	910	0
Bourguignonne seasoning (*Knorr*), 1 tbsp.	35	<1.0	6.0	1.0	0	360	0
Bowtie dishes, mix:							
and beans w/herb sauce (*Knorr*), ⅔ cup	260	12.0	47.0	2.0	<5	790	6.0
Italian cheese (*Lipton* Pasta & Sauce), ½ pkg.	230	8.0	37.0	5.0	10	790	1.0

Food and Measure	cal.	prot. (gms)	carbo. (gms)	fat (gms)	chol. (mgs)	sod. (mgs)	fiber (gms)
Bowtie entree, frozen, 1 pkg.:							
and chicken (*Lean Cuisine* Cafe Classics)	270	19.0	34.0	6.0	60	550	5.0
mushrooms Marsala (*Weight Watchers*)	280	13.0	36.0	9.0	10	560	5.0
Boysenberry, ½ cup:							
fresh, see "Blackberry"							
canned, heavy syrup	113	1.3	28.6	.2	0	4	3.3
frozen, unsweetened	33	.7	8.1	.1	0	1	2.6
Boysenberry drink, 8 fl. oz.:							
(*Farmer's Market*) . .	120	0	30.0	0	0	0	0
cider (*Heinke's*) . . .	120	0	30.0	0	0	25	0
Boysenberry syrup (*Knott's Berry Farm*), 2 tbsp. . . .	120	0	30.0	0	0	0	0
Brains, 4 oz.:							
beef, fried	222	14.3	0	18.0	2262	179	0
lamb, fried	310	19.2	0	25.2	2840	178	0
pork, braised	156	13.8	0	10.8	2894	103	0
veal, fried	242	16.4	0	19.0	2404	200	0
Bran, see "Cereal" and specific grains							
Bratwurst:							
(*Boar's Head*), 4 oz.	300	19.0	0	25.0	75	650	0
(*Jones Dairy Farm* Dinner), 1 cooked link	230	10.0	0	21.0	50	470	0
pork, cooked 1 oz.	85	4.0	.6	7.3	17	158	0
Braunschweiger:							
(*Jones Dairy Farm* Chub), 2 oz.	150	9.0	1.0	12.0	130	520	0
(*Jones Dairy Farm* Chunk), 2 oz. . . .	180	8.0	1.0	16.0	110	460	0
(*Oscar Mayer*), 1-oz. slice	100	4.0	1.0	9.0	50	320	0

Food and Measure	cal.	prot. (gms)	carbo. (gms)	fat (gms)	chol. (mgs)	sod. (mgs)	fiber (gms)
Braunschweiger *(cont.)*							
w/bacon (*Jones Dairy*							
Farm Chub), 2 oz.	150	9.0	1.0	12.0	120	560	0
light, 2 oz.:							
(*Boar's Head*) . . .	120	9.0	0	8.0	50	450	0
(*Jones Dairy Farm*							
Chub)	100	10.0	1.0	6.0	140	500	0
(*Jones Dairy Farm*							
Chunk)	100	10.0	1.0	6.0	110	330	0
w/onion (*Jones Dairy*							
Farm Chub), 2 oz.	150	9.0	2.0	12.0	120	560	0
sliced:							
(*Jones Dairy Farm*),							
1.2-oz. slice . . .	110	5.0	1.0	10.0	70	280	0
(*Jones Dairy Farm*),							
2 slices, 1.6 oz.	150	6.0	1.0	13.0	90	370	0
spread (*Oscar Mayer*),							
2 oz.	190	8.0	2.0	17.0	90	630	0
Brazil nuts, shelled,							
1 oz., 6 large or 8							
medium kernels . .	186	4.1	3.6	18.8	0	<1	1.6
Bread, 1 slice, except							
as noted:							
(*Arnold Bran'nola*							
Country)	90	4.0	18.0	2.5	0	115	3.0
(*Arnold/Brownberry*							
Bran'nola Original)	90	4.0	18.0	2.0	0	125	3.0
apple honey wheat							
(*Brownberry*) . . .	60	2.0	12.0	1.0	0	105	1.0
apple walnut (*Pepper-*							
idge Farm)	80	2.0	14.0	2.0	0	120	1.0
bran:							
honey (*Pepperidge*							
Farm)	90	3.0	17.0	1.0	0	160	2.0
light (*August Bros./*							
Brownberry							
Bakery Country),							
2 slices	80	4.0	21.0	1.0	0	180	5.0
whole (*Brownberry*)	60	2.0	12.0	1.0	0	140	2.0

Food and Measure	cal.	prot. (gms)	carbo. (gms)	fat (gms)	chol. (mgs)	sod. (mgs)	fiber (gms)
buttermilk (*Arnold*)	100	4.0	18.0	2.0	0	170	1.0
cinnamon:							
(*Brownberry*) . . .	80	2.0	14.0	2.0	0	115	<1.0
(*Pepperidge Farm*)	80	3.0	14.0	2.5	0	115	2.0
cranberry (*Arnold*)	70	2.0	14.0	1.0	0	80	1.0
date nut (*Thomas'*),							
1 oz.	80	1.0	16.0	2.0	<5	135	1.0
French:							
(*Arnold Francisco*),							
1 oz.	70	3.0	14.0	1.0	0	140	<1.0
(*Pepperidge Farm*),							
⅑ loaf	130	4.0	25.0	1.5	0	280	1.0
(*Pepperidge Farm*							
sliced), ⅑ loaf . .	120	4.0	24.0	1.5	0	260	1.0
twin (*Brownberry*							
Francisco Intl.)	80	2.0	18.0	1.0	0	140	1.0
golden:							
light (*Brownberry*							
Bakery), 2 slices	80	4.0	20.0	.5	0	180	5.0
swirl (*Pepperidge*							
Farm Vermont							
Maple)	90	2.0	15.0	2.5	0	100	<1.0
Italian:							
(*Arnold Francisco*),							
2 slices	110	4.0	23.0	1.0	0	240	1.0
(*Arnold Savoni's*)	60	2.0	13.0	.5	0	125	<1.0
brown and serve							
(*Pepperidge*							
Farm), ⅑ loaf . .	130	4.0	24.0	2.0	0	260	1.0
light (*Arnold/*							
Brownberry							
Bakery), 2 slices	80	4.0	21.0	1.0	0	200	5.0
stick (*Arnold Fran-*							
cisco 10 oz.),							
1 oz.	70	3.0	14.0	1.0	0	135	1.0
stick, sliced (*Arnold*							
Francisco 1 lb.)	70	2.0	15.0	.5	0	140	<1.0

Food and Measure	cal.	prot. (gms)	carbo. (gms)	fat (gms)	chol. (mgs)	sod. (mgs)	fiber (gms)
Bread, Italian *(cont.)*							
thick (*Brownberry Francisco Intl*), 2 slices	110	3.0	23.0	1.0	0	250	1.0
kamut, sprout (*Shiloh Farms* Egyptian) . .	90	6.0	18.0	1.0	0	115	3.0
mixed/multigrain:							
(*Brownberry* Hearth)	90	4.0	17.0	1.5	0	190	2.0
(*Roman Meal* Round Top)	70	3.0	13.0	1.0	0	140	1.0
(*Roman Meal* Sun)	70	3.0	12.0	1.5	0	140	1.0
5, sprouted (*Shiloh Farms*)	90	5.0	19.0	.5	0	110	3.0
5, sprouted (*Shiloh Farms* No Salt)	90	5.0	19.0	.5	0	0	4.0
7 (*Roman Meal*) . .	70	3.0	16.0	1.0	0	180	1.0
7, hearty (*Pepperidge Farm*)	100	3.0	18.0	1.5	0	180	2.0
7, light (*Pepperidge Farm*), 3 slices	140	6.0	28.0	1.0	0	320	5.0
7, light (*Roman Meal*), 2 slices	80	4.0	19.0	1.0	0	205	5.0
7, sprouted (*Breads for Life/Shiloh Farms*)	90	5.0	19.0	.5	0	130	3.0
7, sprouted (*Shiloh Farms* No Salt)	90	5.0	19.0	.5	0	0	3.0
7, white (*Arnold/ Brownberry Bran'nola*)	90	4.0	18.0	2.0	0	120	3.0
9 (*Pepperidge Farm*)	90	4.0	16.0	1.0	0	170	2.0
12 (*Arnold Bran'nola*)	90	4.0	18.0	2.0	0	135	3.0
12 (*Brownberry*), 2 slices	110	4.0	20.0	2.5	0	180	2.0
12 (*Roman Meal*)	70	3.0	12.0	1.5	0	145	1.0
crunchy (*Pepperidge Farm*)	90	4.0	15.0	1.5	0	130	2.0

Food and Measure	cal.	prot. (gms)	carbo. (gms)	fat (gms)	chol. (mgs)	sod. (mgs)	fiber (gms)
w/oat bran (*Roman Meal*)	70	3.0	13.0	1.0	0	140	1.0
nutty (*Arnold Bran'nola*)	90	4.0	18.0	2.5	0	95	3.0
nutty (*Brownberry Bran'nola*)	90	4.0	18.0	2.5	0	105	3.0
sprouted (*Shiloh Farms* Sandwich)	80	4.0	17.0	.5	0	100	3.0
whole (*Pepperidge Farm* 100%) . . .	90	4.0	15.0	1.0	0	160	2.0
nut (*Brownberry* Natural Health)	70	2.0	13.0	1.5	0	130	1.0
oat:							
(*Brownberry Bran'nola*)	90	3.0	18.0	2.5	0	115	3.0
(*Roman Meal*) . . .	70	3.0	13.0	1.0	0	145	1.0
crunchy, hearty (*Pepperidge Farm*)	100	4.0	17.0	2.0	0	180	2.0
oat bran:							
honey (*Roman Meal*)	70	3.0	13.0	1.0	0	220	1.0
honey nut (*Roman Meal*)	70	3.0	13.0	1.5	0	145	1.0
light (*Roman Meal*), 2 slices	80	4.0	19.0	2.0	0	195	5.0
oatmeal:							
(*Brownberry* Natural)	70	2.0	13.0	1.0	0	135	1.0
(*Pepperidge Farm*)	80	3.0	15.0	1.0	0	200	1.0
light (*Arnold/ Brownberry Bakery*), 2 slices	80	4.0	20.0	1.0	0	200	4.0
light (*Pepperidge Farm*), 3 slices	140	7.0	27.0	1.0	0	310	5.0
soft (*Brownberry*)	70	3.0	14.0	1.5	0	105	1.0
soft (*Pepperidge Farm*)	60	2.0	12.0	.5	0	n.a.	0
thin (*Pepperidge Farm*)	60	2.0	11.0	1.0	0	160	1.0

Food and Measure	cal.	prot. (gms)	carbo. (gms)	fat (gms)	chol. (mgs)	sod. (mgs)	fiber (gms)
Bread *(cont.)*							
orange raisin							
(*Brownberry*) . . .	70	2.0	14.0	1.0	0	70	0
pita/pocket, 1 pc.:							
(*Arnold*), 2 oz. . . .	140	5.0	29.0	.5	0	230	<1.0
(*Arnold*), 3 oz. . . .	210	8.0	44.0	1.0	0	340	<1.0
(*Pepperidge Farm*)	150	6.0	30.0	1.0	0	290	2.0
(*Pepperidge Farm* Mini), 1 oz. . . .	70	3.0	15.0	0	0	140	<1.0
(*Thomas' Sahara*), 2 oz.	150	6.0	31.0	1.0	0	290	1.0
(*Thomas' Sahara*), 3 oz.	220	8.0	48.0	1.0	0	440	2.0
(*Thomas' Sahara* Mini), 1 oz. . . .	70	3.0	15.0	0	0	140	<1.0
garlic (*Arnold*) . . .	160	6.0	30.0	2.0	0	230	<1.0
oat bran (*Thomas' Sahara*)	130	6.0	30.0	1.0	0	300	3.0
onion (*Arnold*) . . .	150	5.0	28.0	2.0	0	220	<1.0
onion (*Thomas' Sahara*)	140	5.0	31.0	.5	0	270	2.0
salsa (*Thomas' Sahara*)	170	6.0	36.0	1.5	0	350	3.0
sourdough (*Thomas' Sahara*)	150	5.0	33.0	.5	0	320	2.0
wheat (*Arnold 4"*), 1 oz.	70	3.0	14.0	0	0	115	2.0
wheat (*Arnold*), 2 oz.	140	6.0	29.0	1.0	0	230	3.0
wheat (*Arnold*), 3 oz.	200	9.0	42.0	1.5	0	350	5.0
wheat (*Thomas' Sahara*), 2 oz. . . .	130	7.0	28.0	1.0	0	310	5.0
wheat (*Thomas' Sahara* Mini), 1 oz.	60	3.0	14.0	.5	0	140	2.0
white (*Arnold 4"*), 1 oz.	70	3.0	15.0	0	0	115	0
poppy seed, hazelnut (*Roman Meal*) . . .	110	4.0	16.0	4.0	0	180	1.0

Food and Measure	cal.	prot. (gms)	carbo. (gms)	fat (gms)	chol. (mgs)	sod. (mgs)	fiber (gms)
potato:							
(*Arnold* Country)	100	3.0	18.0	2.0	0	150	1.0
hearty (*Pepperidge*							
Farm Russet) . .	90	4.0	18.0	1.5	<5	260	3.0
pumpernickel:							
(*Arnold*)	80	3.0	16.0	1.0	0	150	1.0
(*Arnold August*							
Bros. 1 lb.) . . .	80	3.0	16.0	1.0	0	150	<1.0
(*Arnold August*							
Bros. 24 oz.) . .	90	3.0	19.0	1.0	0	170	1.0
(*Arnold Levy's*) . .	80	3.0	16.0	.5	0	150	1.0
dark (*Pepperidge*							
Farm)	80	3.0	15.0	1.0	0	230	1.0
party (*Pepperidge*							
Farm), 8 slices	110	6.0	22.0	1.5	0	320	4.0
rye (*Brownberry*)	70	2.0	14.0	.5	0	150	1.0
raisin:							
(*Arnold Sunmaid*)	70	2.0	14.0	1.0	0	85	0
cinnamon (*Arnold*)	70	2.0	14.0	1.0	0	90	0
cinnamon							
(*Brownberry*) . .	70	2.0	14.0	1.0	0	110	<1.0
cinnamon (*Pepper-*							
idge Farm)	80	3.0	14.0	1.5	0	105	1.0
walnut (*Brownberry*)	80	2.0	13.0	2.5	0	75	1.0
whole wheat (*Shiloh*							
Farms), 2 slices	140	7.0	30.0	1.0	0	160	3.0
rye:							
(*Arnold* Deli)	80	3.0	16.0	1.0	0	150	<1.0
(*Brownberry* Hearth)	90	4.0	18.0	1.5	0	190	2.0
Dijon (*Arnold* Real							
Jewish)	80	3.0	16.0	1.0	0	200	1.0
Dijon, thin (*Pepper-*							
idge Farm),							
2 slices	100	4.0	18.0	1.5	5	340	2.0
dill (*Arnold*)	80	3.0	16.0	1.0	0	160	2.0
dill (*Brownberry*)	70	2.0	15.0	1.0	0	150	1.0
onion (*Arnold Au-*							
gust Bros.) . . .	80	3.0	16.0	1.0	0	140	1.0

Food and Measure	cal.	prot. (gms)	carbo. (gms)	fat (gms)	chol. (mgs)	sod. (mgs)	fiber (gms)
Bread, rye *(cont.)*							
onion, w/seeds (*Arnold August Bros.*)	90	3.0	18.0	1.0	0	160	1.0
onion (*Pepperidge Farm*)	80	3.0	15.0	1.0	0	210	1.0
party (*Pepperidge Farm*), 8 slices	110	6.0	22.0	1.5	0	410	3.0
seeded (*Arnold August Bros.* 1 lb.)	80	3.0	16.0	1.0	0	140	<1.0
seeded (*Arnold/ Levy's* Real Jewish)	70	3.0	16.0	1.0	0	150	1.0
seeded (*Brownberry* Natural)	70	3.0	15.0	1.0	0	160	1.0
seeded or unseeded (*Arnold August Bros.* 24 oz.) . .	90	3.0	18.0	1.0	0	170	1.0
seeded or unseeded (*Pepperidge Farm*)	80	3.0	15.0	1.0	0	210	1.0
soft (*Arnold* Country)	70	3.0	13.0	1.0	0	140	<1.0
soft, light (*Arnold/ Brownberry Bakery*), 2 slices	80	4.0	20.0	1.0	0	180	4.0
soft, seeded (*Arnold Bakery*)	80	3.0	15.0	1.0	0	170	1.0
soft, unseeded (*Arnold Bakery*) . . .	80	3.0	15.0	1.0	0	160	<1.0
thin (*Arnold Levy's Melba*), 2 slices	90	3.0	19.0	1.0	0	180	2.0
thin (*Arnold Levy's Melba*), 2 slices	90	3.0	19.0	1.0	0	190	1.0
unseeded (*Arnold August Bros.* 1 lb.)	80	3.0	16.0	1.0	0	150	<1.0
unseeded (*Arnold* Real Jewish 1 lb.)	70	3.0	16.0	1.0	0	150	1.0

Food and Measure	cal.	prot. (gms)	carbo. (gms)	fat (gms)	chol. (mgs)	sod. (mgs)	fiber (gms)
unseeded (*Arnold* Real Jewish 2 lb.)	70	3.0	15.0	.5	0	140	<1.0
unseeded (*Arnold Levy's* Real Jewish)	70	3.0	16.0	.5	0	150	1.0
unseeded (*Brownberry* Natural)	70	2.0	15.0	1.0	0	160	1.0
unseeded, thin (*Arnold August Bros.*), 2 slices	90	3.0	19.0	1.0	0	180	1.0
unseeded, thin (*Brownberry*), 2 slices	100	3.0	20.0	1.0	0	250	1.0
rye and pump (*Arnold August Bros.*) . . .	90	3.0	18.0	1.0	0	170	1.0
sourdough:							
(*Arnold August Bros.*)	110	4.0	23.0	1.0	0	260	1.0
(*Arnold Francisco*)	90	3.0	19.0	1.0	0	250	1.0
brown and serve (*Arnold Francisco*), 1 oz. . . .	70	2.0	14.0	.5	0	240	1.0
light (*Arnold*), 2 slices	80	4.0	20.0	.5	0	180	4.0
light (*Pepperidge Farm*), 3 slices	130	6.0	27.0	1.0	0	320	4.0
thick (*Brownberry Francisco Intl.*)	90	3.0	19.0	1.0	0	250	1.0
whole grain (*Roman Meal*)	70	3.0	13.0	1.0	0	220	1.0
spelt (*Shiloh Farms*)	100	4.0	21.0	1.0	0	140	2.0
stick, sliced:							
(*Arnold August Bros.*), 2 slices	110	4.0	22.0	1.0	0	230	1.0
(*Brownberry Francisco*)	100	3.0	21.0	0	0	180	1.0
toast, Texas (*Arnold August Bros.*) . . .	150	5.0	28.0	3.0	0	260	1.0

Food and Measure	cal.	prot. (gms)	carbo. (gms)	fat (gms)	chol. (mgs)	sod. (mgs)	fiber (gms)
Bread (cont.)							
Vienna:							
light (*Pepperidge Farm*), 3 slices	130	6.0	28.0	1.0	0	300	5.0
thick (*Pepperidge Farm*)	70	3.0	12.0	1.0	0	150	<1.0
wheat:							
(*Arnold* Brick Oven)	80	3.0	14.0	2.0	0	110	2.0
(*Arnold* Brick Oven 8 oz.), 2 slices	110	5.0	20.0	2.5	0	160	3.0
(*Arnold* Brick Oven 1 lb.), 2 slices . .	110	5.0	21.0	3.0	0	170	3.0
(*Arnold Sunny Valley*), 2 slices . . .	100	4.0	20.0	1.5	0	220	2.0
(*Arnold/Brownberry* Country)	90	4.0	18.0	1.5	0	170	1.0
(*Brownberry* Hearth)	90	4.0	18.0	1.0	0	190	2.0
(*Brownberry* Natural)	80	3.0	17.0	1.0	0	210	2.0
(*Pepperidge Farm*)	90	3.0	16.0	1.5	0	190	1.0
(*Pepperidge Farm* Family)	70	2.0	13.0	1.0	0	135	1.0
(*Pepperidge Farm* Natural)	90	4.0	16.0	1.5	0	170	1.0
(*Roman Meal* Natural)	90	4.0	12.0	1.0	0	140	2.0
(*Shiloh Farms* Homestyle), ½" slice, 2 oz.	160	7.0	29.0	1.5	<5	115	<1.0
cracked, thin (*Pepperidge Farm*) . .	70	2.0	12.0	1.0	0	140	<1.0
dark (*Arnold/ Brownberry Bran'nola*)	90	4.0	16.0	2.0	0	130	3.0
hearty (*Arnold/ Brownberry Bran'nola*)	90	4.0	16.0	3.0	0	130	3.0
light (*Pepperidge Farm*), 3 slices	130	7.0	28.0	1.0	0	290	5.0

Food and Measure	cal.	prot. (gms)	carbo. (gms)	fat (gms)	chol. (mgs)	sod. (mgs)	fiber (gms)
light (*Roman Meal*), 2 slices	80	4.0	20.0	1.0	0	210	5.0
light, golden (*Arnold*), 2 slices . .	80	4.0	20.0	.5	0	180	5.0
light, hearty (*Roman Meal* Light), 2 slices	80	4.0	19.0	1.0	0	205	5.0
sesame, hearty (*Pepperidge Farm*)	100	4.0	18.0	1.5	0	190	2.0
soft (*Brownberry*)	80	3.0	14.0	2.0	0	135	1.0
soft (*Brownberry* 16 oz.), 2 slices	110	4.0	21.0	2.0	0	180	2.0
very thin (*Pepperidge Farm*), 3 slices	110	4.0	22.0	2.0	0	230	4.0
wheat, whole:							
(*Arnold* Stoneground 1 lb. 4 oz.) . . .	60	3.0	12.0	1.0	0	115	2.0
(*Arnold* Stoneground 2 lb.), 2 slices	100	5.0	19.0	1.5	0	170	3.0
(*Roman Meal*) . . .	60	3.0	13.0	1.0	0	140	2.0
(*Shiloh Farms*), 2 slices	140	7.0	26.0	1.5	0	260	4.0
(*Shiloh Farms* No Salt), 2 slices . .	140	7.0	26.0	1.5	0	0	3.0
light (*Roman Meal*), 2 slices	80	5.0	18.0	1.0	0	210	5.0
soft (*Pepperidge Farm*)	60	2.0	11.0	.5	0	210	5.0
thin (*Pepperidge Farm*)	60	3.0	11.0	1.0	0	120	<1.0
wheatberry, honey:							
(*Arnold*)	70	3.0	16.0	1.0	0	160	3.0
(*Arnold Bran'nola*)	90	3.0	19.0	1.5	0	150	3.0
(*Roman Meal*) . . .	70	3.0	13.0	1.0	0	140	1.0
hearty (*Pepperidge Farm*)	100	3.0	18.0	1.5	0	200	2.0

Food and Measure	cal.	prot. (gms)	carbo. (gms)	fat (gms)	chol. (mgs)	sod. (mgs)	fiber (gms)
Bread, wheatberry, honey *(cont.)*							
light (*Roman Meal*), 2 slices	80	4.0	15.0	1.0	0	210	5.0
white:							
(*Arnold* Brick Oven)	80	2.0	16.0	1.5	0	170	<1.0
(*Arnold* Brick Oven 8 oz.), 2 slices	120	3.0	24.0	2.5	0	220	1.0
(*Arnold* Brick Oven 1 lb.), 2 slices . .	130	3.0	24.0	2.5	0	250	1.0
(*Arnold* Country)	100	3.0	19.0	1.5	0	190	<1.0
(*Arnold Sunny Valley*), 2 slices . . .	100	4.0	21.0	1.5	0	210	1.0
(*Brownberry* Country)	90	3.0	19.0	1.5	0	180	<1.0
(*Brownberry* Natural), 2 slices . . .	120	4.0	24.0	1.5	0	160	1.0
hearty (*Pepperidge Farm*)	90	3.0	19.0	1.0	0	190	2.0
hearty (*Pepperidge Farm* Country) . .	90	3.0	19.0	1.0	0	190	2.0
light (*Arnold/ Brownberry Bakery*), 2 slices	80	4.0	21.0	.5	0	200	4.0
light (*Roman Meal*), 2 slices	80	4.0	20.0	1.0	0	210	5.0
sandwich (*Pepperidge Farm*), 2 slices	130	4.0	23.0	2.0	0	260	<1.0
sandwich (*Roman Meal*), 2 slices	110	5.0	21.0	21.5	0	225	2.0
soft (*Arnold* Country)	80	2.0	16.0	1.5	0	150	<1.0
soft (*Brownberry*)	80	2.0	14.0	1.5	0	120	1.0
soft (*Brownberry* 16 oz.), 2 slices	110	4.0	21.0	2.0	0	200	1.0
toasting (*Pepperidge Farm*)	90	3.0	16.0	3.0	0	200	0
thin (*Pepperidge Farm*)	80	2.0	13.0	1.5	0	135	0

Food and Measure	cal.	prot. (gms)	carbo. (gms)	fat (gms)	chol. (mgs)	sod. (mgs)	fiber (gms)
thin (*Pepperidge Farm* Large Family)	80	2.0	14.0	1.5	0	160	0
very thin (*Pepperidge Farm*), 3 slices	110	4.0	23.0	1.5	0	270	2.0
Bread, brown, canned:							
(*B&M/Friend's*), ½" slice	130	3.0	29.0	.5	0	390	2.0
(*S&W*), ½ slice . . .	90	3.0	21.0	1.0	0	220	2.0
raisin (*B&M/Friend's*), ½" slice	130	3.0	29.0	.5	0	360	2.0
Bread, frozen (*Pepperidge Farm*), ⅛ loaf:							
cheddar, two	210	5.0	21.0	11.0	50	280	1.0
garlic	160	5.0	14.0	10.0	30	250	1.0
garlic mozzarella . . .	200	6.0	21.0	10.0	40	280	1.0
garlic Parmesan . . .	160	6.0	19.0	7.0	10	260	2.0
garlic sourdough . .	180	5.0	20.0	9.0	10	220	2.0
Monterey Jack/ jalapeño cheese . .	200	5.0	22.0	10.0	40	280	1.0
Bread, refrigerated:							
(*Pillsbury Pipin' Hot*), ⅙ loaf	110	4.0	22.0	.5	0	350	<1.0
corn bread twists (*Pillsbury*), 1 twist	130	3.0	17.0	6.0	0	320	0
French (*Pillsbury*), ⅕ loaf	150	6.0	28.0	1.0	0	370	<1.0
Bread, stuffed (*Stuffed Breads*), 6 oz.:							
broccoli and cheese	450	19.0	54.0	17.0	25	830	7.0
pepperoni and cheese	610	26.0	45.0	36.0	75	1230	7.0
Bread crumbs, ¼ cup or 1 oz., except as noted:							
(*Contadina*), ⅓ cup	100	3.0	19.0	1.5	0	700	1.0

Food and Measure	cal.	prot. (gms)	carbo. (gms)	fat (gms)	chol. (mgs)	sod. (mgs)	fiber (gms)
Bread crumbs *(cont.)*							
(Devonsheer/Old London)	100	4.0	20.0	1.5	0	230	2.0
(Progresso)	100	4.0	19.0	1.5	0	210	1.0
Italian:							
(Devonsheer) . . .	100	4.0	19.0	2.0	0	590	2.0
(Progresso)	110	4.0	20.0	1.5	0	430	1.0
lemon herb							
(Progresso)	100	3.0	20.0	1.0	0	480	2.0
seasoned *(Old London)*	100	4.0	19.0	2.0	0	590	2.0
tomato basil							
(Progresso)	120	4.0	22.0	1.5	0	750	2.0
Bread cubes, see "Stuffing"							
Bread dough, see "Bread, frozen" and "Bread, refrigerated"							
Bread mix (see also "Bread mix, sweet"), dry, except as noted:							
beer:							
(Buckeye), ¹/₁₄ pkg.	130	3.0	27.0	1.0	0	310	1.0
whole wheat *(Buckeye)*, ¹/₁₄ pkg. . .	120	4.0	26.0	0	0	370	2.0
cheddar cheese *(Dromedary)*,							
¹/₉ pkg.	140	4.0	25.0	2.5	2	280	1.0
corn bread:							
(Arrowhead Mills),							
¼ cup	120	5.0	24.0	1.0	0	270	4.0
(Aunt Jemima Easy Mix), ¹/₃ cup . . .	150	2.0	19.0	4.0	0	450	1.0
(Ballard), ¹/₁₈ pkg.	110	2.0	21.0	1.5	0	500	<1.0
(Buckeye), ¹/₁₆ pkg.	130	2.0	29.0	0	0	260	1.0
(Dromedary),							
¹/₁₀ pkg.	140	3.0	26.0	2.5	0	550	1.0
herb, Italian *(Dromedary)*, ¹/₉ pkg. . . .	140	4.0	25.0	2.5	0	250	1.0

Food and Measure	cal.	prot. (gms)	carbo. (gms)	fat (gms)	chol. (mgs)	sod. (mgs)	fiber (gms)
kamut (*Arrowhead* *Mills*), ⅓ cup . . .	140	7.0	31.0	1.0	0	190	5.0
multigrain (*Arrowhead* *Mills*), ⅓ cup . . .	160	6.0	31.0	1.0	0	190	3.0
oatmeal, honey (*Dromedary*), ⅑ pkg.	150	4.0	27.0	2.0	0	200	1.0
rye (*Arrowhead Mills*), ⅓ cup	160	5.0	33.0	.5	0	190	3.0
sourdough:							
(*Buckeye*), ¹⁄₁₄ pkg.	130	3.0	27.0	0	0	260	1.0
(*Dromedary*), ⅑ pkg.	140	4.0	27.0	2.0	0	210	1.0
spelt (*Arrowhead* *Mills*), ⅓ cup . . .	150	6.0	31.0	1.0	0	190	5.0
wheat:							
cracked (*Pillsbury* Bread Machine), ¹⁄₁₂ loaf*	130	4.0	25.0	2.0	0	260	2.0
stoneground (*Drom-edary*), ⅑ pkg.	140	4.0	26.0	2.0	0	200	2.0
whole (*Arrowhead* *Mills*), ⅓ cup . .	150	7.0	31.0	1.0	0	190	5.0
white:							
(*Arrowhead Mills*), ⅓ cup	150	4.0	31.0	.5	0	170	2.0
country (*Drome-dary*), ⅑ pkg. . .	140	4.0	28.0	1.0	0	250	1.0
crusty (*Pillsbury* Bread Machine), ¹⁄₁₂ loaf*	130	4.0	25.0	2.0	0	250	<1.0
Bread mix, sweet, dry, except as noted:							
(*Buckeye*), ¹⁄₁₆ pkg.	110	2.0	26.0	0	0	200	0
apple cinnamon:							
(*Dromedary*), ⅑ pkg.	140	3.0	27.0	2.0	0	220	1.0
(*Pillsbury*), ¹⁄₁₂ pkg.	140	2.0	30.0	1.5	0	170	1.0

Food and Measure	cal.	prot. (gms)	carbo. (gms)	fat (gms)	chol. (mgs)	sod. (mgs)	fiber (gms)
Bread mix, sweet, apple cinnamon *(cont.)*							
(*Pillsbury*), ¹/₁₂ loaf*	180	2.0	30.0	6.0	20	170	1.0
banana, ¹/₁₂ pkg.:							
(*Pillsbury*)	130	2.0	26.0	1.5	0	190	<1.0
(*Pillsbury*)*	170	3.0	26.0	6.0	35	200	<1.0
blueberry, ¹/₁₂ pkg.:							
(*Pillsbury*)	140	2.0	29.0	1.5	0	160	<1.0
(*Pillsbury*)*	180	2.0	29.0	6.0	20	160	<1.0
carrot, ¹/₁₂ pkg.:							
(*Pillsbury*)	110	2.0	22.0	1.0	0	150	<1.0
(*Pillsbury*)*	140	2.0	22.0	5.0	25	150	<1.0
corn bread, see "Bread mix"							
cranberry, ¹/₁₂ pkg.:							
(*Pillsbury*)	140	2.0	30.0	1.5	0	150	<1.0
(*Pillsbury*)*	160	2.0	30.0	4.0	20	150	<1.0
date, ¹/₁₂ pkg.:							
(*Pillsbury*)	150	2.0	32.0	1.5	0	150	1.0
(*Pillsbury*)*	180	3.0	32.0	4.0	20	160	1.0
nut (*Dromedary*) . .	180	2.0	10.0	7.0	0	550	.5
gingerbread:							
(*Dromedary*), ¹/₆ pkg.	260	4.0	52.0	4.0	10	420	3.0
(*Pillsbury* Bread Machine), ¹/₈ loaf*	220	3.0	40.0	5.0	0	340	<1.0
nut, ¹/₁₂ pkg.:							
(*Pillsbury*)	180	3.0	27.0	3.5	0	180	1.0
(*Pillsbury*)*	190	3.0	27.0	6.0	20	190	1.0
pumpkin, ¹/₁₂ pkg.:							
(*Pillsbury*)	130	2.0	26.0	1.5	0	190	<1.0
(*Pillsbury*)*	170	3.0	27.0	6.0	35	200	<1.0
Bread snack (*Pepperidge Farm*):							
crisps, swirl, 1 oz.:							
cinnamon raisin . .	130	2.0	19.0	5.0	0	100	3.0
garlic butter	140	3.0	16.0	8.0	5	230	<1.0
sticks, 9 pcs.:							
cheese, three . . .	140	4.0	20.0	5.0	<5	410	<1.0
pretzel	130	3.0	23.0	3.0	0	440	<1.0

Food and Measure	cal.	prot. (gms)	carbo. (gms)	fat (gms)	chol. (mgs)	sod. (mgs)	fiber (gms)
pumpernickel/ses- ame	150	3.0	20.0	6.0	0	340	1.0
Breadfruit:							
½ cup	114	1.2	29.8	.3	0	2	5.4
¼ small, 3.4 oz. . . .	99	1.0	26.0	.2	0	2	4.7
Breadfruit nuts (*Goya* Pana de Pepita), 4 nuts	40	1.0	7.0	.5	0	110	2.0
Breadfruit seeds:							
boiled, shelled, 1 oz.	48	1.5	9.1	.7	0	n.a.	n.a.
roasted, shelled, 1 oz.	59	1.8	11.4	.8	0	n.a.	n.a.
Breadstick, 1 stick, except as noted:							
(*Pepperidge Farm* Brown and Serve)	150	7.0	28.0	1.5	0	290	1.0
(*Pillsbury*)	110	3.0	18.0	2.5	0	290	<1.0
(*Stella D'Oro*)	40	1.0	7.0	1.0	0	40	0
(*Stella D'Oro* Fat Free Original), 5 sticks	60	2.0	12.0	0	0	130	<1.0
(*Stella D'Oro* Fat Free Traditional), 2 sticks	70	2.0	15.0	0	0	150	1.0
(*Stella D'Oro* No So- dium)	45	1.0	7.0	1.0	0	0	0
cheddar, thin (*Pepper- idge Farm*), 7 sticks	70	2.0	11.0	2.5	0	120	<1.0
w/cheese (*Handi- Snacks*)	130	4.0	11.0	7.0	15	340	0
garlic:							
(*Stella D'Oro*) . . .	40	1.0	7.0	1.0	0	60	<1.0
(*Stella D'Oro* Fat Free), 2 sticks . .	70	2.0	14.0	0	0	150	1.0
(*Stella D'Oro* Fat Free Deli), 5 sticks	60	2.0	12.0	0	0	120	<1.0
onion:							
(*Stella D'Oro*) . . .	40	1.0	6.0	1.0	0	35	0
thin (*Pepperidge Farm*), 7 sticks	70	2.0	11.0	2.0	0	115	<1.0

Food and Measure	cal.	prot. (gms)	carbo. (gms)	fat (gms)	chol. (mgs)	sod. (mgs)	fiber (gms)
Breadstick *(cont.)*							
sesame:							
(*Stella D'Oro*) . . .	50	1.0	7.0	2.5	0	45	<1.0
(*Stella D'Oro* Low							
Fat), 2 pieces . .	70	2.0	14.0	1.0	0	90	1.0
(*Stella D'Oro* No So-							
dium)	50	1.0	7.0	2.5	0	0	<1.0
thin (*Pepperidge*							
Farm), 7 sticks	60	2.0	11.0	1.5	0	125	<1.0
snack, see "Bread							
snack"							
wheat (*Stella D'Oro*)	40	1.0	6.0	1.0	0	20	<1.0
Breakfast dishes, see							
specific listings							
Breakfast syrup, see							
"Maple syrup" and							
"Pancake syrup"							
Broad beans:							
raw, ½ cup	40	3.1	6.4	.4	0	28	2.3
boiled, drained, 4 oz.	64	5.4	11.5	.6	0	47	<3.0
Broad beans, mature,							
dried:							
(*Frieda's* Fava							
Beans), 1 oz. . .	15	1.6	1.9	.2	0	14	n.a.
(*Goya*), ¼ cup . . .	150	10.0	26.0	0	0	15	10.0
boiled, ½ cup	93	6.5	16.7	.3	0	4	4.6
canned, ½ cup:							
w/liquid	91	7.0	15.9	.3	0	580	n.a.
(*Progresso* Fava							
Beans)	110	6.0	20.0	.5	0	250	5.0
Broccoli, fresh:							
raw:							
8.7-oz. stalk	42	4.5	7.9	.5	0	40	4.5
chopped, ½ cup . .	12	1.3	2.3	.2	0	12	1.3
(*Dole*), 1 stalk . . .	40	5.0	4.0	1.0	0	75	5.0
florets (*Dole*), 3 oz.	25	3.0	2.0	.5	0	40	3.0
boiled, drained:							
1 stalk, 6.3 oz. . .	51	5.4	9.1	.6	0	46	5.2
chopped, ½ cup . .	22	2.3	3.9	.2	0	20	2.3

Food and Measure	cal.	prot. (gms)	carbo. (gms)	fat (gms)	chol. (mgs)	sod. (mgs)	fiber (gms)
Broccoli, frozen:							
spears:							
10-oz. pkg.	84	8.7	15.2	1.0	0	49	8.5
(*Green Giant*), 3 oz.	25	2.0	4.0	0	0	25	2.0
(*Green Giant Harvest Fresh*),							
3.5 oz.	25	2.0	4.0	0	0	125	2.0
florets:							
(*Green Giant*),							
1⅓ cup	25	2.0	4.0	0	0	25	2.0
(*Stilwell*), 4 florets	25	2.0	4.0	0	0	20	2.0
cut:							
(*Green Giant*),							
1 cup	25	2.0	4.0	0	0	25	2.0
(*Green Giant Harvest Fresh*),							
⅔ cup	25	2.0	4.0	0	0	150	2.0
(*Stilwell*), ½ cup	25	2.0	4.0	0	0	20	2.0
chopped:							
10-oz. pkg.	75	8.0	13.6	.8	0	68	8.5
(*Green Giant*),							
¾ cup	25	2.0	4.0	0	0	25	2.0
(*Seabrook*), ¾ cup,							
3 oz.	25	2.0	4.0	0	0	20	2.0
butter sauce, spears							
(*Green Giant*), 4 oz.	50	2.0	7.0	2.0	<5	330	2.0
cheese sauce (*Green Giant*), ⅔ cup . . .	70	3.0	9.0	2.5	<5	520	3.0
Broccoli combinations, frozen:							
and cauliflower							
(*Stilwell*), ½ cup	25	2.0	4.0	0	0	25	2.0
cauliflower/carrots:							
(*Green Giant Harvest Fresh*), 1 cup	30	2.0	5.0	0	0	125	3.0
cheese sauce (*Green Giant*), ⅔ cup . .	80	3.0	11.0	2.5	<5	560	2.0

Food and Measure	cal.	prot. (gms)	carbo. (gms)	fat (gms)	chol. (mgs)	sod. (mgs)	fiber (gms)
Broccoli combinations, cauliflower/carrots *(cont.)*							
w/corn and peas, butter sauce (*Green Giant*), ¾ cup	60	2.0	8.0	2.0	<5	300	2.0
pasta, peas, corn, and peppers, butter sauce (*Green Giant*), ¾ cup	70	3.0	11.0	2.0	<5	280	2.0
stir-fry: (*Bird's Eye*), 1 cup	30	2.0	5.0	0	0	30	2.0
(*Green Giant Create-A-Meal*), 2⅓ cup	120	5.0	16.0	3.5	0	1100	4.0
Broccoli pocket, and cheddar, frozen (*Ken & Robert's Veggie Pockets*), 1 pc.	250	9.0	38.0	8.0	0	460	4.0
Broccoli pot pie, w/cheddar, frozen (*Amy's*), 7.5 oz. . . .	430	11.0	46.0	22.0	45	630	4.0
Broccoli-cheese in pastry (*Pepperidge Farm*), 1 pc.	240	6.0	24.0	14.0	50	430	3.0
Broiling sauce, see "Grilling sauce" and specific listings							
Broth, see "Bouillon" and "Soup"							
Broth concentrate (*Knorr*), 2 tsp.:							
beef flavor	15	2.0	1.0	0	0	850	0
chicken flavor	5	<1.0	<1.0	0	0	740	0
vegetable flavor . . .	15	1.0	4.0	0	0	730	0
Brown gravy, ¼ cup:							
w/onions (*Franco-American*)	25	2.0	4.0	1.0	<5	340	0
savory (*Heinz*)	25	1.0	3.0	1.0	5	360	0

Food and Measure	cal.	prot. (gms)	carbo. (gms)	fat (gms)	chol. (mgs)	sod. (mgs)	fiber (gms)
mix*:							
(*Durkee/French's*)	10	0	3.0	.5	0	250	0
(*Knorr* Classic) . .	20	<1.0	3.0	.5	0	400	0
(*Loma Linda Gravy*							
Quik)	20	<1.0	4.0	0	0	370	0
(*McCormick*)	20	<1.0	3.0	5	0	340	0
(*Pillsbury*)	10	0	3.0	0	0	270	0
(*Weight Watcher's*)	5	0	0	0	0	270	0
(*Tone's* Cook Up)	15	0	2.0	0	0	230	0
herb (*Durkee/*							
French's)	15	1.0	3.0	.5	0	350	0
Brown gravy sauce							
(*La Choy*), ¼ cup	275	3.0	66.0	0	0	320	0
Brownie, 1 pc., ex-							
cept as noted:							
(*Hostess* Light),							
2 pcs., 2.8 oz. . . .	290	3.0	56.0	5.0	20	150	3.0
chocolate:							
(*Awrey's* Decadent)	230	2.0	30.0	12.0	30	120	1.0
(*Little Debbie* Low							
Fat)	190	3.0	39.0	3.0	0	200	1.0
Bavarian (*Awrey's*)	250	3.0	29.0	15.0	60	110	1.0
peanut (*Awrey's*							
Sensation)	230	3.0	27.0	13.0	30	135	1.0
fudge:							
(*Entenmann's* Fat							
Free), ⅒ strip . .	110	2.0	27.0	0	0	140	1.0
(*Little Debbie*) . . .	310	3.0	46.0	15.0	15	190	1.0
w/out nuts (*Aw-*							
rey's)	200	2.0	30.0	9.0	30	120	1.0
fudge nut:							
(*Awrey's*)	190	2.0	23.0	11.0	25	130	<1.0
(*Drake's* Reduced							
Fat)	170	3.0	33.0	2.5	0	230	1.0
chewy (*Awrey's*) . .	210	2.0	28.0	11.0	25	115	1.0
fudge walnut							
(*Tastykake*)	370	5.0	52.0	17.0	80	150	1.0
mini, 5 pcs.:							
(*Hostess Bites*) . .	260	4.0	32.0	14.0	50	125	2.0

Food and Measure	cal.	prot. (gms)	carbo. (gms)	fat (gms)	chol. (mgs)	sod. (mgs)	fiber (gms)
Brownie, mini *(cont.)*							
walnut *(Hostess*							
Bites)	270	4.0	31.0	15.0	50	140	2.0
Brownie, refriger-							
ated, fudge *(Pills-*							
bury), ¹⁄₂₀ pkg. . . .	160	2.0	24.0	6.0	0	110	<1.0
Brownie mix, 1 pc.*							
except as noted:							
(Arrowhead Mills) .	110	2.0	27.0	0	0	100	2.0
(Arrowhead Mills Fat							
Free)	120	2.0	28.0	0	0	110	2.0
(Arrowhead Mills							
Wheat Free)	120	3.0	26.0	2.0	0	110	2.0
chocolate *(Pillsbury)*	180	2.0	28.0	7.0	10	110	<1.0
fudge:							
(Betty Crocker), ¹⁄₁₈							
pkg.	140	1.0	28.0	2.5	0	120	0
(Betty Crocker							
Light), ¹⁄₁₈ pkg.	130	2.0	26.0	2.5	0	110	1.0
(Pillsbury, 15 oz.)	150	1.0	22.0	6.0	15	95	<1.0
(Pillsbury, 21.5 oz.)	180	2.0	25.0	8.0	10	105	<1.0
(Pillsbury Lovin'							
Lites)	160	2.0	29.0	5.0	15	125	0
hot *(Pillsbury)* . . .	160	1.0	24.0	7.0	10	100	<1.0
cream cheese swirl							
(Pillsbury Deluxe)	180	2.0	22.0	9.0	25	95	<1.0
walnut:							
(Betty Crocker Su-							
preme), ¹⁄₁₈ pkg.	140	2.0	23.0	4.0	0	95	1.0
(Pillsbury)	180	2.0	22.0	14.0	10	90	1.0
Browning sauce							
(Gravy Master),							
¹⁄₄ tsp.	10	0	2.0	0	0	110	0
Brussels sprouts:							
fresh:							
raw, ¹⁄₂ cup	19	1.5	3.9	.1	0	11	1.8
boiled, .7-oz. sprout	8	.5	1.8	.1	0	4	.9
boiled, drained,							
¹⁄₂ cup	30	2.0	6.8	.4	0	17	3.4

Food and Measure	cal.	prot. (gms)	carbo. (gms)	fat (gms)	chol. (mgs)	sod. (mgs)	fiber (gms)
frozen:							
boiled, drained,							
½ cup	33	2.8	6.5	.3	0	18	1.4
(*Stilwell*), 6 sprouts	35	3.0	5.0	0	0	25	3.0
baby, in butter							
sauce (*Green Gi-*							
ant), ⅔ cup . . .	60	3.0	4.0	1.5	<5	270	4.0
Buckwheat:							
whole grain, 1 oz. . .	97	3.8	20.3	1.0	0	<1	2.8
whole grain, 1 cup	584	22.5	121.6	5.8	0	1	17.0
Buckwheat flour:							
1 oz.	95	3.6	20.0	.9	0	n.a.	11.4
1 cup	402	15.1	84.7	3.7	0	n.a.	12.0
(*Arrowhead Mills*),							
¼ cup	100	3.0	25.0	1.0	0	0	3.0
Buckwheat groats:							
brown (*Arrowhead*							
Mills), ¼ cup . . .	140	5.0	30.0	1.0	0	0	3.0
roasted:							
dry, 1 oz.	98	3.3	21.2	.8	0	3	n.a.
cooked, 1 cup . . .	182	6.7	39.5	1.2	0	8	n.a.
Bulgur (see also							
"Tabouli"):							
dry:							
1 oz.	97	3.5	21.5	.4	0	5	5.2
1 cup	479	17.2	106.2	1.9	0	23	25.6
(*Arrowhead Mills*),							
¼ cup	150	5.0	33.0	.5	0	0	4.0
cooked, 1 cup	152	5.6	33.8	.4	0	9	8.2
Bulgur pilaf mix							
(*Casbah*), 1 oz. . .	100	4.0	20.0	0	0	280	<1.0
Bun, see "Roll"							
Bun, sweet (see also							
"Danish"), 1 bun:							
apple (*Entenmann's*							
Fat Free)	150	3.0	33.0	0	0	140	1.0
cheese:							
blueberry (*Enten-*							
mann's Fat Free)	140	4.0	31.0	0	0	150	1.0

Food and Measure	cal.	prot. (gms)	carbo. (gms)	fat (gms)	chol. (mgs)	sod. (mgs)	fiber (gms)
Bun, sweet, cheese *(cont.)*							
pineapple (*Entenmann's* Fat Free)	140	4.0	30.0	0	0	150	<1.0
raspberry (*Entenmann's* Fat Free)	160	4.0	36.0	0	0	135	1.0
cinnamon:							
(*Entenmann's*) . . .	220	4.0	31.0	10.0	55	190	<1.0
raisin (*Entenmann's* Fat Free)	160	3.0	36.0	0	0	125	1.0
cinnamon roll:							
(*Hostess*)	220	4.0	39.0	6.0	25	260	1.0
(*Hostess* Home Baked)	150	4.0	23.0	5.0	0	200	1.0
(*Weight Watchers*)	200	4.0	33.0	5.0	5	200	2.0
honey:							
(*Aunt Fanny's*), 3 oz.	360	5.0	41.0	20.0	0	300	2.0
(*Aunt Fanny's*), 4 oz.	500	5.0	53.0	29.0	0	420	3.0
(*Grandma's*)	410	7.0	48.0	21.0	10	290	1.0
(*Little Debbie*), 3 oz.	380	4.0	39.0	23.0	0	190	4.0
(*Morton*), 2.3 oz.	290	3.0	35.0	10.0	0	160	2.0
(*Morton* Mini), 1.3 oz.	160	2.0	19.0	8.0	0	100	1.0
applesauce filled (*Aunt Fanny's*) . .	330	6.0	43.0	17.0	0	300	1.0
banana, chocolate, or vanilla creme filled (*Aunt Fanny's*)	350	5.0	32.0	18.0	0	350	2.0
glazed (*Hostess*) . .	320	5.0	35.0	19.0	15	210	2.0
glazed or iced (*Tastykake*)	350	5.0	47.0	17.0	10	210	1.0
iced (*Aunt Fanny's*)	350	5.0	32.0	18.0	0	290	2.0
iced (*Hostess*) . . .	390	5.0	49.0	20.0	15	220	2.0
raspberry filled (*Aunt Fanny's*) . .	350	5.0	45.0	17.0	0	290	2.0
honey, frozen (*Rich's*)	240	3.0	32.0	11.0	10	85	1.0

Food and Measure	cal.	prot. (gms)	carbo. (gms)	fat (gms)	chol. (mgs)	sod. (mgs)	fiber (gms)
pecan roll (*Little Debbie Spinwheels*) . .	220	3.0	32.0	9.0	0	200	1.0
Bun, sweet, frozen or refrigerated, 1 pc.:							
apple cinnamon, iced (*Pillsbury*)	140	2.0	21.0	5.0	0	310	<1.0
caramel (*Pillsbury*)	170	2.0	25.0	7.0	0	330	<1.0
cinnamon:							
(*Pepperidge Farm*)	250	4.0	33.0	12.0	15	220	2.0
iced (*Pillsbury*) . .	140	2.0	21.0	5.0	0	330	0
raisin, iced (*Pillsbury*)	180	2.0	26.0	7.0	0	310	<1.0
orange, iced (*Pillsbury*)	170	2.0	25.0	7.0	0	330	<1.0
Burbot, meat only:							
raw, 4 oz.	102	21.9	0	.9	68	110	0
baked, broiled, or microwaved, 4 oz. . .	130	28.1	0	1.2	87	141	0
Burdock root:							
raw, 7.3-oz. pc. . . .	112	1.3	13.6	.1	0	4	5.1
raw, pieces, ½ cup	43	.9	10.3	.1	0	3	1.9
boiled, 1″ pcs., ½ cup	55	1.3	13.2	.1	0	3	1.1
Burger King, 1 serving:							
breakfast:							
biscuit w/bacon, egg, cheese . . .	510	19.0	39.0	31.0	225	1530	1.0
biscuit w/sausage	590	16.0	41.0	40.0	45	1390	1.0
Croissan'wich, sausage, egg, cheese	600	22.0	25.0	46.0	260	1140	1.0
French toast sticks	500	4.0	60.0	27.0	0	490	1.0
hash browns	220	2.0	25.0	12.0	0	320	2.0
sandwiches:							
BK Big Fish	700	26.0	56.0	41.0	90	980	3.0
BK Broiler chicken	550	30.0	41.0	29.0	80	480	2.0
cheeseburger:							
regular	380	23.0	28.0	19.0	65	770	1.0
double	600	41.0	28.0	36.0	135	1060	1.0
double w/bacon	640	44.0	28.0	39.0	145	1240	1.0

Food and Measure	cal.	prot. (gms)	carbo. (gms)	fat (gms)	chol. (mgs)	sod. (mgs)	fiber (gms)
***Burger King*, sandwiches** *(cont.)*							
chicken sandwich	710	26.0	54.0	43.0	60	1400	2.0
Double Whopper:							
regular	870	46.0	45.0	56.0	170	940	3.0
w/cheese	960	52.0	46.0	63.0	195	1420	3.0
hamburger	330	20.0	28.0	55.0	55	530	1.0
Whopper	640	27.0	45.0	39.0	90	870	3.0
Whopper w/cheese	730	33.0	46.0	46.0	115	1350	3.0
Whopper Jr.	420	21.0	29.0	24.0	60	530	2.0
Whopper Jr. w/cheese	460	23.0	29.0	28.0	75	770	2.0
Chicken Tenders, 6 pcs.	230	16.0	14.0	12.0	35	530	2.0
dipping sauces, 1 oz.:							
A.M. Express . . .	80	0	21.0	0	0	20	0
barbecue	35	0	9.0	0	0	400	0
Bull's Eye	20	0	5.0	0	0	140	0
honey	90	0	23.0	0	0	10	0
ranch	170	0	2.0	17.0	0	200	0
sweet and sour . .	45	0	11.0	0	0	50	0
side dishes:							
fries, medium . . .	370	5.0	43.0	20.0	0	240	3.0
onion rings	310	4.0	41.0	14.0	0	810	6.0
salad, w/out dressing:							
chicken, broiled . .	200	21.0	7.0	10.0	60	110	3.0
garden	100	6.0	7.0	5.0	15	110	3.0
side	60	3.0	4.0	3.0	5	55	2.0
salad dressings, ½ oz.:							
blue cheese	160	2.0	1.0	16.0	30	260	<1
French	140	0	11.0	10.0	0	190	0
Italian, light	15	0	3.0	.5	0	50	0
ranch	180	<1	2.0	19.0	10	170	<1
Thousand Island . .	140	0	7.0	12.0	15	190	<1
desserts and shakes:							
Dutch apple pie . .	300	3.0	39.0	15.0	0	230	2.0
shakes, medium:							
chocolate	320	9.0	54.0	7.0	20	230	3.0

Food and Measure	cal.	prot. (gms)	carbo. (gms)	fat (gms)	chol. (mgs)	sod. (mgs)	fiber (gms)
chocolate							
w/syrup . . .	440	10.0	84.0	7.0	20	430	2.0
strawberry							
w/syrup . . .	420	9.0	83.0	6.0	20	260	1.0
vanilla	300	9.0	53.0	6.0	20	230	1.0
Burrito, frozen,							
1 pc. or pkg.:							
bean, black (*Amy's*)	320	9.0	54.0	8.0	0	480	4.0
bean and cheese:							
(*Old El Paso*) . . .	290	12.0	44.0	9.0	15	840	3.0
(*Tina's*)	340	12.0	52.0	9.0	4	600	8.0
bean and rice:							
(*Amy's*)	250	9.0	44.0	5.0	0	450	6.0
and cheese (*Amy's*)	280	10.0	43.0	8.0	10	460	6.0
beef:							
(*Hormel Quick*							
Meal)	300	9.0	37.0	13.0	40	550	3.0
(*Tina's* Red Hot) . .	370	11.0	49.0	15.0	10	640	7.0
nacho (*Patio Britos*),							
6 oz.	410	13.0	48.0	18.0	20	520	5.0
beef and bean:							
(*Patio Britos*), 6 oz.	420	11.0	51.0	19.0	20	800	7.0
hot (*Old El Paso*)	320	12.0	45.0	10.0	15	850	3.0
medium (*Old El*							
Paso)	320	12.0	46.0	10.0	15	800	3.0
mild (*Old El Paso*)	330	12.0	48.0	9.0	15	690	4.0
steak (*Don Miguel*)	370	17.0	55.0	8.0	25	970	5.0
cheese:							
(*Hormel Quick*							
Meal)	250	9.0	41.0	6.0	30	640	4.0
nacho (*Patio Britos*)	360	10.0	52.0	13.0	15	500	3.0
chicken:							
(*Don Miguel*) . . .	360	17.0	54.0	8.0	35	920	5.0
and cheese, spicy							
(*Patio Britos*) . .	400	13.0	52.0	16.0	25	640	3.0
con queso (*Healthy*							
Choice)	280	12.0	43.0	6.0	10	600	5.0
chili, red (*Hormel*							
Quick Meal)	280	9.0	37.0	11.0	35	560	3.0

Food and Measure	cal.	prot. (gms)	carbo. (gms)	fat (gms)	chol. (mgs)	sod. (mgs)	fiber (gms)
Burrito *(cont.)*							
pizza:							
cheese (*Old El Paso*)	320	13.0	27.0	9.0	20	430	0
pepperoni (*Old El Paso*)	260	12.0	31.0	10.0	20	510	0
sausage (*Old El Paso*)	260	11.0	32.0	9.0	15	420	0
Burrito, breakfast, frozen, 1 pkg.:							
black bean (*Amy's*)	230	9.0	38.0	5.0	0	480	5.0
egg, scrambled:							
(*Swanson Great Starts* Original)	200	12.0	25.0	8.0	60	510	2.0
w/bacon (*Swanson Great Starts*) . . .	250	17.0	27.0	11.0	90	540	1.0
ham and cheese (*Swanson Great Starts*)	210	9.0	29.0	6.0	60	440	2.0
hot and spicy (*Swanson Great Starts*)	220	11.0	30.0	7.0	55	490	3.0
pizza, w/cheese, pepperoni (*Swanson Great Starts*)	240	14.0	28.0	9.0	60	410	2.0
sausage (*Swanson Great Starts*)	240	18.0	24.0	12.0	90	500	1.0
Burrito dinner, frozen, 15 oz.:							
beef (*Chi-Chi's* Burro)	570	25.0	73.0	19.0	55	2280	9.0
chicken (*Chi-Chi's* Burro)	530	26.0	73.0	16.0	80	2260	9.0
Burrito entree, see "Burrito"							
Burrito mix (*Old El Paso* Dinner), 1 pc.*	280	n.a.	35.0	7.0	66	840	3.0
Burrito sauce (*Hunt's Manwich*), ¼ cup	25	1.0	5.0	0	0	560	1.0

Food and Measure	cal.	prot. (gms)	carbo. (gms)	fat (gms)	chol. (mgs)	sod. (mgs)	fiber (gms)
Burrito seasoning mix:							
(*Durkee* Pouch),							
1/10 pkg.	35	1.0	5.0	1.0	0	240	2.0
(*Lawry's*), 1 tbsp. . . .	35	1.0	6.0	.5	0	720	0
(*Old El Paso*), 2 tsp.	20	<1.0	3.0	0	0	290	1.0
Butter:							
regular, unsalted:							
1 stick or 4 oz. . . .	813	1.0	0	92.0	248	12	0
1 tbsp.	100	.1	0	11.4	31	1	0
1 tsp.	34	<.1	0	3.8	10	<1	0
regular, salted:							
1 stick or 4 oz. . . .	813	1.0	0	92.0	248	937	0
1 tbsp.	100	.1	0	11.4	31	115	0
1 tsp.	34	<.1	0	3.8	10	39	0
whipped, unsalted:							
1/2 cup or 1 stick	542	.6	<.1	61.3	165	8	0
1 tbsp.	67	.1	tr.	7.6	20	1	0
1 tsp.	23	tr.	tr.	2.6	7	<1	0
whipped, salted:							
1/2 cup or 1 stick	542	.6	<.1	61.3	165	625	0
1 tbsp.	67	.1	tr.	7.6	20	78	0
1 tsp.	23	tr.	tr.	2.6	7	26	0
Butter salt (*Durkee*),							
1/2 tsp.	0	0	0	0	0	340	0
Butterbeans, see "Lima beans"							
Butterbur:							
fresh:							
raw, .2-oz. stalk . .	1	<.1	.2	<.1	0	<1	<1.0
boiled, drained,							
4 oz.	9	.3	2.4	<.1	0	5	n.a.
canned, chopped,							
1/2 cup	2	.1	.2	.1	0	3	n.a.
Butterfish, meat only:							
raw, 4 oz.	166	19.6	0	9.1	74	100	0
baked, broiled, or microwaved, 4 oz. . . .	212	25.1	0	11.7	94	129	0

Food and Measure	cal.	prot. (gms)	carbo. (gms)	fat (gms)	chol. (mgs)	sod. (mgs)	fiber (gms)
Buttermilk, see "Milk"							
Butternut, dried:							
in shell, 1 lb.	750	30.5	14.8	69.8	0	1	5.8
shelled, 1 oz.	174	7.1	3.4	16.2	0	<1	1.3
Butternut squash:							
fresh, ½ cup:							
raw, cubed	32	.7	8.1	.1	0	3	1.1
baked, cubed . . .	41	.9	10.7	.1	0	4	2.9
frozen:							
12-oz. pkg.	192	6.0	49.0	.3	0	8	4.4
boiled, drained, mashed, ½ cup	47	1.5	12.1	.1	0	2	n.a.
Butterscotch chips, baking (*Nestlé* Morsels), 1 tbsp. . . .	80	0	10.0	4.0	0	15	0
Butterscotch topping, 2 tbsp.:							
(*Kraft*)	130	<1.0	28.0	1.5	<5	150	0
(*Smucker's* Sundae)	110	0	27.0	0	0	70	1.0
caramel:							
(*Smucker's* Nonfat)	130	0	31.0	0	0	110	1.0
(*Smucker's* Special Recipe)	130	1.0	30.0	1.0	5	70	<1.0

C

Food and Measure	cal.	prot. (gms)	carbo. (gms)	fat (gms)	chol. (mgs)	sod. (mgs)	fiber (gms)
Cabbage (see also "Coleslaw"):							
raw:							
5¾″ head, 2½ lbs.	228	13.1	49.3	2.4	0	164	20.9
shredded, ½ cup	9	.5	1.9	.1	0	6	.8
boiled, drained, shred-							
ded, ½ cup	17	.8	3.4	.3	0	6	2.1
Cabbage, Chinese:							
bok choy:							
raw, whole, 1 lb.	52	6.0	8.7	.8	0	257	4.0
raw, shredded,							
½ cup	5	.5	.8	.1	0	23	.4
boiled, drained,							
shredded, ½ cup	10	1.3	1.5	.1	0	29	1.4
pe-tsai:							
raw, whole, 1 lb.	68	5.1	13.6	.8	0	38	4.2
raw, shredded,							
½ cup	6	.5	1.2	.1	0	3	.4
boiled, drained,							
shredded, ½ cup	8	.9	1.4	.1	0	6	1.0
Cabbage, napa, raw:							
(*Frieda's*), 1 oz. . . .	4	.3	.9	<.1	0	7	<1.0
shredded (*Dole*), 3 oz.	6	.5	1.0	.1	0	3	1.0
Cabbage, red, fresh:							
raw, whole, 1 lb. . .	100	5.0	22.2	.9	0	38	7.3
raw, shredded, ½ cup	10	.5	2.1	.1	0	4	.7
boiled, drained, shred-							
ded, ½ cup	16	.8	3.5	.2	0	6	1.5
Cabbage, red, sweet and sour, in jars:							
(*Greenwood*), ½ cup	100	1.0	24.0	0	0	380	0

Food and Measure	cal.	prot. (gms)	carbo. (gms)	fat (gms)	chol. (mgs)	sod. (mgs)	fiber (gms)
Cabbage, red, sweet and sour *(cont.)*							
(*S&W*), 2 tbsp. . . .	15	0	3.0	0	0	160	0
Cabbage, savoy:							
raw, whole, 1 lb. . .	100	7.3	22.1	.4	0	102	11.2
raw, shredded, ½ cup	10	.7	2.1	<.1	0	10	1.1
boiled, drained, shred-							
ded, ½ cup	18	1.3	4.0	.1	0	17	n.a.
Cabbage, stuffed,							
frozen, w/potato							
(*Lean Cuisine*),							
9½ oz.	220	11.0	27.0	7.0	25	460	5.0
Cactus, marinated							
(*Goya* Napalitos),							
2–3 pcs.	20	1.0	3.0	0	0	1180	3.0
Cactus leaves							
(*Frieda's*), ¾ cup,							
3 oz.	20	1.0	4.0	0	0	5	1.0
Cactus pear, see							
"Prickly pear"							
Caesar salad, see							
"Salad blend mix"							
Cajun seasoning:							
(*Tone's*), ¼ tsp. . . .	0	0	0	0	0	45	0
fish (*Durkee*), ¼ tsp.	0	0	0	0	0	80	0
meat (*Durkee*), ¼ tsp.	0	0	0	0	0	70	0
poultry (*Durkee*),							
¼ tsp.	0	0	0	0	0	60	0
Cake, ⅛ cake, except							
as noted:							
angel food ring (*Host-*							
ess), ⅙ cake	150	2.0	29.0	3.0	<5	220	0
apple-spice crumb							
(*Entenmann's* Fat							
Free)	130	2.0	30.0	0	0	140	2.0
banana:							
(*Awrey's* Sheet),							
1/24 cake	350	3.0	40.0	20.0	55	290	<1.0
(*Entenmann's* Fat							
Free)	150	2.0	34.0	0	0	190	1.0

Food and Measure	cal.	prot. (gms)	carbo. (gms)	fat (gms)	chol. (mgs)	sod. (mgs)	fiber (gms)
chocolate chip (Awrey's Marquise), 1/16 cake	310	2.0	40.0	17.0	30	190	<1.0
crunch (Entenmann's)	220	2.0	32.0	9.0	40	280	<1.0
crunch (Entenmann's Fat Free)	140	2.0	33.0	0	0	150	2.0
Black Forest torte (Awrey's), 1/12 cake	350	3.0	38.0	22.0	45	330	1.0
blueberry crunch (Entenmann's Fat Free)	140	2.0	32.0	0	0	200	2.0
Boston creme (Awrey's), 1/16 cake . .	190	2.0	30.0	7.0	25	230	0
butter:							
French crumb (Entenmenn's) . . .	210	3.0	29.0	10.0	60	240	0
(Entenmann's), 1/6 loaf	220	3.0	31.0	10.0	80	290	0
carrot:							
(Entenmann's) . . .	290	3.0	35.0	16.0	35	240	0
(Entenmann's Fat Free)	170	3.0	40.0	0	0	230	1.0
cream cheese iced (Awrey's), 1/16 cake	390	4.0	44.0	22.0	40	300	1.0
supreme (Awrey's Sheet), 1/24 cake	400	5.0	47.0	23.0	50	350	2.0
cherries cordial (Awrey's Marquise), 1/16 cake	240	2.0	30.0	14.0	25	190	<1.0
chocolate:							
crunch (Entenmann's Fat Free)	130	2.0	32.0	0	0	170	2.0
fudge (Entenmann's), 1/6 cake	310	3.0	47.0	14.0	45	260	2.0
fudge iced (Entenmann's Fat Free), 1/6 cake . .	210	3.0	51.0	0	0	270	2.0

Food and Measure	cal.	prot. (gms)	carbo. (gms)	fat (gms)	chol. (mgs)	sod. (mgs)	fiber (gms)
Cake, chocolate *(cont.)*							
German (*Awrey's* Sheet), 1/24 cake	340	4.0	41.0	19.0	45	290	0
German, layer (*Awrey's*), 1/16 cake	360	4.0	46.0	19.0	40	290	<1.0
loaf (*Entenmann's* Fat Free)	130	3.0	30.0	0	0	250	1.0
mocha iced (*Entenmann's* Fat Free), 1/6 cake . .	200	3.0	46.0	0	0	270	1.0
peanut (*Awrey's* Marquise), 1/16 cake	330	5.0	38.0	19.0	25	270	<1.0
tropical (*Awrey's* Marquise), 1/16 cake	230	3.0	34.0	11.0	25	210	<1.0
white iced, layer (*Awrey's*), 1/16 cake	270	3.0	34.0	15.0	40	290	1.0
chocolate, double: (*Awrey's*), 1/12 cake	340	3.0	52.0	15.0	35	320	2.0
(*Awrey's* Sheet), 1/24 cake	310	4.0	48.0	13.0	40	330	2.0
3 layer (*Awrey's*), 1/16 cake	310	3.0	48:0	13.0	40	320	2.0
2 layer (*Awrey's*), 1/16 cake	250	3.0	38.0	11.0	35	280	1.0
coconut buttercream: (*Awrey's* Sheet), 1/24 cake	380	3.0	43.0	22.0	55	360	0
layer (*Awrey's*), 1/16 cake	360	3.0	41.0	21.0	45	320	0
coffee: (*Awrey's* Long John), 1/12 cake	190	2.0	21.0	12.0	10.0	75	0
cheese (*Entenmann's*), 1/9 cake	190	4.0	24.0	8.0	30	160	0
cheese, crumb (*Entenmann's*) . .	210	4.0	25.0	10.0	40	190	<1.0

Food and Measure	cal.	prot. (gms)	carbo. (gms)	fat (gms)	chol. (mgs)	sod. (mgs)	fiber (gms)
cinnamon apple (*Entenmann's* Fat Free), ⅑ cake . .	130	2.0	29.0	0	0	110	2.0
crumb (*Entenmann's*), ¹⁄₁₀ cake	250	4.0	33.0	12.0	15	210	1.0
crunch, Louisiana:							
(*Entenmann's*), ⅑ cake	310	3.0	45.0	13.0	50	420	<1.0
(*Entenmann's* Fat Free), ⅙ cake . .	220	3.0	51.0	0	0	220	<1.0
danish cake, ⅑ cake:							
Black Forest (*Entenmann's* Fat Free)	130	3.0	32.0	0	0	115	2.0
raspberry cheese (*Entenmann's* Fat Free)	140	3.0	32.0	0	0	110	1.0
danish ring:							
cinnamon filbert (*Entenmann's*), ⅙ ring	270	4.0	27.0	17.0	30	190	1.0
pecan (*Entenmann's*)	230	3.0	23.0	15.0	25	160	1.0
walnut (*Entenmann's*)	230	4.0	23.0	14.0	25	160	1.0
danish twist:							
apricot (*Entenmann's* Fat Free)	150	3.0	34.0	0	0	110	<1.0
cinnamon apple (*Entenmann's* Fat Free)	150	3.0	35.0	0	0	110	<1.0
lemon (*Entenmann's* Fat Free)	130	3.0	31.0	0	0	140	1.0
raspberry (*Entenmann's*)	220	3.0	28.0	11.0	20	170	<1.0
raspberry (*Entenmann's* Fat Free)	140	3.0	33.0	0	0	125	2.0

Food and Measure	cal.	prot. (gms)	carbo. (gms)	fat (gms)	chol. (mgs)	sod. (mgs)	fiber (gms)
Cake *(cont.)*							
devil's food, marsh-mallow iced (*Entenmann's*), ⅙ cake	350	3.0	45.0	18.0	45	290	1.0
espresso, French (*Awrey's* Marquise), 1/16 cake	320	2.0	30.0	22.0	30	210	<1.0
fruit cake:							
(*Hostess* 2 lb.), ⅙ cake	490	4.0	93.0	14.0	10	410	3.0
(*Hostess* 3 lb.), 1/12 cake	370	3.0	70.0	10.0	5	310	2.0
golden:							
crumb, French (*Entenmann's* Fat Free)	140	2.0	35.0	0	0	150	2.0
fudge, thick (*Entenmann's*), ⅙ cake	330	3.0	48.0	16.0	50	270	2.0
fudge iced (*Entenmann's* Fat Free), ⅙ cake . .	220	3.0	52.0	0	0	200	2.0
golden loaf:							
(*Entenmann's* Fat Free)	120	2.0	28.0	0	0	160	<1.0
chocolately chip (*Entenmann's* Fat Free)	130	3.0	31.0	0	0	220	1.0
lemon layer (*Awrey's*), 1/16 cake	320	2.0	38.0	19.0	45	320	0
marble loaf:							
(*Entenmann's*) . . .	200	2.0	25.0	10.0	65	230	<1.0
(*Entenmann's* Fat Free)	130	2.0	29.0	0	0	190	1.0
Neapolitan (*Awrey's*), 1/12 cake	360	3.0	41.0	21.0	45	330	0
orange:							
frosty (*Awrey's* Sheet), 1/24 cake	350	3.0	43.0	18.0	45	340	0

Food and Measure	cal.	prot. (gms)	carbo. (gms)	fat (gms)	chol. (mgs)	sod. (mgs)	fiber (gms)
layer (*Awrey's*),							
¹/₁₆ cake	330	2.0	41.0	18.0	35	280	0
peach, Georgia (*Awrey's* Marquise),							
¹/₁₆ cake	260	2.0	34.0	14.0	30	240	0
pound:							
(*Hostess*), ¹/₅ cake	350	5.0	48.0	16.0	55	360	1.0
golden (*Awrey's*),							
¹/₆ cake	250	4.0	37.0	10.0	45	280	<1.0
raisin loaf:							
(*Entenmann's*) . . .	220	3.0	32.0	9.0	50	200	<1.0
(*Entenmann's* Fat Free)	140	2.0	33.0	0	0	150	1.0
raspberry, ¹/₁₆ cake:							
and creme (*Awrey's* Marquise)	260	2.0	34.0	14.0	25	210	0
nut (*Awrey's* Marquise)	310	3.0	38.0	17.0	30	180	0
sour cream chip-nut loaf (*Entenmann's*)	240	3.0	28.0	14.0	50	150	<1.0
sponge, uniced (*Awrey's*), ¹/₂₄ cake . .	190	3.0	28.0	8.0	28	320	0
strawberry supreme:							
(*Awrey's* Marquise),							
¹/₁₆ cake	240	2.0	36.0	11.0	5	290	<1.0
torte (*Awrey's*),							
¹/₁₂ cake	270	3.0	37.0	12.0	40	290	<1.0
yellow:							
lemon iced, 2 layer (*Awrey's*),							
¹/₁₆ cake	290	2.0	34.0	17.0	40	300	0
white iced (*Awrey's* Sheet), ¹/₂₄ cake	360	3.0	42.0	21.0	55	370	0
Cake, frozen, ¹/₈ cake, except as noted:							
Boston creme:							
(*Mrs. Smith's*) . . .	170	2.0	29.0	5.0	25	140	0
(*Pepperidge Farm*)	260	3.0	42.0	9.0	45	120	<1.0

Food and Measure	cal.	prot. (gms)	carbo. (gms)	fat (gms)	chol. (mgs)	sod. (mgs)	fiber (gms)
Cake, frozen *(cont.)*							
carrot (*Pepperidge Farm* Deluxe) . . .	310	2.0	39.0	16.0	40	320	1.0
cheesecake, straw-berry:							
(*Amy's*), 4 oz. . . .	290	6.0	38.0	13.0	40	190	2.0
French (*Sara Lee*), ⅙ cake	320	4.0	43.0	14.0	20	230	1.0
chocolate:							
double, layer (*Sara Lee*)	260	3.0	33.0	13.0	25	180	2.0
fudge (*Amy's*), 3.25 oz.	320	3.0	60.0	9.0	60	400	1.0
fudge layer (*Pepper-idge Farm*), ⅙ cake	300	2.0	38.0	16.0	35	230	2.0
fudge stripe layer (*Pepperidge Farm*), ⅙ cake . .	290	2.0	38.0	14.0	35	150	2.0
German, layer (*Pep-peridge Farm*), ⅙ cake	300	2.0	37.0	16.0	35	280	2.0
mousse (*Pepperidge Farm*)	250	2.0	35.0	10.0	25	120	2.0
coconut layer (*Pep-peridge Farm*), ⅙ cake	300	2.0	41.0	14.0	40	200	1.0
coffee cake (*Sara Lee*)	220	3.0	32.0	9.0	15	210	<1.0
devil's food layer (*Pepperidge Farm*), ⅙ cake	290	2.0	40.0	14.0	35	220	2.0
golden layer (*Pepper-idge Farm*), ⅙ cake	290	3.0	40.0	14.0	50	230	2.0
lemon mousse (*Pep-peridge Farm*) . . .	250	2.0	34.0	12.0	40	100	<1.0
pineapple cream (*Pep-peridge Farm*), ⅑ cake	240	2.0	38.0	10.0	30	120	<1.0

Food and Measure	cal.	prot. (gms)	carbo. (gms)	fat (gms)	chol. (mgs)	sod. (mgs)	fiber (gms)
pound:							
(*Goya*), ¼ cake . .	280	4.0	37.0	13.0	85	270	0
butter (*Pepperidge Farm*), ⅕ cake . .	290	5.0	39.0	13.0	110	280	<1.0
strawberry:							
cream (*Pepperidge Farm*), ⅑ cake . .	230	2.0	38.0	9.0	30	115	1.0
stripe layer (*Pepperidge Farm*), ⅙ cake	310	2.0	47.0	13.0	65	150	<1.0
vanilla layer (*Pepperidge Farm*), ⅙ cake	290	2.0	41.0	13.0	45	190	<1.0
Cake, mix, 1/12 pkg., except as noted:							
angel food*:							
(*Betty Crocker*) . .	150	3.0	34.0	0	0	300	0
(*Pillsbury Moist Supreme*)	140	3.0	10.0	0	0	330	0
(*Pillsbury Plus*), 1/10 cake	150	3.0	34.0	0	0	360	0
banana:							
(*Pillsbury Moist Supreme*)	180	2.0	35.0	4.0	0	260	0
(*Pillsbury Moist Supreme*)*	260	3.0	36.0	11.0	55	280	0
(*Pillsbury Plus*) . .	180	2.0	35.0	4.0	0	270	0
(*Pillsbury Plus*)* . .	260	3.0	36.0	11.0	55	280	0
butter pecan (*Betty Crocker SuperMoist*)	180	1.0	34.0	3.5	0	280	0
butter recipe:							
(*Pillsbury Moist Supreme*)	170	1.0	35.0	3.0	0	270	0
(*Pillsbury Moist Supreme*)*	260	3.0	36.0	12.0	75	360	0
(*Pillsbury Plus*) . .	170	1.0	35.0	3.0	0	270	0
(*Pillsbury Plus*)* . .	260	3.0	36.0	12.0	75	370	0
chocolate (*Pillsbury Moist Supreme*)	180	2.0	33.0	4.0	0	260	1.0

Food and Measure	cal.	prot. (gms)	carbo. (gms)	fat (gms)	chol. (mgs)	sod. (mgs)	fiber (gms)
Cake, mix, butter recipe *(cont.)*							
chocolate (*Pillsbury Moist Supreme*)*	260	4.0	33.0	13.0	75	330	1.0
chocolate (*Pillsbury Plus*)	180	2.0	33.0	4.0	0	420	2.0
chocolate (*Pillsbury Plus*)*	270	4.0	33.0	13.0	75	430	2.0
carrot:							
(*Betty Crocker SuperMoist*), ¹⁄₁₀ pkg.	210	2.0	41.0	4.0	0	340	0
(*Pillsbury Moist Supreme*)	180	2.0	35.0	4.0	0	280	<1.0
(*Pillsbury Moist Supreme*)*	260	3.0	35.0	12.0	55	290	<1.0
(*Pillsbury Plus*) . .	190	2.0	35.0	4.5	0	280	<1.0
(*Pillsbury Plus*)* . .	260	3.0	35.0	12.0	55	300	<1.0
cheesecake, ¹⁄₆ cake*							
(*Jell-O* Homestyle)	360	7.0	49.0	15.0	5	550	<1.0
(*Jell-O* Real)	350	7.0	46.0	16.0	5	510	<1.0
blueberry (*Jell-O*)	320	5.0	49.0	12.0	5	390	<1.0
cherry (*Jell-O*) . . .	330	5.0	51.0	12.0	5	390	<1.0
strawberry (*Jell-O*)	340	5.0	52.0	12.0	5	400	<1.0
chocolate:							
(*Betty Crocker SuperMoist*) . . .	180	2.0	33.0	4.5	0	370	0
(*Pillsbury Moist Supreme*)	180	2.0	35.0	4.0	0	270	<1.0
(*Pillsbury Moist Supreme*)*	250	3.0	35.0	11.0	35	280	<1.0
(*Pillsbury Plus*) . .	180	2.0	34.0	4.5	0	320	<1.0
(*Pillsbury Plus*)* . .	260	3.0	34.0	12.0	55	330	<1.0
caramel nut (*Pillsbury Bundt*), ¹⁄₁₆ cake	180	2.0	28.0	7.0	0	200	<1.0
chip (*Pillsbury Moist Supreme/ Plus*)	190	2.0	35.0	5.0	0	270	<1.0

Food and Measure	cal.	prot. (gms)	carbo. (gms)	fat (gms)	chol. (mgs)	sod. (mgs)	fiber (gms)
chip (*Pillsbury Moist Supreme/ Plus*)*	240	3.0	35.0	10.0	35	280	<1.0
dark (*Pillsbury Moist Supreme*)	180	2.0	34.0	4.0	0	320	1.0
dark (*Pillsbury Moist Supreme*)*	250	3.0	34.0	11.0	55	340	1.0
dark (*Pillsbury Plus*)	180	2.0	33.0	4.5	0	330	1.0
dark (*Pillsbury Plus*)*	250	3.0	33.0	12.0	55	340	1.0
chocolate, German:							
(*Betty Crocker SuperMoist*) . . .	180	2.0	34.0	4.0	0	390	<1.0
(*Pillsbury Moist Supreme/Plus*) . . .	180	2.0	34.0	4.0	0	270	<1.0
(*Pillsbury Moist Supreme*)*	250	3.0	34.0	11.0	35	280	<1.0
(*Pillsbury Plus*)* . .	250	3.0	34.0	11.0	55	280	<1.0
cinnamon streusel:							
(*Pillsbury Streusel Swirl*), 1/16 pkg.	210	2.0	38.0	4.0	0	210	0
(*Pillsbury Streusel Swirl*), 1/16 cake*	260	3.0	38.0	11.0	35	220	0
coffee (*Aunt Jemima Easy Mix*), 1/3 cup	170	2.0	12.0	5.0	0	240	1.0
date nut roll (*Dromedary*), 1/3 pkg. . . .	200	4.0	31.0	7.0	0	670	4.0
devil's food:							
(*Betty Crocker SuperMoist*) . . .	180	2.0	34.0	4.0	0	360	0
(*Pillsbury Moist Supreme/Plus*) . . .	180	2.0	33.0	4.0	0	320	1.0
(*Pillsbury Moist Supreme/Plus*)* . .	270	4.0	33.0	14.0	55	340	1.0
(*Pillsbury Moist Supreme/Plus Lovin' Lites*), 1/10 pkg.	210	2.0	41.0	4.5	0	410	2.0

Food and Measure	cal.	prot. (gms)	carbo. (gms)	fat (gms)	chol. (mgs)	sod. (mgs)	fiber (gms)
Cake, mix, devil's food *(cont.)*							
(*Pillsbury Moist Supreme/Plus Lovin' Lites*), ¹/₁₀ cake*	230	4.0	41.0	5.0	45	420	2.0
fudge:							
double hot (*Pillsbury Bundt*), ¹/₁₆ cake	180	2.0	32.0	5.0	0	210	<1.0
swirl (*Pillsbury Moist Supreme*)	200	2.0	37.0	4.5	0	280	1.0
swirl (*Pillsbury Moist Supreme*)*	250	3.0	37.0	10.0	55	290	1.0
swirl (*Pillsbury Plus*)	200	2.0	37.0	5.0	0	280	<1.0
swirl (*Pillsbury Plus*)*	270	3.0	37.0	12.0	55	300	<1.0
gingerbread, see "Bread mix, sweet"							
lemon, ¹/₁₀ pkg.:							
(*Pillsbury Moist Supreme*)	210	2.0	42.0	4.0	0	330	1.0
(*Pillsbury Moist Supreme*)*	300	4.0	42.0	13.0	65	350	1.0
(*Pillsbury Plus*) . .	210	2.0	42.0	4.0	0	320	<1.0
(*Pillsbury Plus*)* . .	310	4.0	43.0	13.0	65	340	<1.0
(*Pillsbury Moist Supreme/Plus Funfetti*)	190	2.0	36.0	4.5	0	280	<1.0
(*Pillsbury Moist Supreme/Plus Funfetti*)*	240	3.0	36.0	9.0	0	290	<1.0
pound, ¹/₈ pkg.:							
(*Betty Crocker*) . .	270	2.0	40.0	11.0	0	230	0
(*Dromedary*)	260	2.0	38.0	10.0	0	270	.5
strawberry:							
(*Pillsbury Plus*) . .	180	1.0	36.0	4.0	0	290	0
(*Pillsbury Plus*)* . .	260	3.0	36.0	11.0	55	310	0
cream cheese (*Pillsbury Bundt*), ¹/₁₆ cake	190	1.0	34.0	5.0	<5	180	0

Food and Measure	cal.	prot. (gms)	carbo. (gms)	fat (gms)	chol. (mgs)	sod. (mgs)	fiber (gms)
swirl (*Betty Crocker SuperMoist*), ¹/₁₀ pkg.	200	2.0	42.0	3.0	0	320	0
vanilla, French:							
(*Betty Crocker SuperMoist*) . . .	180	2.0	35.0	3.0	0	260	0
(*Pillsbury Moist Supreme*), ¹/₁₀ pkg.	220	2.0	42.0	5.0	0	330	1.0
(*Pillsbury Moist Supreme*), ¹/₁₀ cake*	300	3.0	42.0	13.0	45	350	1.0
(*Pillsbury Plus*), ¹/₁₀ pkg.	230	2.0	41.0	6.0	0	340	<1.0
(*Pillsbury Plus*), ¹/₁₀ cake*	320	4.0	41.0	15.0	65	360	<1.0
vanilla, sunshine:							
(*Pillsbury Moist Supreme/Plus*) . . .	190	1.0	34.0	5.0	0	280	<1.0
(*Pillsbury Moist Supreme/Plus*)* . .	260	3.0	34.0	12.0	55	300	<1.0
white:							
(*Betty Crocker SuperMoist*) . . .	180	2.0	35.0	3.5	0	280	0
(*Pillsbury Moist Supreme/Plus*), ¹/₁₀ pkg.	220	2.0	41.0	5.0	0	330	<1.0
(*Pillsbury Moist Supreme/Plus*), ¹/₁₀ cake*	280	3.0	41.0	11.0	0	350	<1.0
(*Pillsbury Moist Supreme/Plus Lovin' Lites*), ¹/₁₀ cake	210	2.0	42.0	4.0	0	340	1.0
(*Pillsbury Moist Supreme/Plus Lovin' Lites*), ¹/₁₀ cake*	230	3.0	42.0	5.0	45	350	1.0
white 'n fudge swirl:							
(*Pillsbury Moist Supreme*)	200	2.0	37.0	4.5	0	280	<1.0
(*Pillsbury Moist Supreme*)*	250	3.0	37.0	10.0	35	290	<1.0

Food and Measure	cal.	prot. (gms)	carbo. (gms)	fat (gms)	chol. (mgs)	sod. (mgs)	fiber (gms)
Cake, mix, white 'n fudge swirl *(cont.)*							
(*Pillsbury Plus*) . .	200	2.0	37.0	4.5	0	290	<1.0
(*Pillsbury Plus*)* . .	250	3.0	37.0	10.0	35	300	<1.0
yellow:							
(*Betty Crocker SuperMoist*) . . .	170	2.0	34.0	3.0	0	280	0
(*Pillsbury Moist Supreme*)	180	2.0	35.0	4.0	0	280	<1.0
(*Pillsbury Moist Supreme*)*	240	3.0	35.0	10.0	55	290	<1.0
(*Pillsbury Plus*) . .	180	2.0	35.0	4.0	0	290	<1.0
(*Pillsbury Plus*)* . .	250	3.0	35.0	11.0	35	300	<1.0
(*Pillsbury Moist Supreme/Plus Lovin' Lites*), ¹/₁₀ pkg.	220	2.0	43.0	4.0	0	370	1.0
(*Pillsbury Moist Supreme/Plus Lovin' Lites*), ¹/₁₀ cake*	230	3.0	43.0	5.0	45	380	1.0
butter recipe (*Betty Crocker SuperMoist*) . . .	170	1.0	37.0	2.0	0	240	0
Cake, snack (see also specific listings), 1 pc., except as noted:							
(*Tastykake Koffee Kake*), 2.5 oz.	270	4.0	43.0	9.0	40	220	1.0
(*Tastykake Kreme Krimpies*), 2 pcs.	230	2.0	37.0	8.0	40	160	0
all varieties (*Health Valley* Healthy Tarts)	150	3.0	35.0	0	0	30	3.0
almond twirl (*Aunt Fanny's*)	110	2.0	16.0	4.0	0	80	0
apple bar (*Health Valley*)	140	3.0	35.0	0	0	0	3.0
apple, date, or raisin (*Health Valley* Bakes)	70	2.0	18.0	0	0	30	2.0

Food and Measure	cal.	prot. (gms)	carbo. (gms)	fat (gms)	chol. (mgs)	sod. (mgs)	fiber (gms)
apple filled (*Tastykake Krimpets* Low Fat), 2 pcs.	160	3.0	36.0	1.5	5	200	1.0
apricot bar (*Health Valley*)	140	3.0	35.0	0	0	5	4.0
banana:							
(*Little Debbie* Twins)	250	2.0	39.0	10.0	10	170	0
(*Suzy Q's*)	220	3.0	32.0	10.0	25	280	<1.0
(*Tastykake* Creamies)	170	1.0	27.0	7.0	10	125	0
(*Twinkies*), 2 pcs.	300	4.0	42.0	13.0	35	370	<1.0
Boston creme (*Drake's*)	170	2.0	25.0	8.0	0	105	2.0
brownie, fudge filled (*Health Valley*) . . .	110	3.0	26.0	0	0	30	4.0
butterscotch iced (*Tastykake Krimpets*), 2 pcs.	210	2.0	40.0	5.0	50	170	1.0
cheesecake:							
(*Boar's Head* New York), 4 oz. . . .	380	6.0	21.0	30.0	135	220	0
bar, all varieties (*Health Valley*) . .	160	3.0	34.0	1.5	0	30	3.0
chocolate:							
(*Devil Dogs*), 1.6 oz.	170	2.0	28.0	7.0	0	150	2.0
(*Ding Dongs*), 1.3 oz.	160	1.0	21.0	9.0	5	110	<1.0
(*Funny Bones*), 2 pcs.	300	5.0	42.0	12.0	0	220	4.0
(*Ho-Hos*)	130	1.0	17.0	6.0	10	75	<1.0
(*Hostess Choco-Diles*)	210	2.0	31.0	10.0	20	160	1.0
(*Hostess Choco Licious*)	170	2.0	28.0	6.0	10	190	1.0
(*Ring Dings*), 2 pcs.	320	2.0	42.0	14.0	0	210	2.0
(*Suzy Q's*)	220	2.0	35.0	9.0	10	270	2.0
(*Tastykake* Creamies)	180	2.0	26.0	7.	15	120	0
(*Tastykake* Juniors)	360	4.0	57.0	13.0	70	270	2.0

Food and Measure	cal.	prot. (gms)	carbo. (gms)	fat (gms)	chol. (mgs)	sod. (mgs)	fiber (gms)
Cake, snack, chocolate *(cont.)*							
(*Tastykake Kandy*							
Kakes), 3 pcs. . . .	270	3.0	35.0	13.0	5	120	2.0
(*Yodels*), 2 pcs. . . .	280	2.0	35.0	16.0	0	150	2.0
fingers (*Aunt*							
Fanny's), 2 pcs.	290	4.0	47.0	10.0	20	430	2.0
chocolate chip (*Little*							
Debbie)	280	2.0	37.0	15.0	10	180	1.0
cinnamon twirl (*Aunt*							
Fanny's)	110	2.0	16.0	4.0	5	80	0
coconut covered:							
(*Sno Balls*)	160	2.0	29.0	5.0	0	180	1.0
(*Tastykake* Juniors)	320	4	59.0	8.0	65	260	1.0
(*Tastykake Kandy*							
Kakes), 3 pcs. . . .	260	3.0	34.0	13.0	5	110	2.0
coconut twirl (*Aunt*							
Fanny's)	110	2.0	17.0	4.0	0	80	1.0
coffee cake:							
(*Drake's*)	130	1.0	18.0	6.0	5	80	1.0
(*Drake's* Low Fat)	100	1.0	20.0	1.5	10	105	0
(*Little Debbie*) . . .	230	2.0	39.0	7.0	10	190	1.0
crumb, 2 pcs.:							
(*Hostess*)	210	2.0	33.0	8.0	15	135	1.0
(*Hostess* Light) . .	150	2.0	35.0	1.0	0	190	<1.0
cupcake, 2 pcs.:							
(*Tastykake Kreme*							
Kup)	190	2.0	31.0	6.0	10	250	1.0
(*Yankee Doodles*)	220	2.0	32.0	9.0	0	200	2.0
apple filled (*Tas-*							
tykake Koffee							
Kake Low Fat) . .	160	2.0	33.0	2.0	0	220	0
buttercreme, iced							
(*Tastykake*) . . .	250	3.0	42.0	8.0	10	280	2.0
buttercreme, iced,							
mini (*Tastykake*)	110	1.0	18.0	4.0	5	120	1.0
creme (*Tastykake*							
Koffee Kake) . . .	80	3.0	35.0	9.0	35	150	0

Food and Measure	cal.	prot. (gms)	carbo. (gms)	fat (gms)	chol. (mgs)	sod. (mgs)	fiber (gms)
creme, mini (Tastykake Koffee Kake)	110	1.0	16.0	4.0	15	65	0
lemon filled (Tastykake Koffee Kake Low Fat) . .	160	3.0	34.0	2.0	0	230	0
raspberry filled (Tastykake Koffee Kake Low Fat) . .	160	2.0	34.0	2.0	0	220	0
cupcake, chocolate: (Aunt Fanny's), 2 pcs.	310	3.0	49.0	12.0	20	560	3.0
(Hostess)	170	2.0	28.0	5.0	<5	260	<1.0
(Hostess Light) . .	120	2.0	26.0	1.5	0	170	<1.0
(Tastykake), 2 pcs.	220	3.0	39.0	6.0	10	270	2.0
(Tastykake), 3 pcs.	330	4.0	58.0	9.0	15	390	3.0
creme (Tastykake Low Fat), 2 pcs.	200	3.0	42.0	2.5	0	250	1.0
iced, creme (Tastykake), 2 pcs.	250	3.0	41.0	8.0	10	270	2.0
iced, creme, mini (Tastykake), 2 pcs.	110	1.0	18.0	4.0	5	115	1.0
iced, creme, vanilla, mini (Tastykake), 2 pcs.	110	1.0	17.0	4.0	10	105	1.0
cupcake, orange: (Aunt Fanny's), 2 pcs.	310	3.0	50.0	12.0	15	370	1.0
(Hostess)	160	1.0	28.0	5.0	10	160	0
cupcake, vanilla, creme (Tastykake Low Fat), 2 pcs. . . .	210	2.0	44.0	3.0	0	260	1.0
date bar (Health Valley)	140	3.0	34.0	0	0	5	3.0
devil's food: (Little Debbie Devil Cremes)	370	3.0	56.0	16.0	5	320	1.0
(Twinkies), 2 pcs.	300	3.0	47.0	12.0	15	360	2.0

Food and Measure	cal.	prot. (gms)	carbo. (gms)	fat (gms)	chol. (mgs)	sod. (mgs)	fiber (gms)
Cake, snack *(cont.)*							
frosty (*Tastykake Kandy Kakes*), 3 pcs.	260	1.0	38.0	11.0	5	105	1.0
fruit loaf (*Hostess*)	350	3.0	67.0	10.0	5	290	2.0
fudge:							
frosted (*Little Debbie*)	270	2.0	37.0	14.0	10	200	1.0
rounds (*Little Debbie*)	290	2.0	48.0	12.0	5	180	1.0
golden, creme filled:							
(*Hostess* Dessert Cup)	90	2.0	18.0	1.5	10	170	0
(*Hostess Lil Angels*)	90	1.0	17.0	2.0	<5	130	0
(*Hostess Tiger Tails*)	160	2.0	26.0	6.0	15	190	<1.0
(*Little Debbie Golden Cremes*)	280	2.0	42.0	12.0	5	290	0
(*Sunny Doodles*), 2 pcs.	220	2.0	33.0	8.0	5	170	1.0
(*Sunny Doodles* Reduced Fat), 2 pcs.	180	2.0	33.0	4.5	10	160	1.0
(*Twinkies*), 1.4 oz.	140	1.0	25.0	4.0	15	180	0
(*Twinkies* Light), 1.4 oz.	120	2.0	24.0	1.5	0	200	0
jelly filled, 2 pcs.:							
(*Tastykake Krimpets*)	190	2.0	38.0	3.0	45	170	1.0
(*Tastykake Krimpets* Low Fat)	180	3.0	40.0	1.5	5	200	1.0
lemon filled (*Tastykake Krimpets* Low Fat), 2 pcs. . . .	180	3.0	38.0	2.0	15	220	1.0
peanut butter (*Tastykake Kandy Kakes*), 3 pcs. . . .	280	5.0	32.0	14.0	20	120	1.0
pecan twirl (*Aunt Fanny's*)	100	1.0	16.0	4.0	0	100	0
pound:							
(*Aunt Fanny's*) . . .	250	4.0	37.0	10.0	10	280	1.0

Food and Measure	cal.	prot. (gms)	carbo. (gms)	fat (gms)	chol. (mgs)	sod. (mgs)	fiber (gms)
(*Tastykake*)	320	5.0	46.0	13.0	85	380	1.0
raisin bar (*Health Valley* Fat Free)	140	2.0	35.0	0	0	5	3.0
raspberry fingers (*Aunt Fanny's*), 2 pcs.	280	4.0	49.0	8.0	5	360	2.0
sprinkled (*Tastykake* Creamies)	150	1.0	25.0	6.0	25	115	0
stick, dunking:							
(*Aunt Fanny's*), 1.4 oz.	190	2.0	21.0	11.0	10	150	1.0
(*Aunt Fanny's*), 1.65 oz.	230	2.0	26.0	13.0	25	180	1.0
(*Little Debbie*) . . .	250	2.0	30.0	15.0	5	250	1.0
(*Tastykake* Stix) . .	190	3.0	45.0	11.0	5	150	1.0
cherry (*Aunt Fanny's*)	180	1.0	21.0	11.0	5	150	1.0
chocolate (*Aunt Fanny's*)	180	2.0	21.0	12.0	5	140	1.0
twin sticks (*Awrey's*), 2.75 oz.	330	4.0	32.0	21.0	20	390	<1.0
strawberry:							
(*Twinkies* Fruit 'n Creme)	150	2.0	30.0	3.0	20	200	<1.0
iced (*Tastykake* Krimpets*), 2 pcs.	210	2.0	39.0	5.0	45	180	1.0
strawberry shortcake (*Little Debbie*) . . .	290	1.0	49.0	11.0	15	200	0
Swiss roll (*Little Debbie*)	320	2.0	48.0	14.0	20	220	1.0
vanilla:							
(*Little Debbie*) . . .	380	2.0	53.0	19.0	0	210	0
(*Tastykake* Creamies)	190	1.0	26.0	8.0	30	125	0
fingers (*Aunt Fanny's*), 2 pcs.	290	4.0	47.0	10.0	10	430	2.0
yellow (*Hostess* Baseball)	160	1.0	32.0	3.0	<5	160	0
zebra (*Little Debbie*)	380	2.0	53.0	19.0	0	210	0

Food and Measure	cal.	prot. (gms)	carbo. (gms)	fat (gms)	chol. (mgs)	sod. (mgs)	fiber (gms)
Cake, snack, mix							
(see also specific listings): dry, except as noted:							
(*Betty Crocker Easy Layer Bar*), ¹⁄₁₆ pkg.	120	1.0	20.0	4.0	0	85	0
apple cinnamon (*Sweet Rewards*), ¹⁄₈ pkg.	170	1.0	39.0	0	0	260	0
apple streusel bar:							
(*Pillsbury*), ¹⁄₂₄ pkg.	130	1.0	22.0	4.5	0	40	<1.0
(*Pillsbury*), 1 bar*	150	1.0	23.0	6.0	0	55	<1.0
banana (*Sweet Rewards*), ¹⁄₈ pkg. . .	170	2.0	39.0	0	0	270	0
chocolate bar:							
(*Sweet Rewards*), ¹⁄₈ pkg.	160	2.0	38.0	0	0	400	1.0
chip (*Pillsbury Chips Ahoy!*), ¹⁄₁₈ pkg.	140	1.0	26.0	6.0	0	100	<1.0
chip (*Pillsbury Chips Ahoy!*), 1 bar*	180	2.0	26.0	7.0	0	125	<1.0
chunk (*Betty Crocker*), ¹⁄₃₂ pkg.	80	1.0	17.0	1.5	0	60	0
peanut butter (*Betty Crocker*), ¹⁄₂₀ pkg.	140	2.0	22.0	5.0	0	125	0
chocolate cookie bar:							
(*Pillsbury Oreo*), ¹⁄₂₄ pkg.	130	<1.0	22.0	4.0	0	125	<1.0
(*Pillsbury Oreo*), 1 bar*	150	1.0	22.0	6.0	10	130	<1.0
date bar (*Betty Crocker*), ¹⁄₁₂ pkg.*	150	1.0	23.0	6.0	0	90	1.0
fudge swirl cookie:							
(*Pillsbury*), ¹⁄₂₀ pkg.	150	1.0	25.0	5.0	0	105	<1.0
(*Pillsbury*), 1 bar*	180	1.0	25.0	8.0	10	110	<1.0
gingerbread (*Betty Crocker*), ¹⁄₈ pkg.	220	2.0	37.0	7.0	0	360	0

Food and Measure	cal.	prot. (gms)	carbo. (gms)	fat (gms)	chol. (mgs)	sod. (mgs)	fiber (gms)
lemon bar:							
(*Sweet Rewards*),							
⅛ pkg.	170	1.0	39.0	0	0	280	0
(*Betty Crocker Sun-*							
kist) ¹⁄₁₆ pkg. . .	130	1.0	24.0	3.5	0	80	0
lemon cheesecake							
bar:							
(*Pillsbury*), ¹⁄₂₄ pkg.	170	1.0	20.0	9.0	10	45	0
(*Pillsbury*), 1 bar*	180	2.0	20.0	10.0	25	50	0
peanut butter bar:							
(*Pillsbury Nutter*							
Butter), ¹⁄₁₈ pkg.	150	2.0	26.0	6.0	0	140	0
(*Pillsbury Nutter*							
Butter), 1 bar*	180	3.0	26.0	7.0	15	170	0
raspberry (*Betty*							
Crocker), ¹⁄₂₀ pkg.	150	2.0	26.0	4.0	0	130	0
Cake decoration (see							
also "Frosting"),							
1 tsp., except as							
noted:							
(*Dec-A-Cake*							
Dec-A-Cone)	20	0	3.0	.5	0	5	0
confetti or nonpareils							
(*Dec-A-Cake*) . . .	15	0	3.0	0	0	0	0
hearts, bats, or pump-							
kins (*Dec-A-Cake*)	20	0	4.0	0	0	0	0
party imperials or fruit							
cocktail							
(*Dec-A-Cake*), 9 pcs.	15	0	4.0	0	0	0	0
rainbow (*Dec-A-Cake*)	15	0	4.0	.5	0	5	0
sprinkles:							
(*Hershey's* Cookies							
'n Mint), 2 tbsp.	100	1.0	11.0	6.0	<5	30	<1.0
chocolate, milk							
(*Hershey's*),							
2 tbsp.	140	2.0	22.0	5.0	5	20	<1.0
fun (*Dec-A-Cake*)	20	0	4.0	0	0	0	0
holiday							
(*Dec-A-Cake*) . .	15	0	3.0	.5	0	0	0

Food and Measure	cal.	prot. (gms)	carbo. (gms)	fat (gms)	chol. (mgs)	sod. (mgs)	fiber (gms)
Cake decoration, sprinkles *(cont.)*							
peanut butter							
(*Reese's*), 2 tbsp.	160	4.0	17.0	8.0	<5	45	1.0
sugar crystals							
(*Dec-A-Cake*) . . .	15	0	3.0	0	0	0	0
trims, chocolate:							
(*Dec-A-Cake*) . . .	15	0	2.0	.5	0	10	0
mint (*Dec-A-Cake*)	15	0	3.0	.5	0	5	0
Calves liver, see "Liver"							
Calzone, refrigerated, 6-oz. pc.:							
cheese (*Stefano's*) . .	510	24.0	43.0	27.0	49	860	4.0
pepperoni (*Stefano's*)	520	23.0	46.0	27.0	52	1100	3.0
spinach (*Stefano's*)	440	21.0	46.0	19.0	35	820	4.0
Canary beans, dry (*Goya*), ¼ cup . . .	190	12.0	35.0	0	0	0	15.0
Candy:							
(*Baby Ruth*), 2.1-oz. bar	280	4.0	38.0	12.0	0	135	2.0
(*Baby Ruth* Fun Size), 2 bars	200	3.0	27.0	9.0	0	95	1.0
(*Bar None*), 1.65-oz. bar	250	4.0	25.0	15.0	5	55	1.0
(*Buncha Crunch*), 1.4 oz.	200	2.0	26.0	10.0	5	95	<1.0
butter rum, 2 pcs.:							
(*Lifesavers*)	20	0	5.0	0	0	20	0
(*Pearson Nips*) . .	60	0	12.0	1.5	0	35	0
buttercrunch/almond (*Almond Roca*), 4 pcs.	280	2.0	25.0	20.0	20	170	0
(*Butterfinger*), 2.1-oz. bar	280	4.0	41.0	11.0	0	120	1.0
(*Butterfinger* Fun Size), 2 bars	200	3.0	30.0	8.0	0	85	1.0
(*Butterfinger BB's*), 1.7-oz. bag	230	2.0	34.0	10.0	0	90	1.0

Food and Measure	cal.	prot. (gms)	carbo. (gms)	fat (gms)	chol. (mgs)	sod. (mgs)	fiber (gms)
butterscotch (*Brach's* Disks), 3 pcs. . . .	70	0	17.0	0	0	95	0
candy corn (*Heide/ Heide Indian*), 1 oz.	110	0	7.0	0	0	40	0
caramel:							
(*Kraft*), 5 pcs. . . .	170	2.0	32.0	3.0	<5	110	0
(*Pearson Nips*), 2 pcs.	60	0	12.0	1.5	0	40	0
caramel, chocolate:							
(*Milk Duds*), 1.85 oz.	230	1.0	38.0	8.0	0	115	0
(*Pom Poms*), 1.5 oz.	200	1.0	35.0	6.0	<5	70	2.0
(*Rolo*), 1.9 oz. . . .	260	2.0	35.0	12.0	10	95	<1.0
caramel, w/cookies:							
(*Twix*), 1-oz. pc. . .	140	1.0	19.0	7.0	0	60	0
(*Twix Fun Size*), 1 pc.	80	1.0	10.0	4.0	0	30	0
(*Twix* Single), 2 pcs.	280	3.0	37.0	14.0	5	115	0
cherry, chocolate coated (*Perugina*), 1.21 oz.	160	1.0	26.0	6.0	0	0	1.0
chocolate:							
w/hazelnuts (*Ferraro Rocher*), 3 pcs.	220	4.0	17.0	15.0	0	35	1.0
milk, see "choco- late, milk," below							
parfait (*Pearson Nips*), 2 pcs. . .	60	<1.0	11.0	2.0	0	35	0
chocolate, candy coated, 1½ oz.:							
(*M&M's*)	200	2.0	30.0	9.0	5	30	1.0
w/almonds (*M&M's*)	220	4.0	24.0	12.0	5	20	2.0
peanut butter (*M&M's*)	220	4.0	24.0	12.0	5	90	2.0
w/peanuts (*M&M's*)	220	4.0	25.0	11.0	5	20	2.0
chocolate, dark:							
(*Dove*), ¼ of 6-oz. bar	230	2.0	26.0	14.0	5	0	3.0

Food and Measure	cal.	prot. (gms)	carbo. (gms)	fat (gms)	chol. (mgs)	sod. (mgs)	fiber (gms)
Candy, chocolate, dark *(cont.)*							
(*Dove* Mini), 7 pcs.	220	2.0	26.0	14.0	5	0	2.0
(*Dove* Single),							
1.3 oz.	200	2.0	22.0	12.0	5	0	2.0
(*Ghirardelli*), 1½ oz.	210	2.0	26.0	14.0	0	0	0
(*Ghirardelli*), 1¼-oz.							
bar	180	2.0	22.0	11.0	0	0	0
(*Hershey's Special*							
Dark), 1.45-oz.							
bar	230	2.0	25.0	13.0	0	0	2.0
w/almonds							
(*Ghirardelli*),							
1½-oz. bar . . .	220	3.0	23.0	15.0	0	0	1.0
bittersweet (*Tobler-*							
one), ⅓ of 3½-oz.							
bar	180	0	21.0	10.0	0	0	2.0
w/raspberries							
(*Ghirardelli*),							
4 pcs.	210	2.0	26.0	13.0	0	0	1.0
chocolate, milk:							
(*Cadbury's Dairy*							
Milk), 1.4 oz. . .	220	3.0	24.0	12.0	10	45	<1
(*Dove*), ¼ of 6-oz.							
bar	230	3.0	25.0	13.0	10	30	1.0
(*Dove* Mini), 7 pcs.	230	3.0	25.0	13.0	10	30	1.0
(*Dove* Single),							
1.3-oz. bar	200	2.0	22.0	12.0	5	25	1.0
(*Ghirardelli*), 1½ oz.	220	3.0	25.0	14.0	10	30	0
(*Ghirardelli*), 1¼-oz.							
bar	190	2.0	21.0	11.0	5	25	0
(*Hershey's*), 1½ oz.	200	3.0	21.0	12.0	10	30	1.0
(*Hershey's Hugs*),							
8 pcs.	210	3.0	22.0	12.0	10	35	<1.0
(*Hershey's Nuggets*)							
4 pcs.	210	3.0	23.0	12.0	10	35	1.0
(*Hershey's Kisses*),							
8 pcs.	210	3.0	23.0	12.0	10	35	1.0
(*Nestlé*), 1.45-oz.							
bar	220	4.0	23.0	13.0	10	30	2.0

Food and Measure	cal.	prot. (gms)	carbo. (gms)	fat (gms)	chol. (mgs)	sod. (mgs)	fiber (gms)
(Symphony), 1.4 oz.	220	3.0	22.0	13.0	10	35	<1.0
w/almonds (Cadbury), 1.4 oz.	220	4.0	21.0	13.0	10	80	1.0
w/almonds (Ghirardelli), 1¼-oz. bar . . .	170	3.0	19.0	12.0	5	25	0
w/almonds (Ghirardelli), 1½ oz.	230	4.0	22.0	15.0	5	25	1.0
w/almonds (Ghirardelli), 2.1-oz. bar	320	5.0	32.0	21.0	10	85	1.0
w/almonds (Hershey's), 3 blocks, 1.3 oz.	210	4.0	19.0	13.0	5	30	1.0
w/almonds (Hershey Nuggets), 4 pcs.	210	4.0	20.0	13.0	5	30	1.0
w/almonds (Hershey's Kisses), 8 pcs.	210	4.0	19.0	13.0	5	25	1.0
w/almonds, toffee (Symphony), 1.4 oz.	220	4.0	20.0	14.0	10	55	1.0
w/caramel (Caramello), 1.6-oz. bar	220	3.0	29.0	10.0	10	60	<1.0
cookies and cream (Ghirardelli), 1.3 oz.	190	2.0	22.0	11.0	5	65	0
cookies and cream (Hershey's Nuggets), 4 pcs.	200	4.0	22.0	11.0	5	75	0
w/crisps (Crunch), 1.55-oz. bar . . .	230	3.0	28.0	12.0	5	60	1.0
w/crisps (Crunch Fun Size), 4 bars	200	8.0	25.0	10.0	5	55	1.0
w/crisps (Ghirardelli), 1¼-oz. bar	180	2.0	22.0	10.0	5	25	0

Food and Measure	cal.	prot. (gms)	carbo. (gms)	fat (gms)	chol. (mgs)	sod. (mgs)	fiber (gms)
Candy, chocolate, milk *(cont.)*							
w/crisps (*Ghirardelli*), 2.1-oz. bar	300	4.0	37.0	17.0	10	95	0
w/crisps (*Ghirardelli*), 2½-oz. bar . . .	360	5.0	44.0	20.0	10	115	0
w/crisps (*Krackel*), 2.6-oz. bar	390	5.0	45.0	21.0	10	110	1.0
w/fruit and nuts (*Chunky*), 1.4-oz. bar	200	3.0	22.0	11.0	<5	20	2.0
w/hazelnuts (*Mon Cheri*), 3 pcs. . .	260	4.0	20.0	18.0	5	25	1.0
w/honey and nougat (*Toblerone*), ⅓ of 3½-oz. bar . . .	180	3.0	20.0	10.0	5	25	0
w/macadamias (*Ghirardelli*), 1¼-oz. bar . . .	190	2.0	19.0	13.0	5	25	0
w/peanuts (*Mr. Goodbar*), 1¾-oz. bar	270	5.0	25.0	17.0	<5	20	2.0
w/pecans (*Ghirardelli*), 4 pcs., 1½ oz. . .	230	3.0	22.0	16.0	5	25	1.0
w/raisins and almonds (*Cadbury's* Fruit & Nut), 1.4 oz.	210	3.0	24.0	11.0	5	45	1.0
thins (*Lindt* Swiss), 15 pcs., 1½ oz.	230	2.0	22.0	15.0	5	35	0
w/toffee (*Ghirardelli*), 4 pcs., 1½ oz. . .	220	2.0	26.0	13.0	10	45	0
wafers (*Ghirardelli*), 11 pcs., 1½ oz.	210	3.0	29.0	12.0	10	30	0
chocolate mint:							
(*Ghirardelli*), 1½ oz.	220	2.0	26.0	14.0	5	15	0

Food and Measure	cal.	prot. (gms)	carbo. (gms)	fat (gms)	chol. (mgs)	sod. (mgs)	fiber (gms)
(*Ghirardelli*), 2.1-oz. bar	310	3.0	37.0	19.0	5	20	0
(*Pearson Nips*), 2 pcs.	60	<1.0	11.0	1.5	0	40	0
cookies and (*Hershey's*), 1.55-oz. bar	230	3.0	27.0	12.0	10	80	1.0
cookies and (*Hershey's* Nuggets), 4 pcs.	200	3.0	24.0	10.0	5	70	1.0
candy coated (*M&M's*), 1½ oz.	200	2.0	30.0	9.0	5	30	1.0
wafers (*Ghirardelli*), 11 pcs., 1½ oz.	210	2.0	27.0	12.0	5	15	0
chocolate, white, raspberry cream (*Ghirardelli*), 4 pcs., ⅓ oz.	200	2.0	21.0	12.0	5	35	0
coconut, w/chocolate: (*Mounds*), 1.9-oz. bar	250	2.0	31.0	13.0	0	80	3.0
w/almonds (*Almond Joy*), 1.76-oz. bar	240	2.0	28.0	13.0	0	65	2.0
coffee (*Pearson Nips*), 2 pcs.	60	0	12.0	1.5	0	45	0
fruit flavor: (*Skittles* Original), 1½ oz.	170	0	38.0	2.0	0	5	0
(*Skittles* Singles Original), 2.2-oz. bag . . .	250	0	55.0	2.5	0	10	0
chews (*Starburst*), 8 pcs.	160	0	33.0	3.0	0	20	0
tropical or wild berry: (*Skittles*), 1½ oz.	170	0	38.0	1.5	0	5	0
(*Skittles* Single), 2.2-oz. bag . . .	250	0	56.0	2.5	0	10	0

Food and Measure	cal.	prot. (gms)	carbo. (gms)	fat (gms)	chol. (mgs)	sod. (mgs)	fiber (gms)
Candy *(cont.)*							
fruit flavor, gummed:							
(*Amazin' Fruit*),							
1.9 oz.	180	3.0	41.0	0	0	60	0
(*Brach's Fruit*							
Bunch), 3 pcs.,							
1.6 oz.	150	0	37.0	0	0	15	0
(*Gummi Savers*),							
1½ oz.	130	2.0	32.0	0	0	0	0
fudge (*Kraft* Fudgies),							
5 pcs., 1.4 oz. . . .	180	1.0	32.0	5.0	0	140	0
gum, chewing, all							
flavors, 1 pc.:							
(*Beech-Nut*)	10	0	2.0	0	0	0	0
(*Big Red*)	10	0	2.0	0	0	0	0
(*Care*Free*)	10	0	2.0	0	0	0	0
(*Doublemint/Winter-*							
fresh/Wrigley's							
Spearmint) . . .	10	0	2.0	0	0	0	0
(*Extra/Winterfresh*							
Sugarfree)	5	0	2.0	0	0	0	0
(*Freedent*)	10	0	2.0	0	0	0	0
(*Fruit Stripe*)	10	0	2.0	0	0	0	0
(*Juicy Fruit*)	10	0	2.0	0	0	0	0
gum, bubble, 1 pc.:							
(*Bubble Yum*) . . .	25	0	6.0	0	0	0	0
(*Bubble Yum*							
Sugarless)	15	0	3.0	0	0	0	0
(*Care*Free*)	10	0	2.0	0	0	0	0
stick (*Care*Free*)	5	0	2.0	0	0	0	0
hard, all flavors:							
(*Brach's Sparklers*),							
3 pcs., .6 oz. . .	70	0	17.0	0	0	30	0
(*Lifesavers*), 2 pcs.	20	0	5.0	0	0	0	0
(*Pez*), .3-oz. roll . .	35	0	9.0	0	0	0	0
(*Pez* Sugar Free),							
.3-oz. roll	30	0	8.0	0	0	0	0

Food and Measure	cal.	prot. (gms)	carbo. (gms)	fat (gms)	chol. (mgs)	sod. (mgs)	fiber (gms)
chocolate dipped (*Bogdon's* Reception Sticks), 1 pc.	16	0	3.0	.5	0	2	0
honey (*Bit-O-Honey*), 1.7-oz. bar	200	1.0	41.0	3.5	0	105	0
jelly/jelled:							
(*Jujubes*), 1.4 oz., approx. 58 pcs.	160	0	32.0	0	0	30	0
(*Jujyfruits*), 1.4 oz., approx. 15 pcs.	160	0	33.0	0	0	30	0
spearmint leaves (*Brach's*), 5 pcs.	130	0	34.0	0	0	15	0
licorice:							
(*Pearson Nips*), 2 pcs.	60	0	12.0	1.5	0	40	0
(*Twizzler Nibs*), 2¼ oz.	210	2.0	48.0	1.5	0	340	0
(*Twizzlers*), 4 pcs.	140	1.0	33.0	.5	0	230	0
cherry (*Twizzler Pull-n-Peel*), 1.3-oz. pc.	110	1.0	23.0	1.0	0	85	1.0
cherry (*Twizzler Nibs*), 2¼-oz. pkg.	220	2.0	49.0	1.5	0	135	0
strawberry (*Twizzlers*), 4 pcs., 1½ oz.	140	1.0	33.0	.5	0	105	0
licorice, candy coated:							
(*Good & Fruity*), 1.8-oz. box . . .	150	0	35.0	.5	0	80	2.0
(*Good & Plenty*), 1.4 oz.	130	1.0	33.0	0	0	80	0
lollipop, all flavors, 1 pop:							
(*Astro Pops*), 1 oz.	108	0	27.0	0	0	0	0
(*Dum-Dums*), .6 oz.	71	0	18.0	0	0	0	0
(*Lifesavers*), .4 oz.	40	0	11.0	0	0	0	0

Food and Measure	cal.	prot. (gms)	carbo. (gms)	fat (gms)	chol. (mgs)	sod. (mgs)	fiber (gms)
Candy, lollipop *(cont.)*							
(*Save-A-Sucker/*							
Suck An Egg),							
1 oz.	110	0	27.0	0	0	13	0
(*Save-A-Sucker*),							
2 oz.	200	0	54.0	0	0	25	0
malted milk balls							
(*Whoppers*), 1.4 oz.	190	1.0	30.0	7.0	0	105	0
(*Mars*), 1.76-oz. bar	240	3.0	31.0	13.0	5	70	1.0
(*Mars Fun Size*),							
2 bars	190	3.0	23.0	10.0	5	55	1.0
marshmallow:							
(*Funmallows*),							
4 pcs.	110	<1.0	26.0	0	0	20	0
(*Kraft* Jet-Puffed),							
5 pcs., 1.2 oz. . .	110	<1.0	27.0	0	0	40	0
mini (*Funmallows*),							
½ cup	100	<1.0	25.0	0	0	20	0
mini (*Kraft*), ½ cup	100	<1.0	25.0	0	0	30	0
peanut (*Spangler*),							
6 pcs.	163	0	41.0	0	0	0	0
(*Milky Way*), 2.15-oz.							
bar	280	2.0	43.0	11.0	5	90	1.0
(*Milky Way Fun Size*),							
2 bars	180	2.0	28.0	7.0	5	60	0
(*Milky Way* Dark),							
1.76-oz. bar	220	1.0	36.0	8.0	5	85	1.0
(*Milky Way Fun Size*							
Dark), .7-oz. bar . .	90	1.0	14.0	3.0	0	35	0
mint:							
(*Lifesavers*							
Cryst-O-Mint),							
2 pcs.	20	0	5.0	0	0	0	0
(*Pez* Peppermint),							
3 pcs.	10	0	2.0	0	0	0	0
all flavors (*Lifesav-*							
ers), 3 pcs. . . .	20	0	5.0	0	0	0	0

Food and Measure	cal.	prot. (gms)	carbo. (gms)	fat (gms)	chol. (mgs)	sod. (mgs)	fiber (gms)
all flavors, except iced and vanilla (*Breath Savers*), 1 pc.	0	0	2.0	0	0	0	0
butter (*Kraft*), 7 pcs.	60	0	14.0	0	0	25	0
chocolate coated (*After Eight*), 5 pcs.	190	0	32.0	6.0	5	10	1.0
chocolate coated (*Junior* Mint), 1.6 oz.	190	<1.0	38.0	4.0	0	10	<1.0
chocolate coated (*York Peppermint Pattie*), 1½-oz. pc.	170	1.0	33.0	4.0	0	15	0
chocolate coated (*York Peppermint Pattie* Mini), 3 pcs., 1.4 oz. . . .	160	<1.0	33.0	3.0	0	10	0
iced/vanilla (*Breath Savers*), 1 pc. . . .	10	0	2.0	0	0	0	0
party (*Kraft*), 7 pcs.	60	0	14.0	0	0	35	0
(*Nestlé Turtles*), 2 pcs.	160	2.0	20.0	9.0	<5	30	1.0
nonpareils:							
(*Ghirardelli*), 1.4 oz.	190	2.0	29.0	9.0	0	0	0
(*Sno-Caps*), 2.3 oz.	300	2.0	48.0	13.0	0	0	3.0
nougat (*Brach's*), 4 pcs.	170	0	38.0	2.0	0	55	0
nougat bar, chocolate coated, 1.9-oz. bar:							
chocolate (*Charleston Chew*)	230	3.0	40.0	6.0	0	50	1.0
strawberry (*Charleston Chew*)	230	1.0	42.0	6.0	0	60	<1.0
vanilla (*Charleston Chew*)	230	2.0	40.0	7.0	0	50	1.0
(*Oh Henry!*), 1.8-oz. bar	230	6.0	32.0	9.0	<5	125	2.0

Food and Measure	cal.	prot. (gms)	carbo. (gms)	fat (gms)	chol. (mgs)	sod. (mgs)	fiber (gms)
Candy *(cont.)*							
(*100 Grand*), 1½-oz.							
bar	200	2.0	30.0	8.0	10	75	<1.0
(*Pay Day*), 1.85-oz.							
bar	250	7.0	30.0	13.0	0	190	2.0
peanut:							
(*Planters*), 1.6-oz.							
bar	230	6.0	22.0	14.0	0	70	2.0
chocolate coated							
(*Goobers*),							
1.38 oz.	210	4.0	19.0	13.0	<5	20	3.0
peanut brittle (*Kraft*),							
1.3 oz.	170	3.0	29.0	5.0	0	310	1.0
peanut butter, choco-late:							
(*5th Avenue*), 2-oz.							
bar	280	5.0	38.0	12.0	<5	95	1.0
candy coated							
(*Reese's Pieces*),							
1.4 oz.	190	5.0	24.0	8.0	0	65	0
w/cookie (*Twix*),							
.9 oz.	130	3.0	13.0	8.0	0	70	1.0
peanut butter cup:							
(*Reese's*),							
1½-oz. pkg. . . .	250	5.0	25.0	14.0	<5	140	1.0
(*Reese's*), 2 pcs.,							
1.2 oz.	190	4.0	19.0	11.0	0	100	1.0
(*Reese's* Mini),							
5 pcs.	210	4.0	22.0	12.0	<5	115	1.0
peanut butter parfait							
(*Pearson Nips*),							
2 pcs.	60	<1.0	11.0	2.0	0	40	0
popcorn, caramel, see "Popcorn"							
raisins, chocolate							
coated (*Raisinets*),							
1.58 oz.	200	2.0	31.0	8.0	<5	15	2.0

Food and Measure	cal.	prot. (gms)	carbo. (gms)	fat (gms)	chol. (mgs)	sod. (mgs)	fiber (gms)
raisins, yogurt coated:							
strawberry or vanilla							
(*Del Monte*),							
.9 oz.	110	2.0	20.0	3.0	0	25	<1.0
vanilla (*Del Monte*),							
1 oz.	120	2.0	22.0	3.0	0	25	<1.0
rock (*Brach's*), 1 oz.	110	0	27.0	0	0	10	0
(*Snickers*), 2.07-oz.							
bar	280	4.0	36.0	14.0	10	150	1.0
(*Snickers Fun Size*),							
2 bars	190	3.0	24.0	9.0	5	100	1.0
(*Snickers* Mini),							
4 pcs.	170	3.0	22.0	8.0	5	90	1.0
(*Snickers* Peanut But-							
ter), 2-oz. bar . . .	310	6.0	28.0	20.0	5	150	1.0
(*Snickers Munch*),							
1.4 oz.	230	6.0	17.0	15.0	10	150	2.0
(*3 Musketeers*),							
2.13-oz. bar	260	2.0	46.0	8.0	5	110	1.0
(*3 Musketeers Fun*							
Size), 2 bars	140	1.0	25.0	4.0	5	60	0
toffee (*Brach's* Trea-							
sures), 3 pcs. . . .	80	0	15.0	2.0	10	95	0
toffee bar, 1.4 oz.:							
(*Heath*)	210	2.0	25.0	13.0	20	180	0
(*Skor*)	220	2.0	23.0	13.0	20	110	<1.0
(*Tootsie Roll* Midges),							
6 pcs., 1.4 oz. . . .	160	<1.0	40.0	3.0	0	40	<1.0
wafer, chocolate							
coated (*Kit Kat*),							
1½-oz. bar	220	3.0	26.0	12.0	5	35	<1.0
(*Whatchamacallit*),							
1.7-oz. bar	250	4.0	29.0	13.0	5	125	1.0
Cane syrup, 1 tbsp.	52	0	13.4	0	0	<1	0
Cannellini beans, see							
"Kidney beans"							
Cannelloni dinner,							
frozen (*Amy's*),							
10 oz.	260	11.0	32.0	11.0	20	560	5.0

Food and Measure	cal.	prot. (gms)	carbo. (gms)	fat (gms)	chol. (mgs)	sod. (mgs)	fiber (gms)
Cannelloni entree,							
frozen, cheese (*Lean*							
Cuisine), 9⅛ oz. . . .	240	19.0	29.0	5.0	22	590	4.0
Cantaloupe:							
pulp, cubed, ½ cup	29	.7	6.7	.2	0	7	.6
½ of 5″ melon	94	2.3	22.3	.7	0	23	2.1
Cantaloupe cocktail							
(*Snapple*), 8 fl. oz.	130	0	32.0	0	0	10	0
Capers:							
(*Crosse & Blackwell*),							
1 tbsp.	5	0	1.0	0	0	350	0
(*Krinos*), 1 tsp. . . .	0	0	0	0	0	170	0
(*Progresso*), 1 tsp.	5	0	0	0	0	105	0
w/pimientos (*Goya*),							
¼ cup	25	0	0	2.5	0	330	0
Capon, see "Chicken"							
Caponata, see "Arti-							
choke appetizer" and							
"Eggplant appetizer"							
Cappacola, see "Ham							
lunch meat"							
Cappuccino (see also							
"Coffee, flavored,							
mix"), iced, 8 fl. oz.,							
except as noted:							
(*Jamaican Gold*),							
11 oz.	145	3.0	29.0	2.5	0	40	0
coffee (*Maxwell*							
House)	130	2.0	24.0	2.5	5	120	0
mocha (*Maxwell*							
House)	140	2.0	27.0	2.5	5	115	0
vanilla (*Maxwell*							
House)	140	2.0	27.0	2.5	5	110	0
Cappuccino bar, fro-							
zen (*Frozfruit*), 1 bar	140	1.0	18.0	6.0	25	20	0
Carambola:							
fresh:							
1 medium, 4.7 oz.	42	.7	9.9	.4	0	2	3.4
(*Frieda's*), 3.5 oz.	35	.7	8.0	.5	0	2	n.a.

Food and Measure	cal.	prot. (gms)	carbo. (gms)	fat (gms)	chol. (mgs)	sod. (mgs)	fiber (gms)
dried:							
(*Frieda's*), 1 oz. . .	77	.7	19.6	.5	0	3	0
(*Sonoma*), 1.4 oz.	140	1.0	34.0	0	0	0	0
Caramel dip, 2 tbsp.:							
(*Marie's*)	150	4.0	24.0	5.0	5	75	1.0
(*Marie's* Low Fat) . .	140	1.5	29.0	2.0	5	90	0
Caramel topping,							
2 tbsp.:							
(*Kraft*)	120	2.0	28.0	0	0	90	0
(*Smucker's* Sundae)	110	0	27.0	0	0	70	1.0
butterscotch, see							
"Butterscotch top-							
ping"							
hot (*Smucker's*) . . .	120	1.0	29.0	3.0	0	60	0
Caraway seed:							
1 tsp.	7	.4	1.1	.3	0	<1	<1.0
(*McCormick*), ¼ tsp.	4	.2	.3	.2	0	<1	.3
Carbonara sauce mix							
(*Knorr*), 2 tbsp. . . .	70	4.0	5.0	3.5	5	760	0
Cardamom:							
(*McCormick*), ¼ tsp.	2	0	.4	0	0	<1	.2
ground (*Tone's*),							
1 tsp.	6	.2	1.3	.1	0	<1	.2
seed (*Spice Islands*),							
1 tsp.	6	.2	1.3	.1	0	<1	.2
Cardoon:							
raw, shredded, ½ cup	18	.6	4.4	.1	0	151	1.4
boiled, drained, 4 oz.	25	.9	6.0	.1	0	200	n.a.
Carissa:							
1 medium, .8 oz. . .	12	.1	2.7	.3	0	1	n.a.
sliced, ½ cup	46	.4	10.2	1.0	0	2	n.a.
Carl's Jr., 1 serving:							
breakfast:							
bacon, 2 strips . .	40	3.0	0	3.5	10	125	0
burrito, breakfast	430	22.0	29.0	26.0	460	810	<1.0
English muffin, w/							
margarine	230	5.0	30.0	10.0	0	330	2.0
French toast dips,							
w/out syrup . . .	410	6.0	40.0	25.0	0	380	3.0

Food and Measure	cal.	prot. (gms)	carbo. (gms)	fat (gms)	chol. (mgs)	sod. (mgs)	fiber (gms)
Carl's Jr., breakfast *(cont.)*							
quesadilla, breakfast	300	14.0	27.0	14.0	225	750	1.0
sausage, 1 patty . .	200	7.0	0	18.0	35	530	0
scrambled eggs . .	160	13.0	1.0	11.0	425	125	0
Sunrise Sandwich	370	14.0	31.0	21.0	225	710	2.0
table syrup, 1 oz.	90	0	22.0	0	0	5	0
chicken stars, 6 pcs.	230	13.0	11.0	14.0	85	450	0
sauces:							
barbecue sauce . .	50	<1	11.0	0	0	270	0
honey sauce	90	0	23.0	0	0	5	0
mustard sauce . . .	45	0	10.0	.5	0	150	0
salsa	10	0	2.0	0	0	160	0
sweet 'n sour sauce	50	0	11.0	0	0	60	0
sandwiches:							
Big Burger	470	25.0	46.0	20.0	55	810	2.0
Carl's Catch Fish							
Sandwich	560	17.0	54.0	30.0	60	1220	5.0
chicken bacon							
Swiss	670	28.0	57.0	36.0	80	1480	3.0
chicken, barbequed	310	31.0	34.0	6.0	55	830	3.0
chicken club	550	35.0	37.0	29.0	85	1160	3.0
chicken, ranch . . .	580	23.0	56.0	29.0	60	1140	3.0
chicken, Santa Fe	530	30.0	36.0	30.0	85	1230	3.0
double cheese-							
burger, ⅓ lb. . .	660	34.0	37.0	42.0	110	1060	2.0
Double Western Ba-							
con Cheeseburger	970	56.0	58.0	57.0	145	1810	2.0
Famous Big Star							
hamburger	610	26.0	42.0	38.0	70	890	2.0
hamburger	200	11.0	23.0	8.0	25	500	1.0
Hot & Crispy sand-							
wich	400	14.0	35.0	22.0	45	980	2.0
Super Star ham-							
burger	820	43.0	41.0	53.0	120	1020	1.0
Western Bacon							
Cheeseburger . .	870	34.0	59.0	35.0	90	1490	2.0
"Great Stuff" potato:							
bacon and cheese	630	20.0	76.0	29.0	40	1720	6.0
broccoli and cheese	530	11.0	76.0	22.0	15	930	8.0

Food and Measure	cal.	prot. (gms)	carbo. (gms)	fat (gms)	chol. (mgs)	sod. (mgs)	fiber (gms)
potato, plain	290	6.0	68.0	0	0	40	6.0
sour cream and							
chive	430	8.0	70.0	14.0	10	160	6.0
Entree Salads-to-Go:							
chicken	260	28.0	11.0	9.0	70	530	4.0
garden	50	3.0	4.0	3.0	5	75	2.0
salad dressing, 2 oz.:							
blue cheese	310	2.0	1.0	34.0	25	360	0
French, fat free . .	70	0	18.0	0	0	760	1.0
house	220	1.0	3.0	22.0	20	440	0
Italian, fat free . . .	15	0	4.0	0	0	800	0
Thousand Island . .	250	<1	7.0	24.0	20	540	0
side dishes:							
CrissCut Fries, large	550	7.0	55.0	34.0	0	1280	3.0
fries, regular	370	4.0	44.0	20.0	0	240	3.0
hash brown nuggets	270	3.0	27.0	17.0	0	410	2.0
onion rings	520	8.0	63.0	26.0	0	840	3.0
zucchini	380	7.0	38.0	23.0	0	1040	3.0
bakery products:							
blueberry muffin . .	340	5.0	49.0	14.0	40	340	1.0
bran muffin	370	7.0	61.0	13.0	45	410	7.0
cheese danish . . .	400	5.0	49.0	22.0	15	390	1.0
cheesecake, straw-							
berry swirl	300	6.0	31.0	17.0	55	220	0
chocolate cake . . .	300	3.0	49.0	10.0	23	260	4.0
chocolate chip							
cookie	370	3.0	49.0	19.0	25	350	1.0
cinnamon roll . . .	420	9.0	68.0	13.0	15	570	4.0
shake, small:							
chocolate	390	9.0	74.0	7.0	30	280	0
strawberry	400	9.0	77.0	7.0	30	240	0
vanilla	330	11.0	54.0	8.0	35	250	0
Carob drink mix,							
powder, 3 tsp. . . .	45	.2	11.2	tr.	0	12	<1.0
Carob flour, 1 cup	395	4.8	91.6	.7	0	36	41.0
Carp, meat only:							
raw, 4 oz.	144	20.2	0	6.4	75	58	0
baked, broiled, or mi-							
crowaved, 4 oz. . .	184	25.9	0	8.1	95	71	0

Food and Measure	cal.	prot. (gms)	carbo. (gms)	fat (gms)	chol. (mgs)	sod. (mgs)	fiber (gms)
✓**Carrot,** fresh:							
raw:							
whole, 7½" long,							
2.8 oz.	31	.7	7.3	.1	0	25	2.2
shredded, ½ cup	24	.6	5.6	.1	0	19	1.7
shredded (*Dole*),							
3 oz.	50	1.0	9.0	1.0	0	45	1.0
baby, 1 medium,							
2¾" long	4	.1	.8	.1	0	3	n.a.
mini (*Frieda's*),							
1 oz.	12	.3	2.7	.1	0	13	n.a.
mini, peeled (*Dole*),							
3 oz.	50	1.0	9.0	1.0	0	45	1.0
boiled, drained, sliced,							
½ cup	35	.9	8.2	.1	0	52	2.6
Carrot, canned,							
½ cup, except as							
noted:							
all varieties (*S&W*)	25	1.0	6.0	.5	0	250	2.0
baby, whole (*Green							
Giant LeSueur*) . .	35	<1.0	8.0	0	0	410	3.0
whole or sliced							
(*Stokely*), 4.5 oz.	30	0	5.0	0	0	390	2.0
sliced:							
w/liquid	28	.8	6.2	.2	0	297	1.1
drained	17	.5	4.0	.1	0	176	1.1
(*Allens/Crest Top*)	35	0	8.0	.5	0	230	3.0
(*Del Monte*)	35	0	8.0	0	0	300	3.0
(*Goya*)	30	0	6.0	0	0	420	2.0
(*Green Giant*) . . .	25	<1.0	6.0	0	0	380	2.0
(*Stokely* No Salt)	30	0	5.0	0	0	60	2.0
Carrot, frozen:							
boiled, drained, sliced,							
½ cup	26	.9	6.0	.1	0	43	2.6
baby, whole (*Stilwell*),							
⅔ cup	35	1.0	6.0	0	0	45	2.0
baby cut:							
(*Green Giant*),							
¾ cup	30	<1.0	7.0	0	0	40	3.0

Food and Measure	cal.	prot. (gms)	carbo. (gms)	fat (gms)	chol. (mgs)	sod. (mgs)	fiber (gms)
(Green Giant Harvest Fresh),							
²/₃ cup	20	0	5.0	0	0	70	2.0
crinkle *(Stilwell)*,							
²/₃ cup	35	1.0	6.0	0	0	45	2.0
Carrot juice, canned,							
8 fl. oz.	98	2.3	22.8	.4	0	72	2.0
Carvel, 4 fl. oz.:							
ice cream, soft serve:							
chocolate	180	4.0	21.0	10.0	40	55	0
chocolate, no fat . .	90	3.0	19.0	0	0	70	0
vanilla	190	5.0	21.0	10.0	50	70	0
vanilla, no fat . . .	120	5.0	24.0	0	5	95	0
sherbet, all flavors . .	150	1.0	33.0	1.0	5	35	0
yogurt, soft serve, vanilla, no sugar . . .	100	4.0	12.0	1.5	10	70	0
novelties, 1 pc.:							
Brown Bonnet cone	380	6.0	43.0	21.0	40	150	n.a.
Chipsters	380	6.0	50.0	18.0	30	240	n.a.
Flying Saucer . . .	240	5.0	33.0	10	40	150	n.a.
ice cream cupcake	210	4.0	27.0	12.0	35	95	0
Casaba:							
¹/₁₀ of 7³/₄″ melon . .	43	1.5	10.2	.2	0	20	1.3
pulp, cubed, ½ cup	23	.8	5.3	.1	0	10	.7
Cashew, 1 oz., except as noted:							
(Frito-Lay), 1.5 oz.	270	9.0	9.0	22.0	0	260	1.0
whole *(Paradise/White Swan)*, ¼ cup,							
1.2 oz.	210	8.0	8.0	17.0	0	90	5.0
dry-roasted:							
1 oz. or 18 medium	163	4.4	9.3	13.2	0	4	.9
whole or halves,							
1 cup	787	21.0	44.8	63.5	0	21	4.1
oil-roasted:							
1 oz. or 18 medium	163	4.6	8.1	13.7	0	5	1.1
whole or halves,							
1 cup	748	21.0	37.1	62.7	0	22	4.9
(Master Choice) . .	170	5.0	8.0	14.0	0	150	1.0

Food and Measure	cal.	prot. (gms)	carbo. (gms)	fat (gms)	chol. (mgs)	sod. (mgs)	fiber (gms)
Cashew, oil-roasted *(cont.)*							
(*Planters*),							
1-oz. pkg.	160	5.0	8.0	14.0	0	20	1.0
(*Planters*),							
1.5-oz. pkg. . . .	250	7.0	12.0	21.0	0	240	2.0
(*Planters* Fancy) . .	170	5.0	8.0	14.0	0	120	1.0
(*Planters* Fancy),							
2-oz. pkg.	340	9.0	16.0	29.0	0	240	3.0
(*Planters* Halves)	170	5.0	8.0	14.0	0	120	2.0
(*Planters* Halves							
Lightly Salted) . .	160	4.0	9.0	13.0	0	55	2.0
(*Planters Munch 'N*							
Go Singles),							
2-oz. pkg.	330	10.0	16.0	28.0	0	240	3.0
honey-roasted:							
(*Planters*)	150	4.0	11.0	12.0	0	120	1.0
(*Planters/Planters*							
Munch 'N Go),							
2-oz. pkg.	310	9.0	23.0	24.0	0	240	3.0
and peanuts (*Plant-*							
ers)	150	5.0	10.0	12.0	0	125	2.0
Cashew butter							
(*Roaster Fresh*),							
1 oz.	165	4.0	9.0	14.0	0	4	0
Cassava (see also							
"Yuca"), 1 oz. . . .	34	.9	7.6	.1	0	2	<.1
Catfish, channel:							
farmed, meat only:							
raw, 4 oz.	153	17.7	0	8.6	15	60	0
baked, broiled, or							
microwaved, 4 oz.	172	21.2	0	9.1	73	91	0
wild, meat only:							
raw, 4 oz.	108	18.6	0	3.2	66	49	0
baked, broiled, or							
microwaved, 4 oz.	119	20.9	0	3.2	82	57	0
Catfish, frozen, 4 oz.:							
fillets (*Delta Pride*)	90	15.0	0	3.5	60	200	0
nuggets (*Delta Pride*)	170	17.0	0	11.0	82	125	0
steaks (*Delta Pride*)	170	17.0	0	11.0	72	80	0

Food and Measure	cal.	prot. (gms)	carbo. (gms)	fat (gms)	chol. (mgs)	sod. (mgs)	fiber (gms)
whole (*Delta Pride*)	130	19.0	0	6.0	72	105	0
Catjang, boiled,							
½ cup	100	7.0	17.5	.6	0	16	n.a.
Catsup, see							
"Ketchup"							
Cauliflower, fresh:							
raw:							
3 flowerets	14	1.1	2.9	.1	0	17	1.4
1″ pcs., ½ cup . .	13	1.0	2.6	.1	0	15	1.3
florets (*Dole*), 3 oz.	20	2.0	2.0	.5	0	35	2.0
boiled, drained,							
1″ pcs., ½ cup . .	14	1.1	2.6	.3	0	9	1.7
green:							
raw, ⅕ head	28	2.7	5.7	.3	0	22	3.0
raw (*Dole*), ⅕ head	35	3.0	7.0	0	0	30	2.0
raw, 1″ pcs., ½ cup	16	1.5	3.0	.2	0	12	1.6
boiled, drained,							
1″ pcs., ½ cup	20	1.9	3.9	.2	0	14	2.0
Cauliflower, frozen:							
boiled, drained,							
1″ pcs., ½ cup . .	17	1.5	3.4	.2	0	16	2.0
(*Stilwell*), 1 cup . . .	20	2.0	3.0	0	0	25	2.0
florets (*Green Giant*),							
1 cup	25	2.0	4.0	0	0	25	2.0
w/broccoli, see "Broc-							
coli combinations"							
in cheese sauce							
(*Green Giant*),							
½ cup	60	2.0	8.0	2.5	<5	510	2.0
Cauliflower, pickled,							
sweet (*Vlasic*), 1 oz.	35	0	9.0	0	0	260	n.a.
Cavatelli, frozen							
(*Celentano*), 3.2 oz.	400	16.0	79.0	1.5	15	15	9.0
Caviar (see also							
"Roe"), 1 tbsp.:							
black or red	40	3.9	.6	2.9	94	240	0
carp roe (*Krinos*							
Tarama)	20	3.0	0	.5	50	700	0

Food and Measure	cal.	prot. (gms)	carbo. (gms)	fat (gms)	chol. (mgs)	sod. (mgs)	fiber (gms)
Caviar *(cont.)*							
lumpfish, black or red							
(*Romanoff*)	15	1.0	0	1.0	50	380	0
salmon, red (*Roma-*							
noff)	35	3.0	0	1.5	55	310	0
whitefish, black (*Ro-*							
manoff)	25	1.0	1.0	1.5	45	300	0
Caviar spread (*Krinos*							
Taramosalata),							
1 tbsp.	90	1.0	0	10.0	15	115	0
Cayenne, see "Pep-							
per"							
Ceci, see "Chickpeas"							
Celeriac, fresh, raw:							
trimmed, 4 oz.	44	1.7	10.4	.3	0	113	2.0
trimmed, ½ cup . . .	31	1.2	7.2	.2	0	78	1.4
Celery:							
raw:							
7½"-stalk, 1.6 oz.	6	.3	1.5	.1	0	35	.7
diced, ½ cup . . .	10	.5	2.2	.1	0	52	1.0
boiled, drained, diced,							
½ cup	13	.6	3.0	.1	0	68	1.2
Celery, dried:							
flakes or seeds							
(*Tone's*), 1 tsp. . .	9	.4	.9	.5	0	4	.3
seeds (*McCormick*),							
¼ tsp.	2	.1	.2	.1	0	<1	.2
Celery salt (*Tone's*),							
1 tsp.	6	.3	.6	.4	0	1584	.2
Cellophane noodles,							
see "Noodle, Chi-							
nese"							
Celtus, raw, trimmed,							
1 oz.	6	.2	1.0	.1	0	3	<1.0

Food and Measure	cal.	prot. (gms)	carbo. (gms)	fat (gms)	chol. (mgs)	sod. (mgs)	fiber (gms)
Cereal, ready-to-eat (see also specific grains), 1 cup, except as noted:							
amaranth flakes (*Arrowhead Mills*) . . .	130	4.0	21.0	2.0	0	0	3.0
bran (see also "oat bran," below):							
(*Kellogg's All-Bran*), ½ cup	80	4.0	22.0	1.0	0	280	10.0
(*Kellogg's All-Bran Extra Fiber*), ½ cup	50	4.0	22.0	1.0	0	150	15.0
(*Kellogg's Bran Buds*), ⅓ cup . .	70	3.0	24.0	1.0	0	210	11.0
(*Kellogg's Frosted Bran*), ¾ cup . .	100	2.0	26.0	0	0	200	3.0
(*Kellogg's Fruitful Bran*), 1¼ cups	170	4.0	44.0	1.0	0	330	6.0
(*Post Bran'nola*), ½ cup	200	4.0	43.0	3.0	0	240	5.0
(*Nabisco 100% Bran*), ⅓ cup . .	80	4.0	23.0	.5	0	120	8.0
(*Quaker* Crunchy), ¾ cup	90	2.0	23.0	1.0	0	250	5.0
flakes (*Arrowhead Mills*)	100	5.0	22.0	1.0	0	80	4.0
flakes (*Kellogg's Complete*), ¾ cup	100	3.0	25.0	.5	0	230	5.0
flakes (*Malt-O-Meal*), ¾ cup	100	3.0	24.0	.5	0	210	5.0
flakes (*New Morning Multi-Bran*) . . .	110	4.0	21.0	1.0	0	0	5.0
flakes (*Post*), ⅔ cup	90	3.0	22.0	.5	0	210	6.0
raisin (*Kellogg's*)	170	5.0	43.0	1.0	0	310	7.0
raisin (*Malt-O-Meal*)	180	5.0	43.0	1.0	0	260	7.0
raisin (*New Morning Multi-Bran*) . . .	90	3.0	22.0	.5	0	0	6.0

Food and Measure	cal.	prot. (gms)	carbo. (gms)	fat (gms)	chol. (mgs)	sod. (mgs)	fiber (gms)
Cereal, ready-to-eat, bran *(cont.)*							
raisin (*Post*)	190	4.0	46.0	1.0	0	300	8.0
raisin (*Post Bran'nola*) ½ cup	200	4.0	44.0	3.0	0	220	5.0
corn:							
(*Arrowhead Mills Maple Corns*) . .	190	5.0	43.0	3.0	0	140	6.0
(*Barbara's Frosted Funnies*)	110	2.0	27.0	0	0	100	4.0
(*Barbara's Puffins*), ¾ cup	90	2.0	23.0	1.0	0	190	5.0
(*Cocoa Comets*), ¾ cup	120	1.0	27.0	1.0	0	190	0
(*Corn Bursts*) . . .	110	1.0	27.0	0	0	95	1.0
(*Kellogg's Corn Pops*)	110	1.0	27.0	0	0	95	1.0
(*Nut & Honey Crunch*), 1¼ cup	220	4.0	45.0	4.0	0	370	1.0
(*Perky's Nutty Rice*), ¾ cup	220	4.0	50.0	1.0	0	135	6.0
(*Post Toasties*) . . .	100	2.0	24.0	0	0	270	1.0
almond raisin (*New Morning Crunchy*), ¾ cup	110	2.0	22.0	2.0	0	0	3.0
flakes (*Arrowhead Mills*)	100	5.0	30.0	0	0	65	2.0
flakes (*Barbara's*)	110	2.0	26.0	0	0	130	2.0
flakes (*Kellogg's Corn Flakes*) . . .	110	2.0	26.0	0	0	330	1.0
flakes (*Kellogg's Frosted Flakes*), ¾ cup	120	1.0	28.0	0	0	200	0
flakes (*Malt-O-Meal*)	110	2.0	26.0	0	0	310	1.0
flakes (*Malt-O-Meal Frosted*), ¾ cup	110	1.0	27.0	0	0	200	0
flakes (*New Morning*)	120	2.0	26.0	1.0	0	15	1.0

Food and Measure	cal.	prot. (gms)	carbo. (gms)	fat (gms)	chol. (mgs)	sod. (mgs)	fiber (gms)
flakes, honey frosted (*New Morning*), ⅔ cup	120	2.0	25.0	1.0	0	2	1.0
honey roasted pecan (*Kellogg's Temptations*)	120	2.0	24.0	2.5	0	240	1.0
puffed (*Arrowhead Mills*)	80	3.0	16.0	0	0	0	1.0
puffed, honey (*Health Valley*) . .	80	2.0	20.0	0	0	0	2.0
corn and oat, ¾ cup:							
cinnamon (*Kellogg's* Mini Buns) . . .	120	1.0	27.0	.5	0	210	1.0
vanilla almond (*Kellogg's Temptations*)	120	2.0	24.0	2.0	0	210	1.0
corn and rice:							
(*Kellogg's Crispix*)	110	2.0	26.0	0	0	230	1.0
(*Kellogg's Double Dip Crunch*), ¾ cup	110	2.0	27.0	0	0	160	0
granola, ½ cup, except as noted:							
(*C.W. Post* Hearty), ⅔ cup	280	5.0	45.0	9.0	0	150	4.0
(*Heartland*)	290	9.0	41.0	11.0	0	160	4.0
(*Heartland* Lowfat)	290	9.0	41.0	11.0	0	160	4.0
(*Kellogg's* Lowfat)	210	5.0	43.0	3.0	0	120	3.0
(*New Morning Oatiola*), ¾ cup . . .	200	5.0	42.0	2.0	0	0	3.0
almond (*Sun Country*)	270	7.0	38.0	9.0	0	20	3.0
blueberries, milk (*Mountain House*), ⅓ cup	120	4.0	18.0	4.0	0	30	2.0
carob cashew (*Roman Meal*) . . .	190	5.0	37.0	4.0	0	90	3.0
figs and filberts (*Roman Meal*) . .	190	5.0	39.0	3.0	0	80	3.0

Food and Measure	cal.	prot. (gms)	carbo. (gms)	fat (gms)	chol. (mgs)	sod. (mgs)	fiber (gms)
Cereal, ready-to-eat, granola *(cont.)*							
honey nut (*Roman Meal*)	210	6.0	37.0	5.0	0	85	3.0
raisin (*Heartland*)	290	8.0	42.0	10.0	0	140	4.0
raisin (*Kellogg's Low Fat*), ⅔ cup	210	5.0	43.0	3.0	0	135	3.0
raisin and date (*Sun Country*)	260	6.0	43.0	8.0	0	15	4.0
raisin nut (*Roman Meal*)	210	6.0	37.0	5.0	0	85	4.0
kamut:							
(*New Morning Kamutios*)	120	5.0	23.0	1.0	0	90	1.0
flakes (*Arrowhead Mills*)	120	4.0	25.0	1.0	0	65	3.0
puffed (*Arrowhead Mills*)	50	2.0	19.0	0	0	0	1.0
millet, puffed (*Arrowhead Mills*)	90	3.0	19.0	.5	0	0	1.0
mixed/multigrain:							
(*Apple Jacks*) . . .	110	2.0	27.0	0	0	135	1.0
(*Arrowhead Mills* Crispy Puffs) . .	80	2.0	16.0	1.0	0	0	1.0
(*Barbara's* Shredded Spoonfuls), ¾ cup	120	5.0	23.0	1.5	0	200	4.0
(*Barbara's High 5*), ¾ cup	100	3.0	23.0	.5	0	180	5.0
(*Froot Loops*) . . .	120	1.0	26.0	.5	0	150	1.0
(*Fruiteo's*)	120	2.0	25.0	1.0	0	0	2.0
(*Grape-Nuts*), ½ cup	200	6.0	47.0	1.0	0	350	5.0
(*Grape-Nuts* Flakes), ¾ cup	100	3.0	24.0	1.0	0	140	3.0
(*Just Right* Crunchy Nuggets)	200	4.0	46.0	1.5	0	340	3.0
(*Kellogg's Mueslix* Crispy), ⅔ cup	200	4.0	42.0	3.0	0	190	4.0

Food and Measure	cal.	prot. (gms)	carbo. (gms)	fat (gms)	chol. (mgs)	sod. (mgs)	fiber (gms)
(*Kellogg's Mueslix Golden Crunch*), ¾ cup	210	6.0	40.0	5.0	0	280	6.0
(*Product 19*)	110	3.0	25.0	0	0	280	1.0
(*Quaker Life*), ¾ cup	120	3.0	25.0	1.5	0	170	2.0
(*Team* Flakes), 1¼ cups	220	4.0	49.0	0	0	360	1.0
(*Tootie Fruities*) . .	110	2.0	26.0	1.0	0	150	0
all varieties (*Granola O's*), ¾ cup . . .	120	3.0	26.0	0	0	10	3.0
all varieties (*Health Valley* Honey Clusters & Flakes), ¾ cup	130	3.0	31.0	0	0	20	4.0
brown sugar cinnamon (*Pop-Tarts Crunch*), ¾ cup	120	1.0	26.0	1.0	0	160	1.0
cocoa (*Startoons*)	110	2.0	26.0	.5	0	140	1.0
dates, raisins, walnuts (*Fruit & Fibre*)	210	4.0	46.0	3.0	0	260	6.0
honey (*Startoons*)	110	2.0	26.0	0	0	50	2.0
flakes (*Arrowhead Mills*)	140	3.0	29.0	1.5	0	5	3.0
flakes (*Healthy Choice*)	100	3.0	25.0	0	0	210	3.0
fruit-nut (*Just Right*)	210	4.0	46.0	1.5	0	260	3.0
granola, see "granola," above							
peaches, raisins, almonds (*Fruit & Fibre*)	210	4.0	46.0	3.0	0	270	6.0
pecan (*Great Grains*), ⅔ cup	220	5.0	38.0	6.0	0	150	4.0
raisins, dates, pecans (*Great Grains*), ⅔ cup	210	4.0	39.0	5.0	0	150	4.0

Food and Measure	cal.	prot. (gms)	carbo. (gms)	fat (gms)	chol. (mgs)	sod. (mgs)	fiber (gms)
Cereal, ready-to-eat, mixed/multigrain *(cont.)*							
raisins, oats, al-monds (*Healthy Choice*)	200	4.0	45.0	2.0	0	240	4.0
squares (*Healthy Choice*), 1¼ cups	190	5.0	45.0	1.0	0	190	6.0
strawberry (*Pop-Tarts Crunch*), ¾ cup	120	1.0	27.0	1.0	0	125	0
oat:							
(*Alpha-Bits*)	130	3.0	27.0	1.0	0	210	1.0
(*Arrowhead Mills Nature O's*) . . .	130	5.0	24.0	2.0	0	5	3.0
(*Barbara's Breakfast O's*)	120	5.0	22.0	2.0	0	115	2.0
(*Cheerios*)	110	3.0	23.0	2.0	0	280	3.0
(*Honey Bunches of Oats*), ¾ cup . .	120	2.0	25.0	1.5	0	120	1.0
(*Kellogg's Nut & Honey Crunch O's*), ¾ cup . . .	120	3.0	23.0	2.5	0	200	2.0
(*New Morning Oatios* Original) . .	120	4.0	21.0	1.0	0	0	2.0
(*Quaker* Squares)	220	7.0	44.0	3.0	0	260	4.0
(*Toasty O's*)	110	3.0	22.0	2.0	0	280	3.0
almonds (*Honey Bunches of Oats*), ¾ cup	130	3.0	24.0	3.0	0	180	1.0
apple cinnamon (*New Morning Oatios*)	90	3.0	18.0	1.5	0	0	3.0
apple cinnamon (*Toasty O's*), ¾ cup	120	2.0	24.0	1.5	0	190	2.0
blueberry (*New Morning Oatiola*)	200	5.0	41.0	1.5	0	0	4.0
cinnamon (*Quaker Life*)	190	5.0	39.0	2.0	0	220	3.0

Food and Measure	cal.	prot. (gms)	carbo. (gms)	fat (gms)	chol. (mgs)	sod. (mgs)	fiber (gms)
cocoa (*New Morning Oatios*) . . .	170	6.0	37.0	1.5	0	50	7.0
and honey (*Quaker 100% Natural*), ½ cup	220	5.0	32.0	8.0	0	25	3.0
honey almond (*New Morning Oatios*)	100	3.0	22.0	1.0	0	0	3.0
honey graham (*Quaker Oh!s*), ¾ cup	110	1.0	23.0	2.0	0	180	1.0
honey nut (*Toasty O's*)	110	3.0	24.0	1.0	0	270	2.0
honey, raisins (*Quaker 100% Natural*), ½ cup	220	5.0	35.0	8.0	0	20	4.0
marshmallow (*Alpha-Bits*)	120	2.0	25.0	1.0	0	160	1.0
marshmallow (*Mateys*)	120	2.0	25.0	1.0	0	210	1.0
oat bran:							
(*Common Sense*), ¾ cup	110	4.0	23.0	1.0	0	270	4.0
(*Cracklin' Oat Bran*), ¾ cup	230	4.0	40.0	8.0	0	180	6.0
(*New Morning Ultimate Oat Bran*)	110	4.0	20.0	2.0	0	0	4.0
(*Quaker*), 1¼ cup	210	8.0	41.0	3.0	0	210	7.0
flakes (*Arrowhead Mills*)	110	6.0	22.0	2.0	0	60	4.0
rice:							
(*Apple Cinnamon Rice Krispies*), ¾ cup	110	2.0	27.0	0	0	220	1.0
(*Cocoa Krispies*), ¾ cup	120	2.0	27.0	.5	0	190	0
(*Frosted Krispies*), ¾ cup	110	1.0	27.0	0	0	230	0
(*Fruity Marshmallow Krispies*), ¾ cup	110	1.0	27.0	0	0	180	0

Food and Measure	cal.	prot. (gms)	carbo. (gms)	fat (gms)	chol. (mgs)	sod. (mgs)	fiber (gms)
Cereal, ready-to-eat, rice *(cont.)*							
(*Perky's Nutty Rice*),							
¾ cup	210	4.0	46.0	1.5	0	110	2.0
(*Rice Krispies*),							
1¼ cups	110	2.0	26.0	0	0	320	1.0
(*Rice Krispies*							
Treats), ¾ cup	120	1.0	25.0	1.5	0	170	0
(*Special K*)	110	6.0	21.0	0	0	250	1.0
crispy							
(*Malt-O-Meal*) . .	110	2.0	26.0	0	0	250	0
puffed (*Arrowhead*							
Mills)	90	2.0	19.0	0	0	0	1.0
puffed							
(*Malt-O-Meal*) . .	60	1.0	13.0	0	0	0	0
rice, brown, crisp:							
(*Barbara's*)	120	2.0	25.0	1.0	0	125	1.0
(*Health Valley*) . . .	110	1.0	30.0	0	0	0	1.0
(*New Morning*) . .	110	2.0	23.0	1.0	0	0	1.0
frosted (*New Morn-*							
ing)	210	6.0	45.0	1.5	0	40	6.0
rice and corn, almond							
raisin (*Nutri-Grain*),							
1¼ cups	200	4.0	44.0	3.0	0	330	4.0
rice and rye (*Kellogg's*							
Apple Raisin Crisp)	180	3.0	46.0	0	0	340	4.0
spelt flakes (*Arrow-*							
head Mills)	100	5.0	22.0	1.0	0	60	3.0
wheat:							
(*Golden Puffs*),							
¾ cup	120	2.0	26.0	0	0	40	1.0
(*Kellogg's Apple*							
Cinnamon/Blue-							
berry Squares),							
¾ cup	180	4.0	44.0	1.0	0	15	5.0
(*Kellogg's Frosted*							
Mini-Wheats) . .	190	5.0	45.0	1.0	0	0	6.0
(*Kellogg's Raisin*							
Squares), ¾ cup	180	4.0	44.0	1.0	0	210	5.0

Food and Measure	cal.	prot. (gms)	carbo. (gms)	fat (gms)	chol. (mgs)	sod. (mgs)	fiber (gms)
(*Kellogg's Smacks*), ¾ cup	110	2.0	26.0	.5	0	75	1.0
(*Kellogg's Strawberry Squares*), ¾ cup	180	4.0	44.0	1.0	0	10	5.0
(*Nabisco Frosted Wheat Bites*) . . .	190	4.0	44.0	1.0	0	10	5.0
(*Nutri-Grain Golden*), ¾ cup	100	3.0	24.0	.5	0	240	4.0
blueberry or strawberry (*Nabisco Wheat Bites*), ¾ cup	170	4.0	41.0	.5	0	15	4.0
honey grahams (*New Morning*), 2 pcs.	120	2.0	24.0	3.0	0	80	2.0
puffed (*Arrowhead Mills*)	90	3.0	20.0	.5	0	0	2.0
puffed (*Malt-O-Meal*) . .	50	2.0	11.0	0	0	0	1.0
raisin (*Nutri-Grain Golden*), 1¼ cups	180	4.0	45.0	1.0	0	310	6.0
raspberry (*Nabisco Wheat Bites*), ¾ cup	160	4.0	40.0	.5	0	15	4.0
wheat, shredded:							
(*Barbara's*), 2 pcs.	140	4.0	31.0	1.0	0	0	5.0
(*Nabisco*), 2 pcs.	160	5.0	38.0	.5	0	0	5.0
(*Nabisco Shredded Wheat 'n Bran*), 1¼ cups	200	7.0	47.0	1.0	0	0	8.0
(*Nabisco Spoon Size*)	170	5.0	41.0	.5	0	200	5.0
(*Quaker*), 3 pcs. . .	220	7.0	50.0	1.5	0	0	7.0
wheat and barley (*Perky's Nutty Wheat & Barley*), ¾ cup	220	5.0	47.0	.5	0	135	3.0

Food and Measure	cal.	prot. (gms)	carbo. (gms)	fat (gms)	chol. (mgs)	sod. (mgs)	fiber (gms)
Cereal, cooking/hot							
(see also specific grains), uncooked, 1 pkt., except as noted:							
barley (*Arrowhead Mills Bits O Barley*), ⅓ cup	140	5.0	35.0	1.0	0	0	6.0
farina, see "wheat," below							
mixed/multigrain:							
(*Mothers*), ½ cup	130	5.0	29.0	1.5	0	160	5.0
(*Pritikin*)	160	5.0	34.0	1.5	0	150	4.0
(*Roman Meal*) . . .	130	6.0	25.0	2.5	0	0	6.0
(*Roman Meal* Instant)	100	3.0	21.0	1.5	0	5	2.0
4 grain, w/flax (*Arrowhead Mills*), ¼ cup	150	6.0	28.0	2.0	0	0	6.0
7 grain (*Arrowhead Mills*), ⅓ cup . .	140	6.0	25.0	1.5	0	0	5.0
7 grain (*Arrowhead Mills* Wheat Free), ¼ cup	120	4.0	25.0	1.5	0	0	2.0
apple cinnamon (*Roman Meal*). .	120	4.0	24.0	2.5	0	5	4.0
apple cinnamon (*Roman Meal* Instant)	110	4.0	24.0	1.5	0	5	3.0
raisin date-nut (*Roman Meal*) . . .	140	5.0	26.0	2.5	0	0	4.0
raisin date-nut (*Roman Meal* Instant)	120	4.0	25.0	2.0	0	5	3.0
oat bran:							
(*Mothers*), ½ cup	150	8.0	24.0	3.0	0	230	6.0
(*Quaker*), ½ cup . .	150	8.0	24.0	3.0	0	230	6.0
oat flakes, raisin and spice (*H-O* Instant)	150	4.0	32.0	2.0	0	180	3.0

Food and Measure	cal.	prot. (gms)	carbo. (gms)	fat (gms)	chol. (mgs)	sod. (mgs)	fiber (gms)
oatmeal, instant:							
(*Arrowhead Mills*)	110	4.0	19.0	2.0	0	0	2.0
(*H-O*), ½ cup . . .	150	5.0	27.0	3.0	0	0	4.0
(*Maypo*), ⅓ cup . .	150	5.0	27.0	2.0	0	0	3.0
(*Mothers*), ½ cup	150	5.0	27.0	3.0	0	150	4.0
(*Quaker*)	130	4.0	22.0	2.5	0	95	3.0
(*Roman Meal* Premium)	220	10.0	40.0	4.0	0	0	6.0
w/apples and cinnamon (*Quaker*) . .	130	4.0	26.0	1.5	0	105	3.0
apple, raisin, and walnut (*Quaker*)	140	3.0	27.0	2.5	0	160	3.0
cinnamon, raisin, almond (*Arrowhead Mills*)	130	5.0	24.0	2.0	0	0	2.0
cinnamon spice (*Quaker*)	170˙	4.0	36.0	2.0	0	290	3.0
cinnamon toast (*Quaker*)	130	3.0	27.0	2.0	0	160	2.0
fruit and cream (*Quaker*)	130	3.0	27.0	2.5	0	140	2.0
honey nut (*Quaker*)	130	3.0	25.0	3.0	0	210	3.0
maple (*Maypo*), ½ cup	190	6.0	36.0	2.0	0	0	3.0
maple, apple, spice (*Arrowhead Mills*)	130	4.0	25.0	2.0	0	40	2.0
maple brown sugar (*Quaker*)	160	4.0	33.0	2.0	0	240	3.0
peaches and cream (*Quaker*)	130	3.0	27.0	2.0	0	150	3.0
raisin, date, walnut (*Quaker*)	130	3.0	27.0	2.5	0	240	3.0
raisin spice (*Quaker*)	160	5.0	32.0	2.0	0	250	3.0
raspberry (*Quaker*)	150	4.0	29.0	3.0	0	170	3.0
strawberries and cream (*Quaker*)	130	3.0	27.0	2.0	0	160	2.0
strawberries 'n stuff (*Quaker*)	150	3.0	30.0	2.0	0	170	3.0

Food and Measure	cal.	prot. (gms)	carbo. (gms)	fat (gms)	chol. (mgs)	sod. (mgs)	fiber (gms)
Cereal, cooking/hot *(cont.)*							
oats:							
(*H-O* Quick), ½ cup	150	5.0	27.0	3.0	0	0	4.0
(*H-O* Quick Oats 'n							
Fiber)	110	5.0	17.0	2.0	0	140	3.0
cinnamon graham							
(*Quaker* Instant)	150	4.0	30.0	2.5	0	170	3.0
oats, rolled:							
(*H-O* Instant) . . .	110	4.0	18.0	2.5	0	220	3.0
(*H-O* Sweet & Mel-							
low Instant) . . .	150	4.0	30.0	2.0	0	200	2.0
(*Quaker* Quick/Old							
Fashioned),							
½ cup	150	5.0	27.0	3.0	0	140	4.0
banana creme (*H-O*							
Explo Instant) . .	170	4.0	32.0	3.0	5	240	3.0
almond raisin (*H-O*							
Explo Instant) . .	160	5.0	32.0	2.0	0	240	3.0
apple and cinnamon							
(*H-O* Instant) . .	130	3.0	26.0	3.0	0	100	3.0
apple maple spice							
(*H-O* Explo In-							
stant)	170	4.0	33.0	2.0	0	230	3.0
apricot honey (*H-O*							
Explo Instant) . .	170	4.0	33.0	2.0	0	230	3.0
maple and brown							
sugar (*H-O* In-							
stant)	160	4.0	32.0	2.0	0	220	3.0
oats, toasted (*H-O* Old							
Fashioned), ⅓ cup	160	7.0	28.0	2.5	0	0	5.0
rice:							
(*Lundberg* Amber							
Hot 'n Creamy),							
⅓ cup	190	3.0	44.0	1.5	0	0	2.0
(*Lundberg* Organic							
Hot 'n Creamy),							
⅓ cup	190	4.0	43.0	2.0	0	0	3.0

Food and Measure	cal.	prot. (gms)	carbo. (gms)	fat (gms)	chol. (mgs)	sod. (mgs)	fiber (gms)
(*Arrowhead Mills* *Rice & Shine*), ¼ cup	150	3.0	32.0	1.0	0	0	2.0
almond, sweet (*Lundberg* Hot 'n Creamy), ⅓ cup	200	3.0	40.0	3.5	0	0	4.0
cinnamon raisin (*Lundberg* Hot 'n Creamy), ⅓ cup	190	3.0	42.0	1.5	0	0	4.0
rye, cream of:							
(*Roman Meal*) . . .	110	5.0	25.0	1.0	0	0	5.0
(*Roman Meal* Instant)	100	4.0	20.0	1.0	0	0	3.0
wheat:							
(*Arrowhead Mills* *Bear Mush*), ¼ cup	160	5.0	33.0	1.0	0	0	2.0
(*Malt-O-Meal* Quick), 3 tbsp.	120	4.0	26.0	0	0	0	1.0
(*Mothers*), ½ cup	130	5.0	30.0	1.0	0	170	4.0
(*Wheatena*), ⅓ cup	150	5.0	32.0	1.0	0	0	5.0
all varieties (*Malt-O-Meal*), 3 tbsp.	120	3.0	28.0	0	0	0	1.0
n'berries (*Fantastic* Cup), 1.9 oz. . .	210	6.0	44.0	1.0	0	290	4.0
cracked (*Arrowhead Mills*), ¼ cup . .	170	5.0	29.0	.5	0	0	6.0
farina (*H-O*), 3 tbsp.	120	3.0	26.0	0	0	0	1.0
wheat free:							
apple cinnamon (*Fantastic* Cup), 1.9 oz.	210	4.0	42.0	3.0	0	240	3.0
banana nut (*Fantastic* Cup), 1.6 oz.	180	4.0	35.0	2.5	0	230	4.0
cranberry orange (*Fantastic* Cup), 1.9 oz.	210	4.0	42.0	3.0	0	220	3.0

Food and Measure	cal.	prot. (gms)	carbo. (gms)	fat (gms)	chol. (mgs)	sod. (mgs)	fiber (gms)
Cereal bar, see "Granola and cereal bar"							
Cereal beverage, see "Coffee substitute"							
Charcoal seasoning							
(*Durkee*), ¼ tsp. . .	0	0	0	0	0	180	0
Chayote:							
raw:							
1 medium, 7.2 oz.	49	1.8	11.0	.6	0	8	6.1
1" pcs., ½ cup . .	16	.6	3.6	.2	0	3	2.0
(*Frieda's*), 3.5 oz.	28	.6	7.1	.1	0	5	n.a.
boiled, drained,							
1" pcs., ½ cup . .	19	.5	4.1	.4	0	1	n.a.
Cheese (see also "Cheese Food" and "Cheese Product"), 1 oz., except as noted:							
American, processed:							
(*Boar's Head* Loaf)	100	6.0	1.0	9.0	25	380	0
(*Borden*), ⅔-oz. slice	70	4.0	1.0	6.0	20	290	0
(*Borden*), ¾-oz. slice	80	4.0	1.0	7.0	20	320	0
(*Borden* Loaf) . . .	110	6.0	1.0	9.0	30	380	0
(*Harvest Moon*), ⅔-oz. slice . . .	70	4.0	0	6.0	20	320	0
(*Kraft* Deluxe Loaf)	100	6.0	<1.0	9.0	25	430	0
(*Kraft* Deluxe Slice), ⅔-oz. slice . . .	70	4.0	<1.0	6.0	15	310	0
(*Kraft* Deluxe Slice), ¾-oz. slice . . .	80	4.0	<1.0	7.0	20	340	0
(*Kraft* Deluxe Slice), 1-oz. slice	110	5.0	<1.0	9.0	25	460	0
(*Old English* Loaf)	100	6.0	<1.0	9.0	25	440	0
(*Old English* Slice), 1-oz. slice	110	6.0	<1.0	9.0	30	460	0
sharp (*Borden*) . .	110	6.0	1.0	9.0	30	430	0

Food and Measure	cal.	prot. (gms)	carbo. (gms)	fat (gms)	chol. (mgs)	sod. (mgs)	fiber (gms)
(*Bel Paese*):							
medalions, ¾ oz.	65	3.0	1.5	5.5	13	266	0
flavored varieties	110	5.0	1.0	10.0	5	90	1.0
w/basil, sun-dried							
tomatoes	101	6.0	.7	8.0	20	145	1.0
blue:							
(*Kraft*)	100	6.0	<1.0	8.0	30	390	0
crumbled (*Sargento*)							
¼ cup, 1 oz. . .	100	6.0	1.0	8.0	20	380	0
brick (*Kraft*)	110	6.0	0	9.0	30	190	0
Brie	95	5.9	.1	7.9	20	229	0
butterkase, plain or							
smoked (*Boar's*							
Head)	100	6.0	0	9.0	30	180	0
Camembert	85	5.6	,1	6.9	20	239	0
cheddar:							
(*Alpine Lace* Re-							
duced Fat)	80	9.0	1.0	4.5	15	135	0
(*Boar's Head* Double							
Glouster)	110	7.0	0	10.0	35	200	0
(*Cracker Barrel*							
⅓ Less Fat) . . .	80	9.0	<1.0	5.0	20	220	0
(*Dorman*)	110	7.0	1.0	9.0	30	180	0
(*Dorman* Reduced							
Fat)	80	9.0	0	5.0	15	180	0
(*Heluva* Good Low							
Sodium)	110	7.0	0	9.0	25	8	0
(*Kraft Cracker Bar-*							
rel)	110	7.0	<1.0	9.0	30	180	0
mild (*Kraft*							
⅓ Less Fat) . . .	80	9.0	0	5.0	20	220	0
mild (*Heluva* Good							
Reduced Fat) . .	80	7.0	1.0	6.0	15	200	0
mild (*Weight Watch-*							
ers Low Sodium)	80	8.0	1.0	5.0	15	70	0
mild, light, snack							
(*MooTown Snack-*							
ers), .8 oz. pc.	60	7.0	<1.0	4.0	10	170	0

Food and Measure	cal.	prot. (gms)	carbo. (gms)	fat (gms)	chol. (mgs)	sod. (mgs)	fiber (gms)
Cheese, cheddar *(cont.)*							
mild or sharp							
(*Weight Watchers*)	80	8.0	1.0	5.0	15	180	0
mild or sharp							
(*MooTown Snack-*							
ers), .8 oz. pc.	100	5.0	1.0	8.0	25	130	0
mild, sharp, or extra							
sharp (*Heluva*							
Good)	110	7.0	1.0	9.0	30	180	0
sharp (*Boar's Head*							
Slicing)	110	7.0	<1.0	9.0	30	190	0
sharp (*Kraft* Less							
Fat)	80	9.0	<1.0	5.0	20	220	0
sharp (*Sargento*							
Sliced)	110	6.0	1.0	9.0	30	160	0
nacho, w/peppers							
(*Kraft*)	110	7.0	0	9.0	30	250	0
cheddar, shredded:							
(*Kraft*), ¼ cup . . .	120	7.0	<1.0	10.0	30	190	0
fat free (*Kraft*							
Healthy Favorites),							
¼ cup	45	10.0	1.0	0	<5	220	0
fine (*Kraft*), ¼ cup	90	5.0	<1.0	8.0	25	150	0
mild (*Kraft* ⅓ Less							
Fat), ¼ cup . . .	90	10.0	<1.0	6.0	20	230	0
mild (*Sargento Pre-*							
ferred Light),							
¼ cup	70	8.0	<1.0	4.5	10	200	0
mild or sharp							
(*Sargento*), ¼ cup	110	6.0	1.0	9.0	30	160	0
sharp (*Cracker Bar-*							
rel ⅓ Less Fat),							
¼ cup	80	8.0	<1.0	5.0	20	200	0
Cheshire	110	6.6	1.4	8.7	29	198	0
Colby:							
(*Alpine Lace* Re-							
duced Fat)	80	9.0	1.0	5.0	15	115	0
(*Dorman* Sandwich),							
1.1-oz. slice . . .	130	8.0	1.0	10.0	30	200	0

Food and Measure	cal.	prot. (gms)	carbo. (gms)	fat (gms)	chol. (mgs)	sod. (mgs)	fiber (gms)
(*Kraft*)	110	7.0	<1.0	9.0	30	180	0
(*Kraft* ⅓ Less Fat)	80	9.0	0	5.0	20	220	0
(*Sargento* Sliced)	110	6.0	0	9.0	30	190	0
mild (*Heluva* Good							
Longhorn)	117	7.0	0	9.0	30	186	0
Colby Jack:							
(*Heluva* Good) . . .	110	6.0	0	9.0	30	200	0
shredded							
(*Sargento*), ¼ cup	110	6.0	<1.0	9.0	25	190	0
snack (*MooTown*							
Snackers), .8 oz.	90	5.0	<1.0	8.0	20	160	0
Colby Monterey Jack:							
(*Kraft*)	110	7.0	0	9.0	30	190	0
shredded (*Kraft*),							
¼ cup	30	7.0	<1.0	9.0	30	200	0
cottage, 4%, ½ cup:							
(*Breakstone's*) . . .	120	14.0	4.0	5.0	25	400	0
(*Sealtest*)	120	14.0	4.0	5.0	25	400	0
large curd (*Knud-*							
sen)	130	16.0	3.0	5.0	30	340	0
small curd (*Knud-*							
sen)	120	15.0	2.0	5.0	25	400	0
cottage, dry curd							
(*Breakstone's*),							
¼ cup	45	8.0	0	0	5	25	0
cottage, lowfat,							
½ cup, except as							
noted:							
2% (*Breakstone's*)	90	14.0	4.0	2.5	15	380	0
2% (*Knudsen*) . . .	100	16.0	3.0	2.5	15	400	0
2% (*Sealtest*) . . .	90	14.0	4.0	2.5	15	380	0
2% (*Weight Watch-*							
ers)	90	12.0	4.0	2.0	15	460	0
1% (*Light n' Lively*)	80	14.0	4.0	1.5	15	380	0
1% (*Weight Watch-*							
ers)	90	14.0	4.0	1.0	5	460	0
garden salad, 1%							
(*Light n' Lively*)	90	13.0	5.0	1.5	15	410	0

Food and Measure	cal.	prot. (gms)	carbo. (gms)	fat (gms)	chol. (mgs)	sod. (mgs)	fiber (gms)
Cheese, cottage, lowfat *(cont.)*							
peach, 1.5% (*Knudsen*), 4 oz.	110	11.0	12.0	1.5	10	290	0
peach and pineapple, 1% (*Light n' Lively*)	120	12.0	14.0	1.0	10	350	0
pineapple, 1.5% (*Knudsen*), 4 oz.	110	11.0	11.0	1.5	10	290	0
strawberry, 1.5% (*Knudsen*), 4 oz.	110	11.0	12.0	1.5	10	280	0
tropical fruit (*Knudsen*), 4 oz.	120	11.0	15.0	2.0	10	300	0
cottage, nonfat, ½ cup:							
(*Knudsen Free*) . .	80	15.0	4.0	0	10	370	0
(*Light n' Lively Free*)	80	14.0	3.0	0	10	440	0
cream cheese:							
(*Boar's Head*) . . .	100	2.0	2.0	10.0	30	100	0
(*Heluva* Good) . . .	100	2.0	1.0	10.0	30	85	0
(*Philadelphia Brand*)	100	2.0	<1.0	10.0	30	90	0
(*Weight Watchers Light*), 2 tbsp. . .	40	3.0	1.0	2.5	10	105	0
(*Western Creamy*), 2 tbsp., 1.1 oz.	70	2.0	1.0	7.0	15	85	0
(*Western Creamy Light*), 2 tbsp., 1.1 oz.	50	3.0	0	4.5	10	80	0
w/chive or pimiento (*Philadelphia Brand*)	90	2.0	<1.0	9.0	30	150	0
fat free (*Philadelphia Brand*)	25	4.0	2.0	0	<5	135	0
cream cheese, soft (*Philadelphia Brand*), 2 tbsp.:							
plain	100	2.0	1.0	10.0	30	100	0
plain, fat free . . .	30	5.0	2.0	0	<5	160	0
plain, light	70	3.0	2.0	5.0	15	150	0

Food and Measure	cal.	prot. (gms)	carbo. (gms)	fat (gms)	chol. (mgs)	sod. (mgs)	fiber (gms)
w/chives and onion	110	2.0	2.0	10.0	30	110	0
w/herb and garlic	110	1.0	2.0	10.0	30	180	0
w/olive and pimiento	100	2.0	2.0	9.0	30	170	0
w/pineapple	100	2.0	4.0	9.0	30	100	0
w/smoked salmon	100	2.0	1.0	9.0	30	200	0
w/strawberries . . .	100	1.0	5.0	9.0	30	65	0
cream cheese, whipped, 3 tbsp.:							
plain (*Breakstone's Temp-Tee*)	110	3.0	1.0	10.0	30	115	0
plain (*Philadelphia Brand*)	110	2.0	1.0	11.0	35	95	0
w/smoked salmon (*Philadelphia Brand*)	100	2.0	1.0	9.0	30	200	0
Edam:							
(*Boar's Head*) . . .	90	7.0	0	7.0	20	280	0
(*Dorman* Sliced) . .	90	7.0	0	7.0	25	260	0
farmer:							
(*Kraft*)	100	6.0	<1.0	8.0	25	190	0
(*Western Creamy*), 2.3 oz.	100	6.0	2.0	8.0	15	140	0
dry (*Western Creamy* Fat Free), 2 oz.	50	11.0	1.0	0	5	105	0
feta:							
(*Alpine Lace* Reduced Fat)	60	5.0	1.0	4.0	10	370	0
(*Classika* Portions)	100	6.0	2.0	8.0	5	400	1.0
(*Krinos* Imported)	90	5.0	0	8.0	24	430	0
fontina (*Classica*) . .	110	7.0	<1.0	8.5	25	160	0
goat:							
hard type	128	8.7	.6	10.1	30	98	0
semisoft type . . .	103	6.1	.7	8.5	22	146	0
soft type	76	5.3	.3	6.0	13	104	0
Gorgonzola (*Galbani* Dolcelatte)	93	5.0	<1.0	8.0	22	234	0
Gouda:							
(*Boar's Head*) . . .	110	6.0	0	9.0	30	280	0

Food and Measure	cal.	prot. (gms)	carbo. (gms)	fat (gms)	chol. (mgs)	sod. (mgs)	fiber (gms)
Cheese, Gouda *(cont.)*							
(*Dorman* Sliced) . .	100	7.0	0	8.0	30	240	0
(*Kraft*)	110	7.0	<1.0	9.0	25	160	0
Gruyère	117	8.5	.1	9.2	31	95	0
Havarti:							
(*Boar's Head*) . . .	110	6.0	0	10.0	35	210	0
(*Dorman* Sliced) . .	100	7.0	0	8.0	20	180	0
(*Kraft Casino*) . . .	120	6.0	0	11.0	35	240	0
hot pepper (*Alpine Lace*)	80	6.0	2.0	6.0	20	260	0
Italian (*Classica Italiana*)	110	6.0	1.0	10.0	10	90	0
Italian style:							
grated (*Kraft* ⅓ Less Fat), 2 tsp.	25	2.0	1.0	1.0	<5	115	0
shredded (*Sargento Recipe Blend*), ¼ cup	90	7.0	0	7.0	20	180	0
Jarlsberg (*Sargento*), 1.2-oz. slice	120	9.0	1.0	9.0	20	160	0
(*Laughing Cow Babybel* 7 oz.) . . .	100	6.0	0	8.0	25	230	0
(*Laughing Cow Babybel* Mini), ¾-oz. pc.	70	5.0	0	6.0	15	170	0
(*Laughing Cow* Original Wedge)	70	4.0	1.0	6.0	20	370	0
limburger (*Kraft Mohawk Valley*)	90	6.0	0	8.0	25	240	0
mascarpone:							
(*Classica* Domestic)	120	2.0	1.0	12.0	86	14	<1.0
(*Galbani* Imported)	140	2.0	1.0	14.0	31	10	0
Mexican, 4, shredded (*Sargento Recipe Blend*), ¼ cup . . .	110	6.0	<1.0	9.0	25	200	0
Monterey Jack:							
(*Boar's Head*) . . .	100	6.0	0	9.0	25	190	0
(*Dorman*)	100	7.0	0	8.0	30	170	0

Food and Measure	cal.	prot. (gms)	carbo. (gms)	fat (gms)	chol. (mgs)	sod. (mgs)	fiber (gms)
(*Dorman*), 1.2-oz. slice	130	8.0	1.0	10.0	35	210	0
(*Dorman* Reduced Fat)	80	9.0	0	4.5	15	180	0
(*Dorman* Reduced Fat), 1.5-oz. slice	120	14.0	1.0	7.0	25	280	0
(*Heluva* Good) . . .	100	6.0	0	8.0	25	180	0
(*Kraft*)	110	6.0	0	9.0	30	190	0
(*Kraft* ⅓ Less Fat)	80	9.0	0	5.0	20	220	0
(*Sargento* Sliced)	100	6.0	0	9.0	30	190	0
(*Weight Watchers*)	80	8.0	1.0	5.0	15	180	0
shredded (*Dorman*), ⅓ cup, 1 oz. . .	80	9.0	0	5.0	15	190	0
shredded (*Kraft*), ¼ cup	110	7.0	<1.0	9.0	30	200	0
shredded (*Sargento*), ¼ cup	100	6.0	0	9.0	30	190	0
jalapeño (*Boar's Head*)	100	6.0	0	9.0	25	190	0
jalapeño (*Heluva* Good)	100	7.0	0	8.0	25	180	0
jalapeño (*Kraft*) . .	110	7.0	<1.0	9.0	30	190	0
peppers (*Kraft* ⅓ Less Fat) . . .	80	8.0	<1.0	5.0	20	220	0
mozzarella:							
(*Boar's Head*) . . .	90	6.0	<1.0	7.0	25	140	0
(*Polly-O* Fat Free)	35	7.0	<1.0	0	<5	220	0
(*Polly-O* Fior Di Latte)	80	5.0	0	7.0	20	15	0
(*Polly-O* Lite) . . .	60	7.0	<1.0	2.5	10	230	0
whole milk (*Heluva* Good)	80	6.0	<1.0	6.0	20	220	0
whole milk (*Polly-O*)	80	6.0	<1.0	6.0	20	220	0
part skim (*Alpine Lace* Reduced Fat)	70	7.0	1.0	5.0	15	75	0
part skim (*Dorman*)	80	8.0	1.0	5.0	15	170	0
part skim (*Heluva* Good)	70	6.0	<1.0	5.0	15	220	0
part skim (*Kraft*) . .	80	8.0	<1.0	5.0	15	200	0

Food and Measure	cal.	prot. (gms)	carbo. (gms)	fat (gms)	chol. (mgs)	sod. (mgs)	fiber (gms)
Cheese, mozzarella *(cont.)*							
part skim *(Polly-O)*,							
¼ cup	90	8.0	<1.0	6.0	20	210	0
sliced *(Sargento)*,							
1.6-oz. slice . . .	130	11.0	2.0	9.0	25	230	0
sliced *(Sargento Preferred Light)*,							
1.6 oz.	90	11.0	0	5.0	15	230	0
mozzarella, shredded, ¼ cup:							
(Sargento)	80	7.0	1.0	6.0	15	150	0
(Sargento Preferred Light)	70	8.0	<1.0	3.0	10	140	0
whole milk *(Kraft)*	90	6.0	<1.0	7.0	25	210	0
whole milk *(Polly-O)*	90	6.0	<1.0	7.0	20	200	0
part skim *(Kraft)* . .	90	8.0	<1.0	6.0	20	210	0
part skim *(Kraft ⅓ Less Fat)* . . .	80	9.0	<1.0	5.0	15	210	0
part skim *(Polly-O)*	80	8.0	1.0	5.0	15	200	0
part skim, fine *(Kraft)*	70	6.0	<1.0	4.5	15	160	0
fat free *(Kraft Healthy Favorites)*	50	9.0	2.0	0	<5	280	0
fat free *(Polly-O)*	45	10.0	1.0	0	<5	270	<1.0
light *(Polly-O Lite)*	60	8.0	1.0	3.0	15	220	0
Muenster:							
(Alpine Lace Reduced Sodium)	100	7.0	1.0	9.0	25	85	0
(Boar's Head) . . .	100	6.0	0	8.0	25	180	0
(Boar's Head Low Sodium)	100	6.0	0	8.0	20	75	0
(Dorman), 1-oz. slice	100	6.0	0	8.0	25	190	0
(Dorman), 1.5-oz. slice	160	10.0	1.0	13.0	40	290	0
(Dorman Reduced Fat)*, 1.5 oz. . . .	120	12.0	0	8.0	25	250	0
(Dorman Reduced Sodium)*, 1.5 oz.	160	10.0	0	13.0	40	180	0

Food and Measure	cal.	prot. (gms)	carbo. (gms)	fat (gms)	chol. (mgs)	sod. (mgs)	fiber (gms)
(*Heluva* Good) . . .	100	6.0	0	8.0	25	180	0
(*Kraft*)	110	6.0	0	9.0	30	190	0
(*Sargento* Sliced)	100	6.0	<1.0	9.0	25	200	0
Neufchâtel (*Philadel-*							
phia Brand)	70	3.0	<1.0	6.0	20	120	0
Parmesan, grated:							
1 tbsp.	23	2.1	.2	1.5	4	93	0
(*Classica*), 1 tbsp.	20	2.0	0	1.0	0	35	0
(*Kraft*), 2 tsp. . . .	20	2.0	0	1.5	5	85	0
(*Kraft* Italian Blend),							
2 tsp.	25	3.0	0	1.5	<5	95	0
(*Polly-O*), 2 tsp. . .	25	2.0	0	1.5	5	80	0
(*Sargento*), 1 tbsp.	25	2.0	0	1.5	<5	75	0
Parmesan, shredded:							
(*Classica*), 1 tbsp.	20	2.0	0	1.0	0	35	0
(*Kraft*), 2 tsp. . . .	20	2.0	0	1.5	<5	75	0
(*Sargento*), ¼ cup	110	9.0	1.0	7.0	25	300	0
Parmesan-Romano:							
grated (*Sargento*),							
1 tbsp.	25	2.0	0	1.5	<5	70	0
shredded							
(*Sargento*), ¼ cup	110	9.0	1.0	7.0	25	340	0
pimiento, processed							
(*Kraft* Deluxe) . . .	100	6.0	<1.0	8.0	25	430	0
pizza, shredded,							
¼ cup:							
(*Sargento*)	90	7.0	0	6.0	20	210	0
(*Sargento* Pizza							
Double Cheese)	90	7.0	1.0	6.0	20	150	0
cheddar, mild, and							
mozzarella (*Kraft*)	90	6.0	<1.0	7.0	20	170	0
four cheese (*Kraft*)	90	7.0	<1.0	7.0	20	230	0
mozzarella and							
cheddar (*Kraft*)	100	6.0	<1.0	8.0	25	190	0
mozzarella and							
smoke provolone							
(*Kraft*)	90	6.0	<1.0	7.0	20	210	0
Port du Salut	100	6.7	.2	8.0	35	151	0

Food and Measure	cal.	prot. (gms)	carbo. (gms)	fat (gms)	chol. (mgs)	sod. (mgs)	fiber (gms)
Cheese *(cont.)*							
provolone:							
(*Alpine Lace* Reduced Fat)	70	9.0	1.0	5.0	15	120	0
(*Boar's Head*) . . .	100	7.0	1.0	8.0	20	240	0
(*Dorman*)	100	7.0	1.0	8.0	20	240	0
(*Dorman* Reduced Fat), 1.5 oz. . . .	120	13.0	1.0	7.0	30	300	0
(*Sargento* Sliced)	100	7.0	0	8.0	25	190	0
smoke flavor (*Kraft*)	100	7.0	<1.0	7.0	25	240	0
ricotta, ¼ cup, except as noted:							
(*Breakstone's*) . . .	110	7.0	3.0	8.0	25	90	0
(*Polly-O* Light) . . .	70	8.0	3.0	3.0	10	80	0
(*Sargento* Light) . .	60	5.0	3.0	2.5	15	55	0
(*Sargento* Old Fashioned)	90	7.0	3.0	6.0	25	75	0
whole milk	108	7.0	1.9	8.0	32	52	0
whole milk (*Polly-O*)	110	7.0	2.0	8.0	25	60	0
part skim (*Polly-O*)	90	8.0	2.0	6.0	20	65	0
part skim (*Sargento*)	80	7.0	2.0	5.0	20	75	0
fat free (*Polly-O*)	50	10.0	2.0	0	<5	80	0
Romano, grated:							
(*Kraft*), 2 tsp. . . .	25	2.0	0	1.5	5	90	0
dry (*Classica* Pecorino), 1 tbsp.	20	1.0	0	1.5	0	125	0
fresh (*Classica* Pecorino), 1 tbsp.	20	1.0	0	1.5	0	110	0
Romano, shredded (*Classica* Pecorino), 1 tbsp.	20	1.0	0	2.0	0	100	0
Romano-Parmesan, grated (*Polly-O*), 2 tsp.	25	2.0	0	1.5	5	80	0
Roquefort	105	6.1	.6	8.7	26	513	0
string:							
(*Polly-O*)	80	7.0	<1.0	6.0	20	220	0
(*Polly-O* Light Mozzarella)	60	7.0	<1.0	2.5	10	230	0

Food and Measure	cal.	prot. (gms)	carbo. (gms)	fat (gms)	chol. (mgs)	sod. (mgs)	fiber (gms)
string, snack, 1 pc.:							
(*Polly-O*), ¾ oz. . . .	60	6.0	<1.0	4.0	15	160	0
(*Handi-Snacks/Kraft*)	80	7.0	<1.0	6.0	20	240	0
(*MooTown Snack-*							
ers), .8 oz. . . .	70	6.0	<1.0	5.0	15	170	0
light (*MooTown*							
Snackers), .8 oz.	60	7.0	<1.0	3.0	10	200	0
Swiss:							
(*Alpine Lace* Re-							
duced Fat)	90	8.0	1.0	6.0	20	35	0
(*Boar's Head* Do-							
mestic)	100	8.0	<1.0	8.0	25	60	0
(*Boar's Head* Gold							
Label Imported)	110	8.0	<1.0	8.0	20	65	0
(*Boar's Head* No							
Salt)	110	8.0	<1.0	8.0	25	10	0
(*Borden*)	100	7.0	1.0	8.0	25	400	0
(*Dorman*), 1.2-oz.							
slice	130	10.0	1.0	9.0	30	70	0
(*Dorman* Low So-							
dium), 1.2-oz.							
slice	130	10.0	0	10.0	30	10	0
(*Dorman* Reduced							
Fat), 1.2-oz. slice	100	11.0	1.0	5.0	15	55	0
(*Dorman* Sandwich)	100	8.0	1.0	8.0	25	60	0
(*Dorman* Very Low							
Sodium)	110	8.0	0	8.0	25	10	0
(*Kraft*)	110	8.0	0	9.0	30	50	0
(*Sargento* Sliced),							
¾-oz. slice . . .	80	6.0	0	6.0	20	30	0
(*Sargento Preferred*							
Light Sliced) . . .	80	9.0	<1.0	4.0	15	50	0
(*Sargento Wafer*							
Thin Sliced),							
2 slices	110	8.0	0	9.0	25	40	0
baby (*Boar's Head*)	110	7.0	<1.0	9.0	25	135	0
baby (*Kraft Cracker*							
Barrel)	110	7.0	0	9.0	25	110	0

Food and Measure	cal.	prot. (gms)	carbo. (gms)	fat (gms)	chol. (mgs)	sod. (mgs)	fiber (gms)
Cheese, Swiss *(cont.)*							
processed (*Kraft* Deluxe), ¾-oz. slice	70	5.0	0	5.0	20	310	0
processed (*Kraft* Deluxe), 1-oz. slice	90	7.0	<1.0	7.0	25	420	0
Swiss, shredded:							
(*Kraft*), ¼ cup . . .	110	8.0	<1.0	9.0	30	45	0
(*Sargento*), ¼ cup	110	8.0	0	8.0	30	40	0
taco, shredded, ¼ cup:							
(*Sargento*)	110	6.0	1.0	9.0	25	220	0
(*Sargento Preferred Light*)	70	8.0	<1.0	4.5	15	240	0
cheddar and Monterey Jack (*Kraft*)	100	8.0	<1.0	8.0	25	180	0
nacho and taco (*Sargento*)	110	6.0	1.0	9.0	25	240	0
(*Tal-Fino* Taleggio) . .	110	5.0	2.0	9.0	5	90	1.0
"Cheese," substitute and nondairy:							
(*Sandwich-Mate*), .7-oz. slice	60	3.0	1.0	5.0	0	270	0
(*Smart Beat*), ⅔ oz.	25	4.0	3.0	0	0	180	0
all varieties, 1 oz.:							
(*AlmondRella*) . : .	60	5.0	3.0	3.0	0	250	1.0
(*TofuRella*)	80	5.0	2.0	5.0	0	290	0
(*VeganRella*)	60	1.0	7.0	3.0	0	130	.5
(*Zero-FatRella*) . . .	40	7.0	3.0	0	0	250	0
American flavor:							
(*Borden*), 1 slice . .	60	3.0	1.0	5.0	0	260	0
(*Cheeztwo/Sandwich-Mate*), 1 slice	60	3.0	1.0	5.0	0	270	0
(*Golden Image*), ¾ oz.	70	5.0	1.0	5.0	5	270	0
(*Lunchwagon*), ⅔ oz.	60	3.0	<1.0	5.0	0	210	0

Food and Measure	cal.	prot. (gms)	carbo. (gms)	fat (gms)	chol. (mgs)	sod. (mgs)	fiber (gms)
(*Lunchwagon*),							
¾ oz.	70	4.0	1.0	5.0	0	230	0
(*Smart Beat* Fat							
Free), ⅔ oz. . . .	25	4.0	3.0	0	0	180	0
shredded (*Harvest*							
Moon), ¼ cup . .	120	6.0	3.0	9.0	0	500	0
cheddar flavor:							
(*Borden*)	100	4.0	2.0	8.0	0	280	0
(*Borden* Taco Mate)	100	5.0	3.0	8.0	<5	340	0
fortified (*Borden*)	100	5.0	2.0	8.0	<5	310	0
mellow (*Smart*							
Beat), ⅔ oz.	25	4.0	3.0	0	0	180	0
sharp (*Smart Beat*),							
⅔ oz.	25	4.0	3.0	0	0	230	0
shredded (*Harvest*							
Moon), ¼ cup . .	120	6.0	3.0	9.0	0	480	0
shredded							
(*Sargento*), ¼ cup	90	5.0	2.0	7.0	0	420	0
cream cheese, all varieties (*Tofutti Better Than Cream*							
Cheese), 1 oz. . . .	80	1.0	1.0	8.0	0	135	0
Jamaican Jack style							
(*HempRella*), 1 oz.	70	7.0	1.0	3.0	0	170	.2
Monterey Jack (*Borden*)	90	6.0	1.0	7.0	10	340	0
mozzarella, shredded:							
(*Borden*)	90	6.0	1.0	7.0	0	300	0
(*Harvest Moon*),							
¼ cup	110	8.0	1.0	8.0	0	430	0
(*Sargento*), ¼ cup	80	6.0	<1.0	6.0	0	320	0
imitation (*Borden*)	100	4.0	2.0	8.0	0	280	0
Swiss (*Borden*),							
1 slice	60	3.0	1.0	5.0	0	270	0
Cheese dip, 2 tbsp.:							
(*Chi-Chi's* Fiesta) . .	40	1.0	3.0	3.0	10	270	0
and bacon (*Nalley*)	110	1.0	3.0	11.0	10	240	0
blue (*Kraft* Premium)	45	1.0	2.0	4.0	10	200	0

Food and Measure	cal.	prot. (gms)	carbo. (gms)	fat (gms)	chol. (mgs)	sod. (mgs)	fiber (gms)
Cheese dip *(cont.)*							
cheddar:							
mild (*Frito-Lay*) . .	50	2.0	4.0	3.0	5	240	0
mild (*Old Dutch*)	30	<1.0	3.0	3.0	<5	170	0
and mustard							
(*Heluva* Good							
Pretzel)	80	2.0	2.0	6.0	20	230	0
chili (*Fritos*)	45	1.0	3.0	3.0	<5	310	0
hot (*Price's* Fiesta)	80	3.0	2.0	7.0	15	370	0
nacho:							
(*Kraft* Premium) . .	60	2.0	2.0	5.0	15	270	0
(*Knudsen* Premium)	60	2.0	3.0	4.0	15	200	0
(*Nalley*)	120	1.0	3.0	12.0	15	290	0
(*Old Dutch*)	35	<1.0	3.0	4.0	0	260	0
Parmesan garlic							
(*Marie's*)	140	2.0	2.0	14.0	10	140	<1.0
salsa:							
(*Heluva* Good							
Cheese 'N Salsa)	80	3.0	3.0	5.5	10	210	0
(*Old El Paso*) . . .	40	<1.0	3.0	3.0	<5	300	0
(*Tostitos* Con							
Queso)	40	1.0	5.0	2.0	<5	650	<1.0
(*Tostitos* Con Queso							
Low Fat)	40	1.0	5.0	1.5	<5	280	<1.0
Cheese food (see also							
"Cheese" and							
"Cheese spread"),							
1 oz., except as							
noted:							
American:							
(*Borden*), .7-oz.							
slice	70	3.0	2.0	5.0	15	260	0
(*Heluva* Good) . . .	70	4.0	2.0	5.0	15	390	0
(*Kraft* Singles),							
2/3-oz. slice . . .	60	4.0	2.0	4.5	15	260	0
(*Kraft* Singles),							
3/4-oz. slice . . .	70	4.0	2.0	5.0	15	290	0
(*Kraft* Singles),							
1.2-oz. slice . . .	110	6.0	3.0	8.0	30	460	0

Food and Measure	cal.	prot. (gms)	carbo. (gms)	fat (gms)	chol. (mgs)	sod. (mgs)	fiber (gms)
grated (*Kraft*),							
1 tbsp.	25	1.0	1.0	1.5	<5	35	0
sharp (*Borden*) . .	100	5.0	2.0	8.0	25	430	0
cheddar:							
sharp (*Cracker Bar-*							
rel), 2 tbsp. . . .	100	5.0	4.0	8.0	25	290	0
sharp (*Kaukauna*							
Premium Blend)	100	5.0	2.0	7.0	25	170	0
sharp (*Kaukauna*							
Lite 50)	70	5.0	5.0	3.0	15	190	0
sharp or extra sharp							
(*Kaukauna*) . . .	90	5.0	3.0	7.0	20	210	0
extra sharp (*Cracker*							
Barrel), 2 tbsp.	100	5.0	3.0	8.0	25	290	0
w/garlic (*Kraft*) . . .	90	5.0	2.0	7.0	20	370	0
w/jalapeños:							
(*Kraft*)	90	5.0	2.0	7.0	20	370	0
(*Kraft* Mexican Sin-							
gles), ¾-oz. slice	70	4.0	2.0	5.0	15	330	0
w/jalapeños, shred-							
ded:							
hot (*Velveeta* Mexi-							
can), ¼ cup . . .	130	8.0	3.0	9.0	30	540	0
mild (*Velveeta* Mexi-							
can), ¼ cup . . .	130	8.0	3.0	9.0	30	520	0
Monterey (*Kraft* Sin-							
gles), ¾-oz. slice	70	4.0	2.0	5.0	15	290	0
w/pimiento (*Kraft* Sin-							
gles), ⅔-oz. slice	60	4.0	1.0	4.5	15	260	0
w/pimiento (*Kraft* Sin-							
gles), ¾-oz. slice	70	4.0	2.0	5.0	15	290	0
port wine:							
(*Kaukauna*)	90	5.0	4.0	7.0	20	190	0
(*Kaukauna* Premium							
Blend)	100	5.0	2.0	7.0	25	150	0
(*Kaukauna Lite*) . .	70	5.0	5.0	3.0	15	190	0
(*Wispride* Cup),							
2 tbsp.	100	4.0	4.0	7.0	20	230	0

Food and Measure	cal.	prot. (gms)	carbo. (gms)	fat (gms)	chol. (mgs)	sod. (mgs)	fiber (gms)
Cheese food, port wine *(cont.)*							
(*Wispride* Light							
Cup), 2 tbsp. . . .	80	5.0	5.0	3.0	10	200	0
sharp (*Kraft* Singles),							
¾-oz. slice	70	4.0	<1.0	6.0	20	300	0
shredded (*Velveeta*),							
¼ cup	130	8.0	3.0	9.0	30	500	0
smoke flavor:							
(*Kaukauna* Smokey)	90	5.0	3.0	7.0	20	210	0
(*Kaukauna Lite 50*							
Smokey)	70	5.0	5.0	3.0	15	190	0
Swiss:							
(*Borden*), 1 slice . .	70	4.0	1.0	5.0	15	240	0
(*Kraft* Singles),							
¾-oz. slice . . .	70	4.0	1.0	5.0	15	320	0
almond (*Kaukauna*)	90	5.0	3.0	7.0	20	140	0
almond (*Kaukauna*							
Lite 50)	70	5.0	5.0	3.0	15	180	0
Cheese nut log,							
sharp (*Wispride*),							
2 tbsp.	100	4.0	4.0	8.0	20	190	0
Cheese pastry, see							
"Danish"							
Cheese product (see							
also "Cheese							
food"), ¾-oz. slice,							
except as noted:							
all varieties (*Borden*							
Fat Free), 1 slice . .	25	4.0	2.0	0	0	280	0
(*Cheez Whiz Light*),							
2 tbsp.	80	6.0	6.0	3.0	15	540	0
(*Kraft Free* Singles),							
⅔-oz. slice	30	4.0	3.0	0	<5	290	0
(*Kraft Free* Singles)	30	5.0	3.0	0	<5	320	0
(*Velveeta Light*), 1 oz.	60	6.0	3.0	3.0	10	420	0
all varieties (*Lite-*							
Line), 7-oz. slice . .	30	4.0	1.0	1.0	<5	260	0
American flavor:							
(*Alpine Lace*), 1 oz.	80	6.0	2.0	6.0	20	200	0

Food and Measure	cal.	prot. (gms)	carbo. (gms)	fat (gms)	chol. (mgs)	sod. (mgs)	fiber (gms)
(*Alpine Lace* Nonfat), 1 oz. . .	45	8.0	2.0	0	<5	280	0
(*Alpine Lace* Nonfat)	30	5.0	1.0	0	<5	310	0
(*Borden* Fat Free)	45	5.0	1.0	2.5	10	300	0
(*Borden* Light) . . .	45	5.0	1.0	2.5	10	300	0
(*Borden* Lowfat), 1 slice	30	4.0	1.0	1.0	<5	260	0
(*Harvest Moon*), ⅔ oz.	50	4.0	1.0	3.0	10	280	0
(*Kraft* Deluxe 25% Less Fat)	70	4.0	1.0	5.0	15	350	0
(*Kraft* Singles Less Fat)	50	5.0	2.0	3.0	10	330	0
(*Light n' Lively* 50% Less Fat)	50	5.0	2.0	2.5	10	280	0
(*Light n' Lively* White 50% Less Fat)	50	5.0	2.0	2.5	10	300	0
cheddar flavor:							
(*Alpine Lace* Nonfat), 1 oz. . .	45	8.0	2.0	0	<5	280	0
all varieties (*Spreadery*), 2 tbsp. . . .	80	5.0	3.0	4.5	15	290	0
sharp (*Kraft* Singles ⅓ Less Fat) . . .	50	5.0	2.0	3.0	10	300	0
sharp (*Kraft Free* Singles)	30	5.0	3.0	0	<5	290	0
mozzarella (*Alpine Lace* Nonfat), 1 oz.	45	8.0	2.0	0	<5	280	0
Neufchâtel, 2 tbsp.:							
garlic herb (*Spreadery*) . . .	80	3.0	1.0	7.0	20	180	0
ranch (*Spreadery*)	80	3.0	1.0	7.0	20	210	0
vegetable (*Spreadery*) . . .	70	3.0	2.0	6.0	20	230	0
pimiento (*Spreadery*), 2 tbsp.	100	4.0	3.0	8.0	20	320	0

Food and Measure	cal.	prot. (gms)	carbo. (gms)	fat (gms)	chol. (mgs)	sod. (mgs)	fiber (gms)
Cheese product *(cont.)*							
Swiss flavor:							
(*Kraft* Singles Less							
Fat)	50	5.0	2.0	2.5	10	270	0
(*Kraft Free* Singles)	30	5.0	3.0	0	<5	290	0
Cheese sandwich,							
frozen, grilled							
(*Swanson Fun*							
Feast) 1 pkg. . . .	460	31.0	56.0	20.0	30	70	5.0
Cheese sauce,							
2 tbsp., except as							
noted:							
all varieties (*Kaukauna*							
Micro Melt)	80	4.0	2.0	6.0	15	380	0
(*Cheez Whiz* Squeez-							
able)	100	2.0	4.0	8.0	15	470	0
(*Cheez Whiz*							
Zap-A-Pack)	90	3.0	3.0	8.0	20	580	0
(*Franco-American*),							
¼ cup	40	3.0	4.0	2.0	5	390	0
nacho (*Kaukauna*) . .	80	3.0	4.0	6.0	8	330	0
salsa (*Cheez Whiz*							
Zap-A-Pack)	90	3.0	3.0	8.0	25	580	0
Cheese sauce mix:							
(*Durkee*), ¼ pkg. . .	25	1.0	4.0	1.5	2	260	0
(*French's*), ¼ pkg. . .	25	.5	4.0	.5	0	250	0
four (*Knorr*), ⅓ pkg.	70	3.0	4.0	4.0	10	700	0
nacho (*Durkee*),							
⅕ pkg.	25	1.0	2.0	2.0	0	180	0
Cheese spread (see							
also "Cheese" and							
"Cheese product"),							
2 tbsp., except as							
noted:							
(*Cheez Whiz*)	90	5.0	2.0	7.0	20	560	0
(*Squeez-A-Snak*) . . .	90	5.0	<1.0	8.0	25	440	0
(*Velveeta*), 1 oz. . . .	80	5.0	3.0	6.0	20	420	0
(*Velveeta Italiana*),							
1 oz.	80	5.0	2.0	6.0	20	430	0

Food and Measure	cal.	prot. (gms)	carbo. (gms)	fat (gms)	chol. (mgs)	sod. (mgs)	fiber (gms)
American:							
(*Borden*), 1 oz. . .	80	4.0	3.0	6.0	20	360	0
(*Easy Cheese*) . . .	100	6.0	2.0	7.0	25	400	0
(*Harvest Moon*),							
⅔ oz.	60	3.0	2.0	4.0	15	270	0
(*Harvest Moon*),							
¾ oz.	60	3.0	2.0	4.5	15	300	0
(*The Big!*), 1 slice	80	4.0	2.0	6.0	20	310	0
w/bacon (*Kraft*) . . .	90	5.0	<1.0	8.0	25	570	0
blue cheese (*Kraft*							
Roka)	80	3.0	2.0	7.0	20	340	0
cheddar:							
sharp (*Heluva* Good)	90	5.0	3.0	7.0	20	210	0
w/bacon or horse-							
radish (*Heluva*							
Good)	90	5.0	3.0	7.0	20	210	0
regular or bacon							
(*Easy Cheese*) . .	100	5.0	3.0	7.0	25	410	0
sharp (*Easy Cheese*)	100	5.0	3.0	7.0	25	440	0
w/jalapeños:							
(*Cheez Whiz*) . . .	90	5.0	2.0	8.0	25	530	0
(*Kraft*), 1 oz.	80	5.0	2.0	6.0	20	470	0
hot (*Velveeta* Mexi-							
can), 1 oz.	80	5.0	2.0	6.0	20	520	0
mild (*Velveeta* Mexi-							
can), 1 oz.	80	5.0	3.0	6.0	20	440	0
limburger (*Mohawk*							
Valley)	80	4.0	0	7.0	20	500	0
nacho:							
(*Easy Cheese*) . . .	100	5.0	3.0	7.0	25	390	0
(*The Big!*), 1 slice	80	4.0	2.0	6.0	20	340	0
olive and pimiento							
(*Kraft*)	70	2.0	3.0	6.0	20	220	0
Neufchâtel, 1 oz.:							
garden vegetable							
(*Kaukauna*) . . .	80	3.0	1.0	7.0	25	200	0
garlic and herb or							
ranch (*Kaukauna*)	80	3.0	1.0	7.0	25	160	0

Food and Measure	cal.	prot. (gms)	carbo. (gms)	fat (gms)	chol. (mgs)	sod. (mgs)	fiber (gms)
Cheese spread *(cont.)*							
pimiento:							
(*Kraft*)	80	2.0	3.0	6.0	20	170	0
(*Price's*)	80	3.0	2.0	7.0	15	320	0
(*Price's* Light) . . .	60	4.0	3.0	3.5	10	260	0
pineapple (*Kraft*) . . .	70	2.0	4.0	5.0	15	120	0
port wine (*Heluva*							
Good)	90	5.0	3.0	7.0	20	210	0
salsa:							
hot (*Cheez Whiz*)	90	5.0	2.0	7.0	25	540	0
mild (*Cheez Whiz*)	90	5.0	2.0	7.0	25	530	0
sharp (*Old English*)	90	5.0	<1.0	8.0	25	520	0
slices:							
(*Velveeta*), ¾ oz.	60	4.0	2.0	4.5	15	300	0
(*Velveeta*), ⅘ oz.	70	4.0	2.0	4.5	15	310	0
(*Velveeta*), 1.2 oz.	100	6.0	3.0	7.0	25	480	0
Cheese stick, w/corn-							
meal coating (*Goya*							
Surullitos), 7 pcs.	300	6.0	48.0	9.0	10	530	5.0
Cheeseburger, see							
"Beef sandwich"							
Cherimoya (see also							
"Custard apple"):							
1 medium, 1.9 lb. . . .	515	7.1	131.3	2.2	0	n.a.	13.1
(*Frieda's*), 3.5 oz. . .	94	1.3	24.0	.4	0	n.a.	n.a.
Cherry, ½ cup, except							
as noted:							
fresh, sour, red:							
w/pits	26	.5	6.3	.2	0	2	.6
pitted	39	.8	9.4	.2	0	3	.9
fresh, sweet:							
w/pits	52	.9	12.0	.7	0	1	1.7
10 medium, 2.6 oz.	49	.8	11.3	.7	0	<1	1.6
canned, sour, pitted:							
red, water (*Lucky*							
Leaf/Musselman's)	60	0	13.0	0	0	10	1.0
heavy syrup	116	.9	29.8	.1	0	9	1.0
canned, sweet, pitted:							
heavy syrup	107	.8	27.4	.2	0	3	.9

Food and Measure	cal.	prot. (gms)	carbo. (gms)	fat (gms)	chol. (mgs)	sod. (mgs)	fiber (gms)
dark (*Del Monte*)	100	<1.0	24.0	0	0	10	<1.0
dark (*S&W*)	140	1.0	34.0	0	0	10	1.0
light (*S&W* Royal Anne)	140	1.0	33.0	0	0	15	1.0
dried, pitted:							
(*Sonoma*), ¼ cup	140	1.0	34.0	0	0	0	2.0
bing (*Frieda's*), 1 oz.	79	1.4	19.8	.3	0	2	n.a.
frozen, unsweetened:							
dark, sweet (*Big Valley*), ¾ cup . .	90	1.0	20.0	0	0	0	3.0
tart, red (*Stilwell*), 1 cup	60	2.0	14.0	0	0	25	2.0
frozen, sweetened, 4 oz.	101	1.3	25.4	.1	0	1	1.1
Cherry, candied, green or red:							
(*Paradise/White Swan*), .2-oz. pc.	15	0	4.0	0	0	0	0
(*S&W* Glace), 5 pcs.	80	0	20.0	0	0	20	0
and pineapple mix (*Paradise/White Swan*), 2 tbsp., 1.3 oz.	110	0	29.0	0	0	25	1.0
Cherry, maraschino:							
w/liquid, 1 oz.	33	.1	8.3	.1	0	n.a.	<1.0
green or red, 1 pc.:							
(*Haddon House*) . .	10	0	2.0	0	0	0	0
(*S&W*)	10	0	3.0	0	0	0	0
Cherry drink, 8 fl. oz., except as noted:							
(*After the Fall* Very Cherry)	100	0	26.0	0	0	20	0
(*Farmer's Market*) . .	120	0	31.0	0	0	0	0
(*Hi-C*)	130	0	34.0	0	0	30	0
blend (*Tree Top* Not Plain Cherry) . . .	120	0	30.0	0	0	25	0
wild (*Capri Sun*), 6.75 fl. oz.	110	0	30.0	0	0	20	0

Food and Measure	cal.	prot. (gms)	carbo. (gms)	fat (gms)	chol. (mgs)	sod. (mgs)	fiber (gms)
Cherry drink mix*, 8 fl. oz.:							
(*Hi-C*)	100	0	26.0	0	0	35	0
(*Kool-Aid*)	100	0	25.0	0	0	10	0
Cherry glace, see "Cherry, candied"							
Cherry juice, 8 fl. oz.:							
(*Juicy Juice*)	130	1.0	32.0	0	0	10	0
black (*Heinke's*) . . .	180	2.0	43.0	0	0	40	0
black (*R.W. Knudsen*)	180	2.0	43.0	0	0	40	0
Cherry juice blends, 8 fl. oz.:							
(*Apple & Eve Nothin' But Juice*)	120	1.0	29.0	0	0	30	0
(*Dole* Mountain) . . .	120	0	30.0	0	0	30	0
(*Veryfine* Juice-Ups)	150	0	33.0	0	0	15	0
black (*R.W. Knudsen* Concentrate)	130	0	23.0	0	0	15	0
cider:							
(*Heinke's*)	115	0	28.0	0	0	5	0
(*R.W. Knudsen*) . .	130	0	33.0	0	0	35	0
Cherry nectar (*Santa Cruz*), 8 fl. oz. . . .	110	0	26.0	0	0	20	0
Cherry pastry, 1 pc.:							
dumpling, frozen (*Pepperidge Farm*)	280	3.0	47.0	9.0	0	280	2.0
pocket (*Tastykake*) . .	370	3.0	45.0	20.0	55	190	2.0
Cherry syrup, 2 tbsp.:							
black (*Fox's*)	80	0	21.0	0	0	10	0
black (*Fox's No Cal*)	0	0	0	0	0	35	0
Cherries jubilee (*Lucky Leaf/Musselman's*), ¼ cup	80	0	20.0	0	0	10	1.0
Chervil, dried:							
1 tsp.	1	.1	.3	<.1	0	<1	.1
(*McCormick*), ¼ tsp.	<1	.1	.1	0	0	<1	0
Chestnut, Chinese, shelled, 1 oz.:							
dried	103	1.9	22.7	.5	0	2	<1.0

Food and Measure	cal.	prot. (gms)	carbo. (gms)	fat (gms)	chol. (mgs)	sod. (mgs)	fiber (gms)
boiled or steamed . .	44	.8	9.6	.2	0	1	<1.0
roasted	68	1.3	14.9	.3	0	1	<1.0
Chestnut, European:							
raw:							
in shell, 1 lb. . . .	714	8.1	152.8	7.6	0	9	27.2
shelled, w/peel,							
1 cup, 13 kernels	308	3.5	66.0	3.3	0	4	11.7
dried, peeled, 1 oz.	105	1.4	22.3	1.1	0	11	<2.0
boiled, 1 oz.	37	.8	7.9	.4	0	8	<1.0
roasted, peeled:							
1 oz.	70	.9	15.0	.6	0	1	3.3
1 cup, 17 kernels	350	4.3	75.7	3.2	0	3	16.7
Chestnut, Japanese:							
dried, 1 oz.	102	1.5	23.1	.4	0	10	n.a.
boiled or steamed,							
1 oz.	16	.2	3.6	.1	0	1	<1.0
roasted, 1 oz.	57	.8	12.8	.2	0	n.a.	<1.0
Chicken, fresh (see							
also "Chicken, re-							
frigerated or fro-							
zen"), 4 oz., except							
as noted:							
broiler-fryer, roasted:							
w/skin, ½ chicken,							
10½ oz. (15.8 oz.							
w/bone)	715	81.6	0	40.7	263	244	0
w/skin	271	31.0	0	15.4	100	93	0
meat only	215	32.8	0	8.4	101	98	0
meat only, chopped							
or diced, 1 cup	266	40.5	0	10.4	125	120	0
skin only, 1 oz. . .	129	5.8	0	11.5	24	18	0
dark meat only . .	232	31.0	0	11.0	105	105	0
light meat only . .	196	35.1	0	5.1	96	87	0
breast, w/skin,							
½ breast, 3½ oz.							
(8½ oz. w/bone)	193	29.2	0	7.6	83	69	0
drumstick, w/skin,							
1.8 oz. (2.9 oz.							
w/bone)	112	14.1	0	5.8	48	47	0

Food and Measure	cal.	prot. (gms)	carbo. (gms)	fat (gms)	chol. (mgs)	sod. (mgs)	fiber (gms)
Chicken, broiler-fryer, roasted *(cont.)*							
leg, w/skin (5.7 oz. w/bone)	265	29.6	0	15.4	105	99	0
thigh, w/skin, 2.2 oz. (2.9 oz. w/bone)	153	15.5	0	9.6	58	52	0
wing, w/skin, 1.2 oz. (2.3 oz. w/bone)	99	9.1	0	6.6	29	28	0
capon, roasted, w/skin:							
½ capon, 1.4 lbs. (2 lbs. w/bone)	1457	184.5	0	74.2	549	313	0
w/skin	260	32.8	0	13.2	98	56	0
Cornish hen, see "Cornish hen"							
ground, see "Chicken, ground"							
roaster, roasted:							
w/skin, ½ chicken, 1 lb. (1½ lbs. w/bone)	1071	115.0	0	64.3	365	349	0
meat w/skin	253	27.2	0	15.2	86	83	0
stewing, stewed:							
w/skin, ½ chicken, 9.2 oz. (13½ oz. w/bone)	744	70.2	0	49.2	205	190	0
meat w/skin	323	30.5	0	21.4	90	83	0
meat only	269	34.5	0	13.5	94	88	0
meat only, chopped or diced, 1 cup	332	42.6	0	16.6	117	109	0
Chicken, canned, chunk, 2 oz., ¼ cup:							
(*Hormel*)	70	12.0	0	3.0	35	200	0
(*Swanson*)	90	5.0	2.0	3.0	35	200	0
breast (*Hormel*) . . .	60	12.0	0	1.5	25	200	0
breast (*Hormel* No Salt)	60	12.0	0	1.5	30	20	0

Food and Measure	cal.	prot. (gms)	carbo. (gms)	fat (gms)	chol. (mgs)	sod. (mgs)	fiber (gms)
broth (*Swanson* Mixin')	110	11.0	1.0	7.0	45	190	0
water (*Swanson* Premium)	90	5.0	1.0	3.0	55	220	0
white (*Swanson*) . . .	80	3.0	1.0	2.0	40	240	0
white, in water (*Swanson* Premium)	80	3.0	1.0	2.0	35	220	0
Chicken, ground:							
raw, 4 oz.:							
(*Perdue*)	180	17.0	0	12.0	145	65	0
(*Perdue* Burger) . .	180	18.0	0	11.0	120	45	0
cooked, 3 oz.:							
(*Perdue*)	170	17.0	0	12.0	145	55	0
(*Perdue* Burger) . .	170	17.0	0	11.0	120	35	0
Chicken, refrigerated or frozen:							
whole, cooked, 3 oz.:							
dark meat (*Perdue*)	210	17.0	0	15.0	110	55	0
dark meat (*Perdue* Oven Stuffer) . .	200	19.0	0	14.0	105	50	0
white meat (*Perdue*)	160	20.0	0	9.0	85	40	0
white meat (*Perdue* Oven Stuffer) . .	160	22.0	0	8.0	80	45	0
barbecued (*Empire* Kosher), 5 oz. edible	280	31.0	1.0	17.0	110	460	0
breast, raw, 4 oz.:							
halves (*Tyson*) . . .	190	21.0	1.0	12.0	80	40	0
halves, skinless (*Tyson*)	130	25.0	0	3.0	75	70	0
quarters (*Tyson*) . .	210	21.0	1.0	14.0	90	45	0
breast, raw, boneless, 4 oz., except as noted:							
(*Perdue*)	130	25.0	0	2.5	80	35	0
(*Perdue* Family Pack)	130	26.0	0	2.5	80	35	0
(*Perdue Oven Stuffer*)	130	25.0	0	2.0	80	50	0

Food and Measure	cal.	prot. (gms)	carbo. (gms)	fat (gms)	chol. (mgs)	sod. (mgs)	fiber (gms)
Chicken, refrigerated or frozen, breast, raw, boneless *(cont.)*							
tenderloins (*Perdue*)	110	25.0	0	1.0	65	15	0
tenderloins (*Tyson*)	110	26.0	0	.5	55	40	0
thin sliced (*Perdue*), 3 oz.	80	18.0	0	1.0	55	35	0
breast, raw, seasoned, boneless, 4 oz.:							
barbecue (*Perdue*)	130	24.0	8.0	1.0	70	600	0
lemon pepper (*Perdue*)	110	23.0	2.0	1.0	60	700	0
Italian (*Perdue*) . .	110	22.0	4.0	1.0	60	740	0
Oriental (*Perdue*)	120	23.0	5.0	1.0	60	720	0
breast, cooked, 3 oz., except as noted:							
whole (*Perdue*) . .	160	22.0	0	8.0	80	35	0
whole (*Perdue Oven Stuffer*)	150	22.0	0	7.0	75	35	0
boneless (*Perdue*)	120	25.0	0	2.0	70	10	0
boneless (*Perdue Oven Stuffer*) . .	120	24.0	0	2.0	70	25	0
quartered (*Perdue*)	180	21.0	0	10.0	90	35	0
roundelet (*Tyson*), 2.6-oz. pc.	170	10.0	10.0	10.0	5	410	1.0
tenderloins (*Perdue*)	100	23.0	0	1.0	55	25	0
thin sliced (*Perdue*), 2 oz.	80	17.0	0	1.0	50	10	0
breast, cooked, seasoned, boneless, 3 oz.:							
barbecue (*Perdue*)	110	22.0	5.0	.5	60	420	0
lemon pepper (*Perdue*)	90	19.0	2.0	.5	55	520	0
Italian (*Perdue*) . .	100	20.0	2.0	.5	55	520	0
Oriental (*Perdue*)	100	20.0	3.0	1.0	55	550	0
breast, fried, battered and breaded (*Empire* Kosher), 3 oz. edible	170	21.0	3.0	8.0	45	440	<1.0

Food and Measure	cal.	prot. (gms)	carbo. (gms)	fat (gms)	chol. (mgs)	sod. (mgs)	fiber (gms)
breast, roasted:							
(*Perdue*), 6.7-oz.							
half	370	48.0	0	20.0	175	80	0
(*Tyson*), ½ breast	250	34.0	0	13.0	110	670	0
boneless (*Perdue*),							
3.6-oz. half . . .	140	30.0	0	2.5	85	15	0
boneless (*Perdue Fit*							
'*n Easy*), 3.6-oz.							
half	150	30.0	0	3.0	85	35	0
skinless (*Perdue*),							
5.9-oz. half . . .	250	46.0	0	8.0	140	55	0
breast, seasoned,							
4 oz.:							
Cajun (*Chicken By*							
George)	120	20.0	2.0	4.0	55	650	0
Caribbean grill							
(*Chicken By*							
George)	150	21.0	8.0	4.0	55	550	0
garlic and herb							
(*Chicken By*							
George)	120	21.0	3.0	2.5	60	600	0
Italian bleu cheese							
(*Chicken By*							
George)	130	20.0	2.0	5.0	60	790	0
lemon herb (*Chicken*							
By George) . . .	120	19.0	3.0	3.0	50	800	0
lemon oregano							
(*Chicken By*							
George)	130	20.0	3.0	4.0	50	600	0
mesquite barbecue							
(*Chicken By*							
George)	120	20.0	5.0	2.0	50	800	0
mustard dill							
(*Chicken By*							
George)	140	20.0	2.0	5.0	65	650	0˙
roasted (*Chicken By*							
George)	110	20.0	1.0	3.0	55	500	0
teriyaki (*Chicken By*							
George)	130	20.0	6.0	3.0	50	650	0

Food and Measure	cal.	prot. (gms)	carbo. (gms)	fat (gms)	chol. (mgs)	sod. (mgs)	fiber (gms)
Chicken, refrigerated or frozen, breast, seasoned *(cont.)*							
tomato herb w/basil (*Chicken By George*)	140	20.0	5.0	5.0	60	630	0
cutlet, battered or breaded (*Empire* Kosher), 3.3-oz. pc.	200	18.0	11.0	9.0	25	320	2.0
diced (*Tyson*), 9 oz.	130	26.0	0	3.0	80	40	0
drumstick and thigh, fried (*Empire* Kosher), 3 oz. edible	240	16.0	7.0	16.0	80	260	2.0
drumstick, roasted:							
(*Perdue*), 2.2-oz. pc.	110	14.0	0	6.0	85	50	0
(*Perdue Oven Stuffer*), 3.6-oz. pc.	190	25.0	0	11.0	135	80	0
(*Tyson*), 3 pcs. . .	330	40.0	1.0	18.0	225	870	0
skinless (*Perdue* Pick), 2 pcs., 3.5 oz.	150	25.0	0	6.0	135	85	0
ground, see "Chicken, ground"							
leg, whole, roasted:							
(*Perdue*), 5.5 oz.	370	35.0	0	26.0	215	105	0
(*Perdue* Jumbo Family/Value), 5.5 oz.	360	33.0	0	25.0	205	110	0
leg, quarters:							
raw (*Tyson*), 4 oz.	230	19.0	1.0	17.0	115	70	0
cooked (*Perdue*), 3 oz.	210	18.0	0	16.0	115	55	0
nuggets (*Empire* Kosher), 5 pcs., 3 oz.	180	13.0	12.0	9.0	15	370	1.0
sticks (*Empire* Kosher Stix), 4 pcs., 3.1 oz.	180	18.0	6.0	9.0	25	420	2.0
thigh, raw:							
(*Tyson*), 4 oz. . . .	250	17.0	0	20.0	100	80	0
boneless, skinless (*Tyson*), 4 oz. . .	160	19.0	0	10.0	90	75	0

Food and Measure	cal.	prot. (gms)	carbo. (gms)	fat (gms)	chol. (mgs)	sod. (mgs)	fiber (gms)
thigh, roasted:							
(*Perdue*), 3.2-oz. pc.	240	19.0	0	18.0	125	60	0
boneless (*Perdue*),							
2 thighs, 3.6 oz.	200	26.0	0	11.0	130	60	0
boneless (*Perdue Fit*							
'n Easy), 2 pcs.	190	26.0	0	10.0	140	50	0
boneless (*Perdue*							
Oven Stuffer),							
3.3 oz.	170	25.0	0	8.0	125	40	0
skinless (*Perdue*),							
2.7 oz.	160	18.0	0	9.0	100	55	0
skinless (*Tyson*),							
3 oz.	160	18.0	0	10.0	105	470	0
wing, raw, whole (*Tyson*), 4 oz.	250	18.0	1.0	20.0	125	60	0
wing, roasted:							
(*Perdue*), 2 pcs. . .	210	20.0	0	15.0	125	75	0
(*Perdue* Wingettes),							
3 pcs.	200	19.0	0	14.0	120	65	0
(*Perdue Oven Stuffer*							
Drummettes),							
2 pcs.	170	17.0	0	11.0	90	45	0
(*Perdue Oven Stuffer*							
Wingettes), 3 pcs.	220	23.0	0	14.0	120	70	0
"Chicken," vegetarian:							
canned:							
diced (*Worthington*							
Chik), ¼ cup . .	60	5.0	1.0	3.5	0	240	1.0
fried (*Loma Linda*							
Chik'n), 2 pcs. . .	390	21.0	6.0	31.0	5	810	3.0
fried (*Worthington*							
FriChik), 2 pcs.	120	10.0	1.0	8.0	0	430	1.0
sliced (*Worthington*							
Chik), 3 slices . .	90	9.0	1.0	6.0	0	390	1.0
frozen:							
(*Worthington Chik-Stiks*), 1 pc.	110	9.0	3.0	7.0	0	360	2.0

Food and Measure	cal.	prot. (gms)	carbo. (gms)	fat (gms)	chol. (mgs)	sod. (mgs)	fiber (gms)
"Chicken," vegetarian, frozen *(cont.)*							
diced (*Worthington* Meatless), ¼ cup	80	9.0	1.0	4.5	0	360	<1.0
fried (*Loma Linda Chik'n*), 1 pc. . . .	180	11.0	1.0	15.0	<5	500	<1.0
nuggets (*Worthington Chik-Nuggets*), 5 pcs. . . .	240	12.0	13.0	16.0	0	710	5.0
patties (*Morningstar Farms* Chik), 1 patty	170	7.0	13.0	10.0	0	570	2.0
patties (*Worthington Crispy Chik*), 1 patty	170	8.0	15.0	9.0	0	600	4.0
roll (*Worthington*), ⅜" slice	80	9.0	1.0	4.5	0	360	<1.0
roll (*Worthington Chic-Ketts* 1 lb.), 2 slices, ⅜" . . .	120	13.0	2.0	7.0	0	390	2.0
roll (*Worthington Chic-Ketts* 56 oz.), ½" slice	120	13.0	2.0	7.0	0	390	2.0
sliced (*Worthington*), 2 slices . .	80	9.0	1.0	4.5	0	370	<1.0
mix (*Loma Linda* Supreme), ⅓ cup . .	90	15.0	6.0	1.0	0	720	4.0
Chicken dinner, frozen, 1 pkg.:							
barbecue, mesquite:							
(*The Budget Gourmet* Light & Healthy)	280	19.0	37.0	6.0	40	480	6.0
(*Healthy Choice*) . .	320	19.0	55.0	2.0	35	290	6.0
boneless (*Swanson Hungry Man*) . . .	690	42.0	76.0	27.0	105	1390	7.0
breaded, country (*Healthy Choice*) . .	350	18.0	55.0	7.0	45	500	5.0
broccoli Alfredo (*Healthy Choice*) . .	370	23.0	53.0	8.0	45	470	6.0

Food and Measure	cal.	prot. (gms)	carbo. (gms)	fat (gms)	chol. (mgs)	sod. (mgs)	fiber (gms)
Cantonese (*Healthy Choice*)	210	19.0	31.0	.5	30	360	5.0
Dijon (*Healthy Choice*)	280	21.0	41.0	4.0	30	410	9.0
fried:							
(*Banquet* Extra Helping)	790	37.0	72.0	39.0	110	1820	8.0
country, w/gravy (*Marie Callender's*)	610	25.0	67.0	27.0	55	1680	6.0
dark (*Swanson*) . .	550	45.0	50.0	28.0	110	1530	4.0
dark (*Swanson* Budget)	460	32.0	46.0	21.0	85	1480	4.0
dark (*Swanson Hungry Man*)	810	63.0	76.0	41.0	120	1710	9.0
Southern (*Banquet* Extra Helping) . .	750	38.0	67.0	37.0	120	2140	9.0
white (*Banquet* Extra Helping)	820	40.0	72.0	41.0	95	1890	8.0
white (*Swanson*) . .	560	40.0	54.0	26.0	70	1710	5.0
white, mostly (*Swanson Hungry Man*)	810	62.0	77.0	40.0	120	2060	7.0
glazed, Southwestern (*Healthy Choice*) . .	300	20.0	48.0	3.0	45	430	6.0
grilled:							
patties (*Swanson Hungry Man*) . .	580	29.0	67.0	19.0	90	1360	13.0
white, in garlic sauce (*Swanson*)	260	9.0	35.0	6.0	30	660	5.0
herb, country (*Healthy Choice*)	270	20.0	40.0	4.0	35	340	6.0
herbed (*The Budget Gourmet* Light & Healthy)	300	25.0	34.0	8.0	65	620	5.0
honey mustard (*The Budget Gourmet* Light & Healthy) . .	310	20.0	46.0	6.0	50	540	6.0
nuggets (*Swanson*)	440	29.0	48.0	19.0	35	980	4.0

Food and Measure	cal.	prot. (gms)	carbo. (gms)	fat (gms)	chol. (mgs)	sod. (mgs)	fiber (gms)
Chicken dinner, frozen *(cont.)*							
parmigiana:							
(*Banquet* Extra Helping)	650	24.0	64.0	33.0	65	1770	9.0
(*The Budget Gourmet* Light & Healthy)	300	21.0	32.0	10.0	45	480	5.0
(*Healthy Choice*) . .	300	20.0	47.0	4.0	35	490	5.0
(*Marie Callender's*)	620	31.0	63.0	27.0	50	730	9.0
(*Swanson*)	400	29.0	43.0	19.0	35	1160	4.0
(*Swanson* Budget)	340	28.0	33.0	18.0	40	760	4.0
pasta and (*Swanson* Budget)	250	17.0	30.0	11.0	40	660	5.0
picante (*Healthy Choice*)	220	19.0	30.0	2.0	35	330	6.0
roasted, herb:							
(*The Budget Gourmet* Light & Healthy)	240	16.0	29.0	7.0	35	60	4.0
(*Swanson*)	290	9.0	42.0	6.0	30	750	3.0
mashed potatoes (*Marie Callender's*)	670	43.0	32.0	42.0	205	2100	7.0
sweet and sour (*Healthy Choice*) . .	310	23.0	42.0	5.0	50	250	6.0
tenders, platter (*Swanson*)	320	18.0	39.0	12.0	25	790	3.0
teriyaki:							
(*The Budget Gourmet* Light & Healthy)	290	18.0	42.0	6.0	35	800	3.0
(*Healthy Choice*) . .	270	21.0	42.0	2.0	40	420	5.0
Chicken entree, canned:							
à la king:							
(*Swanson* Main Dish), 1 cup . . .	320	34.0	17.0	22.0	60	1080	0
(*Top Shelf*), 10 oz.	380	21.0	47.0	12.0	45	960	2.0

Food and Measure	cal.	prot. (gms)	carbo. (gms)	fat (gms)	chol. (mgs)	sod. (mgs)	fiber (gms)
breast, glazed (*Top Shelf*), 10 oz. . . .	200	22.0	17.0	5.0	50	910	2.0
and broccoli (*Healthy Choice Hearty Handfuls*), 6.1 oz.	320	17.0	51.0	5.0	20	580	5.0
cacciatore (*Top Shelf*), 10 oz.	210	21.0	26.0	2.5	45	850	3.0
chow mein, 1 cup:							
(*La Choy* Bi-Pack)	110	7.5	12.0	4.0	10	1080	4.0
(*La Choy* Entree)	80	8.0	6.0	4.0	10	1350	3.0
and dumplings:							
(*Dinty Moore* Cup), 7½ oz.	190	15.0	20.0	6.0	30	670	1.0
(*Swanson* Main Dish), 1 cup . . .	260	20.0	22.0	13.0	65	1120	0
fiesta (*Top Shelf*), 10 oz.	420	26.0	45.0	16.0	70	1070	2.0
w/mashed potato (*Dinty Moore American Classics*), 10 oz.	220	21.0	25.0	4.0	35	1080	2.0
and noodles (*Dinty Moore American Classics*), 10 oz. . .	260	21.0	26.0	8.0	80	1150	2.0
noodles and, see "Noodle entree"							
Oriental, w/noodles (*La Choy*), 1 cup	150	11.0	17.0	5.0	30	1190	5.0
and pasta (*Chef Boyardee* Bowl), 7½ oz.	150	16.0	21.0	1.0	30	1300	2.0
spicy (*La Choy* Szechwan Bi-Pack), 1 cup	100	8.0	11.0	3.0	20	860	1.0
stew:							
(*Dinty Moore*), 1 cup	220	12.0	16.0	11.0	40	980	2.0
(*Dinty Moore* Cup), 7½ oz.	180	10.0	18.0	8.0	30	920	2.0

Food and Measure	cal.	prot. (gms)	carbo. (gms)	fat (gms)	chol. (mgs)	sod. (mgs)	fiber (gms)
Chicken entree, canned, stew *(cont.)*							
(*Swanson* Main Dish), 1 cup . . .	180	12.0	17.0	8.0	35	1110	2.0
sweet and sour (*La Choy* Bi-Pack), 1 cup	160	8.0	29.0	2.5	25	660	1.0
teriyaki (*La Choy* Bi-Pack), 1 cup	115	8.0	15.0	3.0	25	1250	2.0
Chicken entree, freeze-dried (*Mountain House*), 1 cup:							
à la king and noodles	290	19.0	31.0	10.0	70	1070	1.0
honey lime, w/rice . .	240	9.0	42.0	4.0	40	430	1.0
noodles and	200	11.0	33.0	3.0	40	940	3.0
Polynesian w/rice . .	200	9.0	34.0	4.0	25	770	1.0
rice and	300	8.0	44.0	10.0	15	1150	1.0
stew	220	11.0	24.0	9.0	30	1080	3.0
teriyaki, w/rice	210	10.0	37.0	2.0	20	770	2.0
Chicken entree, frozen (see also "Chicken entree, refrigerated"), 1 pkg., except as noted:							
à la king:							
(*Banquet* Toppers), 4.5-oz. bag . . .	100	9.0	7.0	4.0	40	480	1.0
(*Stouffer's*)	320	15.0	43.0	10.0	55	750	3.0
Alfredo (*Stouffer's Lunch Express*) . .	360	18.0	34.0	17.0	60	620	3.0
au gratin (*The Budget Gourmet* Light & Healthy)	250	18.0	26.0	8.0	45	820	3.0
baked:							
and gravy, whipped potato (*Stouffer's* Homestyle) . . .	270	22.0	19.0	12.0	75	750	2.0
whipped potato (*Lean Cuisine*) . .	250	19.0	30.0	6.0	30	590	2.0

Food and Measure	cal.	prot. (gms)	carbo. (gms)	fat (gms)	chol. (mgs)	sod. (mgs)	fiber (gms)
barbecue:							
glazed (*Weight Watchers*)	230	20.0	33.0	2.5	30	440	4.0
honey, w/potato, vegetables (*Tyson*)	430	20.0	53.0	16.0	35	520	5.0
style (*Banquet*) . .	320	18.0	36.0	12.0	60	800	3.0
w/potato, vegetables (*Tyson* BBQ) . . .	360	18.0	49.0	10.0	30	590	6.0
biryani (*Curry Classics*)	460	28.0	58.0	13.0	n.a.	820	4.0
blackened (*Tyson*) . .	260	17.0	38.0	4.0	30	370	4.0
breaded cutlet, pasta marinara (*Celentano*)	170	19.0	36.0	19.0	50	1040	8.0
breast, breaded, 3 oz.:							
(*Tyson*), 2 pcs. . .	180	12.0	15.0	8.0	25	440	1.0
Southern (*Tyson Breast Fillets*), 2 pcs.	170	13.0	13.0	7.0	30	440	1.0
breast, in wine sauce (*Lean Cuisine* Cafe Classics)	220	16.0	25.0	6.0	35	560	3.0
breast tenders, 3 oz.:							
(*Banquet*), 3 pcs.	260	12.0	16.0	16.0	25	490	2.0
(*Tyson*), 5 pcs. . .	210	13.0	8.0	14.0	40	290	1.0
Southern (*Banquet*), 3 pcs.	260	12.0	16.0	16.0	15	460	1.0
w/broccoli and cheese (*Tyson*)	260	19.0	21.0	11.0	40	630	3.0
cacciatore (*Healthy Choice*)	260	22.0	36.0	3.0	25	510	6.0
calypso (*Lean Cuisine* Cafe Classics) . . .	280	15.0	42.0	6.0	40	590	3.0
carbonara (*Lean Cuisine* Cafe Classics)	290	22.0	32.0	8.0	40	540	4.0
chow mein:							
(*Banquet*)	210	9.0	28.0	7.0	30	650	3.0
(*Chun King*)	370	16.0	45.0	14.0	45	2010	4.0

Food and Measure	cal.	prot. (gms)	carbo. (gms)	fat (gms)	chol. (mgs)	sod. (mgs)	fiber (gms)
Chicken entree, frozen, chow mein *(cont.)*							
(*Lean Cuisine*) . . .	210	13.0	28.0	5.0	35	510	2.0
(*Smart Ones*) . . .	200	12.0	34.0	2.0	25	490	3.0
(*Stouffer's Lunch Express*)	260	13.0	43.0	4.0	30	940	3.0
chunks, breaded:							
(*Country Skillet*), 5 pcs., 3.3 oz. . .	270	12.0	18.0	17.0	20	720	1.0
(*Tyson Breast Chunks*), 6 pcs., 3 oz.	220	13.0	11.0	14.0	36	480	1.0
(*Tyson Chick'n Chunks*), 6 pcs., 3 oz.	280	11.0	14.0	20.0	50	490	2.0
and cheddar (*Banquet*), 4 pcs., 2.9 oz.	280	12.0	13.0	19.0	25	560	1.0
Southern (*Banquet*), 5 pcs., 3.1 oz. . .	270	12.0	16.0	18.0	35	570	2.0
Southern (*Country Skillet*), 5 pcs., 3.3 oz.	250	12.0	16.0	15.0	20	550	1.0
Southern (*Tyson Chick'n Chunks*), 6 pcs., 3 oz. . . .	250	10.0	13.0	17.0	40	450	1.0
Cordon Bleu (*Weight Watchers*)	230	15.0	31.0	4.5	20	650	2.0
creamed (*Stouffer's*)	280	17.0	8.0	20.0	80	720	0
creamy, and broccoli (*Stouffer's*)	320	19.0	26.0	15.0	60	820	2.0
croquettes (*Goya*), 3 pcs.	280	13.0	30.0	12.0	55	520	3.0
drumlets (*Swanson Fun Feast*)	470	35.0	50.0	23.0	60	1110	3.0
and dumplings:							
(*Banquet* Family Size), 1 cup . . .	290	11.0	18.0	14.0	40	1270	2.0
(*Banquet* Home-style)	260	13.0	35.0	8.0	35	780	3.0

Food and Measure	cal.	prot. (gms)	carbo. (gms)	fat (gms)	chol. (mgs)	sod. (mgs)	fiber (gms)
enchilada, see "Enchilada entree"							
escalloped, and noodles (*Stouffer's*) . .	450	17.0	32.0	28.0	50	1170	1.0
fajita, see "Fajita entree"							
fettuccine:							
(*The Budget Gourmet*)	380	20.0	33.0	19.0	85	810	3.0
(*Lean Cuisine*) . . .	270	22.0	33.0	6.0	45	580	2.0
(*Stouffer's* Homestyle)	390	31.0	32.0	15.0	65	1250	3.0
(*Weight Watchers*)	290	19.0	39.0	7.0	50	590	4.0
Alfredo (*Healthy Choice*)	260	22.0	35.0	4.5	40	410	3.0
w/broccoli (*Lean Cuisine Lunch Express*)	290	16.0	38.0	8.0	40	570	3.0
fiesta:							
(*Lean Cuisine*) . . .	260	19.0	35.0	5.0	40	550	3.0
(*Smart Ones*) . . .	220	12.0	38.0	2.0	25	480	5.0
Français (*Tyson*) . . .	260	19.0	23.0	10.0	45	790	6.0
Francesca (*Healthy Choice*)	360	27.0	51.0	5.0	30	500	5.0
French recipe (*The Budget Gourmet Light & Healthy*) . .	200	13.0	19.0	8.0	30	950	4.0
fricassee, w/rice (*Goya*)	810	40.0	118.0	21.0	80	790	5.0
fried:							
(*Banquet* Meal) . .	470	21.0	35.0	27.0	105	980	6.0
(*Kid Cuisine* High Flying)	440	18.0	49.0	19.0	40	940	5.0
(*Morton*)	420	20.0	30.0	25.0	85	1000	4.0
(*Swanson Fun Feast* Frazzlin')	570	46.,0	50.0	30.0	110	1430	4.0
Southern (*Banquet* Meal)	530	22.0	44.0	30.0	85	1610	4.0

Food and Measure	cal.	prot. (gms)	carbo. (gms)	fat (gms)	chol. (mgs)	sod. (mgs)	fiber (gms)
Chicken entree, frozen, fried *(cont.)*							
whipped potato (*Stouffer's* Home-style)	330	18.0	29.0	16.0	55	780	3.0
whipped potatoes (*Swanson*)	400	32.0	34.0	21.0	80	1120	2.0
white meat (*Banquet* Meal)	470	22.0	33.0	28.0	100	1100	6.0
fried, pieces:							
(*Banquet* Original), 3 oz.	270	14.0	13.0	18.0	65	620	1.0
(*Country Skillet*), 3 oz.	270	14.0	13.0	18.0	65	620	1.0
breast (*Banquet Original*), 5.5-oz. pc.	410	23.0	18.0	26.0	85	600	4.0
country (*Banquet*), 3 oz.	270	14.0	13.0	18.0	65	620	1.0
drums and thighs (*Banquet*), 3 oz.	260	15.0	10.0	18.0	65	540	2.0
honey BBQ, skinless (*Banquet*), 3 oz.	210	28.0	7.0	13.0	55	480	2.0
hot 'n spicy (*Ban-quet*), 3 oz. . . .	260	14.0	13.0	18.0	65	590	1.0
skinless (*Banquet*), 3 oz.	210	18.0	7.0	13.0	55	480	2.0
Southern (*Banquet*), 3 oz.	270	14.0	13.0	18.0	65	590	1.0
wing, hot and spicy (*Banquet*), 4 oz., 4 pcs.	230	15.0	5.0	16.0	85	280	1.0
fried rice (*Tyson* Kit), 1 cup	200	11.0	34.0	2.0	20	670	2.0
garlic:							
(*Healthy Choice Hearty Handfuls*), 6.1 oz.	330	20.0	53.0	5.0	25	600	5.0
Milano (*Healthy Choice*)	240	18.0	34.0	4.0	35	510	6.0

Food and Measure	cal.	prot. (gms)	carbo. (gms)	fat (gms)	chol. (mgs)	sod. (mgs)	fiber (gms)
ginger, Hunan							
(*Healthy Choice*) . .	350	24.0	59.0	2.5	25	430	5.0
glazed:							
country (*Healthy*							
Choice)	200	17.0	30.0	1.5	30	480	3.0
w/rice, broccoli, car-							
rots (*Tyson*) . . .	240	16.0	30.0	6.0	30	450	2.0
w/vegetable rice							
(*Lean Cuisine*) . .	240	22.0	24.0	6.0	60	460	2.0
grilled:							
angel hair pasta							
(*Stouffer's Lunch*							
Express)	340	21.0	35.0	13.0	50	650	3.0
w/corn, beans (*Ty-*							
son)	220	18.0	28.0	4.0	30	480	7.0
Italian, w/linguine							
(*Tyson*)	190	21.0	19.0	3.5	30	440	3.0
salsa (*Lean Cuisine*							
Cafe Classics) . .	240	15.0	32.0	6.0	40	550	4.0
gumbo (*Goya*							
Asopao de Pollo)	190	15.0	25.0	3.5	20	1670	3.0
herb, w/radiatore,							
vegetables (*Tyson*)	320	22.0	44.0	6.0	35	610	3.0
honey mustard:							
(*Lean Cuisine* Cafe							
Classics)	270	16.0	39.0	5.0	35	580	3.0
(*Healthy Choice*) . .	260	21.0	40.0	2.0	30	550	4.0
(*Smart Ones*) . . .	200	13.0	33.0	2.0	30	340	6.0
w/gemelli (*Tyson*)	330	22.0	49.0	6.0	30	620	6.0
imperial (*Healthy*							
Choice)	230	17.0	31.0	4.0	40	470	3.0
Italian, w/fettuccine							
(*Lean Cuisine*) . . .	270	22.0	31.0	6.0	40	560	3.0
Kiev (*Tyson*)	440	18.0	36.0	25.0	85	680	2.0
w/linguine (*Stouffer's*							
Lunch Express) . .	300	15.0	36.0	11.0	40	680	5.0
lo mein (*Banquet*) . .	270	11.0	43.0	6.0	20	1060	5.0

Food and Measure	cal.	prot. (gms)	carbo. (gms)	fat (gms)	chol. (mgs)	sod. (mgs)	fiber (gms)
Chicken entree, frozen *(cont.)*							
mandarin:							
(*The Budget Gour-* *met* Light & Healthy)	250	16.0	37.0	5.0	45	850	4.0
(*Lean Cuisine Lunch* *Express*)	270	12.0	41.0	6.0	30	520	2.0
(*Healthy Choice*) . .	280	20.0	44.0	2.5	25	520	4.0
marinara, w/pasta (*Ty-* *son*)	430	27.0	59.0	9.0	35	660	6.0
Marsala:							
(*The Budget Gour-* *met*)	270	18.0	34.0	7.0	80	750	5.0
(*Smart Ones*) . . .	150	10.0	22.0	2.0	25	500	6.0
w/potato, carrots (*Tyson*)	180	15.0	19.0	5.0	30	520	4.0
and vegetables (*Healthy Choice*)	220	22.0	32.0	1.0	30	440	3.0
Mediterranean (*Lean* *Cuisine* Cafe Clas- sics)	250	19.0	35.0	4.0	30	570	4.0
mesquite (*Tyson*) . .	310	23.0	38.0	7.0	40	590	6.0
Mexican, and rice (*Stouffer's Lunch* *Express*)	280	13.0	40.0	8.0	40	540	4.0
Mirabella (*Smart* *Ones*)	170	11.0	26.0	2.0	20	470	6.0
Monterey (*Stouffer's* Homestyle)	410	23.0	35.0	20.0	75	700	4.0
and mushroom (*Healthy Choice* *Hearty Handfuls*), 6.1 oz.	300	17.0	49.0	4.0	20	560	4.0
w/mushroom sauce (*Tyson*)	220	19.0	27.0	3.5	30	460	3.0
nibbles (*Swanson*) . .	340	31.0	31.0	20.0	90	730	2.0
and noodles:							
(*The Budget Gour-* *met*)	410	21.0	30.0	23.0	110	930	3.0

Food and Measure	cal.	prot. (gms)	carbo. (gms)	fat (gms)	chol. (mgs)	sod. (mgs)	fiber (gms)
(*Stouffer's* Home-style)	300	20.0	25.0	13.0	90	950	3.0
noodle casserole:							
(*Swanson*)	290	14.0	33.0	9.0	40	1000	2.0
w/vegetables (*Swanson*)	320	23.0	32.0	15.0	50	980	4.0
nuggets:							
(*Banquet*), 6 pcs., 3 oz.	240	14.0	12.0	15.0	35	540	1.0
(*Banquet*), 6 pcs., 4.5 oz.	320	16.0	25.0	18.0	45	670	2.0
(*Banquet* Home-style), 6.75 oz.	410	18.0	35.0	21.0	45	650	4.0
(*Country Skillet*), 10 pcs., 3.3 oz.	280	14.0	16.0	18.0	25	620	1.0
(*Kid Cuisine* Cosmic)	440	18.0	54.0	16.0	30	1070	5.0
(*Morton*)	320	13.0	30.0	17.0	30	460	3.0
mozzarella (*Banquet*), 6 pcs., 2.9 oz.	250	13.0	18.0	14.0	25	460	2.0
Southern (*Banquet*), 6 pcs., 4.5 oz. . . .	340	16.0	22.0	20.0	45	840	2.0
à l'orange (*Lean Cuisine*)	260	19.0	40.0	2.5	40	260	1.0
orange glazed (*The Budget Gourmet Light & Healthy*) . .	300	15.0	56.0	2.0	30	920	1.0
Oriental:							
(*Banquet*)	260	12.0	34.0	9.0	40	610	4.0
(*The Budget Gourmet* Light & Healthy)	300	18.0	44.0	6.0	20	700	6.0
(*Lean Cuisine*) . . .	260	21.0	30.0	6.0	45	530	3.0
(*Stouffer's Lunch Express*)	370	11.0	55.0	12.0	28	910	3.0
Parmesan (*Lean Cuisine* Cafe Classics)	240	20.0	25.0	7.0	50	580	4.0

Food and Measure	cal.	prot. (gms)	carbo. (gms)	fat (gms)	chol. (mgs)	sod. (mgs)	fiber (gms)
Chicken entree, frozen (cont.)							
parmigiana:							
(*Banquet*)	290	14.0	27.0	15.0	50	900	3.0
(*Banquet* Family Size), 4.7-oz. pc.	240	11.0	18.0	13.0	20	690	2.0
(*Stouffer's* Home-style)	320	27.0	30.0	10.0	75	890	4.0
(*Tyson*)	290	17.0	31.0	11.0	20	680	4.0
(*Weight Watchers*)	310	21.0	39.0	7.0	30	500	4.0
Italian style (*Banquet*), 4.6-oz. pc.	250	12.0	17.0	15.0	45	630	2.0
patties, breaded:							
(*Banquet*)	380	17.0	31.0	21.0	40	1270	4.0
(*Banquet*), 2.3-oz. pc.	180	10.0	10.0	11.0	25	360	<1.0
(*Country Skillet*), 2½-oz. pc.	190	9.0	12.0	12.0	20	500	1.0
(*Morton*)	280	11.0	24.0	15.0	20	840	4.0
(*Tyson Thick'n Crispy*), 2½-oz. pc.	200	10.0	10.0	14.0	40	320	1.0
breaded strips (*Swanson*)	340	29.0	31.0	19.0	30	560	3.0
breast (*Tyson*), 2½-oz. pc.	190	10.0	11.0	12.0	30	230	1.0
breast, Southern (*Tyson*), 2½-oz. pc.	180	11.0	8.0	12.0	30	360	1.0
w/cheddar (*Tyson Chick'n with Cheddar*), 1 pc.	220	11.0	12.0	14.0	40	270	0
Southern (*Tyson Chick'n Chunks*), 6 pcs., 3 oz. . . .	250	10.0	13.0	17.0	40	450	1.0
Southern (*Banquet*), 2.3-oz. pc.	170	10.0	10.0	10.0	20	430	1.0
Southern (*Country Skillet*), 3.3-oz. pc.	190	9.0	12.0	12.0	20	450	1.0

Food and Measure	cal.	prot. (gms)	carbo. (gms)	fat (gms)	chol. (mgs)	sod. (mgs)	fiber (gms)
in peanut sauce (*Lean Cuisine*)	280	23.0	33.0	6.0	45	590	3.0
penne pollo (*Weight Watchers*)	290	22.0	40.0	5.0	35	620	3.0
piccata:							
(*Lean Cuisine* Cafe Classics)	290	15.0	45.0	6.0	30	540	1.0
lemon herb (*Smart Ones*)	190	10.0	34.0	2.0	25	460	3.0
w/potato, broccoli (*Tyson*)	180	15.0	19.0	5.0	30	470	5.0
pie or pot pie:							
(*Banquet*)	350	10.0	36.0	18.0	40	950	3.0
(*Banquet* Family Size), 1 cup . . .	480	14.0	39.0	29.0	35	1010	6.0
(*Empire* Kosher) . .	440	23.0	41.0	21.0	30	960	11.0
(*Lean Cuisine*) . . .	320	18.0	39.0	10.0	35	590	3.0
(*Marie Callender's*), 10-oz. pie	680	17.0	54.0	44.0	30	920	3.0
(*Marie Callender's*), 1 cup, 8½ oz. . . .	620	13.0	49.0	31.0	15	810	1.0
(*Stouffer's*), 10 oz.	560	20.0	40.0	36.0	50	1050	4.0
(*Stouffer's*), ½ of 16-oz. pkg. . . .	540	16.0	40.0	35.0	35	950	4.0
(*Swanson*)	410	34.0	45.0	22.0	30	810	3.0
(*Swanson* Deluxe)	470	32.0	56.0	21.0	20	950	7.0
(*Swanson* Hungry Man)	650	54.0	64.0	35.0	65	1470	3.0
(*Tyson* Meat Lovers), 9-oz. pie . .	600	16.0	48.0	39.0	25	790	1.0
(*Tyson* Meat Lovers), 1 cup, 8.4 oz.	560	15.0	44.0	36.0	20	740	1.0
au gratin (*Marie Callender's*), 10-oz. pie	720	19.0	53.0	48.0	25	1040	4.0
au gratin (*Marie Callender's*), 1 cup, 8½ oz. . . .	740	21.0	46.0	53.0	15	610	6.0

Food and Measure	cal.	prot. (gms)	carbo. (gms)	fat (gms)	chol. (mgs)	sod. (mgs)	fiber (gms)
Chicken entree, frozen, pie or pot pie *(cont.)*							
and broccoli (*Marie Callender's*), 10-oz. pie	780	18.0	88.0	48.0	20	1030	3.0
and broccoli (*Marie Callender's*), 1 cup, 8½ oz. . .	800	20.0	61.0	49.0	20	960	1.0
broccoli and cheese (*Tyson*), 9-oz. pie	580	18.0	48.0	35.0	25	1150	2.0
broccoli and cheese (*Tyson*), 1 cup, 8.4 oz.	560	17.0	47.0	34.0	25	1070	2.0
and vegetables (*Tyson*), 9-oz. pie . .	550	15.0	46.0	35.0	20	740	1.0
and vegetables (*Tyson*), 1 cup, 8.4 oz.	550	14.0	46.0	35.0	20	700	1.0
primavera, w/pasta:							
(*Banquet*)	330	13.0	40.0	13.0	25	930	6.0
(*Tyson*)	390	29.0	52.0	8.0	45	790	6.0
and rice, stir-fry casserole (*Swanson*)	240	5.0	40.0	3.0	20	1200	2.0
w/rice (*Goya* Arroz con Pollo)	750	47.0	79.0	28.0	125	2000	4.0
roast, glazed (*Weight Watchers*)	240	18.0	29.0	6.0	20	550	4.0
roasted:							
herb (*Lean Cuisine Cafe Classics*) . .	210	17.0	25.0	5.0	40	430	4.0
w/linguini, broccoli (*Tyson*)	190	21.0	20.0	3.0	45	460	4.0
sandwich, see "Chicken sandwich"							
sesame:							
(*Healthy Choice*) . .	240	16.0	38.0	3.0	30	600	3.0
Shanghai (*Healthy Choice*)	310	24.0	42.0	5.0	30	460	5.0
stir-fry (*Tyson* Kit), 1 cup	180	10.0	31.0	2.0	20	720	2.0

Food and Measure	cal.	prot. (gms)	carbo. (gms)	fat (gms)	chol. (mgs)	sod. (mgs)	fiber (gms)
supreme, w/potato, green beans (*Tyson*)	230	15.0	24.0	8.0	35	310	5.0
sweet and sour (*The Budget Gourmet*)	330	18.0	55.0	5.0	40	700	4.0
tikka (*Curry Classics Makhanwala*)	480	31.0	15.0	33.0	n.a.	850	6.0
and vegetables (*Lean Cuisine*)	240	19.0	30.0	5.0	35	520	5.0
w/vegetables, garden (*Stouffer's Lunch Express*)	340	15.0	45.0	11.0	30	750	2.0
walnut, crunchy (*Chun King*)	470	19.0	56.0	19.0	35	1820	5.0
wings, 4 pcs.:							
barbecue (*Tyson*)	220	20.0	2.0	15.0	130	160	0
teriyaki (*Tyson*) . .	190	21.0	2.0	12.0	120	210	2.0
Chicken entree, mix, stir-fry (*Tyson*), 1 cup*	150	9.0	22.0	3.0	30	480	2.0
Chicken entree, re-frigerated (see also "Chicken, refriger-ated or frozen"):							
cutlet, breaded (*Per-due*), 3½-oz. pc. . .	230	10.0	18.0	13.0	40	450	2.0
Italian (*Perdue Short Cuts*), 3 oz.	110	22.0	1.0	2.0	55	540	0
lemon pepper (*Perdue Short Cuts*), 3 oz.	110	22.0	2.0	1.5	60	620	0
mesquite (*Perdue Short Cuts*), 3 oz.	110	21.0	2.0	1.5	50	510	0
nuggets, breaded:							
(*Perdue*), 5 pcs., 3 oz.	200	9.0	15.0	12.0	35	390	2.0
and cheese (*Per-due*), 5 pcs., 3 oz.	220	11.0	11.0	15.0	95	550	2.0
oven roasted, 3 oz.:							
(*Perdue Short Cuts*)	110	22.0	2.0	1.5	55	765	0
dark meat (*Perdue*)	170	17.0	0	11.0	110	320	0

Food and Measure	cal.	prot. (gms)	carbo. (gms)	fat (gms)	chol. (mgs)	sod. (mgs)	fiber (gms)
Chicken entree, refrigerated, oven roasted *(cont.)*							
white meat (*Perdue*)	140	19.0	0	7.0	80	320	0
tenderloins, breaded							
(*Perdue*), 3 oz. . . .	160	18.0	7.0	7.0	65	320	2.0
wings, 3 oz.:							
barbecued (*Perdue*)	200	16.0	3.0	13.0	105	600	n.a.
hot and spicy (*Per-*							
due)	190	16.0	2.0	13.0	110	610	n.a.
Chicken fat:							
1 oz.	178	1.1	0	19.3	16	9	0
rendered (*Empire* Ko-							
sher), 1 tbsp. . . .	120	0	<1.0	13.0	10	0	0
Chicken frankfurter							
(see also "Turkey							
frankfurter") (*Em-*							
pire Kosher),							
2-oz. link	100	8.0	1.0	7.0	70	465	0
Chicken giblets,							
simmered:							
4 oz.	178	29.3	1.1	5.4	446	66	0
chopped, 1 cup . . .	228	37.5	1.4	6.9	570	85	0
Chicken gravy,							
¹⁄₄ cup:							
(*Franco-American*) . .	45	6.0	3.0	4.0	5	270	0
(*Heinz* Home Style							
Classic)	20	0	3.0	1.0	0	350	0
cream of (*Pepperidge*							
Farm)	30	2.0	3.0	1.0	5	280	0
giblet (*Franco-Ameri-*							
can)	30	3.0	3.0	2.0	10	310	0
golden, with chicken							
(*Pepperidge Farm*)	25	2.0	3.0	1.0	<5	270	0
rotisserie (*Pepperidge*							
Farm Rotissore) . .	25	2.0	3.0	1.0	5	280	0
Chicken gravy mix,							
¹⁄₄ cup*:							
(*Durkee*)	20	.5	4.0	.5	0	350	0
(*French's*)	25	.5	4.0	.5	0	250	0
(*McCormick*)	20	<1.0	4.0	0	0	310	0

Food and Measure	cal.	prot. (gms)	carbo. (gms)	fat (gms)	chol. (mgs)	sod. (mgs)	fiber (gms)
(*Pillsbury* w/Water)	10	0	3.0	0	0	250	0
(*Pillsbury* w/Water and Skim Milk) . .	20	<1.0	4.0	0	0	260	0
(*Weight Watcher's*)	10	0	1.0	0	0	400	0
roasted (*Knorr*) . . .	30	2.0	3.0	1.0	5	300	0
vegetarian (*Loma Linda Gravy Quik*)	20	1.0	3.0	0	0	410	0
Chicken lunch meat, 2 oz., except as noted:							
breast:							
baked, grilled, or honey glazed (*Louis Rich Carving Board*), 2 slices, 1.6 oz.	40	9.0	0	.5	25	530	0
honey glazed (*Oscar Mayer Deli-Thin*), 4 slices, 1.8 oz.	60	10.0	2.0	1.0	25	740	0
breast, oven roasted:							
(*Boar's Head Golden*)	50	11.0	<1.0	1.0	30	420	0
(*Hebrew National*)	45	10.0	0	.5	25	470	0
(*Hebrew National*), 5 slices, 1.8 oz.	45	10.0	0	.5	20	460	0
(*Louis Rich* Deluxe), 1-oz. slice	30	5.0	1.0	1.0	15	330	0
(*Louis Rich Deli-Thin*), 4 slices, 1.8 oz.	60	9.0	1.0	1.5	25	620	0
(*Oscar Mayer* Fat Free), 4 slices, 1.8 oz.	45	9.0	1.0	0	25	650	0
peppered (*Tyson*), 3 slices, 2.2 oz.	50	11.0	2.0	0	25	720	0
breast, smoked:							
(*Boar's Head* Hickory)	60	11.0	<1.0	1.0	30	440	0

Food and Measure	cal.	prot. (gms)	carbo. (gms)	fat (gms)	chol. (mgs)	sod. (mgs)	fiber (gms)
Chicken lunch meat, breast, smoked *(cont.)*							
(*Tyson* Hickory),							
3 slices, 2.2 oz.	50	10.0	2.0	0	25	680	0
roll, light meat, 1 oz.	45	5.5	.7	2.1	14	166	0
white, sliced:							
(*Tyson*), 3 slices . .	90	10.0	0	6.0	25	440	0
oven roasted (*Louis*							
Rich), 1-oz. slice	40	4.0	1.0	2.5	15	350	0
Chicken pie, see							
"Chicken entree,							
frozen"							
Chicken sandwich,							
frozen, 1 pc.:							
(*Hormel Quick Meal*)	340	14.0	42.0	12.0	60	480	1.0
broccoli and cheddar							
(*Croissant Pockets*)	300	14.0	37.0	11.0	35	640	5.0
and cheddar							
w/broccoli (*Hot*							
Pockets)	300	12.0	37.0	12.0	30	620	<1.0
fajita (*Lean Pockets*)	260	12.0	36.0	8.0	40	770	3.0
glazed, supreme (*Lean*							
Pockets)	240	10.0	34.0	7.0	30	600	<1.0
grilled (*Hormel Quick*							
Meal)	300	20.0	36.0	9.0	60	640	2.0
Parmesan (*Lean*							
Pockets)	260	12.0	34.0	8.0	25	630	<1.0
pastry (*Mrs. Pater-*							
son's Aussie Pie)	460	12.0	45.0	25.0	90	770	2.0
Chicken sauce (see							
also specific list-							
ings), 1 tbsp., ex-							
cept as noted:							
barbecue flavor							
(*Hunt's Chicken*							
Sensations)	35	0	3.0	3.0	0	310	0
Caesar (*Lawry's*),							
2 tbsp.	30	1.0	5.0	.5	0	480	0
Italian garlic (*Hunt's*							
Chicken Sensations)	30	0	1.0	3.0	0	325	1.5

Food and Measure	cal.	prot. (gms)	carbo. (gms)	fat (gms)	chol. (mgs)	sod. (mgs)	fiber (gms)
lemon herb (*Hunt's Chicken Sensations*)	30	0	2.0	3.0	0	375	0
sherried (*Lawry's*) . .	20	1.0	5.0	0	0	210	0
Southwestern (*Hunt's Chicken Sensations*)	30	0	1.0	2.5	0	280	0
Thai, satay (*Lawry's*)	35	1.0	4.0	2.0	0	270	0
wing, 2 tbsp.:							
hot (*Nance's*) . . .	15	0	3.0	0	0	130	0
mild (*Nance's*) . . .	15	0	3.0	0	0	120	0
Chicken sausage, 3.3-oz. link:							
and apricot (*Bilinski*)	120	15.0	8.0	3.0	60	650	1.0
and broccoli (*Bilinski*)	110	15.0	1.0	3.5	65	710	0
Italian, w/pepper and onion (*Bilinski*) . .	120	19.0	1.0	4.0	80	800	0
and jalapeño (*Bilinski*)	130	21.0	1.0	4.0	85	870	0
and pesto (*Bilinski*)	110	17.0	0	4.5	70	740	0
and spinach (*Bilinski*)	100	15.0	2.0	3.0	60	640	1.0
and sun-dried tomato w/basil (*Bilinski*) . .	120	17.0	5.0	3.5	55	770	0
Chicken seasoning and coating mix, ⅛ pkg., except as noted:							
(*Durkee/French's* Roasting Bag), ⅙ pkg.	20	1.0	4.0	0	0	500	0
(*McCormick Bag 'n Season*), 1 tbsp. . . .	20	<1.0	4.0	0	0	460	0
(*Shake'n Bake* Original Recipe)	40	1.0	7.0	1.0	0	230	0
barbecue (*Durkee* Roasting Bag), ⅙ pkg.	30	0	8.0	0	0	570	.5
barbecue glaze (*Shake'n Bake*) . .	45	0	9.0	1.0	0	410	0
Buffalo wing:							
Cajun (*Durkee*) . .	15	0	3.0	0	0	490	0

Food and Measure	cal.	prot. (gms)	carbo. (gms)	fat (gms)	chol. (mgs)	sod. (mgs)	fiber (gms)
Chicken seasoning and coating mix, Buffalo wing *(cont.)*							
garlic and herb (*Durkee*)	15	0	3.0	0	0	590	0
hot or screaming hot (*Durkee*) . . .	20	0	3.0	.5	0	510	0
mild (*Durkee*) . . .	20	0	3.0	.5	0	500	0
cacciatore (*Durkee Easy*), 1/10 pkg. . . .	10	0	3.0	0	0	110	0
coq au vin (*Knorr Recipe*), 1 tbsp. . .	30	<1.0	5.0	1.0	0	250	0
country (*Durkee Roasting Bag*), 1/6 pkg.	35	.5	5.0	1.5	0	360	0
country (*McCormick Bag 'n Season*), 2 tsp.	25	<1.0	3.0	1.0	0	880	0
Dijonne (*Knorr* Recipe), 1/6 pkg.	30	1.0	5.0	1.0	0	360	0
extra crispy (*Oven Fry*)	60	2.0	10.0	1.0	0	420	0
homestyle flour (*Oven Fry*)	40	1.0	7.0	1.0	0	470	0
hot and spicy (*Shake'n Bake*) . .	40	1.0	7.0	1.0	0	190	0
hot, spicy (*McCormick Bag 'n Season*), 1 tbsp.	30	0	5.0	0	0	630	0
Mexican salsa (*Durkee Easy*), 1/10 pkg. . . .	10	0	3.0	0	0	120	0
mushroom (*Durkee Easy*), 1/8 pkg. . . .	15	0	3.0	0	0	200	0
Southwest, marinade (*Lawry's*), 1 tsp. . . .	5	0	1.0	0	0	320	0
sweet and sour (*Durkee Easy*), 1/9 pkg.	20	0	5.0	0	0	70	0

Food and Measure	cal.	prot. (gms)	carbo. (gms)	fat (gms)	chol. (mgs)	sod. (mgs)	fiber (gms)
Chicken spread:							
chunky:							
(*Underwood*),							
¼ cup	120	9.0	2.0	8.0	40	470	0
w/crackers (*Red Devil* Snackers),							
1 pkg.	270	13.0	20.0	16.0	45	720	1.0
salad (*Libby's Spreadables*), ⅓ cup . . .	140	7.0	7.0	9.0	25	340	2.0
Chicken wing sauce,							
see "Chicken sauce"							
Chick-fil-A, 1 serving:							
chicken dishes:							
3.7 oz.	160	21.0	1.0	8.0	45	690	0
chargrilled, 2.8 oz.	130	27.0	0	3.0	30	630	0
Chick-fil-A Nuggets,							
8-pack	290	28.0	12.0	14.0	60	770	0
Chick-n-Strips,							
4 pcs.	230	29.0	10.0	8.0	20	380	0
Chick-n-Strips salad	290	32.0	21.0	9.0	20	430	5.0
salad, chargrilled							
garden	170	26.0	10.0	3.0	25	650	5.0
salad plate	290	21.0	40.0	5.0	35	570	6.0
chicken sandwiches:							
regular	290	24.0	29.0	9.0	50	870	1.0
chargrilled	280	27.0	36.0	3.0	40	640	1.0
chargrilled, deluxe	290	28.0	38.0	3.0	40	640	2.0
chargrilled club, w/out dressing	390	33.0	38.0	12.0	70	980	2.0
Chick-n-Q	370	25.0	36.0	13.0	20	1040	1.0
deluxe	300	25.0	31.0	9.0	50	870	2.0
salad, whole wheat	320	25.0	42.0	5.0	10	810	1.0
side dishes, small:							
carrot raisin salad	150	5.0	28.0	2.0	6	650	2.0
chicken soup, 1 cup	110	16.0	10.0	1.0	45	760	1.0
coleslaw	130	6.0	11.0	6.0	15	430	1.0
tossed salad	70	5.0	13.0	0	0	0	1.0
Waffle fries:							
salted	290	1.0	49.0	10.0	5	960	0

Food and Measure	cal.	prot. (gms)	carbo. (gms)	fat (gms)	chol. (mgs)	sod. (mgs)	fiber (gms)
Chick-fil-A, side dishes, small *(cont.)*							
unsalted	290	1.0	49.0	10.0	5	80	0
desserts:							
brownie, fudge nut	350	10.0	41.0	16.0	30	650	0
cheesecake	270	13.0	7.0	21.0	10	510	0
w/blueberry . . .	290	14.0	9.0	23.0	10	550	0
w/strawberry . .	290	14.0	8.0	23.0	10	580	0
Icedream, small							
cone	140	11.0	16.0	4.0	40	240	0
Icedream, small cup	350	16.0	50.0	10.0	70	390	0
lemon pie	280	1.0	19.0	22.0	5	550	0
Chickpea flour (*Arrowhead Mills*),							
2 oz.	200	12.0	35.0	3.0	0	9	7.4
Chickpeas:							
dry:							
(*Arrowhead Mills*),							
¼ cup	170	10.0	29.0	2.0	0	10	6.0
boiled, ½ cup . . .	134	7.3	22.5	2.1	0	6	2.9
canned, ½ cup:							
w/liquid	143	5.9	27.1	1.4	0	359	5.3
(*Allens/East Texas Fair*)	120	5.0	19.0	2.5	0	330	8.0
(*Eden* Organic) . .	110	6.0	17.0	1.5	0	10	4.0
(*Eden* Organic Jars)	110	7.0	20.0	1.0	0	95	4.0
(*Goya*)	100	6.0	20.0	2.0	0	360	7.0
(*Green Giant/Joan of Arc*)	110	6.0	18.0	1.5	0	380	5.0
(*Old El Paso*) . . .	120	5.0	20.0	2.5	0	280	7.0
(*Progresso*)	120	5.0	20.0	2.5	0	280	7.0
(*Stokely*)	110	6.0	17.0	1.5	0	360	6.0
in tomato sauce							
(*Goya* Guisados)	100	5.0	17.0	1.5	0	520	4.0
Chicory, witloof:							
5–7″ head, 2.1 oz. . .	9	.5	2.1	.1	0	1	1.6
½ cup	8	.4	1.8	<.1	0	1	1.4
Chicory greens:							
trimmed, 1 oz.	7	.5	1.3	.1	0	13	1.1
chopped, ½ cup . . .	21	1.5	4.2	.3	0	41	3.6

Food and Measure	cal.	prot. (gms)	carbo. (gms)	fat (gms)	chol. (mgs)	sod. (mgs)	fiber (gms)
Chicory root:							
1 medium, 2.6 oz. . .	44	.8	10.5	.1	0	30	n.a.
1″ pcs., ½ cup . . .	33	.6	7.9	.1	0	23	n.a.
Chili, canned (see also "Chili base"), 1 cup, except as noted:							
w/beans:							
(*Chi-Chi's* San Antonio)	340	19.0	23.0	19.0	60	900	6.0
(*Gebhardt*)	320	15.5	32.0	15.0	30	675	15.0
(*Hormel*)	340	18.0	30.0	17.0	60	1200	9.0
(*Hormel*), 7½-oz. can	250	15.0	23.0	11.0	50	1000	6.0
(*Hormel* Micro Cup), 1 cont.	250	15.0	23.0	11.0	50	980	6.0
(*Hormel* Micro Cup), 10.5-oz. cont. . .	410	23.0	41.0	17.0	75	1430	12.0
(*Just Rite*)	380	18.0	30.0	25.0	35	1235	13.0
(*Libby's*)	420	16.0	29.0	27.0	50	1210	4.0
(*Libby's Diner*), 7¾ oz.	320	13.0	23.0	22.0	40	1010	9.0
(*Nalley* Real Hearty)	310	20.0	27.0	14.0	30	990	12.0
(*Nalley* Thick) . . .	290	21.0	32.0	9.0	30	1100	11.0
(*Old El Paso*) . . .	200	19.0	15.0	7.0	30	420	6.0
(*Van Camp's*) . . .	350	19.0	28.0	21.0	45	1020	7.0
(*Wolf*)	330	19.0	30.0	18.0	45	1050	9.0
w/beef and hot dogs (*Nalley* Chili Dog)	300	20.0	27.0	12.0	20	1050	8.0
cheddar (*Nalley*) . .	320	23.0	28.0	12.0	35	1250	8.0
chunky (*Hormel*)	330	17.0	30.0	16.0	60	1040	8.0
hot (*Hormel*) . . .	340	18.0	30.0	17.0	60	1200	9.0
hot (*Hormel/Hormel* Micro Cup), 7½ oz.	250	15.0	23.0	11.0	50	980	6.0
jalapeño (*Wolf*) . .	330	19.0	30.0	18.0	45	1050	9.0
jalapeño hot (*Nalley*)	280	20.0	30.0	8.0	25	1010	12.0
w/out beans:							
(*Hormel*)	410	19.0	16.0	30.0	75	950	3.0

Food and Measure	cal.	prot. (gms)	carbo. (gms)	fat (gms)	chol. (mgs)	sod. (mgs)	fiber (gms)
Chili, canned, w/out beans *(cont.)*							
(*Hormel*),							
7½-oz. can . . .	390	18.0	13.0	30.0	65	1030	2.0
(*Hormel Micro Cup*),							
1 cont.	290	18.0	15.0	17.0	65	830	3.0
(*Libby's*)	480	21.0	16.0	37.0	75	1580	1.0
(*Nalley Big Chunk*)	280	25.0	13.0	14.0	50	1040	3.0
(*Wolf*)	420	22.0	20.0	30.0	80	1150	5.0
hot (*Hormel*) . . .	410	19.0	16.0	30.0	75	950	3.0
jalapeño (*Wolf*) . .	420	22.0	20.0	30.0	80	1150	5.0
onion (*Nalley* Walla							
Walla)	300	23.0	20.0	15.0	30	1130	4.0
w/franks, see "Beans and franks"							
turkey:							
w/beans (*Hormel*)	220	18.0	26.0	3.0	50	1170	5.0
w/out beans (*Hormel*)	190	23.0	17.0	3.0	70	1210	3.0
vegetarian:							
(*Hormel*)	200	12.0	38.0	0	0	830	9.0
(*Natural Touch*) . .	270	18.0	21.0	12.0	0	1330	11.0
(*Worthington*) . . .	290	19.0	21.0	15.0	0	420	9.0
all varieties, except burrito flavor (*Health Valley* Nonfat), ½ cup	80	7.0	15.0	0	0	160	7.0
burrito flavor (*Health Valley*), ½ cup	80	7.0	15.0	0	0	180	7.0
w/macaroni:							
(*Hormel* Chili Mac), 7.5-oz. can . . .	200	11.0	17.0	9.0	25	980	2.0
(*Hormel* Chili Mac Micro Cup), 1 cont.	200	11.0	17.0	9.0	25	980	2.0
Chili, freeze-dried:							
w/beef, 1 cup:							
beans (*Mountain House*)	190	11.0	27.0	4.0	10	1090	7.0

Food and Measure	cal.	prot. (gms)	carbo. (gms)	fat (gms)	chol. (mgs)	sod. (mgs)	fiber (gms)
macaroni (*Mountain House*)	220	13.0	30.0	6.0	20	510	6.0
meatless (*AlpineAire Mountain*), 1½ cups	340	24.0	54.0	2.0	n.a.	1334	n.a.
Chili, frozen, 1 pkg.:							
w/beans (*Stouffer's* Entree)	270	15.0	29.0	10.0	35	1130	8.0
w/cornbread (*Marie Callender's* Dinner)	350	14.0	45.0	13.0	30	1380	5.0
three bean (*Lean Cuisine* Entree)	210	8.0	32.0	6.0	10	460	7.0
vegetarian (*Tabachnik* Side Dish)	210	12.0	28.0	6.0	0	530	10.0
Chili, mix, 1 pkg., except as noted:							
all varieties (*Health Valley* Chili in a Cup), ⅓ cup	120	10.0	21.0	1.0	0	290	6.0
4 bean (*Knorr* Cup)	230	7.0	53.0	1.5	0	970	7.0
3 bean (*Spice Islands* Quick Meal)	180	9.0	34.0	1.0	0	640	10.0
vegetarian (*Spice Islands* Quick Meal)	180	9.0	32.0	2.0	0	500	7.0
Chili base, canned ½ cup:							
(*Hunt's* Homestyle Fixings)	85	5.5	18.5	1.0	0	860	6.0
(*S&W* Chili Makin's)	80	5.0	20.0	5.0	0	790	5.0
black bean (*S&W* Chili Makin's)	80	6.0	19.0	0	0	750	6.0
homestyle (*S&W* Chili Makin's)	80	7.0	19.0	0	0	630	6.0
Santa Fe (*S&W* Chili Makin's)	80	6.0	18.0	0	0	870	5.0
Chili beans (see also "Mexican beans"), canned, ½ cup:							
(*Gebhardt*)	135	7.0	30.0	1.0	0	630	7.0
(*Hunt's*)	85	6.0	17.0	1.0	0	600	6.0

Food and Measure	cal.	prot. (gms)	carbo. (gms)	fat (gms)	chol. (mgs)	sod. (mgs)	fiber (gms)
Chili beans *(cont.)*							
(*S&W*)	110	7.0	23.0	1.0	0	580	6.0
(*Stokely*)	120	7.0	21.0	.5	0	550	6.0
(*Sun-Vista*)	110	7.0	24.0	1.0	0	360	7.0
(*Van Camp's* Mexican)	110	7.0	21.0	2.0	0	430	8.0
hot (*S&W* Chipotle)	90	7.0	21.0	0	0	570	6.0
spicy (*Green Giant/ Joan of Arc*)	110	6.0	20.0	1.0	0	490	5.0
zesty (*Campbell's*) . .	130	5.0	21.0	3.0	5	490	6.0
Chili dinner or entree, see "Chili, frozen"							
Chili dip, green (*La Victoria*), 2 tbsp.	10	0	2.0	0	0	140	0
Chili dip mix, caliente (*Knorr*), ½ tsp. . .	5	0	1.0	0	0	80	0
Chili pepper, see "Pepper, chili"							
Chili powder:							
1 tbsp.	24	.9	4.1	1.3	0	76	2.6
1 tsp.	8	.3	1.4	.4	0	26	.9
(*Gebhardt*), ¼ tsp.	1	0	.1	0	0	<1	0
(*Tone's*), ¼ tsp. . . .	0	0	0	0	0	35	0
Chili sauce (see also "Pepper sauce" and "Szechuan sauce"):							
(*Del Monte*), 1 tbsp.	20	0	5.0	0	0	480	0
(*Las Palmas*), ¼ cup	15	0	2.0	.5	0	310	1.0
(*Nance's*), 2 tbsp. . .	25	0	5.0	0	0	150	0
(*S&W* Steakhouse), 1 tbsp.	15	0	4.0	0	0	180	0
hot dog:							
(*Gebhardt*), ¼ cup	60	3.0	6.0	3.0	<5	260	2.0
(*Just Rite*), 2 oz.	50	2.0	5.0	3.0	<5	265	2.0
(*Wolf*), 1 tbsp. . . .	15	1.0	2.0	1.0	0	90	0
w/beef (*Stenger*), ¼ cup	70	2.0	7.0	4.0	5	370	2.0
Chili seasoning mix:							
(*Durkee*), ⅕ pkg. . .	30	0	7.0	0	0	660	0

Food and Measure	cal.	prot. (gms)	carbo. (gms)	fat (gms)	chol. (mgs)	sod. (mgs)	fiber (gms)
(*Durkee* Pot-O),							
⅛ pkg.	30	0	7.0	0	0	380	0
(*Gebhardt Chili Quik*),							
2 tbsp.	30	1.0	5.5	.5	0	410	0
(*Lawry's*), 1 tbsp. . . .	25	<1.0	5.0	.5	0	460	0
(*Lawry's* Tex-Mex),							
2 tbsp.	50	1.0	8.0	1.5	0	750	3.0
(*McCormick*), approx.							
4 tsp.	30	1.0	5.0	.5	0	310	2.0
(*Mick Fowler's*							
2-*Alarm* Kit), 3 tbsp.	60	2.0	10.0	1.5	0	980	0
(*Mick Fowler's*							
2-*Alarm* Family),							
2 tbsp.	50	2.0	9.0	1.5	0	980	0
(*Old El Paso*), 1 tbsp.	25	<1.0	4.0	.5	0	770	1.0
mild (*Durkee*), ⅕ pkg.	30	1.0	5.0	.5	0	380	0
Texas red (*Durkee*),							
⅓ pkg.	45	2.0	2.0	1.0	0	910	0
Chimichanga, frozen:							
beef (*Old El Paso*),							
4.5-oz. pc.	370	9.0	37.0	20.0	10	470	3.0
beefsteak and bean							
(*Don Miguel*), 7 oz.	410	17.0	55.0	12.0	25	970	5.0
chicken:							
(*Don Miguel*), 7 oz.	400	17.0	54.0	12.0	35	910	5.0
(*Old El Paso*),							
4.5-oz. pc.	350	11.0	39.0	16.0	20	540	2.0
Chimichanga dinner,							
frozen, 15 oz.:							
beef (*Chi-Chi's*) . . .	630	26.0	70.0	27.0	55	2050	10.0
chicken (*Chi-Chi's*)	600	20.0	74.0	23.0	60	2280	9.0
Chimichanga entree,							
frozen (*Banquet*),							
9.5 oz.	470	13.0	56.0	10.0	20	1580	9.0
Chitterlings, pork,							
simmered, 4 oz. . . .	344	11.6	0	32.6	162	44	0
Chives:							
fresh:							
1 oz.	9	.9	1.2	.2	0	1	.9

Food and Measure	cal.	prot. (gms)	carbo. (gms)	fat (gms)	chol. (mgs)	sod. (mgs)	fiber (gms)
Chives, fresh *(cont.)*							
chopped, 1 tbsp.	1	.1	.1	<.1	0	<1	.1
freeze-dried:							
¼ cup	2	.2	.5	<.1	0	24	<1.0
1 tbsp.	1	<.1	.1	<.1	0	6	<1.0
(McCormick),							
¼ tsp.	<1	0	0	0	0	<1	0
(Tone's), ¼ tsp. . . .	0	0	0	0	0	0	0
Chocolate, see							
"Candy"							
Chocolate, baking:							
(Choco Bake), ½ oz.	80	1.0	5.0	8.0	0	0	3.0
bar, 3 sqs., 1.5 oz.,							
except as noted:							
bittersweet							
(Ghirardelli) . . .	210	3.0	24.0	15.0	0	0	1.0
milk *(Ghirardelli)* . .	220	3.0	25.0	14.0	10	30	0
milk *(Ghirardelli)*,							
1 oz.	140	2.0	17.0	8.0	5	20	0
semisweet *(Baker's)*,							
1 oz.	130	2.0	17.0	9.0	0	0	<1.0
semisweet							
(Ghirardelli) . . .	210	2.0	25.0	14.0	5	0	0
semisweet *(Nestlé)*,							
½ oz.	70	<1.0	9.0	4.0	0	0	2.0
sweet *(Baker's Ger-*							
man), ½ oz.	60	1.0	8.0	3.5	0	0	<1.0
sweet, dark							
(Ghirardelli) . . .	210	2.0	26.0	14.0	0	0	0
unsweetened							
(Baker's), 1 oz.	140	3.0	9.0	14.0	0	0	4.0
unsweetened							
(Ghirardelli) . . .	210	5.0	12.0	23.0	0	0	1.0
unsweetened *(Nes-*							
tlé), ½ oz.	80	2.0	5.0	7.0	0	0	3.0
white *(Baker's)*,							
1 oz.	160	2.0	17.0	9.0	5	25	0
white *(Ghirardelli)*	240	2.0	25.0	15.0	5	40	0

Food and Measure	cal.	prot. (gms)	carbo. (gms)	fat (gms)	chol. (mgs)	sod. (mgs)	fiber (gms)
white (*Nestlé*),							
½ oz.	80	1.0	8.0	5.0	<5	15	0
chips or morsels,							
½ oz. or 1 tbsp.:							
(*Ghirardelli Flicket-*							
tes)	70	1.0	10.0	4.0	<1	15	0
milk (*Baker's*) . . .	70	1.0	9.0	4.0	0	10	0
milk (*Ghirardelli*) . .	70	0	10.0	4.0	0	10	0
milk (*Hershey's*							
Bake Shoppe) . .	80	<1.0	9.0	4.5	<5	10	0
milk (*M&M's*) . . .	70	7.0	10.0	3.0	5	0	0
milk (*Nestlé*)	70	0	10.0	4.0	0	0	0
mint (*Nestlé*)	70	0	9.0	4.0	0	0	2.0
raspberry (*Hershey's*							
Bake Shoppe) . .	80	<1.0	10.0	4.0	0	0	0
semisweet							
(*Ghirardelli*) . . .	70	0	10.0	4.0	0	0	0
semisweet (*Her-*							
shey's Bake							
Shoppe)	80	<1.0	10.0	4.0	0	0	0
white (*Ghirardelli*)	80	1.0	10.0	4.0	0	15	0
white (*Hershey's*							
Bake Shoppe) . .	80	1.0	9.0	4.0	0	30	0
semisweet, ½ oz.:							
(*Baker's* Real) . . .	60	1.0	9.0	3.5	0	0	<1.0
(*M&M's*)	70	1.0	9.0	3.5	0	0	1.0
flavor (*Baker's*) . .	70	0	10.0	3.0	0	10	<1.0
plain or mint (*Nes-*							
tlé)	70	0	9.0	4.0	0	0	2.0
Chocolate drink							
(*Yoo-Hoo*):							
bottled, 9 fl. oz. . . .	150	2.0	33.0	1.0	0	200	0
canned, 11 fl. oz. . .	180	3.0	40.0	1.5	0	240	0
Chocolate flavor							
drink:							
canned, 10 fl. oz.:							
(*Sego* Lite)	150	12.0	21.0	3.0	0	400	0
creamy milk (*Nestlé*							
Instant Breakfast)	220	12.0	37.0	2.5	5	230	1.0

Food and Measure	cal.	prot. (gms)	carbo. (gms)	fat (gms)	chol. (mgs)	sod. (mgs)	fiber (gms)
Chocolate flavor drink, canned *(cont.)*							
fudge, mocha, or raspberry truffle *(Sweet Success)*	200	12.0	38.0	3.0	5	220	6.0
regular or malt *(Sego)*	240	13.0	44.0	1.5	5	310	0
regular or Dutch *(Sego* Lite) . . .	150	12.0	21.0	3.0	0	400	0
rich almond or creamy milk *(Sweet Success)*	200	12.0	38.0	3.0	5	240	6.0
refrigerated, 12 fl. oz.: creamy milk or almond *(Sweet Success)*	220	14.0	45.0	1.5	<5	300	6.0
fudge *(Sweet Success)*	220	14.0	45.0	1.5	<5	310	6.0
Chocolate flavor drink mix, 1 pkt., except as noted:							
(Nestlé Quik), 2 tbsp.	90	1.0	19.0	.5	0	30	1.0
(Nestlé Quik No Sugar), 2 tbsp. . .	40	0	7.0	.5	0	45	2.0
(Pillsbury Instant Breakfast)	140	10.0	28.0	1.0	<5	190	0
almond, creamy milk, fudge, or mocha *(Sweet Success)* . .	90	7.0	19.0	1.5	<5	210	6.0
chocolate chip *(Sweet Success)*	90	7.0	19.0	2.0	<5	170	6.0
creamy milk *(Carnation Instant Breakfast)*	130	4.0	28.0	1.0	<5	100	1.0
creamy milk or malt *(Carnation Instant Breakfast* No Sugar)	70	4.0	12.0	1.0	<5	100	1.0
malt, classic *(Carnation Instant Breakfast)*	130	4.0	28.0	1.0	<5	130	1.0

Food and Measure	cal.	prot. (gms)	carbo. (gms)	fat (gms)	chol. (mgs)	sod. (mgs)	fiber (gms)
raspberry truffle							
(*Sweet Success*) . .	90	7.0	19.0	1.5	<5	230	6.0
shake (*Weight Watchers*)	80	6.0	12.0	1.0	0	140	2.0
Chocolate fruit dip, see "Fruit dip"							
Chocolate milk, 1 cup, except as noted:							
(*Nestlé Quik*)	230	7.0	31.0	9.0	30	120	0
lowfat:							
(*Hershey's*)	190	8.0	30.0	4.5	15	130	1.0
(*Nestlé Quik*)	190	8.0	29.0	5.0	20	150	0
(*Nestlé Quik*), 8 fl. oz.	200	8.0	30.0	5.0	20	130	0
shake, see "Chocolate shake"							
Chocolate pastry (see also specific listings),							
dark (*Pepperidge Farm* Clouds), 2 pcs.	580	6.0	53.0	38.0	25	380	4.0
milk (*Pepperidge Farm* Clouds), 2 pcs.	580	6.0	54.0	38.0	55	400	6.0
Chocolate shake:							
(*Nestlé Killer*), 14 oz.	470	14.0	65.0	17.0	60	320	6.0
(*Nestlé Quik*), 9 oz.	300	9.0	41.0	11.0	40	200	4.0
Chocolate syrup, 2 tbsp.:							
(*Fox's No Cal*)	0	0	0	0	0	35	0
(*Fox's U-Bet*)	120	1.0	29.0	0	0	35	0
(*Hershey's*)	100	1.0	24.0	0	0	25	0
(*Smucker's* Sundae)	110	0	27.0	0	0	70	1.0
(*Yoo-Hoo*)	110	0	25.0	.5	0	50	0
malt (*Hershey's*) . . .	100	1.0	25.0	0	0	55	0

Food and Measure	cal.	prot. (gms)	carbo. (gms)	fat (gms)	chol. (mgs)	sod. (mgs)	fiber (gms)
Chocolate topping, 2 tbsp.:							
(*Kraft*) . . . . all varieties	110	2.0	26.0	0	0	30	1.0
(*Smucker's Magic Shell*)	220	1.0	16.0	16.0	0	25	0
caramel (*Hershey's*)	100	<1.0	25.0	0	0	95	0
cherry Melba (*Dickinson's Black Forest*)	130	<1.0	26.0	2.5	0	70	1.0
double (*Hershey's*)	110	<1.0	26.0	0	0	25	0
fudge: chocolate (*Smucker's*) . . .	130	0	28.0	1.5	0	60	1.0
double (*Hershey's*)	120	2.0	24.0	2.0	<5	75	<1.0
hot (*Hershey's*) . .	130	2.0	20.0	4.5	<5	180	<1.0
hot, fat free (*Hershey's*)	100	1.0	23.0	0	0	135	1.0
hot (*Kraft*)	140	1.0	24.0	4.0	10	100	<1.0
hot (*Smucker's*) . .	140	2.0	24.0	4.0	0	60	1.0
hot (*Smucker's* Special Recipe) . . .	140	2.0	22.0	4.0	0	70	<1.0
hot, light (*Smucker's*) . . .	90	2.0	23.0	0	0	90	2.0
mint (*Hershey's*) . . .	110	<1.0	25.0	0	0	25	0
Chorizo (*Goya*), 1.6-oz. stick	160	11.0	2.0	13.0	45	910	0
Chow chow (*Crosse & Blackwell*), 1 tbsp.	10	0	1.0	0	0	105	<1.0
Chow mein, see specific entree listings							
Chrysanthemum garland, ½ cup:							
raw, 1″ pcs.	2	.2	.5	<.1	0	7	.4
boiled, drained, 1″ pcs.	10	.8	2.2	.1	0	27	1.2

Food and Measure	cal.	prot. (gms)	carbo. (gms)	fat (gms)	chol. (mgs)	sod. (mgs)	fiber (gms)
Church's Chicken,							
1 serving:							
chicken, edible portion:							
breast, 2.8 oz. . . .	200	19.0	4.3	12.4	65	510	0
leg, 2 oz.	140	12.7	2.4	9.1	45	160	0
Tender Strip, 1.1 oz.	80	6.0	4.5	4.0	15	140	.5
thigh, 2.8 oz. . . .	230	16.2	5.3	16.2	80	520	0
wing, 3.1 oz.	250	18.5	7.7	16.1	60	540	0
sides:							
biscuit	250	2.2	25.6	16.4	<5	640	1.0
Cajun rice	130	1.3	15.6	7.0	5	260	<1.0
coleslaw	92	4.2	8.4	5.5	0	230	2.0
corn on cob	139	4.4	23.5	3.2	0	15	9.0
fries	210	3.3	28.5	10.5	0	60	2.0
okra	210	2.7	19.1	16.1	0	520	4.0
potatoes and gravy	90	1.2	14.0	3.3	0	520	1.0
apple pie	280	2.3	40.5	12.3	<5	340	1.0
Churro, cinnamon							
(*Tio Pepe's*), 1 oz.	110	1.0	14.0	5.0	15	100	2.0
Chutney, 1 tbsp.:							
mango (*Patak's* Major							
Grey's)	50	0	12.0	.5	0	230	0
tomato, dried (*Scnoma*)	35	0	9.0	0	0	0	0
tropical fruit and nut							
(*Patak's*)	60	0	12.0	1.0	0	80	0
Cilantro, see "Coriander"							
Cinnamon:							
ground, 1 tsp.	6	.1	2.1	.1	0	1	1.4
(*McCormick*), ¼ tsp.	2	0	.4	0	0	0	.3
(*Tone's*), ¼ tsp. . . .	5	0	1.0	0	0	0	0
Cisco, meat only,							
raw, 4 oz.	112	21.5	0	2.2	n.a.	62	0
Citron, candied:							
(*S&W*), 39 pcs.,							
1.1 oz.	90	0	23.0	0	0	25	1.0

Food and Measure	cal.	prot. (gms)	carbo. (gms)	fat (gms)	chol. (mgs)	sod. (mgs)	fiber (gms)
Citron *(cont.)*							
diced (*Paradise/White Swan*), 2 tbsp., .9 oz.	80	0	19.0	0	0	15	1.0
Citrus juice blend (*Pet/Season's Best Medley*), 8 fl. oz.	120	<1.0	31.0	0	0	25	0
Citrus drink, 8 fl. oz.:							
(*Five Alive*)	120	0	30.0	0	0	25	0
punch:							
(*Goya*)	130	0	30.0	0	0	20	0
(*Minute Maid*) . . .	120	0	32.0	0	0	25	0
(*Tropicana*)	140	0	36.0	0	0	15	0
tropical (*Five Alive*)	110	0	29.0	0	0	25	0
frozen*:							
(*Five Alive*)	110	0	30.0	0	0	0	0
punch (*Minute Maid*)	120	0	31.0	0	0	5	0
tropical (*Five Alive*)	110	0	29.0	0	0	5	0
Clam, meat only:							
raw:							
4 oz.	84	14.5	2.9	1.1	39	64	0
9 large or 20 small, 6.3 oz.	133	23.0	4.6	1.8	60	100	0
boiled, poached, or steamed, 4 oz. . . .	168	29.0	5.8	2.2	76	127	0
Clam, canned, ¼ cup or 2 oz.:							
baby, whole (*S&W*)	50	8.0	2.0	1.5	40	260	0
chopped (*S&W*) . . .	20	4.0.	1.0	0	10	360	0
chopped or minced:							
(*Doxsee*)	25	4.0	2.0	0	10	320	0
(*Progresso*)	60	4.0	2.0	0	0	250	0
minced (*S&W*) . . .	20	8.0	1.0	0	10	360	0
smoked (*S&W*) . . .	130	9.0	2.0	10.0	20	220	0
Clam, fried, frozen, 3 oz.:							
(*Gorton's* Crunchy)	260	9.0	17.0	17.0	10	300	0

Food and Measure	cal.	prot. (gms)	carbo. (gms)	fat (gms)	chol. (mgs)	sod. (mgs)	fiber (gms)
(*Mrs. Paul's*)	280	23.0	28.0	15.0	10	480	1.0
Clam chowder, see "Soup"							
Clam dip, 2 tbsp.:							
(*Breakstone's* Chesapeake)	50	1.0	2.0	4.0	30	190	0
(*Heluva* Good New England)	50	1.0	2.0	4.5	20	130	0
(*Kraft*)	60	1.0	3.0	4.0	0	250	0
(*Kraft* Premium) . . .	45	1.0	2.0	4.0	10	210	0
(*Nalley*)	100	1.0	3.0	10.0	10	260	0
Clam juice:							
(*Bookbinder's*), 10.5 oz.	10	2.0	1.0	0	0	71	0
(*Doxsee*), 1 tbsp. . .	0	0	0	0	0	70	0
(*S&W*), 9.6 fl. oz. . .	20	8.0	0	0	0	740	0
Clam sauce, canned, ½ cup:							
creamy (*Progresso*)	100	5.0	8.0	6.0	10	560	0
red (*Progresso*) . . .	80	6.0	8.0	3.0	5	620	1.0
white:							
(*Bookbinder's*) . . .	300	4.0	4.0	30.0	0	860	<1.0
(*Progresso*)	120	10.0	1.0	9.0	15	310	0
(*Progresso* Authentic)	90	5.0	2.0	7.0	10	470	0
Clover seeds, sprouted, raw (*Shaw's*), 2 oz. . .	7	1.0	0	<1.0	0	40	3.0
Clover sprouts (*Jonathan's*), 1 cup, 3 oz.	25	3.0	3.0	.5	0	5	2.0
Cloves, ground:							
1 tbsp.	21	.4	4.0	1.3	0	16	<1.0
1 tsp.	7	.1	1.3	.4	0	5	.2
(*McCormick*), ¼ tsp.	1	0	.2	0	0	1	.1
Cobbler, frozen:							
apple:							
(*Marie Callender's*), 4¼ oz.	350	2.0	45.0	18.0	0	170	2.0

Food and Measure	cal.	prot. (gms)	carbo. (gms)	fat (gms)	chol. (mgs)	sod. (mgs)	fiber (gms)
Cobbler, apple *(cont.)*							
(*Pet-Ritz*), ⅙ pkg.	280	2.0	41.0	12.0	5	380	0
(*Stilwell*), ⅛ pkg.	240	2.0	39.0	9.0	0	370	3.0
(*Stilwell* Lite),							
⅛ pkg.	140	3.0	22.0	4.5	2	290	2.0
crumb (*Pet-Ritz*),							
⅙ pkg.	280	2.0	49.0	9.0	5	270	0
apricot (*Stilwell*),							
⅛ pkg.	240	3.0	39.0	9.0	0	230	3.0
berry:							
(*Marie Callender's*),							
4¼ oz.	390	3.0	41.0	19.0	0	170	1.0
(*Stilwell*), ⅛ pkg.	250	3.0	42.0	9.0	0	250	3.0
(*Stilwell* Lite),							
⅛ pkg.	140	3.0	22.0	4.5	0	140	2.0
blackberry:							
(*Pet-Ritz*), ⅙ pkg.	260	2.0	38.0	11.0	5	230	1.0
(*Stilwell*), ⅛ pkg.	250	3.0	39.0	9.0	0	220	4.0
(*Stilwell* Lite),							
⅛ pkg.	150	3.0	23.0	4.5	2	150	1.0
crumb (*Pet-Ritz*),							
⅙ pkg.	260	3.0	45.0	8.0	5	170	1.0
blueberry:							
(*Marie Callender's*),							
4 oz.	340	3.0	42.0	18.0	0	220	2.0
(*Pet-Ritz*), ⅙ pkg.	280	4.0	42.0	11.0	5	240	0
cherry:							
(*Marie Callender's*),							
4½ oz.	390	3.0	50.0	19.0	0	100	0
(*Pet-Ritz*), ⅙ pkg.	300	2.0	48.0	11.0	5	300	1.0
(*Stilwell*), ⅛ pkg.	250	3.0	39.0	9.0	0	280	3.0
(*Stilwell* Lite),							
⅛ pkg.	150	3.0	23.0	4.5	2	160	1.0
crumb (*Pet-Ritz*),							
⅙ pkg.	280	2.0	54.0	6.0	5	330	0
peach:							
(*Marie Callender's*),							
4¼ oz.	370	3.0	47.0	18.0	0	170	0
(*Pet-Ritz*), ⅙ pkg.	230	1.0	37.0	9.0	5	220	1.0

Food and Measure	cal.	prot. (gms)	carbo. (gms)	fat (gms)	chol. (mgs)	sod. (mgs)	fiber (gms)
(*Stilwell*), ⅛ pkg.	240	3.0	38.0	9.0	0	250	3.0
(*Stilwell* Lite), ⅛ pkg.	140	3.0	22.0	4.5	2	140	1.0
crumb (*Pet-Ritz*), ⅙ pkg.	230	2.0	38.0	7.0	5	170	1.0
strawberry:							
(*Pet-Ritz*), ⅙ pkg.	260	2.0	41.0	9.0	5	330	1.0
(*Stilwell*), ⅛ pkg.	260	3.0	41.0	9.0	0	200	3.0
Cobbler, freeze-dried, apple-blueberry (*AlpineAire*), ½ cup . .	210	2.0	46.0	2.0	0	2	n.a.
Cocktail sauce, see "Seafood sauce"							
Cocoa, baking:							
unsweetened, 1 tbsp.:							
(*Hershey's*)	20	1.0	3.0	.5	0	0	1.0
(*Ghirardelli*)	35	2.0	5.0	3.0	0	0	3.0
(*Nestlé* Baking) . .	15	1.0	3.0	1.0	0	0	2.0
sweetened (*Ghirardelli*), 2½ tbsp. . .	80	1.0	19.0	1.5	0	30	0
Cocoa mix, hot, 1 pkt., except as noted:							
(*Carnation* Fat Free)	25	2.0	4.0	0	0	135	1.0
(*Carnation* No Sugar)	50	4.0	8.0	0	<5	140	<1.0
(*Carnation* 70)	70	3.0	15.0	0	0	140	<1.0
(*Swiss Miss*)	140	2.0	27.0	3.0	<5	130	<1.0
(*Swiss Miss* Diet) . .	20	2.0	4.0	0	0	205	<1.0
(*Swiss Miss* Fat Free)	50	3.0	9.0	0	0	200	<1.0
(*Swiss Miss* Lite) . .	70	1.0	17.0	<1.0	0	200	2.0
(*Swiss Miss* Sugar Free), ¼ cup	70	3.0	13.0	0	0	240	1.0
(*Weight Watchers*) . .	70	6.0	10.0	0	0	160	1.0
almond mocha (*Swiss Miss* Premiere) . .	140	2.0	28.0	3.0	<5	210	1.5
chocolate:							
(*Land O Lakes*) . .	160	4.0	25.0	5.0	0	180	0

Food and Measure	cal.	prot. (gms)	carbo. (gms)	fat (gms)	chol. (mgs)	sod. (mgs)	fiber (gms)
Cocoa mix, chocolate *(cont.)*							
(*Swiss Miss* Sensa-							
tions)	150	2.0	27.0	4.0	0	170	1.5
cinnamon or rasp-							
berry (*Land O*							
Lakes)	160	4.0	25.0	5.0	0	180	0
double (*Ghirardelli*)	90	1.0	21.0	1.5	0	35	1.0
hazelnut (*Ghirardelli*)	90	1.0	21.0	1.5	0	35	1.0
Irish creme (*Nestlé*),							
3 tbsp.	90	2.0	16.0	1.5	0	85	<1.0
milk (*Carnation*),							
3 tbsp.	110	2.0	24.0	1.0	<5	95	<1.0
milk (*Swiss Miss*)	110	1.0	24.0	1.0	<5	140	<1.0
milk (*Swiss Miss*							
Sugar Free) . . .	50	2.0	10.0	0	0	180	<1.0
mint (*Land O Lakes*)	160	4.0	25.0	5.0	0	220	0
mocha (*Ghirardelli*)	90	1.0	21.0	2.0	0	35	1.0
raspberry truffle							
(*Swiss Miss* Pre-							
miere)	140	2.0	28.0	3.0	<5	220	1.5
rich (*Carnation*),							
3 tbsp.	110	1.0	24.0	1.0	<5	100	<1.0
rich (*Swiss Miss*)	110	2.0	24.0	1.0	0	170	<1.0
rich, w/marshmallow							
(*Carnation*),							
3 tbsp.	110	1.0	24.0	1.0	<5	95	<1.0
rich, w/ or w/out							
marshmallow							
(*Nestlé*)	110	1.0	24.0	1.0	0	60	<1.0
Suisse truffle (*Swiss*							
Miss Premiere)	140	2.0	28.0	2.0	<5	225	1.5
Swiss truffle (*Nes-*							
tlé), 3 tbsp. . . .	90	1.5	17.0	1.0	0	65	<1.0
toffee, English							
(*Swiss Miss* Pre-							
miere)	140	2.0	29.0	2.0	<5	225	0
white (*Ghirardelli*),							
2 tbsp.	90	0	23.0	0	0	0	0
white (*Swiss Miss*)	110	3.0	21.0	1.0	0	130	0

Food and Measure	cal.	prot. (gms)	carbo. (gms)	fat (gms)	chol. (mgs)	sod. (mgs)	fiber (gms)
and cream (*Swiss Miss*)	150	2.0	25.0	5.0	10	160	1.0
mini-marshmallow:							
(*Swiss Miss*)	110	1.0	24.0	1.0	0	150	<1.0
(*Swiss Miss* No Sugar)	50	1.0	11.0	<1.0	0	160	<1.0
Coconut:							
fresh, shelled:							
1 oz.	100	.9	4.3	9.5	0	6	2.6
shredded or grated, 1 cup not packed	283	2.7	12.2	26.8	0	16	7.2
canned, flaked:							
sweetened, ⅓ cup	114	.9	10.5	8.1	0	5	1.2
(*Angel Flake*), 2 tbsp.	70	1.0	7.0	5.0	0	0	1.0
(*Durkee*), 2 tbsp.	80	.5	6.0	6.09	0	25	2.0
dried, toasted, 1 oz.	168	1.5	12.6	13.4	0	11	.7
packaged, flaked:							
sweetened, ⅓ cup	117	.8	11.8	7.9	0	63	1.1
(*Angel Flake*), 2 tbsp.	70	1.0	7.0	4.5	0	45	1.0
(*Mounds*), 2 tbsp.	70	<1.0	8.0	4.5	0	45	1.0
shredded (*Baker's Premium*), 2 tbsp.	60	0	6.0	4.0	0	35	1.0
Coconut cream, canned:							
1 tbsp.	36	.5	1.6	3.4	0	10	.4
(*Coco Casa*), 3 tbsp.	170	0	35.0	3.0	0	90	1.0
(*Coco Goya*), 1 tbsp.	140	0	22.0	5.0	0	15	0
(*Coco Lopez*), 3 tbsp.	170	0	35.0	3.0	0	90	1.0
Coconut milk[1], 1 tbsp.	35	.3	.8	3.6	0	2	.3
Coconut milk, canned:							
(*Goya*), 1 tbsp. . . .	50	1.0	1.0	5.0	0	5	0
(*Taste of Thai*), ¼ cup	110	1.0	2.0	11.0	0	15	0

[1] *Liquid expressed from mixture of grated coconut and water.*

Food and Measure	cal.	prot. (gms)	carbo. (gms)	fat (gms)	chol. (mgs)	sod. (mgs)	fiber (gms)
Coconut milk, canned *(cont.)*							
light *(Taste of Thai)*,							
¼ cup	36	0	2.0	3.0	0	22	0
Coconut nectar							
(R. W. Knudsen),							
8 fl. oz.	140	1.0	26.0	0	0	5	0
Coconut water[1],							
1 tbsp.	3	.1	.6	<.1	0	16	.2
Cod, meat only:							
Atlantic:							
raw, 4 oz.	93	20.2	0	.8	49	62	0
baked, broiled, or							
microwaved, 4 oz.	119	25.9	0	1.0	62	88	0
Pacific:							
raw, 4 oz.	93	20.3	0	.7	42	81	0
baked, broiled, or							
microwaved, 4 oz.	119	26.0	0	.9	53	103	0
Cod, canned, Atlantic,							
w/liquid, 4 oz. . . .	119	25.8	0	1.0	62	247	0
Cod, dried, Atlantic,							
salted, 1 oz.	81	17.6	0	.7	42	1968	0
Cod, frozen, Pacific,							
loins *(Peter Pan)*,							
4 oz.	90	22.0	0	.5	35	85	0
Cod entree, frozen,							
breaded, 1 fillet:							
(Mrs. Paul's Pre-							
mium)	240	17.0	23.0	11.0	40	440	2.0
(Van de Kamp's Light)	220	14.0	19.0	10.0	35	410	n.a.
Cod liver oil, see							
"Oil"							
Codfish fritter mix,							
see "Bacalaitos"							
Coffee:							
brewed, 6 fl. oz. . . .	4	.1	.8	0	0	4	0
instant, regular,							
1 rounded tsp.* . .	4	.2	.7	tr.	0	1	0

[1] *Liquid from coconuts.*

Food and Measure	cal.	prot. (gms)	carbo. (gms)	fat (gms)	chol. (mgs)	sod. (mgs)	fiber (gms)
Coffee, flavored, see "Coffee, iced" and "Cappuccino"							
Coffee, flavored, mix, 8 fl. oz.*, except as noted:							
cafe Amaretto (*General Foods International*)	60	<1.0	8.0	3.0	0	105	0
cafe Français (*General Foods International*)	60	<1.0	7.0	3.5	0	25	0
cafe Vienna: (*General Foods International*)	70	<1.0	11.0	2.5	0	110	0
cappuccino: (*Nestlé* Instant), 1 pkt.	80	2.0	16.0	1.5	0	30	0
cinnamon (*Maxwell House*)	90	2.0	16.0	1.5	0	70	0
coffee (*Maxwell House*)	90	1.0	18.0	1.0	0	65	0
Italian (*General Foods International*)	50	<1.0	10.0	1.5	0	50	0
mocha (*Maxwell House*)	100	2.0	17.0	2.5	0	70	0
mocha (*Nestlé*), 1 pkt.	110	3.0	21.0	2.0	0	30	<1.0
orange (*General Foods International*)	70	<1.0	11.0	2.0	0	100	0
vanilla (*Maxwell House*)	90	1.0	19.0	1.0	0	65	0
chocolate, Viennese (*General Foods International*)	60	<1.0	10.0	2.0	0	30	0
hazelnut, Belgian (*General Foods International*)	70	<1.0	12.0	2.0	0	65	0

Food and Measure	cal.	prot. (gms)	carbo. (gms)	fat (gms)	chol. (mgs)	sod. (mgs)	fiber (gms)
Coffee, flavored, mix (cont.)							
Kahlua Cafe (General Foods International)	60	<1.0	10.0	2.0	0	55	0
mocha, cafe (Carnation Instant Breakfast)	130	4.0	28.0	.5	<5	100	<1.0
mocha, Suisse (General Foods International)	60	<1.0	8.0	2.5	0	50	0
vanilla, French (General Foods International)	60	<1.0	10.0	2.5	0	55	0
Coffee, iced (see also "Cappuccino"), canned, 11-oz. can:							
(Jamaican Gold) . . .	140	3.0	29.0	2.5	0	40	0
latte (Jamaican Gold)	140	3.0	27.0	2.5	0	40	0
Coffee creamer, see "Creamer, nondairy"							
Coffee substitute, cereal grain:							
1 tsp.	9	.1	1.9	.1	0	2	0
(Kaffree Roma), 1 tsp.	10	0	2.0	0	0	0	0
regular or coffee flavor (Postum Instant)	10	0	3.0	0	0	110	0
Cold cuts, see specific listings							
Coleslaw, salad blend mix (Dole), 3.5 oz.	30	1.0	5.0	.5	0	35	2.0
Collard greens, ½ cup, except as noted:							
fresh:							
raw, 1 oz.	9	.4	2.0	.1	0	6	1.0
raw, chopped . . .	6	.3	1.3	<.1	0	4	.7
boiled, drained, chopped	17	.9	3.9	.1	0	10	1.3

Food and Measure	cal.	prot. (gms)	carbo. (gms)	fat (gms)	chol. (mgs)	sod. (mgs)	fiber (gms)
canned (*Allens/Sunshine*)	30	1.0	5.0	.5	0	20	3.0
frozen, chopped, boiled, drained . . .	31	2.5	6.1	.4	0	42	n.a.
Cookie, 1 pc., except as noted:							
almond:							
(*Archway* Crescents), 2 pcs., .8 oz.	100	1.0	17.0	3.5	<5	75	<1.0
(*Stella D'Oro* Breakfast Treats), .8-oz. pc.	100	1.0	16.0	3.0	10	80	<1.0
(*Stella D'Oro* Chinese Dessert), 1.2-oz. pc.	170	2.0	21.0	2.0	5	90	<1.0
(*Sunshine* Crescents), 4 pcs., 1.1 oz.	150	2.0	22.0	6.0	0	105	<1.0
toast (*Stella D'Oro* Mandel), 2 pcs., 1 oz.	110	2.0	21.0	2.5	30	85	1.0
amaretti di Saronno, chocolate dipped (*Lazzaroni*), 4 pcs., 1.1 oz.	140	1.0	22.0	5.0	0	10	0
animal, 1.1 oz.:							
(*Barnum's Animals*)	140	2.0	23.0	4.0	0	160	1.0
(*Sunshine*)	140	2.0	24.0	4.0	0	125	<1.0
animal, vanilla (*Barbara's*), 8 pcs., 1 oz.	130	2.0	20.0	5.0	0	105	1.0
anisette:							
(*Stella D'Oro* Sponge), 2 pcs., 1 oz.	90	2.0	19.0	1.0	40	80	<1.0
(*Stella D'Oro* Toast), 3 pcs., 1.2 oz. . . .	130	2.0	27.0	1.0	35	150	<1.0

Food and Measure	cal.	prot. (gms)	carbo. (gms)	fat (gms)	chol. (mgs)	sod. (mgs)	fiber (gms)
Cookie, anisette *(cont.)*							
(*Stella D'Oro* Toast Jumbo), 1 pc., 1.1 oz.	100	2.0	23.0	.5	15	65	<1.0
apple:							
(*Newtons* Fat Free), 2 pcs., 1 oz. . . .	100	1.0	24.0	0	0	60	1.0
(*Sunshine* Golden Fruit)	80	1.0	15.0	1.5	0	40	<1.0
bar (*Archway* Nonfat)	60	<1.0	15.0	0	0	30	0
bran (*Archway*) . .	130	2.0	27.0	1.5	0	140	2.0
cinnamon bar (*Tastykake*)	180	2.0	29.0	7.0	0	160	1.0
pastry (*Stella D'Oro* Low Sodium) . .	80	1.0	14.0	2.5	<5	5	1.0
and raisin (*Archway*)	130	2.0	20.0	4.5	<5	105	1.0
raisin (*Health Valley* Fat Free Jumbo)	80	2.0	19.0	0	0	35	3.0
raisin bar (*Smart Snackers*)	70	1.0	14.0	2.0	0	60	2.0
spice (*Health Valley* Fat Free), 3 pcs.	100	2.0	24.0	0	0	50	3.0
apricot:							
filled (*Archway*) . .	110	1.0	18.0	4.0	5	90	<1.0
raspberry (*Pepperidge Farm*), 3 pcs., 1.1 oz.	140	2.0	22.0	6.0	5	110	<1.0
apricot or date (*Health Valley* Nonfat), 3 pcs.	100	2.0	24.0	0	0	50	3.0
(*Archway* Bells and Stars), 3 pcs. . . .	150	1.0	19.0	7.0	5	100	<1.0
(*Archway* Old Fashion Windmill)	100	1.0	15.0	4.0	0	95	0
(*Archway* Party Treats), 3 pcs. . . .	140	2.0	20.0	7.0	15	105	0
arrowroot (*National*)	20	0	3.0	.5	0	15	0

Food and Measure	cal.	prot. (gms)	carbo. (gms)	fat (gms)	chol. (mgs)	sod. (mgs)	fiber (gms)
banana bran (*Archway* Low Fat)	120	2.0	27.0	1.5	0	115	2.0
biscotti:							
all varieties (*Health Valley*), 2 pcs. . .	120	3.0	23.0	3.0	0	50	3.0
almond (*Pepperidge Farm Caruso*) . .	90	2.0	12.0	3.5	5	65	<1.0
anise (*Pepperidge Farm La Scala*)	90	2.0	14.0	3.0	5	75	0
chocolate dipped (*Pepperidge Farm Figaro*)	110	2.0	14.0	4.0	10	70	1.0
cranberry pistachio (*Pepperidge Farm Tosca*)	90	2.0	13.0	3.0	5	65	<1.0
biscottini cashews (*Stella D'Oro*) . . .	110	1.0	13.0	6.0	5	50	<1.0
blueberry:							
(*Archway*)	110	1.0	19.0	4.0	5	115	<1.0
(*Fruitastic* Bar) . . .	40	0	13.0	0	0	60	1.0
brown edge wafer (*Nabisco*), 5 pcs.	140	1.0	21.0	9.0	<5	35	<1.0
butter (see also "shortbread," below):							
(*Master Choice* Southern Classics), 10 pcs. . .	150	1.0	20.0	7.0	15	160	0
(*Peak Freans* Petit Beurre), 4 pcs.	130	2.0	22.0	4.0	<5	115	<1.0
(*Pepperidge Farm* Madaillon au Beurre), 4 pcs.	150	2.0	25.0	5.0	15	105	<1.0
(*Pepperidge Farm* Chessman), 3 pcs.	120	2.0	18.0	5.0	20	80	<1.0
(*Sunshine*), 5 pcs.	140	2.0	21.0	6.0	<5	135	<1.0

Food and Measure	cal.	prot. (gms)	carbo. (gms)	fat (gms)	chol. (mgs)	sod. (mgs)	fiber (gms)
Cookie, butter *(cont.)*							
assorted (*Pepperidge Farm* Toy Chest), 3 pcs. . . .	120	2.0	18.0	5.0	20	80	<1.0
sandwich w/fudge (*E. L. Fudge*), 3 pcs.	170	2.0	24.0	8.0	<5	105	<1.0
butter pecan bites (*Barbara's Small Indulgences*), 6 pcs.	140	2.0	16.0	8.0	20	95	0
caramel:							
apple (*Barbara's* Fat Free Mini), 6 pcs.	110	1.0	22.0	0	0	130	0
pecan (*Pepperidge Farm*)	130	2.0	16.0	7.0	20	55	<1. 0
carrot cake (*Archway*)	120	1.0	18.0	5.0	<5	180	0
cherry:							
cobbler (*Pepperidge Farm*)	70	<1.0	11.0	2.5	<5	45	0
filled (*Archway*) . .	110	1.0	19.0	4.0	10	100	<1.0
cherry nougat (*Archway*), 3 pcs.	150	1.0	18.0	9.0	0	40	0
chocolate:							
(*Archway* Fat Free)	90	1.0	19.0	0	0	105	<1.0
(*Pepperidge Farm Goldfish*), 1.1 oz.	140	2.0	22.0	5.0	10	85	2.0
(*Stella D'Oro* Castelets), 2 pcs. . .	130	2.0	19.0	6.0	<5	65	<1.0
(*Stella D'Oro* Margherite), 2 pcs.	150	2.0	18.0	7.0	<5	80	1.0
bits (*Grandma's*), 9 pcs.	170	2.0	24.0	8.0	0	230	1.0
brownie (*Entenmann's* Fat Free), 2 pcs. . . .	80	1.0	20.0	0	0	90	1.0
brownie nut (*Pepperidge Farm*), 3 pcs.	160	2.0	18.0	9.0	15	115	2.0

Food and Measure	cal.	prot. (gms)	carbo. (gms)	fat (gms)	chol. (mgs)	sod. (mgs)	fiber (gms)
caramel or fudge center (*Health Valley* Fat Free), 2 pcs.	70	2.0	17.0	0	0	20	3.0
covered (*Ritz*), 3 pcs.	150	2.0	17.0	9.0	0	95	1.0
dark (*Pepperidge Farm* Espirits Noir)	90	1.0	10.0	5.0	10	50	0
double (*Barbara's* Fat Free Mini), 6 pcs.	90	2.0	20.0	0	0	130	0
fudge (*Dare*)	97	1.1	13.0	4.8	1	38	.5
fudge, iced (*Tastykake*)	170	4.0	25.0	7.0	55	190	1.0
fudge mint (*Grasshopper*), 4 pcs.	150	1.0	20.0	7.0	0	70	<1.0
laced (*Pepperidge Farm Pirouette*), 5 pcs.	180	2.0	20.0	10.0	5	90	<1.0
milk, peanut butter (*Pepperidge Farm Chocolate Heaven*), 2 pcs.	130	2.0	15.0	7.0	<5	50	<1.0
w/nuts (*Pepperidge Farm Geneva*), 3 pcs.	160	2.0	19.0	9.0	0	95	1.0
orange (*Pepperidge Farm* Chocolat a l'Orange), 2 pcs.	150	2.0	23.0	6.0	<5	20	0
snaps (*Nabisco*), 7 pcs.	140	2.0	23.0	5.0	0	180	1.0
wafer (*Nabisco* Famous), 5 pcs. . .	140	2.0	24.0	4.0	<5	230	1.0
wafer, light (*Keebler*), 8 pcs. . . .	130	1.0	25.0	3.5	0	170	0
chocolate chip/chunk: (*Archway*)	130	1.0	19.0	6.0	<5	150	0

Food and Measure	cal.	prot. (gms)	carbo. (gms)	fat (gms)	chol. (mgs)	sod. (mgs)	fiber (gms)
Cookie, chocolate chip/chunk *(cont.)*							
(*Archway* Bag), 3 pcs.	130	1.0	17.0	7.0	10	70	0
(*Archway* Ice Box)	140	1.0	19.0	7.0	5	80	0
(*Barbara's*), 2 pcs.	170	3.0	25.0	7.0	0	90	3.0
(*Chip-A-Roos*), 3 pcs.	190	2.0	23.0	10.0	0	150	1.0
(*Chips Ahoy!* Chewy), 3 pcs.	170	1.0	23.0	8.0	<5	125	<1.0
(*Chips Ahoy!* Chunky)	80	1.0	11.0	4.0	10	60	<1.0
(*Chips Ahoy!* Mini), 14 pcs.	150	2.0	21.0	7.0	0	105	<1.0
(*Chips Ahoy!* Real Chocolate), 3 pcs.	160	2.0	21.0	8.0	0	105	1.0
(*Chips Ahoy!* Reduced Fat), 3 pcs.	150	2.0	23.0	6.0	0	150	1.0
(*Chips Deluxe*) . . .	80	1.0	9.0	4.5	0	60	0
(*Chips Deluxe* Chocolate Lovers) . .	90	<1.0	11.0	5.0	10	75	<1.0
(*Chips Deluxe* Light)	70	<1.0	11.0	3.0	0	70	<1.0
(*Dare*)	77	.9	9.2	4.1	2	42	.4
(*Dare Breaktime*)	37	.4	5.0	1.7	0	37	.1
(*Entenmann's*), 3 pcs.	140	1.0	20.0	7.0	10	90	<1.0
(*Grandma's* Big) . .	190	2.0	25.0	9.0	<5	130	1.0
(*Little Debbie*), 2 pcs.	180	2.0	24.0	9.0	5	130	1.0
(*Pepperidge Farm* Old Fashioned), 3 pcs.	140	2.0	18.0	7.0	10	65	<1.0
(*Pepperidge Farm* Chesapeake) . . .	140	2.0	15.0	8.0	10	100	<1.0
(*Pepperidge Farm* Goldfish), 1.1 oz.	150	2.0	21.0	7.0	20	50	1.0
(*Pepperidge Farm* Nantucket) . . .	130	1.0	16.0	7.0	10	75	<1.0
(*Smart Snackers*), 1.06 oz.	140	2.0	22.0	5.0	0	90	1.0

Food and Measure	cal.	prot. (gms)	carbo. (gms)	fat (gms)	chol. (mgs)	sod. (mgs)	fiber (gms)
(*Snackwell's* Reduced Fat),							
13 pcs.	130	2.0	22.0	3.5	0	170	1.0
(*Tastykake*)	180	2.0	26.0	7.0	10	160	1.0
all varieties (*Health Valley Healthy Chips* Fat Free),							
3 pcs.	100	3.0	24.0	0	0	20	4.0
bar (*Tastykake*) . .	200	2.0	30.0	8.0	5	85	1.0
chocolate (*Barbara's*), 2 pcs. . .	150	3.0	23.0	7.0	0	80	3.0
chocolate, walnut, soft (*Pepperidge Farm*)	130	2.0	16.0	6.0	5	45	1.0
crisps (*Barbara's Small Indulgences*), 6 pcs.	140	2.0	18.0	7.0	15	105	0
drop (*Archway*) . .	140	2.0	11.0	10.0	10	105	<1.0
fudge (*Grandma's Big*)	170	2.0	27.0	6.0	<5	160	1.0
fudge bar (*Grandma's*) . . .	190	2.0	29.0	7.0	10	160	1.0
macadamia (*Pepperidge Farm Sausalito*)	140	2.0	16.0	7.0	10	110	<1.0
macadamia, soft (*Pepperidge Farm*)	130	1.0	16.0	6.0	10	55	1.0
macadamia, white (*Pepperidge Farm Tahoe*)	130	2.0	16.0	7.0	15	110	<1.0
mini (*Sunshine*), 5 pcs.	160	2.0	20.0	8.0	0	120	<1.0
rainbow (*Chips Deluxe*)	80	1.0	10.0	4.0	<5	45	<1.0
snaps (*Nabisco*), 7 pcs.	150	2.0	24.0	5.0	0	115	<1.0
soft (*Chips Deluxe*)	70	1.0	10.0	3.5	5	50	0
soft (*Pepperidge Farm* Chunk) . .	130	1.0	16.0	6.0	10	35	2.0

Food and Measure	cal.	prot. (gms)	carbo. (gms)	fat (gms)	chol. (mgs)	sod. (mgs)	fiber (gms)
Cookie, chocolate chip/chunk *(cont.)*							
sprinkled (*Chips Ahoy!*), 3 pcs. . . .	170	2.0	24.0	8.0	0	120	<1.0
striped (*Chips Ahoy!*)	80	1.0	10.0	4.0	0	45	<1.0
and toffee (*Archway*)	140	1.0	19.0	7.0	<5	120	<1.0
toffee (*Pepperidge Farm Charleston*)	130	1.0	16.0	7.0	20	110	<1.0
walnut (*Pepperidge Farm Beacon Hill*)	130	2.0	16.0	7.0	5	100	<1.0
chocolate sandwich:							
(*Elfin Delights Light*), 2 pcs. . .	110	1.0	19.0	2.5	0	120	<1.0
(*Hydrox*), 3 pcs. . . .	150	2.0	21.0	7.0	0	125	1.0
(*Hydrox* Fat Free), 3 pcs.	130	1.0	24.0	4.0	0	140	1.0
(*Oreo*), 3 pcs. . . .	160	2.0	23.0	7.0	0	220	1.0
(*Oreo* Reduced Fat), 3 pcs.	140	2.0	24.0	6.0	0	70	<1.0
(*Oreo Double Stuf*), 2 pcs.	140	1.0	19.0	7.0	0	150	<1.0
(*Pepperidge Farm Bordeaux*), 4 pcs.	130	2.0	20.0	5.0	10	95	<1.0
(*Pepperidge Farm Brussels*), 3 pcs.	150	2.0	20.0	7.0	5	80	1.0
(*Pepperidge Farm Lido*)	90	<1.0	11.0	4.5	5	45	0
(*Pepperidge Farm Milano*), 3 pcs.	180	2.0	21.0	10.0	10	80	<1.0
(*Smart Snackers*), 1.06 oz.	140	2.0	23.0	3.5	0	160	1.0
(*Snackwell's* Reduced Fat), 2 pcs.	100	1.0	20.0	2.5	0	190	1.0
(*Vienna Fingers* Reduced Fat), 2 pcs.	120	2.0	22.0	3.5	0	115	<1.0
chocolate fudge (*Keebler Classic Collection*)	80	1.0	12.0	3.5	0	75	0

Food and Measure	cal.	prot. (gms)	carbo. (gms)	fat (gms)	chol. (mgs)	sod. (mgs)	fiber (gms)
chocolate fudge, double (*Barbara's Cookies & Creme*), 2 pcs.	120	2.0	17.0	5.0	15	80	<1.0
double (*Pepperidge Farm Milano*), 2 pcs.	150	2.0	17.0	8.0	10	70	<1.0
fudge coated (*Oreo*)	110	1.0	14.0	6.0	0	85	<1.0
hazelnut (*Pepperidge Farm Milano*), 2 pcs. . . .	130	2.0	15.0	7.0	5	65	1.0
milk (*Pepperidge Farm Bordeaux*), 3 pcs.	160	2.0	19.0	9.0	0	95	0
milk (*Pepperidge Farm Milano*), 3 pcs.	180	2.0	21.0	10.0	10	80	<1.0
mint (*Pepperidge Farm Brussels*), 3 pcs.	190	2.0	22.0	10.0	0	100	1.0
mint (*Pepperidge Farm Milano*), 2 pcs.	140	1.0	16.0	8.0	<5	70	<1.0
orange (*Pepperidge Farm Milano*), 2 pcs.	140	1.0	16.0	8.0	5	70	<1.0
raspberry or vanilla (*Barbara's Cookies & Creme*), 2 pcs.	120	2.0	18.0	5.0	15	80	<1.0
white fudge coated (*Oreo*)	110	1.0	14.0	6.0	0	70	<1.0
cinnamon:							
apple (*Archway*) . .	110	1.0	20.0	3.5	5	135	<1.0
honey heart (*Archway* Fat Free), 3 pcs.	100	1.0	24.0	0	0	115	<1.0
snaps (*Archway*), 5 pcs.	150	1.0	20.0	7.0	<5	120	0

Food and Measure	cal.	prot. (gms)	carbo. (gms)	fat (gms)	chol. (mgs)	sod. (mgs)	fiber (gms)
Cookie (cont.)							
cocoa:							
Dutch (*Archway*) . .	120	1.0	19.0	4.0	<5	110	0
mocha (*Barbara's Fat Free Mini*),							
6 pcs.	100	2.0	21.0	0	0	130	0
coconut:							
(*Dare Breaktime*)	35	.5	5.2	1.4	0	15	.1
macaroon (*Archway*)	90	1.0	14.0	5.0	0	55	2.0
coffee cake crunch (*Barbara's Small Indulgences*), 6 pcs.	130	2.0	18.0	6.0	20	140	0
cranberry bar:							
(*Archway* Fat Free)	70	<1.0	16.0	0	0	25	<1.0
(*Newtons* Fat Free), 2 pcs.	100	1.0	23.0	0	0	95	1.0
(*Sunshine* Golden Fruit)	70	1.0	15.0	1.0	0	55	<1.0
Danish (*Nabisco* Import), 5 pcs.	170	2.0	22.0	8.0	0	80	1.0
devil's food cake (*Snackwell's* Fat Free)	50	1.0	13.0	0	0	25	<1.0
egg biscuit:							
(*Stella D'Oro* Jumbo), 2 pcs.	90	2.0	18.0	1.0	30	60	<1.0
(*Stella D'Oro* Low Sodium), 3 pcs.	120	4.0	20.0	3.0	40	15	1.0
Roman (*Stella D'Oro*)	140	2.0	21.0	5.0	20	125	<1.0
fig:							
(*Archway* Fat Free)	80	<1.0	15.0	0	0	40	<1.0
(*Fig Newtons*), 2 pcs.	110	1.0	20.0	2.5	0	120	1.0
(*Fig Newtons* Fat Free), 2 pcs. . . .	100	1.0	22.0	0	0	115	2.0
(*Smart Snackers*)	70	1.0	16.0	0	0	50	0
(*Sunshine* Bar), 2 pcs.	110	1.0	20.0	2.5	0	60	1.0

Food and Measure	cal.	prot. (gms)	carbo. (gms)	fat (gms)	chol. (mgs)	sod. (mgs)	fiber (gms)
(*Sunshine* Golden Fruit Fat Free) . .	60	<1.0	13.0	0	0	50	<1.0
fortune (*La Choy*), 4 pcs.	110	2.0	26.0	0	0	10	<1.0
fruit:							
bar (*Archway* Fat Free), ½ pc. . . .	90	2.0	21.0	0	0	95	0
cake (*Archway*), 3 pcs.	140	2.0	20.0	7.0	0	100	2.0
Hawaiian (*Health Valley* Fat Free), 3 pcs.	100	2.0	24.0	0	0	50	3.0
honey bar (*Archway*)	110	1.0	18.0	4.0	5	120	<1.0
slices (*Stella D'Oro* Fat Free)	50	1.0	12.0	0	0	50	1.0
fudge:							
(*Stella D'Oro* Swiss), 2 pcs. . .	130	1.0	17.0	6.0	15	65	<1.0
bar (*Tastykake*) . .	190	2.0	29.0	7.0	5	100	1.0
double, cake (*Snackwell's* Fat Free)	50	1.0	12.0	0	0	70	<1.0
fudge filled (*Keebler* Truffles), 3 pcs.	180	1.0	22.0	10.0	0	105	<1.0
mint patties (*Sunshine*), 2 pcs. . .	130	1.0	16.0	7.0	0	60	<1.0
nut bar (*Archway*)	110	2.0	17.0	4.5	<5	120	<1.0
nutty (*Grandma's* Big)	190	3.0	25.0	8.0	<5	150	1.0
ginger:							
(*Dare Breaktime*)	34	.4	5.7	1.1	0	<15	n.a.
(*Pepperidge Farm* Gingerman), 4 pcs.	120	2.0	21.0	3.5	10	95	<1.0
ginger snaps:							
(*Archway*), 5 pcs.	140	1.0	18.0	5.0	0	110	0
(*Nabisco*), 4 pcs.	120	1.0	22.0	2.5	0	170	<1.0
(*Sunshine*), 7 pcs.	130	2.0	22.0	4.5	0	150	<1.0

Food and Measure	cal.	prot. (gms)	carbo. (gms)	fat (gms)	chol. (mgs)	sod. (mgs)	fiber (gms)
Cookie *(cont.)*							
gingerbread, iced:							
(*Archway*), 3 pcs.	140	1.0	23.0	5.0	5	130	0
(*Sunshine*), 5 pcs.	130	2.0	19.0	6.0	5	135	<1.0
golden bar (*Stella D'Oro*)	110	2.0	17.0	3.5	20	65	0
graham:							
(*Bugs Bunny*), 10 pcs.	140	2.0	23.0	5.0	0	180	1.0
(*Keebler*), 8 pcs. . . .	130	2.0	23.0	3.0	0	135	<1.0
(*Nabisco*), 8 pcs.	120	2.0	22.0	3.0	0	180	1.0
(*Pepperidge Farm Goldfish*), 1.1 oz.	150	2.0	20.0	7.0	15	150	2.0
amaranth or oat bran (*Health Valley* Fat Free), 11 pcs.	100	4.0	23.0	0	0	30	3.0
chocolate (*Bugs Bunny*), 13 pcs.	140	2.0	22.0	5.0	0	180	1.0
chocolate (*Keebler*), 8 pcs.	140	2.0	22.0	5.0	0	125	<1.0
chocolate (*Nabisco Pure*), 3 pcs. . .	160	2.0	21.0	8.0	0	90	1.0
chocolate (*Teddy Grahams* Snacks), 24 pcs.	140	2.0	22.0	5.0	0	150	1.0
chocolate-coated (*Dunkaroos*), 1-oz. tray	120	1.0	20.0	4.5	0	85	<1.0
cinnamon (*Bugs Bunny*), 13 pcs.	140	2.0	23.0	4.5	0	160	<1.0
cinnamon (*Honey Maid*), 10 pcs.	140	2.0	26.0	3.0	0	210	1.0
cinnamon (*Keebler Light*), 8 pcs. . .	110	2.0	24.0	1.5	0	190	1.0
cinnamon (*Pepperidge Farm Goldfish*), 1.1 oz.	150	2.0	20.0	7.0	10	140	2.0

Food and Measure	cal.	prot. (gms)	carbo. (gms)	fat (gms)	chol. (mgs)	sod. (mgs)	fiber (gms)
cinnamon (*Snackwell's* Fat Free Snacks), 20 pcs.	110	2.0	26.0	0	0	90	1.0
cinnamon (*Sunshine*), 2 pcs. . .	140	2.0	22.0	6.0	0	150	<1.0
cinnamon (*Teddy Grahams* Snacks), 24 pcs.	140	2.0	23.0	4.0	0	150	1.0
French vanilla (*Keebler* Light), 8 pcs.	110	2.0	24.0	1.5	0	140	<1.0
fudge coated (*Keebler* Deluxe), 3 pcs.	140	1.0	19.0	7.0	0	105	<1.0
fudge coated (*Nabisco* Family Favorites), 3 pcs.	140	2.0	19.0	7.0	0	125	1.0
fudge coated, marshmallow filled (*Keebler* S'mores), 3 pcs.	150	1.0	21.0	7.0	0	90	<1.0
fudge dipped (*Sunshine*), 4 pcs. . .	170	2.0	21.0	9.0	0	75	1.0
honey (*Honey Maid*), 8 pcs. . .	120	2.0	22.0	3.0	0	180	1.0
honey (*Keebler* Light), 9 pcs. . .	120	2.0	25.0	1.5	0	210	1.0
honey (*Sunshine*), 2 pcs.	120	2.0	20.0	4.0	0	130	1.0
honey (*Teddy Grahams* Snacks), 24 pcs.	140	2.0	22.0	4.0	0	150	1.0
granola: (*Archway* Fat Free), 2 pcs.	100	1.0	24.0	0	0	120	1.0
soft (*Grandma's* Bar)	180	3.0	29.0	6.0	15	260	2.0
hazelnut (*Pepperidge Farm*), 3 pcs. . . .	160	2.0	21.0	8.0	0	135	<1.0

Food and Measure	cal.	prot. (gms)	carbo. (gms)	fat (gms)	chol. (mgs)	sod. (mgs)	fiber (gms)
Cookie *(cont.)*							
hermits *(Archway Cookie Jar)*	110	1.0	19.0	3.0	<5	160	<1.0
(Heyday Bar)	110	2.0	13.0	5.0	0	40	<1.0
kichel *(Stella D'Oro Low Sodium),* 21 pcs.	150	4.0	13.0	9.0	80	25	<1.0
lemon:							
(Sunshine Coolers), 5 pcs.	140	1.0	21.0	6.0	0	100	<1.0
almond *(Barbara's Small Indul-gences),* 6 pcs.	140	2.0	18.0	6.0	20	135	0
bits *(Grandma's),* 9 pcs.	150	2.0	21.0	6.0	<5	90	<1.0
creme *(Dare)* . . .	95	1.0	13.0	4.5	1	36	.2
drop *(Archway)* . .	110	1.0	18.0	3.5	5	120	0
frosty *(Archway)* . .	120	1.0	19.0	5.0	0	110	0
nuggets *(Archway Fat Free),* 5 pcs.	100	1.0	22.0	0	0	130	0
nut crunch *(Pepper-idge Farm),* 3 pcs.	170	2.0	18.0	9.0	15	60	2.0
sandwich *(Barbara's Cookies & Creme),* 2 pcs.	120	1.0	18.0	5.0	15	75	0
snaps *(Archway),* 5 pcs.	150	1.0	20.0	7.0	<5	115	0
marshmallow:							
chocolate *(Mal-lomars),* 2 pcs.	120	1.0	17.0	5.0	0	35	1.0
chocolate *(Pin-wheels)*	130	1.0	21.0	5.0	0	35	<1.0
fudge puffs *(Nabisco)*	90	1.0	14.0	4.0	0	45	0
fudge twirls *(Nabisco)*	130	1.0	20.0	6.0	0	75	<1.0
mint sandwich *(Mys-tic Mint)*	90	1.0	11.0	4.0	0	65	0

Food and Measure	cal.	prot. (gms)	carbo. (gms)	fat (gms)	chol. (mgs)	sod. (mgs)	fiber (gms)
molasses:							
(*Archway*)	110	1.0	20.0	3.5	10	150	<1.0
(*Archway* Low Fat)	100	2.0	22.0	1.0	0	95	1.0
(*Archway* Old Fashion)	120	1.0	20.0	3.0	5	150	0
(*Archway* Super Pak)	110	1.0	20.0	3.5	10	170	<1.0
(*Grandma's* Old Time Big)	160	2.0	29.0	4.0	<5	230	<1.0
crisps (*Pepperidge Farm*), 5 pcs. . .	150	2.0	20.0	6.0	0	140	<1.0
dark (*Archway*) . .	110	1.0	20.0	3.5	<5	150	<1.0
drop, soft (*Archway*)	110	1.0	18.0	3.5	<5	160	<1.0
iced (*Archway* Iowa)	140	1.0	20.0	4.0	5	135	<1.0
iced (*Archway* Ohio)	110	1.0	19.0	3.5	0	170	<1.0
iced (*Archway* Super Pak)	120	2.0	19.0	5.0	<5	85	1.0
mud pie (*Archway*)	110	2.0	18.0	4.0	<5	110	2.0
New Orleans cake (*Archway*)	110	1.0	18.0	4.0	<5	105	<1.0
nut:							
(*Archway* Nutty Nougat), 3 pcs.	160	1.0	18.0	10.0	0	60	0
(*Little Debbie Nutty Bars*), 2 pcs. . .	180	3.0	18.0	12.0	0	75	2.0
oatmeal:							
(*Archway*)	110	2.0	19.0	3.0	<5	95	<1.0
(*Dare Breaktime*)	35	.5	5.0	1.3	0	27	.2
(*Nabisco* Family Favorites)	80	1.0	12.0	3.0	0	65	<1.0
(*Ruth's*)	120	2.0	19.0	4.5	<5	135	<1.0
(*Ruth's* Golden) . .	120	2.0	19.0	5.0	<5	135	<1.0
(*Sunshine* Country), 3 pcs.	170	2.0	24.0	7.0	0	160	1.0
apple filled (*Archway*)	110	1.0	18.0	3.0	<5	105	0
apple spice (*Grandma's* Big)	170	2.0	26.0	6.0	<5	220	2.0

Food and Measure	cal.	prot. (gms)	carbo. (gms)	fat (gms)	chol. (mgs)	sod. (mgs)	fiber (gms)
Cookie, oatmeal *(cont.)*							
apple spice bar							
(*Grandma's*) . . .	170	2.0	28.0	5.0	10	270	1.0
butterscotch (*Pepperidge Farm*),							
3 pcs.	170	2.0	22.0	9.0	10	110	1.0
chewy (*Master Choice*)	80	2.0	9.0	4.0	2	65	<1.0
chocolate chip (*Entenmann's* Fat Free), 2 pcs. . . .	80	1.0	19.0	0	0	110	1.0
chocolate chip (*Sunshine*), 3 pcs. . .	170	3.0	23.0	8.0	0	130	2.0
date filled (*Archway*)	110	2.0	18.0	4.0	<5	120	<1.0
iced (*Archway*) . . .	120	2.0	19.0	5.0	<5	85	1.0
iced (*Sunshine*), 2 pcs.	120	2.0	18.0	5.0	0	90	<1.0
Irish (*Pepperidge Farm*), 3 pcs. . .	130	2.0	19.0	6.0	<5	70	2.0
pecan (*Archway*) . .	120	2.0	18.0	5.0	<5	100	1.0
raspberry (*Archway Fat Free*)	100	1.0	24.0	0	0	170	<1.0
oatmeal raisin:							
(*Archway*)	110	2.0	19.0	4.0	<5	115	<1.0
(*Archway* Bag), 3 pcs.	130	2.0	19.0	6.0	10	55	1.0
(*Archway* Fat Free)	100	1.0	23.0	0	0	170	<1.0
(*Barbara's*), 2 pcs.	160	3.0	24.0	7.0	0	70	2.0
(*Barbara's* Fat Free Mini), 6 pcs. . .	110	2.0	22.0	0	0	130	0
(*Entenmann's* Fat ·Free), 2 pcs. . . .	80	1.0	18.0	0	0	120	<1.0
(*Health Valley* Fat Free), 3 pcs. . . .	100	2.0	24.0	0	0	50	3.0
(*Little Debbie*), 2 pcs.	170	2.0	25.0	7.0	0	170	1.0
(*Pepperidge Farm* Old Fashioned), 3 pcs.	160	2.0	23.0	6.0	10	150	1.0

Food and Measure	cal.	prot. (gms)	carbo. (gms)	fat (gms)	chol. (mgs)	sod. (mgs)	fiber (gms)
(*Pepperidge Farm Soft*)	110	1.0	17.0	4.0	15	60	1.0
(*Pepperidge Farm Santa Fe*)	120	2.0	18.0	4.5	<5	110	<1.0
(*Smart Snackers*), 1.1 oz.	120	2.0	22.0	2.0	0	90	1.0
(*Snackwell's* Reduced Fat), 2 pcs.	110	2.0	20.0	2.5	0	135	1.0
(*Tastykake* Bar) . .	190	3.0	28.0	7.0	15	180	1.0
bran (*Archway*) . .	110	2.0	19.0	3.5	<5	100	<1.0
iced (*Tastykake*) . .	170	3.0	27.0	6.0	25	150	1.0
peach tart (*Pepperidge Farm*), 2 pcs.	120	1.0	23.0	3.0	0	115	<1.0
peach-apricot (*Stella D'Oro* Sodium Free)	80	1.0	13.0	3.0	<5	0	<1.0
peanut:							
(*Archway* Jumble)	130	3.0	17.0	7.0	<5	90	1.0
crunch (*Archway*), 6 pcs.	150	2.0	18.0	8.0	10	120	0
peanut butter:							
(*Archway*)	140	3.0	16.0	7.0	10	125	<1.0
(*Archway* Ol' Fashion)	130	3.0	17.0	6.0	10	160	<1.0
(*Grandma's* Big) . .	190	4.0	22.0	9.0	<5	180	1.0
(*Little Debbie* Bar)	250	4.0	30.0	14.0	0	180	1.0
bits (*Grandma's*), 9 pcs.	150	3.0	21.0	6.0	0	135	1.0
chip (*Archway*) . .	140	3.0	16.0	7.0	5	115	<1.0
chocolate chip (*Grandma's* Bar)	210	4.0	24.0	10.0	10	150	1.0
chocolate chip (*Grandma's* Big)	190	4.0	23.0	10.0	<5	170	1.0
chunky (*Tastykake* Bar)	240	2.0	18.0	11.0	5	110	<1.0
fudge (*P. B. Fudgebutters*), 2 pcs.	130	2.0	14.0	7.0	<5	90	<1.0
patties (*Nutter Butter*), 5 pcs. . . .	160	4.0	17.0	9.0	0	80	1.0

Food and Measure	cal.	prot. (gms)	carbo. (gms)	fat (gms)	chol. (mgs)	sod. (mgs)	fiber (gms)
Cookie, peanut butter *(cont.)*							
sandwich							
(*Grandma's*),							
5 pcs.	210	4.0	29.0	9.0	0	190	1.0
sandwich (*Nutter*							
Butter), 2 pcs. . .	130	3.0	19.0	6.0	<5	110	1.0
sandwich (*Nutter*							
Butter Bites),							
10 pcs.	150	3.0	20.0	7.0	<5	125	1.0
pecan:							
(*Archway* Ice Box)	140	1.0	17.0	8.0	10	100	0
malted nougat							
(*Archway*), 3 pcs.	160	2.0	17.0	10.0	0	60	2.0
shortbread, see							
"shortbread," be-							
low							
pound cake (*Aunt*							
Bea's)	110	1.0	17.0	4.0	10	95	0
prune pastry (*Stella*							
D'Oro)	90	1.0	14.0	3.0	<5	0	1.0
raisin:							
(*Dare Sun•Maid*)	52	1.0	7.5	2.5	5	30	.3
(*Health Valley* Fat							
Free Jumbo) . . .	80	2.0	19.0	0	0	35	3.0
oatmeal, see							
"oatmeal raisin,"							
above							
raspberry:							
(*Health Valley* Fat							
Free Jumbo) . . .	80	2.0	19.0	0	0	35	3.0
(*Fruitastic* Bar) . . .	40	0	13.0	0	0	65	1.0
(*Newtons* Fat Free),							
2 pcs.	100	1.0	23.0	0	0	115	<1.0
(*Sunshine Oh!*							
Berry), 3 pcs. . .	120	<1.0	20.0	4.5	0	30	2.0
centers (*Health Val-*							
ley Fat Free) . . .	70	2.0	18.0	0	0	20	2.0
filled (*Archway*) . .	110	1.0	18.0	4.0	5	90	<1.0

Food and Measure	cal.	prot. (gms)	carbo. (gms)	fat (gms)	chol. (mgs)	sod. (mgs)	fiber (gms)
filled (*Pepperidge Farm Linzer*) . . .	100	1.0	15.0	4.0	5	65	<1.0
filled (*Smart Snackers*)	70	1.0	16.0	0	0	90	1.0
hazelnut (*Pepperidge Farm Chantilly*)	80	<1.0	12.0	3.0	5	50	<1.0
rocky road:							
(*Archway* Iowa) . .	120	2.0	19.0	4.5	10	75	1.0
(*Archway* Ohio) . .	130	2.0	18.0	6.0	10	85	<1.0
sesame (*Stella D'Oro* Regina), 3 pcs. . .	150	2.0	21.0	6.0	10	85	1.0
shortbread:							
(*Lorna Doone*), 4 pcs.	140	2.0	19.0	7.0	5	130	<1.0
(*Pepperidge Farm*), 2 pcs.	140	2.0	16.0	7.0	10	105	<1.0
(*Simply Sandies*)	80	1.0	9.0	4.5	10	75	0
butter (*Dare*)	63	.7	7.0	3.7	5	45	.2
fudge coated (*Nabisco* Family Favorites), 3 pcs.	160	2.0	22.0	8.0	0	140	1.0
fudge striped (*Keebler*), 3 pcs. . . .	160	1.0	21.0	8.0	0	140	<1.0
fudge striped (*Sunshine*), 3 pcs. . .	160	2.0	20.0	9.0	0	85	1.0
pecan (*Pecan Passion*)	90	<1.0	9.0	5.0	<5	35	0
pecan (*Pecan Sandies*)	80	<1.0	9.0	5.0	<5	75	<1.0
pecan (*Pepperidge Farm*), 2 pcs. . .	140	1.0	14.0	9.0	<5	85	1.0
(*Social Tea*), 6 pcs.	120	2.0	20.0	4.0	5	105	<1.0
spice, pfeffernusse:							
(*Archway*), 2 pcs.	140	1.0	32.0	1.0	0	100	<1.0
drops (*Stella D'Oro*), 3 pcs.	120	1.0	21.0	3.0	15	55	0
sprinkles (*Dare Breaktime*)	36	.3	5.0	1.6	0	46	n.a.

Food and Measure	cal.	prot. (gms)	carbo. (gms)	fat (gms)	chol. (mgs)	sod. (mgs)	fiber (gms)
Cookie *(cont.)*							
(Stella D'Oro Angelica Goodies)	100	2.0	15.0	4.0	15	45	0
(Stella D'Oro Angel Wings), 2 pcs. . . .	140	2.0	13.0	9.0	<5	80	<1.0
(Stella D'Oro Anginetti), 4 pcs.	140	2.0	23.0	4.0	40	10	<1.0
(Stella D'Oro Como Delights), 1.1 oz.	140	2.0	18.0	7.0	40	60	<1.0
strawberry:							
(Newtons Fat Free), 2 pcs.	100	1.0	23.0	0	0	115	<1.0
(Pepperidge Farm), 3 pcs.	140	2.0	22.0	5.0	10	105	<1.0
(Sunshine Oh! Berry Fat Free), 1 oz.	100	<1.0	20.0	0	0	40	0
filled *(Archway)* . .	100	1.0	16.0	3.5	<5	80	<1.0
filled *(Archway* Ohio)	110	1.0	18.0	4.0	<5	90	<1.0
sugar:							
(Archway)	120	2.0	20.0	4.0	<5	190	0
(Archway Fat Free)	70	<1.0	17.0	0	0	85	0
(Dare)	39	.4	6.0	1.4	0	13	n.a.
(Keebler Classic Collection), 2 pcs.	140	2.0	18.0	7.0	25	150	0
(Pepperidge Farm), 3 pcs.	140	2.0	20.0	6.0	15	90	<1.0
soft *(Archway)* . . .	110	1.0	18.0	4.0	5	110	0
wafer *(Biscos)*, 8 pcs.	140	<1.0	21.0	6.0	0	40	<1.0
wafer, chocolate *(Sunshine)*, 3 pcs.	130	2.0	30.0	7.0	0	30	<1.0
wafer, peanut butter *(Sunshine)*, 4 pcs.	170	3.0	19.0	9.0	0	75	1.0
wafer, vanilla *(Sunshine)*, 3 pcs. . .	130	1.0	18.0	6.0	0	20	<1.0
waffle *(Biscos)*, 4 pcs.	180	<1.0	35.0	6.0	0	40	<1.0

Food and Measure	cal.	prot. (gms)	carbo. (gms)	fat (gms)	chol. (mgs)	sod. (mgs)	fiber (gms)
(*Sunshine Jingles*), 6 pcs.	150	2.0	22.0	5.0	0	115	<1.0
vanilla:							
(*Pepperidge Farm Goldfish*), 1.1 oz.	150	2.0	21.0	7.0	20	50	1.0
(*Stella D'Oro* Margherite), 2 pcs.	140	2.0	22.0	5.0	15	90	<1.0
bits (*Grandma's*), 9 pcs.	150	2.0	21.0	7.0	<5	80	<1.0
raspberry tart (*Pepperidge Farm Wholesome Choice*), 2 pcs.	120	1.0	23.0	3.0	0	115	<1.0
wafer (*Archway*), 5 pcs.	130	2.0	22.0	4.0	<5	140	0
wafer (*Keebler*), 8 pcs.	150	1.0	20.0	7.0	0	120	<1.0
wafer (*Keebler Light*), 8 pcs. . .	130	2.0	25.0	3.5	0	140	<1.0
wafer (*Nilla*), 8 pcs.	140	2.0	24.0	5.0	5	105	0
wafer (*Sunshine*), 7 pcs.	150	2.0	20.0	7.0	3	110	<1.0
vanilla sandwich:							
(*Cameo*), 2 pcs. . .	130	1.0	21.0	5.0	0	105	<1.0
(*Cookie Break*), 3 pcs.	160	1.0	23.0	6.0	0	115	<1.0
(*Grandma's*), 5 pcs.	210	3.0	30.0	9.0	<5	110	1.0
(*Nabisco* Family Favorites), 3 pcs.	170	2.0	25.0	8.0	0	120	0
(*Smart Snackers*), 1.1 oz.	140	1.0	25.0	3.0	0	80	1.0
(*Snackwell's* Reduced Fat), 2 pcs.	110	1.0	21.0	2.5	0	95	1.0
(*Vienna Fingers*), 2 pcs.	130	1.0	23.0	3.5	0	95	<1.0
French (*Keebler Classic Collection*)	80	1.0	12.0	3.5	0	65	0

Food and Measure	cal.	prot. (gms)	carbo. (gms)	fat (gms)	chol. (mgs)	sod. (mgs)	fiber (gms)
Cookie, vanilla sandwich *(cont.)*							
raspberry or vanilla (*Barbara's Cookies & Creme*),							
2 pcs.	120	1.0	18.0	5.0	15	75	0
wafer, fudge (*Keebler Fudge Sticks*),							
3 pcs.	150	1.0	20.0	8.0	0	55	<1.0
walnut, black (*Archway* Ice Box) . . .	120	1.0	15.0	6.0	5	75	0
Cookie, refrigerated:							
candy (*Pillsbury*),							
1 oz.	130	1.0	18.0	6.0	<5	80	<1.0
chocolate chip, 1 oz.:							
(*Pillsbury*)	130	1.0	17.0	6.0	<5	85	<1.0
chocolate (*Pillsbury*)	130	1.0	17.0	6.0	0	65	<1.0
oatmeal (*Pillsbury*)	120	1.0	16.0	6.0	<5	95	<1.0
peanut butter (*Pillsbury*), 1 oz.	110	2.0	15.0	5.0	<5	135	0
sugar (*Pillsbury*),							
2 pcs.	130	1.0	19.0	5.0	<5	125	0
Cookie crumbs, see "Pie crust"							
Cookie mix, 1 pc.*:							
chocolate chip:							
(*Arrowhead Mills*)	80	1.0	16.0	1.5	0	110	0
(*Arrowhead Mills* Wheat Free) . . .	80	2.0	14.0	2.0	0	105	0
espresso chip (*Arrowhead Mills*)	80	1.0	16.0	1.5	0	50	0
oatmeal (*Arrowhead Mills*)	70	1.0	16.0	0	0	110	1.0
Cooking sauce, see specific listings							
Coquito nut, shelled, (*Frieda's*), 1 oz. . .	180	2.3	5.0	17.0	0	n.a.	3.4
Coriander:							
fresh, ¼ cup	1	.1	.1	<.1	0	1	.1

Food and Measure	cal.	prot. (gms)	carbo. (gms)	fat (gms)	chol. (mgs)	sod. (mgs)	fiber (gms)
dried:							
(*McCormick*),							
¼ tsp.	<1	.1	.1	0	0	1	0
ground (*McCor-*							
mick), ¼ tsp. . . .	2	.1	.2	.1	0	<1	.2
leaf, 1 tsp.	2	.1	.3	<.1	0	1	.1
seeds, 1 tsp.	5	.2	1.0	.3	0	1	.5
seeds (*McCormick*),							
¼ tsp.	3	.1	.4	.1	0	<1	.4
(*Tone's* Cilantro),							
¼ tsp.	0	0	0	0	0	0	0
Corkscrew pasta, see "Pasta"							
Corn, fresh, kernels, boiled, drained,							
½ cup	89	2.7	20.6	1.1	0	14	2.3
Corn, canned, ½ cup, except as noted:							
baby:							
(*Haddon House*) . .	30	1.0	3.0	1.5	0	30	4.0
(*Roland*)	25	2.0	4.0	0	0	280	2.0
kernel:							
(*Del Monte*)	90	2.0	18.0	1.0	0	360	3.0
(*Del Monte* Super-sweet No Salt)	60	2.0	11.0	1.0	0	10	3.0
(*Del Monte* Super-sweet No Sugar)	60	2.0	11.0	1.0	0	360	3.0
(*Del Monte* Super-sweet Vac Pack)	70	2.0	13.0	1.0	0	270	3.0
(*Del Monte* Super-sweet Vac Pack No Salt)	70	2.0	13.0	1.0	0	10	3.0
(*Del Monte* Fiesta)	50	2.0	12.0	1.0	0	310	2.0
(*Goya*)	100	3.0	21.0	.5	0	430	2.0
(*Green Giant*) . . .	80	2.0	18.0	1.0	0	360	2.0
(*Green Giant* Less Salt)	80	2.0	17.0	1.0	0	180	2.0
(*Green Giant* Niblets), ⅓ cup	70	2.0	15.0	0	0	230	2.0

Food and Measure	cal.	prot. (gms)	carbo. (gms)	fat (gms)	chol. (mgs)	sod. (mgs)	fiber (gms)
Corn, canned, kernel *(cont.)*							
(*Green Giant Niblets* Extra Sweet), ⅓ cup	50	2.0	10.0	1.0	0	200	2.0
(*Green Giant Niblets* Less Sodium), ⅓ cup	60	2.0	14.0	0	0	115	1.0
(*Green Giant Niblets* No Salt/Sugar), ⅓ cup	60	2.0	13.0	0	0	0	2.0
(*S&W*)	90	2.0	14.0	1.0	0	340	2.0
(*S&W* Sweet 'n Crisp), ⅓ cup . .	70	2.0	12.0	1.5	0	170	2.0
(*Stokely*)	90	2.0	14.0	1.0	0	340	2.0
(*Stokely* No Salt)	90	2.0	14.0	1.0	0	20	2.0
(*Stokely* Vac Pack), ⅓ cup	80	2.0	14.0	1.0	0	240	2.0
(*Stokely* Vac Pack No Salt), ⅓ cup	70	2.0	14.0	1.0	0	10	2.0
gold/white (*Del Monte* Super- sweet)	80	2.0	18.0	.5	0	360	2.0
white (*Del Monte*)	80	2.0	17.0	0	0	360	2.0
white (*Green Giant*), ⅓ cup	80	2.0	16.0	1.0	0	220	1.0
white (*Stokely*) . .	90	2.0	14.0	1.0	0	340	2.0
white (*Stokely* No Salt)	90	2.0	14.0	1.0	0	20	2.0
kernel, w/peppers:							
(*Green Giant Mex- icorn*), ⅓ cup . .	60	2.0	14.0	0	0	430	2.0
(*Stokely*), ⅓ cup . .	80	2.0	16.0	1.0	0	240	2.0
cream style:							
(*Del Monte*)	90	2.0	20.0	.5	0	360	2.0
(*Del Monte* No Salt)	90	2.0	20.0	.5	0	10	2.0
(*Del Monte* Super- sweet)	60	1.0	14.0	.5	0	360	2.0
(*Del Monte* Super- sweet No Salt)	60	1.0	14.0	.5	0	10	2.0

Food and Measure	cal.	prot. (gms)	carbo. (gms)	fat (gms)	chol. (mgs)	sod. (mgs)	fiber (gms)
(*Green Giant*) . . .	100	2.0	22.0	1.0	0	430	1.0
(*S&W*)	100	2.0	24.0	1.0	0	340	1.0
(*Stokely*)	100	2.0	21.0	1.0	0	400	1.0
white (*Del Monte*)	100	2.0	21.0	1.0	0	360	2.0
Corn, freeze-dried, ½ cup:							
(*AlpineAire*)	85	3.0	20.0	1.0	0	n.a.	2.0
(*Mountain House*) . .	80	2.0	17.0	1.0	0	0	2.0
Corn, frozen:							
on the cob, 1 ear:							
(*John Cope's*) . . .	120	4.0	22.0	1.5	0	5	5.0
(*Green Giant* Extra Sweet)	120	4.0	7.0	2.0	0	0	3.0
(*Green Giant Nib- blers*)	70	2.0	5.0	.5	0	5	1.0
(*Green Giant Niblets*)	160	4.0	11.0	1.5	0	10	3.0
(*Ore-Ida Mini-Gold*)	80	3.0	18.0	1.0	0	10	1.0
white (*John Cope's*)	150	4.0	31.0	1.5	0	5	3.0
kernel:							
(*Green Giant Harvest Fresh Niblets*), ⅔ cup	80	3.0	17.0	1.0	0	60	3.0
(*Green Giant Niblets*), ⅔ cup	80	2.0	17.0	.5	0	5	2.0
(*Green Giant Niblets Extra Sweet*), ⅔ cup	70	2.0	13.0	1.0	0	0	2.0
(*Stilwell*), ⅔ cup	80	3.0	19.0	1.0	0	10	1.0
white (*Green Giant*), ¾ cup	100	3.0	20.0	1.0	0	0	3.0
white (*Green Giant* Extra Sweet), ⅔ cup	50	2.0	10.0	.5	0	0	3.0
white (*Green Giant Harvest Fresh*) . .	70	2.0	14.0	1.0	0	45	2.0
white (*John Cope's*), ⅓ cup	80	2.0	17.0	.5	0	0	1.0

Food and Measure	cal.	prot. (gms)	carbo. (gms)	fat (gms)	chol. (mgs)	sod. (mgs)	fiber (gms)
Corn, frozen *(cont.)*							
cream style:							
(*Green Giant*) . . .	110	2.0	23.0	1.0	0	330	2.0
white (*John Cope's* Sweet 'N Creamy), ⅓ cup	100	3.0	17.0	2.5	<5	120	1.0
in butter sauce:							
(*Green Giant Niblets*), ⅔ cup	130	3.0	23.0	3.0	<5	350	3.0
white (*Green Giant*), ¾ cup	120	3.0	21.0	2.5	<5	320	3.0
Corn, dried (*John Cope's*), ¼ cup . .	130	2.0	15.0	1.0	0	0	1.0
Corn, whole grain:							
1 oz.	103	2.7	21.1	1.3	0	10	n.a.
1 cup	605	15.6	123.3	7.9	0	58	n.a.
Corn bran, crude:							
1 oz.	64	2.4	24.3	.3	0	2	24.0
1 cup	170	6.4	65.1	.7	0	5	64.3
Corn bread, see "Bread mix"							
Corn chips, puffs, and similar snacks see also "Snack chips and crisps"), 1 oz., except as noted:							
(*Barbara's* Pinta Chips)	130	2.0	19.0	6.0	0	70	2.0
(*Barrel O'Fun* Chip), 1.1 oz.	160	2.0	18.0	10.0	0	275	0
(*Bugles*), 1⅓ cups . .	160	2.0	18.0	9.0	0	310	<1.0
(*Bugles* Light), 1½ cups	130	2.0	23.0	3.5	0	350	0
(*Dipsey Doodles*) . .	160	1.0	16.0	10.0	0	180	1.0
(*Fritos* King Size) . .	160	2.0	15.0	10.0	0	150	1.0
(*Fritos* Original/Wild 'N Mild)	160	2.0	15.0	10.0	0	170	1.0
(*Fritos* Scoops) . . .	150	2.0	16.0	9.0	0	135	1.0

Food and Measure	cal.	prot. (gms)	carbo. (gms)	fat (gms)	chol. (mgs)	sod. (mgs)	fiber (gms)
(*Old Dutch* Chips), 1.1 oz.	170	2.0	16.0	10.0	0	180	2.0
(*Old Dutch* Chips), 1¼-oz. bag	200	3.0	16.0	12.0	0	213	2.0
(*Old Dutch Puffcorn* Curls), 1.1 oz. . . .	180	1.0	14.0	14.0	0	240	<1.0
(*Planters* Chips) . . .	160	2.0	16.0	10.0	0	170	2.0
(*Sunchips* Original)	140	2.0	18.0	7.0	0	160	2.0
barbecue:							
(*Fritos*)	150	2.0	16.0	9.0	0	310	1.0
(*Old Dutch*), 1.1 oz.	165	3.0	16.0	10.0	0	200	2.0
(*Old Dutch*), 1¼-oz. bag . . .	190	3.0	19.0	12.0	0	230	2.0
(*Smart Snackers* Curls), ½ oz. . .	60	1.0	11.0	1.5	0	110	1.0
blue corn:							
(*Barbara's*), 1.1 oz.	140	3.0	16.0	7.0	0	40	<1.0
(*Barbara's* Pinta Blues)	130	3.0	17.0	7.0	0	100	3.0
light salt (*Barbara's* Amazing Bakes)	100	2.0	24.0	1.0	0	75	1.0
picante (*Barbara's* Pinta)	130	3.0	17.0	7.0	0	240	3.0
salsa (*Barbara's* Pinta)	130	2.0	19.0	6.0	0	210	2.0
caramel coated (*Old Dutch Puffcorn*) . .	120	0	24.0	2.5	0	100	0
cheese:							
(*Cheese Doodles*)	150	2.0	17.0	8.0	0	360	0
(*Chee • tos* Cheesy Checkers)	150	2.0	15.0	10.0	<5	350	<1.0
(*Chee • tos* Crunchy)	150	2.0	16.0	9.0	0	300	<1.0
cheddar (*Sunchips* Harvest)	140	2.0	18.0	7.0	0	180	2.0
chili, w/corn shell (*Combos*)	140	2.0	17.0	6.0	0	420	1.0
fried (*Cheese Doo- dles*)	150	2.0	16.0	9.0	0	190	0

Food and Measure	cal.	prot. (gms)	carbo. (gms)	fat (gms)	chol. (mgs)	sod. (mgs)	fiber (gms)
Corn chips, puffs, and similar snacks, cheese *(cont.)*							
hot (*Chee • tos* Flamin')	160	2.0	16.0	9.0	0	240	<1.0
nacho (*Barbara's* Pinta)	130	2.0	18.0	6.0	0	180	2.0
nacho (*Doodle Twisters*)	160	2.0	15.0	10.0	0	270	1.0
nacho, w/tortilla shell (*Combos*)	140	2.0	17.0	6.0	0	380	1.0
nacho, w/tortilla shell (*Combos*), 1.7-oz. bag . . .	230	4.0	30.0	11.0	0	640	1.0
and pepperoni (*Combos*)	140	2.0	17.0	7.0	5	280	0
cheese balls:							
(*Barrel O'Fun*), 1.1 oz.	160	2.0	16.0	11.0	0	280	0
(*Planters* Cheez) . .	150	2.0	15.0	10.0	<5	300	1.0
(*Planters* Cheez), 1-oz. bag	150	2.0	15.0	10.0	<5	330	1.0
puffed (*Chee • tos*)	160	2.0	13.0	10.0	<5	370	<1.0
cheese curls:							
(*Barrel O'Fun* Baked), 1.1 oz.	160	2.0	18.0	10.0	0	280	0
(*Barrel O'Fun* Crunchy), 1.1 oz.	160	2.0	17.0	10.0	0	225	0
(*Chee • tos*)	150	2.0	16.0	9.0	0	280	1.0
(*Old Dutch* Crunchy)	130	2.0	19.0	6.0	0	230	0
(*Planters* Cheez) . .	150	2.0	15.0	10.0	<5	310	1.0
(*Planters* Cheez), 1¼-oz. pkg. . . .	190	2.0	19.0	12.0	<5	380	1.0
(*Smart Snackers*), ½ oz.	70	1.0	10.0	2.5	0	85	0
cheese puffs:							
(*Barbara's* Original)	150	2.0	16.0	10.0	0	130	0
(*Barbara's* Bakes)	160	2.0	13.0	11.0	0	190	1.0
(*Barrel O'Fun* Light), 1.1 oz.	125	2.0	24.0	3.0	0	300	1.0
(*Chee • tos*)	160	2.0	15.0	10.0	0	370	<1.0

Food and Measure	cal.	prot. (gms)	carbo. (gms)	fat (gms)	chol. (mgs)	sod. (mgs)	fiber (gms)
cheddar (*No Fries*)	110	3.0	23.0	0	0	250	1.0
cheddar, New York (*Barbara's* Less Fat)	140	2.0	18.0	6.0	0	210	<1.0
jalapeño (*Barbara's*)	150	2.0	15.0	9.0	0	250	1.0
Monterey Jack and green chili (*Barbara's* Less Fat)	140	2.0	19.0	5.0	0	160	1.0
chili cheese (*Fritos*)	160	2.0	15.0	10.0	0	260	1.0
onion, French (*Sunchips*)	140	2.0	18.0	7.0	0	115	2.0
onion flavor rings (*Borden*), 1-oz. bag	140	0	20.0	6.0	0	420	0
pizza curls (*Smart Snackers*), ½ oz.	60	1.0	11.0	2.0	0	125	1.0
ranch:							
(*Combos*)	140	2.0	17.0	7.0	5	350	1.0
(*Smart Snackers*), ½ oz.	60	1.0	10.0	2.0	0	170	1.0
puffs (*No Fries*) . .	110	3.0	23.0	0	0	310	1.0
sour cream and onion (*Bugles*), 1⅓ cup	160	2.0	18.0	9.0	0	260	0
taco (*Taco Bell* Supreme)	140	2.0	18.0	7.0	0	200	1.0
tortilla:							
(*Doritos* Dunkers)	140	2.0	19.0	6.0	0	80	1.0
(*Doritos* Toasted)	140	2.0	19.0	6.0	0	65	1.0
(*Mesa*)	150	2.0	16.0	1.0	0	160	1.0
(*Nachips*)	150	3.0	17.0	8.0	0	85	2.0
(*No Fries* Natural)	100	2.0	22.0	1.0	0	160	1.0
(*Old Dutch* Restaurant)	140	2.0	18.0	6.0	0	123	1.0
(*Santitas* Chips) . .	140	2.0	19.0	6.0	0	75	1.0
(*Santitas* Strips) . .	140	2.0	19.0	6.0	0	40	1.0
(*Tostitos* Baked) . .	110	2.0	24.0	1.0	0	200	2.0
(*Tostitos* Bite Size)	140	2.0	17.0	8.0	0	110	1.0
(*Tostitos* Crispy Round)	150	2.0	17.0	8.0	0	85	1.0

Food and Measure	cal.	prot. (gms)	carbo. (gms)	fat (gms)	chol. (mgs)	sod. (mgs)	fiber (gms)
Corn chips, puffs, and similar snacks, tortilla *(cont.)*							
(*Tostitos* Restaurant/ Santa Fe Gold)	140	2.0	19.0	6.0	0	80	1.0
(*Tyson*), 1.2 oz. . .	170	2.0	22.0	7.0	0	75	2.0
(*Tyson* Yellow Corn), 1.1 oz. . .	150	2.0	21.0	7.0	0	5	2.0
crisps (*Mr. Phipps*)	130	2.0	21.0	4.0	0	130	3.0
crisps (*Pepperidge Farm*), 1.1 oz. . .	130	4.0	18.0	6.0	<5	290	2.0
5 grain (*Kettle* Tias)	140	2.0	18.0	6.0	0	80	2.0
hot (*Doritos* Flamin')	140	2.0	17.0	8.0	0	270	1.0
lime and chili (*Kettle* Tias)	140	2.0	18.0	6.0	0	210	2.0
lime and chili (*Tostitos*)	150	2.0	19.0	6.0	0	80	1.0
pizza (*Doritos* Cravers)	140	2.0	18.0	7.0	0	170	1.0
ranch (*Doritos* Cooler)	140	2.0	18.0	7.0	0	160	1.0
ranch (*Doritos* Cooler Reduced Fat)	130	2.0	19.0	5.0	0	200	1.0
ranch (*No Fries*), 1.1 oz.	110	3.0	24.0	0	0	240	1.0
ranch (*Tostitos* Baked)	120	2.0	21.0	3.0	3	170	1.0
salsa crisps (*Pepperidge Farm*), 1.1 oz.	130	3.0	18.0	7.0	<5	350	3.0
salsa and sour cream (*No Fries*), 1.1 oz.	110	3.0	25.0	0	0	200	1.0
tomato basil (*Kettle* Tias)	140	2.0	18.0	6.0	0	150	2.0
tostados (*Old Dutch*), 1.1 oz.	150	3.0	19.0	7.0	0	200	1.0
tortilla, blue corn:							
(*Barbara's* Less Fat)	120	2.0	21.0	4.0	0	95	1.0
(*Kettle Tias*)	140	3.0	18.0	6.0	0	80	2.0

Food and Measure	cal.	prot. (gms)	carbo. (gms)	fat (gms)	chol. (mgs)	sod. (mgs)	fiber (gms)
hot salsa (*Barbara's* Less Fat)	120	2.0	20.0	4.0	0	170	1.0
cheddar jalapeño (*No Fries*), 1.1 oz.	110	3.0	25.0	0	0	170	1.0
tortilla, cheese:							
(*Doritos Chester's*)	140	2.0	18.0	7.0	0	160	1.0
cheddar, white (*Barbara's* Less Fat)	120	2.0	20.0	4.0	0	170	1.0
chili crisps (*Pepperidge Farm*),							
1.1 oz.	130	4.0	18.0	7.0	<5	340	2.0
nacho (*Barrel O'Fun*)	130	2.0	18.0	6.0	0	150	1.0
nacho (*Borden*) . .	150	2.0	17.0	8.0	0	170	1.0
nacho (*Doritos* Cheesier)	140	2.0	18.0	7.0	0	170	1.0
nacho (*Doritos* Cheesier Reduced Fat)	130	3.0	19.0	5.0	0	210	1.0
nacho (*Old Dutch*), 1-oz. bag	140	2.0	17.0	7.0	0	230	1.0
nacho (*Old Dutch*), 2¼-oz. bag . . .	320	5.0	39.0	16.0	0	520	3.0
nacho (*Tyson*) . . .	140	2.0	19.0	6.0	0	180	2.0
nacho, crisps (*Mr. Phipps*) . . .	130	2.0	20.0	4.0	0	150	3.0
tortilla, flour:							
cheese and salsa (*Barrel O'Fun*) . .	140	3.0	19.0	6.0	0	110	.5
nacho (*Barrel O'Fun*)	140	2.0	19.0	5.0	0	240	0
white (*Barrel O'Fun*)	140	2.0	20.0	6.0	0	50	0
white, mini-rounds (*Barrel O'Fun*) . .	150	1.0	19.0	7.0	0	260	0
yellow (*Barrel O'Fun* Tostada)	130	2.0	20.0	5.0	0	160	0
yellow, mini (*Barrel O'Fun* Tostada)	140	2.0	19.0	7.0	0	265	1.0
tortilla, white corn:							
(*Barbara's* Less Fat)	120	2.0	21.0	4.0	0	95	1.0
(*Kettle* Tias)	140	2.0	18.0	6.0	0	80	2.0

Food and Measure	cal.	prot. (gms)	carbo. (gms)	fat (gms)	chol. (mgs)	sod. (mgs)	fiber (gms)
Corn chips, puffs, and similar snacks, tortilla, white corn *(cont.)*							
(*Old Dutch*), 1.1 oz.	150	3.0	20.0	7.0	0	135	2.0
(*Old El Paso*) . . .	140	2.0	16.0	8.0	0	60	1.0
(*Santitas* 100%) . .	140	2.0	19.0	6.0	0	75	1.0
ranch (*Barbara's* Less Fat)	120	2.0	20.0	4.0	0	170	<1.0
Corn flake crumbs							
(*Kellogg's*), 2 tbsp.	40	1.0	9.0	0	0	120	0
Corn flour:							
whole grain, 1 oz. . . .	102	2.0	21.8	1.1	0	1	3.8
whole grain, 1 cup	422	8.1	89.9	4.5	0	6	15.7
masa, 1 oz.	103	2.6	21.6	1.1	0	1	2.7
masa, 1 cup	416	10.7	87.0	4.3	0	6	10.9
Corn fritter, frozen							
(*Mrs. Paul's*), 1 pc.	130	11.0	16.0	7.0	5	310	1.0
Corn grits, dry:							
(*Albers* Quick Hominy), ¼ cup . .	140	3.0	31.0	.5	0	0	1.0
(*Goya*), ¼ cup	180	4.0	39.0	0	0	0	0
instant, 1-oz. pkt.:							
(*Quaker* Original)	100	2.0	22.0	0	0	300	1.0
bacon bits (*Quaker*)	100	2.0	22.0	.5	0	340	1.0
butter flavor (*Quaker*)	100	2.0	21.0	1.5	0	320	1.0
cheddar (*Quaker*)	100	3.0	21.0	1.5	0	520	1.0
cheddar, zesty (*Quaker*)	100	2.0	20.0	1.5	0	460	1.0
ham bits (*Quaker*)	90	2.0	21.0	.5	0	530	1.0
sausage bits (*Quaker*)	100	2.0	21.0	1.0	0	480	2.0
white, ¼ cup:							
(*Arrowhead Mills*)	140	3.0	30.0	0	0	0	<1.0
(*Quaker* Hominy)	140	3.0	32.0	.5	0	60	2.0
(*Quaker* Quick Hominy)	130	3.0	27.0	.5	0	55	2.0
yellow, ¼ cup:							
(*Arrowhead Mills*)	130	3.0	29.0	0	0	0	1.0
(*Quaker* Quick Hominy)	120	3.0	26.0	.5	0	60	2.0

Food and Measure	cal.	prot. (gms)	carbo. (gms)	fat (gms)	chol. (mgs)	sod. (mgs)	fiber (gms)
Corn pudding mix							
(*Goya*), ½ cup* . .	100	1.0	23.0	.5	0	45	1.0
Corn relish:							
(*Green Giant*), 1 tbsp.	20	0	5.0	0	0	40	0
(*Nance's*), 2 tbsp. . . .	25	0	6.0	0	0	75	0
(*Pickle Eater's*),							
1 tbsp.	20	0	5.0	0	0	0	0
Corn soufflé, frozen							
(*Stouffer's*), 4.8 oz.	170	5.0	21.0	7.0	65	490	1.0
Corn syrup, 2 tbsp.:							
dark (*Karo*)	120	0	30.0	0	0	45	0
light (*Karo*)	120	0	30.0	0	0	35	0
Cornish hen:							
cooked, 3 oz.:							
dark meat (*Perdue*)	200	17.0	0	15.0	130	45	0
white meat (*Perdue*)	170	21.0	0	9.0	100	40	0
roasted, half, 6.5 oz.:							
dark meat (*Perdue*)	210	18.0	0	15.0	130	45	0
white meat (*Perdue*)	200	24.0	0	11.0	115	45	0
Cornmeal (see also							
"Corn flour" and							
"Polenta"):							
blue or hi-lysine (*Ar-*							
rowhead Mills),							
¼ cup	130	3.0	25.0	1.5	0	0	3.0
blue and red							
(*Frieda's*), ½ cup	214	5.3	44.0	2.0	0	<1	n.a.
coarse (*Goya*), 3 tbsp.	110	2.0	25.0	0	0	0	1.0
fine (*Goya*), 3 tbsp.	100	2.0	23.0	0	0	0	1.0
self-rising, 3 tbsp.:							
white (*Aunt Je-*							
mima)	90	2.0	20.0	.5	0	360	1.0
white (*Aunt Jemima*							
Mix)	80	2.0	19.0	.5	0	340	1.0
white, buttermilk							
(*Aunt Jemima*							
Mix)	80	2.0	18.0	.5	0	440	1.0
yellow (*Aunt Je-*							
mima Mix)	90	2.0	19.0	.5	0	310	1.0

Food and Measure	cal.	prot. (gms)	carbo. (gms)	fat (gms)	chol. (mgs)	sod. (mgs)	fiber (gms)
Cornmeal *(cont.)*							
white (*Arrowhead Mills*), ¼ cup . . .	120	3.0	23.0	1.0	0	0	3.0
white (*Goya*), 2½ tbsp.	100	2.0	22.0	0	0	0	0
white or yellow (*Albers*), 3 tbsp. . . .	110	2.0	34.0	0	0	0	<1.0
yellow (*Arrowhead Mills*), ¼ cup . . .	120	3.0	27.0	1.0	0	0	3.0
yellow (*Goya*), 2½ tbsp.	110	3.0	25.0	0	0	0	0
Cornstarch (*Argo/ Kingsford*), 1 tbsp.	30	0	7.0	0	0	0	0
Cottonseed kernels, roasted, 1 tbsp. . .	51	3.3	2.2	3.6	0	3	.6
Cottonseed meal, partially defatted, 1 oz.	104	13.9	10.9	1.4	0	10	<1.0
Country gravy mix:							
(*Durkee*), 1½ tbsp.	35	1.0	5.0	2.0	0	570	0
(*French's*), ¼ cup*	35	1.0	5.0	2.0	0	370	0
(*Loma Linda Gravy Quik*), 1 tbsp. . . .	25	<1.0	4.0	.5	0	260	0
Couscous:							
dry, ¼ cup:							
(*Arrowhead Mills*)	170	6.0	35.0	0	0	0	<1.0
(*Fantastic Foods*)	210	7.0	43.0	0	0	5	3.0
whole wheat (*Fantastic Foods*) . .	180	5.0	42.0	.5	0	10	5.0
cooked, ½ cup . . .	101	3.4	20.9	.1	0	4	1.3
Couscous mix, 1 pkg., except as noted:							
(*Near East* Moroccan), 1¼ cups*	260	8.0	46.0	6.0	0	65	2.0
almond chicken, vegetarian (*Casbah*) . .	160	5.0	29.0	1.5	0	470	<1.0

Food and Measure	cal.	prot. (gms)	carbo. (gms)	fat (gms)	chol. (mgs)	sod. (mgs)	fiber (gms)
asparagus au gratin							
(*Casbah*)	150	4.0	28.0	2.0	<5	420	1.0
black bean salsa (*Fantastic* Cup)	240	11.0	46.0	1.5	0	450	8.0
cheddar:							
broccoli, creamy							
(*Casbah*)	130	11.0	23.0	2.0	<5	470	<1.0
nacho (*Fantastic* Cup)	200	8.0	36.0	3.0	0	590	6.0
corn, sweet (*Fantastic* Cup)	180	7.0	36.0	1.0	0	510	6.0
w/lentils (*Fantastic Only A Pinch* Cup)	220	12.0	26.0	.5	0	540	4.0
pilaf (*Casbah*), 1 oz.	100	4.0	20.0	0	0	280	<1.0
savory pilaf (*Fantastic Foods*), 1 cup . . .	240	9.0	50.0	1.0	0	450	4.0
tomato Parmesan (*Casbah*)	170	7.0	34.0	1.5	<5	490	2.0
vegetable, creole (*Fantastic* Cup)	220	10.0	41.0	1.5	0	590	6.0
Cowpeas, ½ cup, except as noted:							
fresh:							
raw, trimmed . . .	65	2.1	13.6	.3	0	3	3.6
boiled, drained . . .	79	2.6	16.7	.3	0	3	4.1
fresh, leafy tips:							
raw, chopped . . .	5	.7	.9	<.1	0	1	n.a.
boiled, drained, 4 oz.	25	5.3	3.2	.1	0	7	n.a.
fresh, pods, w/seeds:							
raw, trimmed . . .	21	1.6	4.5	.1	0	2	n.a.
boiled, drained . . .	16	1.2	3.3	.1	0	1	n.a.
mature, boiled	100	6.7	17.9	.5	0	3	5.6
canned, see "Black-eyed peas"							
frozen, boiled, drained	112	7.2	20.2	.6	0	5	4.3
Cowpeas, catjang, see "Catjang"							

Food and Measure	cal.	prot. (gms)	carbo. (gms)	fat (gms)	chol. (mgs)	sod. (mgs)	fiber (gms)
Crab, meat only:							
Alaska king:							
raw, 4 oz.	95	20.8	0	.7	47	948	0
boiled, poached, or							
steamed, 4 oz.	110	21.9	0	1.7	60	1216	0
blue:							
raw, 4 oz.	99	20.5	.1	1.2	89	332	0
boiled, poached, or							
steamed, 4 oz.	116	22.9	0	2.0	113	316	0
dungeness:							
raw, 4 oz.	98	19.8	.8	1.1	67	335	0
boiled, poached, or							
steamed, 4 oz.	125	25.3	1.1	1.4	86	429	0
queen:							
raw, 4 oz.	102	21.0	0	1.4	62	611	0
boiled, poached, or							
steamed, 4 oz.	130	26.9	0	1.7	81	784	0
Crab, canned:							
blue, 4 oz.	112	23.3	0	1.4	101	378	0
dungeness (*S&W*),							
⅓ cup, 3 oz.	80	18.0	0	1.0	60	310	0
"Crab," imitation,							
frozen or refriger-							
ated:							
(*Peter Pan*), 3 oz. . .	70	6.0	13.0	0	20	480	1.0
from surimi, 1 oz. . .	29	3.4	3.0	.4	6	238	0
flaked, ½ cup, 3 oz.:							
(*Captain Jac Crab*							
Tasties)	100	7.0	15.0	2.0	5	500	1.0
(*Louis Kemp Crab*							
Delights)	80	9.0	10.0	0	5	470	0
(*Pacific Mate*) . . .	90	7.0	14.0	1.0	5	590	0
(*Pacific Mate* Fat							
Free)	90	8.0	15.0	0	5	660	0
(*Seafest*)	100	8.0	14.0	1.5	5	500	1.0
or chunk (*Louis*							
Kemp Crab De-							
lights)	80	9.0	10.0	0	5	470	0

Food and Measure	cal.	prot. (gms)	carbo. (gms)	fat (gms)	chol. (mgs)	sod. (mgs)	fiber (gms)
leg style, 3 legs, 3 oz.:							
(*Louis Kemp Crab Delights*)	80	9.0	10.0	0	10	500	0
w/crab (*Captain Jac Crab Tasties*) . .	100	7.0	15.0	2.0	5	500	1.0
(*Captain Jac* Easy Shreds), ½ cup, 3 oz.	80	8.0	11.0	0	5	670	0
Crab cake, deviled, frozen:							
(*Mrs. Paul's*), 1 pc.	170	11.0	17.0	7.0	20	430	1.0
miniature (*Mrs. Paul's*), 6 pcs., 3.5 oz.	230	17.0	25.0	11.0	15	620	2.0
Crabapple, fresh, w/peel:							
1 oz.	22	.1	5.7	.1	0	<1	n.a.
sliced, ½ cup	42	.2	11.0	.2	0	1	n.a.
(*Frieda's*), 1 oz. . . .	19	.1	5.0	.1	0	<1	n.a.
Crabapple, canned:							
(*S&W*), 1 pc.	35	0	8.0	0	0	15	1.0
spiced (*Apple Time*), 1 pc., 1.1 oz. . . .	40	0	10.0	0	0	0	1.0
Cracker, 1 oz.–1.1 oz., except as noted:							
bacon flavor (*Nabisco*)	160	3.0	19.0	8.0	0	460	<1.0
(*Barbara's* Rite Lite), 5 pcs., ½ oz. . . .	55	3.0	12.0	<1.0	0	150	0
butter/butter flavor:							
(*Goya* Tropical), 4 pcs.	140	4.0	21.0	4.0	0	110	0
(*Hi-Ho*)	160	2.0	19.0	9.0	3	280	<1.0
(*Keebler Club* Partners), 4 pcs., ½ oz.	70	1.0	9.0	3.0	0	160	<1.0
(*Ritz*), 5 pcs., .6 oz.	80	1.0	10.0	4.0	0	135	<1.0

Food and Measure	cal.	prot. (gms)	carbo. (gms)	fat (gms)	chol. (mgs)	sod. (mgs)	fiber (gms)
Cracker, butter/butter flavor *(cont.)*							
(*Ritz* Low Sodium), 5 pcs., .6 oz. . .	80	1.0	10.0	4.0	0	35	<1.0
(*Toasted Complements* Buttercrisp)	140	2.0	19.0	7.0	<5	280	<1.0
(*Town House*), 5 pcs., .6 oz. . .	80	1.0	9.0	4.5	0	150	<1.0
mini (*Ritz Bits*) . .	160	2.0	18.0	9.0	0	250	1.0
thins (*Pepperidge Farm*), 4 pcs., ½ oz.	70	1.0	10.0	3.0	10	95	0
cheese:							
(*Appeteasers* Original)	130	5.0	18.0	4.0	10	250	n.a.
(*Barbara's* Bites Original/Hot & Spicy)	120	3.0	24.0	1.5	0	290	1.0
(*Krispy* Mild Cheddar), 5 pcs., ½ oz.	60	2.0	10.0	2.0	0	180	<1.0
(*Nips*)	150	3.0	18.0	6.0	0	310	<1.0
(*Snackwell's*) . . .	130	4.0	23.0	2.0	0	340	1.0
(*Tid-Bit*)	150	2.0	17.0	8.0	0	420	<1.0
chili (*Munch 'ems*)	130	2.0	23.0	4.0	0	470	1.0
garlic herb (*Appeteasers*)	130	5.0	18.0	4.0	10	370	0
Parmesan (*Goldfish*)	140	4.0	19.0	5.0	0	300	1.0
Swiss (*Nabisco Swiss*)	140	2.0	18.0	7.0	0	350	<1.0
zesty (*Snackwell's*)	120	3.0	23.0	2.0	5	350	1.0
cheese, cheddar:							
(*Better Cheddars*)	150	3.0	18.0	8.0	<5	290	<1.0
(*Better Cheddars* Low Sodium) . .	150	3.0	18.0	7.0	<5	75	<1.0
(*Better Cheddars* Reduced Fat) . .	140	3.0	19.0	6.0	<5	350	<1.0
(*Cheez-It*)	160	4.0	16.0	8.0	0	240	<1.0
(*Cheez-It* Low Sodium)	160	4.0	16.0	8.0	0	70	<1.0

Food and Measure	cal.	prot. (gms)	carbo. (gms)	fat (gms)	chol. (mgs)	sod. (mgs)	fiber (gms)
(*Cheez-It* Reduced Fat)	130	4.0	19.0	4.5	0	280	<1.0
(*Combos*)	140	3.0	16.0	8.0	5	300	0
(*Munch 'ems*) . . .	130	3.0	21.0	4.0	0	330	<1.0
(*Goldfish*)	140	4.0	19.0	6.0	10	200	<1.0
(*Goldfish* Less Sodium)	150	3.0	18.0	6.0	10	140	<1.0
(*Snorkels*)	140	4.0	19.0	5.0	1	200	1.0
double (*Appeteasers*)	130	5.0	17.0	5.0	10	280	0
hot and spicy (*Cheez-It*)	160	3.0	17.0	8.0	0	220	1.0
white (*Cheeze-It*)	160	3.0	17.0	9.0	3	280	<1.0
white (*Wheatables*)	130	3.0	21.0	4.0	0	330	<1.0
cheese sandwich:							
(*Little Debbie*), 1.4 oz.	200	4.0	22.0	11.0	5.0	310	1.0
(*Handi-Snacks* Cheez'n Crackers), 1 pc.	130	4.0	10.0	8.0	15	340	0
(*Ritz*), 1.4-oz. pkg.	210	4.0	21.0	12.0	5	450	1.0
(*Ritz Bits*)	160	3.0	17.0	10.0	5	300	1.0
bacon (*Frito-Lay*), 1 pkg.	200	3.0	24.0	10.0	<5	380	1.0
cheddar, golden toast (*Frito-Lay*), 1 pkg.	230	3.0	25.0	13.0	5	510	1.0
cheddar, jalapeño (*Frito-Lay*), 1 pkg.	200	4.0	24.0	10.0	<5	470	1.0
cream cheese and chive, golden toast (*Frito-Lay*), 1 pkg.	240	3.0	25.0	14.0	<5	490	1.0
peanut butter, see "peanut butter," below							
wheat (*Frito-Lay*), 1 pkg.	200	4.0	24.0	9.0	<5	430	1.0
(*Chicken In A Biskit*)	160	2.0	17.0	9.0	0	270	<1.0

Food and Measure	cal.	prot. (gms)	carbo. (gms)	fat (gms)	chol. (mgs)	sod. (mgs)	fiber (gms)
Cracker *(cont.)*							
cracked pepper, see "flatbread," "saltine," and "water or soda," below							
croissant (*Carr's*), 3 pcs., ½ oz. . . .	70	1.0	10.0	3.0	<5	115	0
flatbread, 1 pc., except as noted:							
(*J.J. Flats* Flavorall)	50	2.0	11.0	1.0	0	120	1.0
(*Lavosh Hawaii* Classic), 1 oz. . . .	120	3.0	19.0	3.0	21	290	0
(*New York*)	45	1.0	7.0	1.0	0	40	1.0
(*New York* Everything)	50	2.0	8.0	1.0	0	40	1.0
(*New York* Fat Free)	40	1.0	8.0	0	0	55	0
Cajun (*New York*)	45	2.0	8.0	1.0	0	105	1.0
caraway rye (*Lavosh Hawaii*), 1 oz. . .	115	3.0	20.0	3.0	21	290	0
cracked pepper (*New York* Fat Free)	40	1.0	8.0	0	0	50	0
garlic (*California Crisps*), 2 pcs., ½ oz.	65	1.4	8.8	2.7	8	130	0
garlic (*J.J. Flats*) . .	50	2.0	11.0	1.0	0	130	1.0
garlic, roasted, or honey cinnamon (*New York* Fat Free)	40	1.0	8.0	0	0	50	0
herb, Italian (*J.J. Flats*)	50	2.0	10.0	1.5	0	70	1.0
multigrain (*J.J. Flats*)	50	1.0	1.0	1.5	0	120	1.0
oat bran (*J.J. Flats*)	50	2.0	11.0	.5	0	65	1.0
onion or poppy (*California Crisps*), 2 pcs., ½ oz. . .	66	1.9	10.2	1.9	10	120	0
onion (*J.J. Flats*)	50	2.0	11.0	1.0	0	120	<1.0

Food and Measure	cal.	prot. (gms)	carbo. (gms)	fat (gms)	chol. (mgs)	sod. (mgs)	fiber (gms)
onion (*New York*)	40	1.0	7.0	1.0	0	40	1.0
onion, slightly (*Lavosh Hawaii*), 1 oz........	120	3.0	19.0	3.0	21	300	0
peppercorn (*Lavosh Hawaii*), 1 oz. . .	115	3.0	20.0	3.0	21	300	0
poppy (*J.J. Flats*)	50	2.0	10.0	1.0	0	120	<1.0
poppy (*New York*)	50	2.0	8.0	1.0	0	45	1.0
pumpernickel (*New York* Fat Free) . .	40	1.0	8.0	0	0	75	0
pumpernickel onion (*New York*) . . .	40	1.0	7.0	1.0	0	45	1.0
pumpernickel sesame (*New York*)	50	1.0	8.0	1.5	0	50	1.0
rosemary garlic (*Lavosh Hawaii*), 1 oz........	125	3.0	19.0	3.0	21	290	0
sesame (*J.J. Flats*)	50	2.0	10.0	1.0	0	120	1.0
sesame (*New York*)	50	2.0	8.0	1.5	0	40	1.0
10 grain (*California Crisps*), 2 pcs., ½ oz.	59	2.2	10.2	1.6	0	120	0
10 grain (*Lavosh Hawaii*), 1 oz. . .	110	4.0	19.0	3.0	0	300	0
vegetable, garden (*New York* Fat Free)	40	1.0	8.0	0	0	55	0
golden (*Snackwell's* Classic), 6 pcs., ½ oz.	60	1.0	11.0	1.0	0	140	0
(*Goldfish* Original) . .	140	3.0	19.0	6.0	0	230	<1.0
(*Goya* Snack), 11 pcs.	140	4.0	21.0	4.0	0	140	0
(*Goya* Tropical), 4 pcs.	140	4.0	21.0	4.0	3	130	0
graham, see "Cookie" matzo:							
(*Manischewitz* Unsalted)	110	3.0	24.0	.5	0	0	0

Food and Measure	cal.	prot. (gms)	carbo. (gms)	fat (gms)	chol. (mgs)	sod. (mgs)	fiber (gms)
Cracker, matzo (cont.)							
(Manischewitz Everything!)	110	3.0	22.0	.5	0	150	1.0
garlic (Manischewitz Savory)	100	3.0	23.0	0	0	200	1.0
rye (Manischewitz)	110	3.0	23.0	0	0	220	1.0
melba rounds/snacks, 5 pcs., ½ oz.:							
plain (Devonsheer)	50	2.0	12.0	0	0	95	1.0
bacon (Old London)	60	2.0	11.0	1.5	0	110	2.0
cheese (Old London)	60	2.0	10.0	1.0	0	160	0
garlic (Devonsheer)	60	2.0	11.0	1.5	0	85	1.0
garlic (Old London)	60	2.0	11.0	1.5	0	105	2.0
herb, savory (Devonsheer) . .	50	2.0	11.0	.5	0	80	1.0
honey bran (Devonsheer)	50	2.0	12.0	0	0	70	1.0
onion (Devonsheer)	50	2.0	11.0	0	0	95	1.0
onion (Old London)	60	2.0	11.0	1.5	0	140	2.0
Mexicali corn (Old London)	60	2.0	10.0	1.5	0	100	2.0
rye (Old London)	60	2.0	11.0	1.5	0	190	1.0
sesame (Devonsheer)	60	2.0	10.0	2.5	0	125	1.0
sesame (Old London)	60	2.0	9.0	3.0	0	110	1.0
12 grain (Devonsheer)	50	2.0	12.0	0	0	90	1.0
vegetable (Devonsheer)	50	2.0	12.0	0	0	90	1.0
white (Old London)	60	2.0	11.0	1.5	0	105	2.0
whole grain (Old London)	60	2.0	11.0	1.5	0	120	2.0
melba toast, 3 pcs., ½ oz.:							
plain, rye, or wheat (Devonsheer) . .	50	2.0	11.0	0	0	85	1.0

Food and Measure	cal.	prot. (gms)	carbo. (gms)	fat (gms)	chol. (mgs)	sod. (mgs)	fiber (gms)
plain or wheat (*Devonsheer* No Salt)	50	2.0	11.0	0	0	0	1.0
onion (*Old London*)	50	2.0	11.0	.5	0	140	1.0
rye (*Devonsheer*)	50	2.0	11.0	0	0	85	1.0
rye (*Old London*)	50	2.0	11.0	.5	0	105	1.0
sesame (*Devon-sheer*)	50	2.0	10.0	1.0	0	90	1.0
sesame (*Devon-sheer/Old London* No Salt)	50	2.0	10.0	1.5	0	0	2.0
sesame (*Old London*)	50	2.0	10.0	1.5	0	140	2.0
12 grain or vegetable (*Devonsheer*)	50	2.0	11.0	0	0	90	1.0
wheat (*Old London*)	50	2.0	11.0	.5	0	100	2.0
white (*Old London*)	50	2.0	11.0	.5	0	105	1.0
whole grain (*Old London*)	45	2.0	11.0	.5	0	120	2.0
whole grain (*Old London* No Salt)	50	2.0	11.0	.5	0	0	2.0
milk (*Royal Lunch*), 1 pc.	50	<1.0	8.0	2.0	0	65	0
multigrain:							
(*Hi-Ho*)	160	2.0	18.0	9.0	0	370	2.0
(*Wheat Thins*) . . .	130	2.0	21.0	4.0	0	290	2.0
5 (*Harvest Crisps*)	130	3.0	23.0	3.5	0	300	1.0
(*Munch 'ems*)	130	3.0	20.0	5.0	0	350	<1.0
oat:							
(*Harvest Crisps*) . .	140	3.0	22.0	4.5	0	300	1.0
(*Oat Thins*)	140	3.0	20.0	6.0	0	190	2.0
onion:							
(*Toasted Comple-ments*)	140	2.0	19.0	6.0	0	310	<1.0
French (*Snackwell's*)	120	2.0	23.0	2.0	0	290	1.0
French (*Wheatables*)	130	3.0	21.0	4.0	0	320	<1.0
peanut butter:							
(*Combos*)	140	4.0	15.0	8.0	0	260	1.0
(*Handi-Snacks*) . .	180	5.0	12.0	12.0	0	150	1.0

Food and Measure	cal.	prot. (gms)	carbo. (gms)	fat (gms)	chol. (mgs)	sod. (mgs)	fiber (gms)
Cracker, peanut butter *(cont.)*							
graham *(Handi-Snacks* Graham-stick)	170	5.0	14.0	10.0	0	130	1.0
peanut butter sandwich:							
(Ritz)	150	4.0	17.0	8.0	0	130	1.0
cheese *(Little Debbie),* 1.4 oz. . . .	200	4.0	22.0	11.0	0	290	1.0
cheese *(Frito-Lay),* 1 pkg.	200	6.0	22.0	10.0	0	400	1.0
cheese *(Nabs),* 1.4 oz.	190	4.0	24.0	10.0	0	390	1.0
cheese *(Planters),* 1.4-oz. pkg. . . .	190	4.0	23.0	10.0	0	380	1.0
toast *(Frito-Lay),* 1 pkg.	190	5.0	23.0	9.0	0	380	1.0
toast *(Little Debbie),* 1.4 oz.	190	4.0	23.0	10.0	0	290	1.0
toast *(Nabs),* 1.4 oz.	190	4.0	24.0	10.0	0	380	1.0
toast *(Planters),* 1.4-oz. pkg. . . .	190	4.0	23.0	10.0	0	370	1.0
toast *(Sunshine),* 1.2-oz. pkg. . . .	180	4.0	18.0	10.0	0	350	1.0
pizza:							
(Goldfish)	140	3.0	19.0	6.0	0	160	1.0
all varieties *(Health Valley),* 6 pcs. . .	50	2.0	11.0	0	0	140	2.0
bites *(Barbara's)* . .	120	3.0	24.0	1.5	0	290	1.0
potato:							
au gratin *(No Fries)*	110	3.0	25.0	0	0	160	1.0
barbecue *(No Fries)*	110	2.0	26.0	0	0	150	1.0
sour cream and chives *(No Fries)*	110	3.0	25.0	0	0	150	1.0
ranch *(Munch 'ems)*	130	3.0	21.0	4.0	0	310	<1.0
rice:							
bran *(Health Valley)*	110	3.0	19.0	3.0	0	70	3.0
brown *(Eden)* . . .	120	3.0	22.0	2.0	0	230	2.0
salsa *(Munch 'ems)*	130	2.0	23.0	4.0	0	260	1.0

Food and Measure	cal.	prot. (gms)	carbo. (gms)	fat (gms)	chol. (mgs)	sod. (mgs)	fiber (gms)
saltines, 5 pcs., ½ oz., except as noted:							
(*Dux*), 2 pcs. . . .	40	1.0	8.0	.5	0	125	0
(*Krispy*)	60	2.0	10.0	1.5	0	180	<1.0
(*Krispy* Fat Free) . .	60	2.0	12.0	0	0	135	<1.0
(*Krispy* Unsalted Top)	60	2.0	10.0	1.5	0	120	<1.0
(*Premium*)	60	1.0	10.0	1.5	0	180	<1.0
(*Premium* Fat Free)	50	1.0	11.0	0	0	130	0
(*Premium* Low Sodium)	60	1.0	10.0	1.0	0	35	<1.0
(*Premium* Unsalted Top)	60	1.0	10.0	1.5	0	135	<1.0
(*Zesta*)	60	1.0	10.0	2.0	0	190	<1.0
cracked pepper (*Krispy*)	60	2.0	10.0	1.5	0	180	<1.0
saltines, mini (*Premium* Bits)	150	2.0	19.0	7.0	0	340	<1.0
sesame:							
(*Breton*), 1½ oz. . .	220	4.0	25.0	11.0	0	400	1.0
(*Pepperidge Farm*), 3 pcs., ½ oz. . .	70	1.0	9.0	2.5	0	95	2.0
(*Toasted Complements*)	140	3.0	19.0	6.0	0	320	<1.0
sesame cheese (*Twigs*)	150	4.0	17.0	7.0	0	300	<1.0
(*Sociables*), 7 pcs., ½ oz.	80	1.0	9.0	4.0	0	150	<1.0
soup and oyster, ½ oz.:							
(*Krispy*)	60	2.0	11.0	1.5	0	200	<1.0
(*Oysterettes*)	60	1.0	10.0	2.5	0	150	<1.0
(*Premium*)	60	1.0	10.0	1.5	0	230	<1.0
sour cream and onion (*Munch 'ems*) . . .	130	2.0	22.0	3.5	0	390	0
(*Uneeda*), 2 pcs., ½ oz.	60	1.0	11.0	1.5	0	110	<1.0

Food and Measure	cal.	prot. (gms)	carbo. (gms)	fat (gms)	chol. (mgs)	sod. (mgs)	fiber (gms)
Cracker *(cont.)*							
vegetable:							
(*Garden Crisps*) . .	130	2.0	22.0	3.5	0	290	1.0
(*Vegetable Thins*)	160	2.0	19.0	9.0	0	310	1.0
water or soda:							
(*Breton*), 1½ oz. . . .	210	5.0	26.0	9.0	0	400	1.0
(*Breton* Less Salt),							
1½ oz.	210	5.0	26.0	10.0	0	150	1.0
(*Breton* Light),							
1½ oz.	200	5.0	33.0	6.0	0	390	n.a.
(*Cabaret*), 1.7 oz.	230	4.0	30.0	11.0	0	450	1.0
(*Carr's Table Water*),							
5 pcs., .6 oz. . .	70	2.0	13.0	1.5	0	100	<1.0
(*Crown Pilot*),							
.6-oz. pc.	70	1.0	13.0	1.5	0	85	<1.0
(*Dux*), 2 pcs. . . .	40	1.0	8.0	.5	0	70	0
(*Hi-Ho*)	160	2.0	18.0	9.0	0	280	<1.0
(*Pepperidge Farm*							
Original), ½ oz.	60	2.0	11.0	1.0	<5	100	<1.0
(*Vivant*), 1½ oz. . . .	210	3.0	27.0	10.0	0	390	1.0
cracked pepper							
(*Carr's Table Wa-*							
ter), 5 pcs., .6 oz.	70	2.0	13.0	1.5	0	100	<1.0
cracked pepper (*Hi-*							
Ho)	160	2.0	18.0	9.0	0	280	<1.0
cracked pepper							
(*Pepperidge*							
Farm), ½ oz. . .	60	2.0	12.0	1.0	<5	90	<1.0
cracked pepper							
(*Snackwell's*),							
½ oz.	60	2.0	13.0	0	0	150	<1.0
poppy sesame							
(*Carr's*), ½ oz.	80	1.0	9.0	4.0	0	80	<1.0
sesame (*Breton*),							
1½ oz.	220	4.0	25.0	11.0	0	400	1.0
sesame (*Carr's Ta-*							
ble Water), 5 pcs.,							
.6 oz.	70	2.0	13.0	1.5	0	95	<1.0

Food and Measure	cal.	prot. (gms)	carbo. (gms)	fat (gms)	chol. (mgs)	sod. (mgs)	fiber (gms)
wheat:							
(*Snackwell's* Fat Free), ½ oz. . . .	60	2.0	12.0	0	0	170	1.0
(*Stoned Wheat Thins*), 2 pcs. . .	60	2.0	10.0	1.5	0	140	<1.0
(*Stoned Wheat Thins* Lower Sodium), 2 pcs. . .	60	2.0	10.0	1.5	0	70	<1.0
(*Toasted Complements*)	140	2.0	19.0	6.0	0	270	<1.0
(*Triscuit*)	140	3.0	21.0	5.0	0	170	4.0
(*Triscuit* Low Sodium)	150	3.0	21.0	6.0	0	50	3.0
(*Triscuit* Reduced Fat)	130	3.0	24.0	3.0	0	180	4.0
(*Waverly*), ½ oz. . .	70	1.0	10.0	3.5	0	135	0
(*Wheat Thins*) . . .	140	2.0	19.0	6.0	0	1709	2.0
(*Wheat Thins* Low Salt)	140	2.0	20.0	6.0	0	75	2.0
(*Wheat Thins* Reduced Fat)	120	2.0	21.0	4.0	0	220	2.0
(*Wheatables*)	150	3.0	18.0	7.0	0	320	1.0
(*Wheatsworth*), .6 oz.	80	2.0	10.0	3.5	0	170	1.0
all varieties (*Barbara's* Wheatines), ½-oz. sq.	60	1.0	11.0	1.0	0	132	0
cracked (*Pepperidge Farm*), 2 pcs., ½ oz.	70	1.0	9.0	2.5	0	150	<1.0
hearty (*Pepperidge Farm*), 3 pcs., ½ oz.	80	2.0	10.0	3.5	0	100	1.0
herb, garden (*Triscuit*)	130	3.0	20.0	4.5	0	130	3.0
and rye (*Triscuit* Deli)	140	3.0	22.0	5.0	0	180	4.0

Food and Measure	cal.	prot. (gms)	carbo. (gms)	fat (gms)	chol. (mgs)	sod. (mgs)	fiber (gms)
Cracker *(cont.)*							
wheat, whole:							
(*Carr's*), 2 pcs.,							
.6 oz.	80	1.0	11.0	3.5	0	100	1.0
(*Health Valley* No							
Salt), 5 pcs. . . .	50	2.0	11.0	0	0	15	2.0
(*Hi-Ho*)	150	3.0	18.0	8.0	0	280	2.0
(*Krispy*), 5 pcs.,							
½ oz.	60	2.0	10.0	1.5	0	130	<1.0
all varieties (*Health*							
Valley), 5 pcs. . .	50	2.0	11.0	0	0	80	2.0
and bran (*Triscuit*)	140	3.0	22.0	8.0	0	170	4.0
(*Zwieback*), .3-oz. pc.	35	1.0	5.0	1.0	0	10	<1.0
Cracker crumbs and							
meal, ¼ cup, ex-							
cept as noted:							
crumbs:							
(*Ritz*), ⅓ cup . . .	140	2.0	17.0	7.0	0	270	1.0
saltine (*Premium* Fat							
Free)	100	3.0	23.0	0	0	0	1.0
matzo meal:							
(*Manischewitz*) . . .	130	3.0	27.0	.5	0	0	0
(*Streit's*)	110	3.0	24.0	.5	0	0	1.0
Cranberry, fresh, raw:							
whole, ½ cup	23	.2	6.0	.1	0	1	2.0
chopped, ½ cup . . .	27	.2	7.0	.1	0	1	2.3
Cranberry, dried (*So-*							
noma), ⅓ cup . . .	120	0	29.0	.5	0	0	2.0
Cranberry bean:							
boiled, ½ cup	120	8.2	21.5	.4	0	1	3.0
canned, ½ cup . . .	108	7.2	19.7	.4	0	431	n.a.
Cranberry drink,							
8 fl. oz., except as							
noted:							
(*Farmer's Market*) . .	120	0	31.0	0	0	0	0
(*Tropicana* Punch) . .	140	0	34.0	0	0	15	0
(*Tropicana* Punch),							
11.5 fl. oz.	200	0	49.0	0	0	15	0
(*Tropicana* Ruby Red)	120	0	30.0	0	0	65	0

Food and Measure	cal.	prot. (gms)	carbo. (gms)	fat (gms)	chol. (mgs)	sod. (mgs)	fiber (gms)
spiced (*J.M.S.* Cooler)	120	0	30.0	0	0	0	0
Cranberry drink blends, 8 fl. oz.:							
hibiscus:							
(*Heinke's*)	120	0	30.0	0	0	35	0
(*R.W. Knudsen*) . .	120	0	30.0	0	0	35	0
lemon (*Santa Cruz*)	120	0	29.0	0	0	35	0
raspberry:							
(*After the Fall*) . . .	90	1.0	23.0	0	0	20	0
(*R.W. Knudsen*) . .	140	0	36.0	0	0	35	0
raspberry-strawberry:							
(*Tropicana Twister*)	120	0	31.0	0	0	5	0
(*Tropicana Twister* Light)	45	<1.0	11.0	0	0	10	0
Cranberry juice, 8 fl. oz., except as noted:							
(*After the Fall* Cape Cod)	100	0	24.0	0	0	20	0
(*After the Fall* Nantucket)	60	1.0	15.0	0	0	25	0
(*Apple & Eve Naturally Cranberry*) . .	120	1.0	30.0	0	0	20	0
(*Heinke's* 100%) . . .	60	0	14.0	0	0	25	0
(*Ocean Spray* Cocktail), 6 fl. oz.	100	0	25.0	0	0	15	0
(*R.W. Knudsen* Concentrate)	70	1.0	13.0	0	0	15	0
(*R.W. Knudsen* Just Cranberry)	60	0	14.0	0	0	25	0
(*R.W. Knudsen* Yankee)	120	1.0	30.0	0	0	25	0
(*Season's Best* Medley)	120	<1.0	29.0	0	0	20	0
(*Snapple*), 10 fl. oz.	150	0	37.0	0	0	25	0
Cranberry juice blends, 8 fl. oz., except as noted:							
apple (*Cranapple*) . .	160	0	40.0	0	0	35	0

Food and Measure	cal.	prot. (gms)	carbo. (gms)	fat (gms)	chol. (mgs)	sod. (mgs)	fiber (gms)
Cranberry juice blends *(cont.)*							
apricot (*Cranicot*) . .	160	0	40.0	0	0	35	0
blueberry							
(*Cran•Blueberry*) . .	160	0	41.0	0	0	35	0
grape:							
(*Apple & Eve*),							
10 fl. oz.	175	1.0	42.0	0	0	31	0
(*Cran•Grape*)	170	0	41.0	0	0	35	0
grapefruit (*After the*							
Fall)	110	1.0	29.0	0	0	10	0
kiwi (*After the Fall*)	100	1.0	26.0	0	0	18	0
mango (*After the Fall*)	100	1.0	26.0	0	0	15	0
orange (*After the Fall*)	110	1.0	28.0	0	0	15	0
punch (*Crantastic*) . .	150	0	37.0	0	0	35	0
raspberry (*After the*							
Fall)	90	1.0	23.0	0	0	20	0
strawberry:							
(*After the Fall*) . . .	100	1.0	26.0	0	0	15	0
(*Ocean Spray*) . . .	140	0	35.0	0	0	35	0
Cranberry nectar,							
8 fl. oz.:							
(*Heinke's*)	120	0	30.0	0	0	5	0
(*R.W. Knudsen*) . . .	150	1.0	38.0	0	0	45	0
(*Santa Cruz*)	110	0	27.0	0	0	25	0
guava (*Santa Cruz*)	110	0	24.0	0	0	25	0
Cranberry sauce:							
(*Ocean Spray*), 2 oz.	80	0	22.0	0	0	10	0
(*R.W. Knudsen*),							
1 tbsp.	25	0	6.0	0	0	0	0
(*S&W*), ¼ cup . . .	100	0	26.0	0	0	15	1.0
Cranberry sauce							
blends, 2 oz.:							
w/orange or raspberry							
(*Cran•Fruit*)	90	0	23.0	0	0	10	0
w/strawberry							
(*Cran•Fruit*)	90	0	22.0	0	0	10	0
Cranberry-orange rel-							
ish, in jars (*New*							
England), ¼ cup	120	0	31.0	0	0	0	0

Food and Measure	cal.	prot. (gms)	carbo. (gms)	fat (gms)	chol. (mgs)	sod. (mgs)	fiber (gms)
Crayfish, mixed species, meat only:							
wild:							
raw, 4 oz.	87	18.1	0	1.1	130	66	0
raw, 8 medium,							
1 oz.	22	4.5	0	.3	32	16	0
boiled or steamed,							
4 oz.	100	19.0	0	1.4	151	107	0
farmed:							
raw, 4 oz.	82	16.9	0	1.1	122	70	0
boiled or steamed,							
4 oz.	99	19.9	0	1.5	155	110	0
Cream:							
half and half:							
1 cup	315	7.2	10.4	27.8	89	98	0
1 tbsp.	20	.4	.6	1.7	6	6	0
light, coffee or table:							
1 cup	469	6.5	8.8	46.3	159	95	0
1 tbsp.	29	.4	.6	2.9	10	6	0
medium (25% fat):							
1 cup	583	5.9	8.3	59.8	209	88	0
1 tbsp.	37	.4	.5	3.8	13	6	0
sour, see "Cream, sour"							
whipping[1], light:							
1 cup	699	5.2	7.1	73.9	265	82	0
1 tbsp.	44	.3	.4	4.6	17	5	0
whipping[1], heavy:							
1 cup	821	4.9	6.6	88.1	326	89	0
1 tbsp.	52	.3	.4	5.6	21	6	0
whipped topping, see "Cream topping"							
Cream, canned, light (*Nestlé* Crema),							
1 tbsp.	30	0	<1.0	3.0	10	10	0

[1] *Unwhipped; volume approximately doubled when whipped.*

Food and Measure	cal.	prot. (gms)	carbo. (gms)	fat (gms)	chol. (mgs)	sod. (mgs)	fiber (gms)
Cream, sour, 2 tbsp., except as noted:							
1 cup	493	7.3	9.8	48.2	102	123	0
(*Breakstone's*)	60	1.0	1.0	5.0	25	15	0
(*Heluva* Good)	60	1.0	2.0	5.0	20	15	0
(*Knudsen Hampshire*)	60	1.0	1.0	6.0	25	15	0
(*Sealtest*)	60	<1.0	1.0	5.0	20	15	0
half and half (*Break-stone's*)	45	1.0	2.0	3.5	15	20	0
light:							
(*Heluva* Good) . . .	40	1.0	3.0	2.5	10	20	0
(*Knudsen Light*) . .	40	2.0	2.0	2.5	10	20	0
(*Sealtest Light*) . .	40	2.0	2.0	2.5	10	20	0
nondairy, plain or flavored (*Sour Supreme*)	50	1.0	1.0	5.0	0	120	0
nonfat:							
(*Breakstone's/Sealtest Free*)	35	2.0	6.0	0	<5	25	0
(*Heluva* Good) . . .	20	1.0	3.0	0	0	45	0
(*Naturally Yours*)	20	2.0	4.0	0	0	25	<1.0
Cream of tartar (*Tone's*), 1 tsp. . .	2	0	.6	0	0	n.a.	0
Cream topping, 2 tbsp.:							
(*Cool Whip* Extra Creamy)	30	0	2.0	2.0	0	5	0
(*Cool Whip* Lite) . . .	20	0	2.0	1.0	0	0	0
(*Cool Whip* Nondairy)	25	0	2.0	1.5	0	0	0
(*Kraft* Real)	20	0	1.0	1.5	5	0	0
(*Kraft* Whipped Topping)	20	0	1.0	1.5	0	0	0
(*La Crema* Lite) . . .	15	0	2.0	1.0	0	10	0
(*Pet Whip*)	30	0	2.0	2.0	0	0	0
(*Rich's*)	25	0	2.0	1.5	0	0	0
pressurized can (*Rich's*)	25	0	2.0	2.0	0	5	0
mix*:							
1 cup	151	2.9	13.2	9.9	0	53	0

Food and Measure	cal.	prot. (gms)	carbo. (gms)	fat (gms)	chol. (mgs)	sod. (mgs)	fiber (gms)
(*D-Zerta*)	10	0	1.0	1.0	0	10	0
(*Dream Whip*) . . .	20	0	2.0	1.0	0	10	0
Creamer, nondairy, 1 tbsp., except as noted:							
(*Coffee-mate*)	20	0	2.0	1.0	0	0	0
(*Coffee-mate* Fat Free)	10	0	2.0	0	0	0	0
(*Coffee-mate* Lite) . .	10	0	1.0	.5	0	5	0
(*Rich's Coffee Rich*)	25	0	3.0	1.5	0	10	0
(*Rich's Coffee Rich* Light)	15	0	1.0	1.0	0	5	0
(*Rich's Farm Rich*)	20	0	1.0	1.5	0	5	0
(*Rich's Farm Rich* Light)	10	0	1.0	1.0	0	5	0
(*Rich's Farm Rich* Fat Free)	10	0	1.0	0	0	5	0
powder, 1 tsp.:							
(*Coffee-mate*) . . .	10	0	1.0	.5	0	0	0
(*Coffee-mate* Lite)	10	0	2.0	0	0	0	0
(*Cremora*)	10	0	1.0	1.0	0	0	0
(*Cremora* Fat Free)	10	0	2.0	0	0	10	0
(*Cremora* Lite) . . .	10	0	2.0	0	0	0	0
Creamer, nondairy, flavored (*Coffee-mate*), all flavors:							
liquid, 1 tbsp.	40	0	5.0	2.0	0	5	0
powdered, 1⅓ tbsp.	60	0	9.0	3.0	0	15	0
Crepe, fresh (*Frieda's*), 1 pc. . .	45	1.0	7.0	1.0	n.a.	80	n.a.
Cress, garden, ½ cup:							
raw	8	.7	1.4	.2	0	4	.3
boiled, drained	16	1.3	2.6	.4	0	5	.5
Cress, water, see "Watercress"							
Croaker, meat only, raw, Atlantic, 4 oz.	119	20.2	0	3.6	69	63	0

Food and Measure	cal.	prot. (gms)	carbo. (gms)	fat (gms)	chol. (mgs)	sod. (mgs)	fiber (gms)
Croissant, 1 pc.:							
butter:							
(*Awrey's*), 1.5 oz.	140	3.0	13.0	9.0	25	230	0
(*Awrey's*), 2 oz. . . .	190	4.0	17.0	12.0	35	310	<1.0
(*Awrey's Tip-to-Tip*)	290	6.0	26.0	18.0	55	470	<1.0
(*Pepperidge Farm* Petite)	130	3.0	13.0	8.0	20	180	<1.0
margarine (*Awrey's Tip-to-Tip*)	140	2.0	14.0	8.0	0	140	0
margarine, sandwich:							
(*Awrey's*), 1.8 oz.	180	3.0	17.0	11.0	0	170	<1.0
(*Awrey's*), 2.5 oz.	250	5.0	23.0	15.0	0	230	<1.0
wheat (*Awrey's*) . .	250	5.0	22.0	15.0	0	220	1.0
frozen (*Sara Lee*) . .	170	4.0	20.0	8.0	<5	200	1.0
Crookneck squash:							
fresh, sliced, ½ cup:							
raw, ends trimmed	12	.6	2.6	.2	0	1	.7
boiled, drained . . .	18	.8	3.9	.3	0	1	1.3
canned, cut, drained, no salt, ½ cup . . .	14	.7	3.2	.1	0	5	1.1
frozen, boiled, sliced, ½ cup	24	1.2	5.3	.2	0	6	1.2
Croutons (see also "Salad toppers"), ¼ oz. or 2 tbsp.:							
Caesar:							
(*Brownberry*) . . .	30	1.0	4.0	1.5	0	70	0
(*Pepperidge Farm*)	35	1.0	4.0	1.5	0	90	0
cheddar (*Brownberry*)	30	1.0	4.0	1.5	0	65	0
cheddar and Romano (*Pepperidge Farm*)	30	1.0	4.0	1.0	0	95	0
cheese and garlic:							
(*Arnold* Crispy) . .	30	1.0	5.0	1.0	0	50	0
(*Brownberry*) . . .	30	1.0	5.0	1.0	0	60	0
(*Pepperidge Farm*)	35	1.0	4.0	1.5	0	80	0
cracked pepper and Parmesan (*Pepperidge Farm*)	35	1.0	4.0	1.5	0	90	0

Food and Measure	cal.	prot. (gms)	carbo. (gms)	fat (gms)	chol. (mgs)	sod. (mgs)	fiber (gms)
garlic (*Old London* Restaurant Style)	30	<1.0	4.0	1.5	0	95	0
herb, fine (*Arnold* Crispy)	30	1.0	5.0	1.0	0	60	0
Italian:							
(*Arnold* Crispy) . .	30	1.0	4.0	1.0	0	65	0
(*Old London* Restaurant Style) . .	30	<1.0	4.0	1.5	0	70	0
zesty (*Pepperidge Farm*)	35	1.0	4.0	1.5	0	65	0
olive oil and garlic (*Pepperidge Farm*)	30	1.0	5.0	1.0	0	80	0
onion and garlic:							
(*Arnold* Crispy) . .	30	1.0	5.0	1.0	0	80	0
(*Brownberry*) . . .	30	1.0	4.0	1.0	0	80	0
(*Pepperidge Farm*)	30	1.0	5.0	1.0	0	80	0
ranch:							
(*Arnold* Crispy) . .	30	<1.0	5.0	1.0	0	75	0
(*Brownberry*) . . .	30	<1.0	4.0	1.0	0	80	0
(*Pepperidge Farm*)	35	1.0	4.0	1.5	<5	65	0
seasoned:							
(*Arnold* Crispy) . .	30	1.0	5.0	1.0	0	60	0
(*Brownberry*) . . .	30	<1.0	4.0	1.0	0	70	0
(*Pepperidge Farm*)	35	1.0	4.0	1.5	0	85	0
sourdough:							
(*Old London* Restaurant Style) . .	30	<1.0	4.0	1.5	0	65	0
cheese (*Pepperidge Farm*)	30	1.0	4.0	1.0	0	80	0
toasted (*Brownberry*)	30	<1.0	5.0	1.0	0	45	0
Cucumber, w/peel:							
1 medium, 8¼″ long	38	2.1	8.3	.4	0	6	2.4
sliced, ½ cup	7	.4	1.4	.1	0	1	.4
hot house, unpeeled (*Frieda's*), 1 oz. . .	4	.2	.8	<.1	0	1	n.a.
Cucumber, pickled, see "Pickle"							

Food and Measure	cal.	prot. (gms)	carbo. (gms)	fat (gms)	chol. (mgs)	sod. (mgs)	fiber (gms)
Cucumber dip, creamy (*Kraft* Premium), 2 tbsp. . .	50	<1.0	2.0	4.0	15	140	0
Cucumber-garlic dip, see "Tzatziki"							
Cucumber salad (*Rosoff/Schorr's*), 1 oz.	12	0	3.0	0	0	220	0
Cumin seed, ground:							
1 tsp.	8	.4	.9	.5	0	4	.2
(*McCormick*), ¼ tsp.	3	.1	.2	.1	0	1	.2
(*Tone's*), ¼ tsp. . . .	0	0	0	0	0	0	0
Cupcake, see "Cake, snack"							
Currant, ½ cup, except as noted:							
fresh, black, Europe	36	.8	8.6	.2	0	1	3.0
fresh, red or white	31	.8	7.7	.1	0	1	2.4
dried, zante	204	2.9	53.3	.2	0	6	4.9
dried, zante (*S&W*), ¼ cup	130	1.0	31.0	0	0	10	2.0
Curry paste (*Patak's*), 2 tbsp.	170	2.0	4.0	16.0	5	900	0
Curry powder:							
1 tbsp.	20	.8	3.7	.9	0	3	1.0
1 tsp.	6	.3	1.2	.3	0	1	.3
(*Tone's*), ¼ tsp. . . .	0	0	0	0	0	15	0
Curry sauce, cooking:							
(*Kylin Thai*), ¼ cup	25	1.0	5.0	.5	0	600	<1.0
hot, ½ cup:							
madras (*Patak's*)	300	4.0	17.0	25.0	5	1330	5.0
tikka masala (*Patak's*)	240	4.0	14.0	18.0	10	1390	3.0
vindaloo (*Patak's*)	320	4.0	16.0	27.0	<5	1540	5.0
jalfrezzi (*Patak's*), ½ cup	160	3.0	15.0	10.0	0	430	4.0
Masala, ¼ cup:							
(*Shahi* Cream) . . .	50	1.0	5.0	4.0	0	550	1.0
(*Shahi* Curry) . . .	50	1.0	4.0	4.0	0	680	1.0

Food and Measure	cal.	prot. (gms)	carbo. (gms)	fat (gms)	chol. (mgs)	sod. (mgs)	fiber (gms)
rogan josh (*Patak's*), ½ cup	190	3.0	12.0	15.0	<5	1270	4.0
Curry sauce mix(*Knorr*), ⅕ pkg.	30	1.0	4.0	1.5	0	220	0
Cusk, meat only:							
raw, 4 oz.	99	21.6	0	.8	47	36	0
baked, broiled, or microwaved, 4 oz. . .	127	27.6	0	1.0	60	45	0
Custard, see "Pudding mix"							
Custard apple, trimmed, 1 oz. . . .	29	.5	7.1	.2	0	1	1.0
Custard marrow, see "Chayote"							
Cuttlefish, meat only:							
raw, 4 oz.	90	18.4	.9	.8	127	422	0
boiled or steamed, 4 oz.	179	36.8	1.9	1.6	254	844	0
Cuttlefish, canned, in ink (*Goya*), ¼ cup	120	8.0	2.0	9.0	15	350	0

D

Food and Measure	cal.	prot. (gms)	carbo. (gms)	fat (gms)	chol. (mgs)	sod. (mgs)	fiber (gms)
Daikon, see "Radish, Oriental"							
Daiquiri mixer:							
bottled:							
(*Holland House/Mr. & Mrs. "T"*),							
4 fl. oz.	150	0	33.0	0	0	120	0
strawberry (*Holland House*), 3.5 fl. oz.	150	0	34.0	0	0	20	0
frozen*, strawberry (*Bacardi*), 8 fl. oz.	140	0	35.0	0	0	0	0
mix (*Bar-Tenders*), 2 pkts., 1.2 oz. . .	30	0	30.0	0	0	90	0
Dairy Queen/Brazier,							
1 serving:							
DQ Homestyle							
burgers:							
cheeseburger . . .	340	20.0	29.0	17.0	55	850	2.0
double cheeseburger	540	35.0	30.0	31.0	115	1130	2.0
deluxe double cheeseburger . .	540	36.0	31.0	31.0	115	1130	2.0
cheeseburger w/bacon, double	610	41.0	31.0	36.0	130	1380	2.0
hamburger	290	17.0	29.0	12.0	45	630	2.0
hamburger, deluxe double	440	30.0	29.0	22.0	90	680	2.0
Ultimate burger . .	670	40.0	29.0	43.0	135	1210	2.0
sandwiches:							
chicken fillet:							
breaded	430	24.0	37.0	20.0	55	760	2.0

Food and Measure	cal.	prot. (gms)	carbo. (gms)	fat (gms)	chol. (mgs)	sod. (mgs)	fiber (gms)
breaded							
w/cheese	480	27.0	38.0	25.0	70	980	2.0
grilled	310	24.0	30.0	10.0	50	1040	3.0
fish fillet	370	16.0	39.0	16.0	45	630	2.0
fish fillet w/cheese	420	19.0	40.0	21.0	60	850	2.0
hot dog:							
plain	240	9.0	19.0	14.0	25	730	1.0
w/cheese	290	12.0	20.0	18.0	40	950	1.0
w/chili	280	12.0	21.0	16.0	35	870	2.0
w/chili and							
cheese	330	14.0	22.0	21.0	45	1090	2.0
chicken strip basket:							
w/gravy	860	35.0	88.0	42.0	55	1820	5.0
w/BBQ sauce . . .	810	33.0	88.0	37.0	55	1590	5.0
side dishes:							
fries, large	390	5.0	52.0	18.0	0	200	6.0
fries, regular	300	4.0	40.0	14.0	0	160	4.0
fries, small	210	3.0	29.0	10.0	0	115	3.0
onion rings, regular	240	4.0	29.0	12.0	0	135	2.0
desserts and shakes:							
banana split	510	8.0	96.0	12.0	30	180	3.0
Blizzard:							
Butterfinger, regu-							
lar	750	16.0	115.0	26.0	50	360	1.0
Butterfinger, small	520	11.0	80.0	18.0	35	250	1.0
chocolate chip							
cookie dough,							
regular	950	17.0	143.0	36.0	75	660	2.0
chocolate chip							
cookie dough,							
small	660	12.0	99.0	24.0	55	440	1.0
chocolate sand-							
wich cookie, reg-							
ular	640	12.0	97.0	23.0	45	500	1.0
chocolate sand-							
wich cookie,							
small	520	10.0	79.0	18.0	40	380	1.0
Heath, regular . .	820	14.0	119.0	33.0	60	580	1.0
Heath, small . . .	560	10.0	82.0	21.0	45	380	1.0

Food and Measure	cal.	prot. (gms)	carbo. (gms)	fat (gms)	chol. (mgs)	sod. (mgs)	fiber (gms)
Dairy Queen/Brazier, desserts and shakes, Blizzard *(cont.)*							
Reese's peanut butter cup, regular	790	19.0	105.0	33.0	55	430	2.0
Reese's peanut butter cup, small	590	14.0	81.0	24.0	45	320	1.0
strawberry, regular	570	12.0	95.0	16.0	50	260	1.0
strawberry, small	400	9.0	66.0	11.0	35	190	1.0
Buster Bar	450	10.0	41.0	28.0	15	280	2.0
cone, chocolate:							
regular	360	9.0	56.0	11.0	30	180	0
small	240	6.0	37.0	8.0	20	115	0
cone, chocolate-dipped:							
regular	510	9.0	63.0	25.0	30	200	1.0
small	340	6.0	42.0	17.0	20	130	1.0
cone, vanilla:							
large	410	10.0	65.0	12.0	40	200	0
regular	350	8.0	57.0	10.0	30	170	0
small	230	6.0	38.0	7.0	20	115	0
DQ cake, un-decorated:							
heart, 1/10 cake . .	270	5.0	41.0	9.0	20	190	1.0
log, 1/8 cake . . .	280	5.0	43.0	9.0	15	220	1.0
round, 8", 1/8 cake	340	7.0	53.0	12.0	25	250	1.0
round, 10", 1/12 cake	360	7.0	55.0	12.0	25	260	1.0
sheet, 1/20 cake . .	350	7.0	54.0	12.0	20	270	1.0
DQ caramel & nut bar	260	5.0	32.0	13.0	15	90	0
DQ fudge bar . . .	50	4.0	13.0	0	0	70	0
DQ Lemon Freez'r, 1/2 cup	80	0	20.0	0	0	10	0
DQ sandwich . . .	150	3.0	24.0	5.0	5	115	1.0
DQ Treatzza Pizza, 1/8 pie:							
Heath	180	3.0	28.0	7.0	5	160	1.0
M&M	190	3.0	29.0	7.0	5	160	1.0

Food and Measure	cal.	prot. (gms)	carbo. (gms)	fat (gms)	chol. (mgs)	sod. (mgs)	fiber (gms)
peanut butter							
fudge	220	4.0	28.0	10.0	5	200	1.0
strawberry-banana	180	3.0	29.0	6.0	5	140	1.0
DQ vanilla orange							
bar	60	2.0	17.0	0	0	40	0
Dilly bar:							
chocolate	210	3.0	21.0	13.0	10	75	0
chocolate mint . .	190	3.0	20.0	12.0	15	100	0
toffee, w/Heath	210	3.0	24.0	12.0	15	100	0
Fudge Nut Bar . . .	410	8.0	40.0	25.0	15	250	2.0
malt, chocolate:							
regular	880	19.0	153.0	22.0	70	500	0
small	650	15.0	111.0	16.0	55	370	0
Misty:							
cooler, strawberry	190	0	49.0	0	0	25	1.0
slush, regular . .	290	0	74.0	0	0	30	0
slush, small . . .	220	0	56.0	0	0	20	0
Peanut Buster par-							
fait	730	16.0	99.0	31.0	35	400	2.0
Queen's Choice Big							
Scoop:							
chocolate	250	4.0	28.0	14.0	55	95	0
vanilla	250	4.0	27.0	14.0	55	100	0
shake, chocolate:							
regular	770	17.0	130.0	20.0	70	420	0
small	560	13.0	94.0	15.0	50	310	0
soft-serve, DQ:							
chocolate, ½ cup	150	4.0	22.0	5.0	15	75	0
vanilla, ½ cup . .	140	3.0	22.0	4.5	15	70	0
Starkiss	80	0	21.0	0	0	10	0
strawberry short-							
cake	430	7.0	70.0	14.0	60	360	1.0
sundae, chocolate:							
regular	410	8.0	73.0	10.0	30	210	0
small	290	6.0	51.0	7.0	25	150	0
yogurt, Breeze:							
Heath, regular . .	710	15.0	123.0	18.0	20	580	1.0
Heath, small . . .	470	11.0	85.0	10.0	10	380	1.0
strawberry, regular	460	13.0	99.0	10.0	10	270	1.0

Food and Measure	cal.	prot. (gms)	carbo. (gms)	fat (gms)	chol. (mgs)	sod. (mgs)	fiber (gms)
Dairy Queen/Brazier, desserts and shakes, yogurt, Breeze *(cont.)*							
strawberry, small	320	10.0	68.0	.5	5	190	1.0
yogurt, frozen:							
DQ nonfat, ½ cup	100	3.0	21.0	0	<5	70	0
regular cup . . .	230	8.0	49.0	.5	5	160	0
cone	280	9.0	59.0	1.0	5	170	0
strawberry sundae	300	9.0	66.0	.5	5	180	1.0
Dandelion greens:							
raw, 1 oz. or ½ cup							
chopped	13	.8	2.6	.2	0	22	1.0
boiled, drained,							
chopped, ½ cup . .	17	1.0	3.3	.3	0	23	1.5
Danish, 1 pc.:							
cake, ring, or twist,							
see "Cake'							
all varieties (*Awrey's*							
Petite)	130	1.0	14.0	8.0	5	85	0
apple:							
(*Awrey's* Grande)	450	4.0	51.0	26.0	15	270	1.0
(*Hostess*)	400	2.0	47.0	22.0	20	340	2.0
(*Hostess* Fruit Roll)	180	4.0	33.0	4.0	<5	170	1.0
(*Hostess* Twist) . .	220	4.0	42.0	4.0	15	270	<1.0
apple, cheese, cinna-							
mon swirl, or straw-							
berry (*Awrey's*) . .	300	3.0	32.0	17.0	10	210	<1.0
caramel pecan swirl							
(*Hostess*)	250	3.0	25.0	15.0	15	130	1.0
cheese:							
(*Awrey's* Grande)	480	5.0	49.0	30.0	20	360	<1.0
(*Tastykake* Pocket)	410	4.0	38.0	27.0	10	210	2.0
cherry or lemon							
(*Awrey's* Mar-							
quise)	350	4.0	38.0	21.0	20	250	<1.0
cinnamon (*Awrey's*							
Marquise)	470	5.0	60.0	24.0	15	310	<1.0
raspberry swirl (*Aw-*							
rey's Grande) . .	400	6.0	51.0	19.0	20	400	1.0
cinnamon swirl (*Aw-*							
rey's Grande) . . .	420	6.0	57.0	21.0	10	410	2.0

Food and Measure	cal.	prot. (gms)	carbo. (gms)	fat (gms)	chol. (mgs)	sod. (mgs)	fiber (gms)
pecan (*Hostess* Spinners)	110	2.0	15.0	5.0	0	65	<1.0
raspberry (*Hostess*)	110	2.0	21.0	2.5	<5	110	<1.0
strawberry (*Awrey's* Grande)	460	4.0	53.0	26.0	15	280	1.0
Danish, frozen or refrigerated, 1 pc.:							
apple or raspberry (*Pepperidge Farm*)	210	4.0	29.0	9.0	15	190	2.0
cheese (*Pepperidge Farm*)	230	6.0	25.0	11.0	55	230	1.0
Dasheen, see "Taro"							
Date, dehydrated, coarse ground (*Dole*), 1 oz.	110	1.0	27.0	0	0	0	2.0
Date, dried, pitted:							
(*Del Monte*), 5–6 pcs., 1.4 oz.	120	1.0	31.0	0	0	0	3.0
(*Dole*), ½ cup	280	8.0	62.0	0	0	0	n.a.
(*Sonoma*), 5–6 pcs., 1.4 oz.	110	1.0	30.0	0	0	15	5.0
chopped:							
(*Del Monte*), 1.4 oz., ¼ cup	120	1.0	33.0	0	0	10	3.0
(*Dole*), ½ cup . . .	230	0	56.0	0	0	5	n.a.
natural, dry, 10 dates, 2.9 oz.	228	1.6	61.0	.4	0	2	6.2
Date nut loaf, see "Bread mix, sweet"							
Date nut pastry (*Awrey's*), 1 pc.	130	1.0	20.0	5.0	10	85	<1.0
Demi-glace sauce mix (*Knorr*), 1 tbsp.	30	1.0	4.0	1.0	0	380	0
Dessert, see specific listings							
Dessert bar mix, see "Cake, snack, mix"							

Food and Measure	cal.	prot. (gms)	carbo. (gms)	fat (gms)	chol. (mgs)	sod. (mgs)	fiber (gms)
Dessert filling, see "Pastry filling" and "Pie filling"							
Dessert mix, no-bake (*Betty Crocker*), ⅑ pkg., except as noted:							
banana cream	160	2.0	31.0	4.0	45	330	0
chocolate French silk, ⅛ pkg.	180	2.0	35.0	4.0	0	150	0
coconut cream	200	2.0	34.0	6.0	50	380	0
cookies 'n creme, ⅙ pkg.	260	3.0	49.0	6.0	0	340	0
lemon supreme . . .	270	1.0	51.0	7.0	30	75	0
Diable sauce (*Escoffier*), 1 tbsp.	20	0	4.0	0	0	160	0
Dill dip, 2 tbsp.:							
(*Bernstein's* Zesty)	120	0	2.0	12.0	20	160	0
(*Marie's*)	190	3.0	3.0	20.0	15	160	0
Dill seed:							
1 tsp.	6	.3	1.2	.3	0	<1	.4
(*McCormick*) ¼ tsp.	3	.1	.4	.1	0	<1	.4
Dill weed:							
fresh:							
5 sprigs	<1	<1.0	.1	<.1	0	1	n.a.
½ cup loose packed	2	.2	.3	.1	0	3	n.a.
dried:							
1 tsp.	3	.2	.6	<.1	0	2	.1
(*McCormick*), ¼ tsp.	1	.1	.1	0	0	3	.1
(*Tone's*), ¼ tsp. . .	0	0	0	0	0	0	0
Dock, boiled, drained, 4 oz.	23	2.1	3.3	.7	0	3	<1.0
Dolphinfish, meat only:							
raw, 4 oz.	97	21.0	0	.8	83	99	0
baked, broiled, or microwaved, 4 oz. . .	124	26.9	0	1.0	107	128	0

Food and Measure	cal.	prot. (gms)	carbo. (gms)	fat (gms)	chol. (mgs)	sod. (mgs)	fiber (gms)
Domino's Pizza, ¼ of 12″ pie (2 slices), except as noted:							
deep dish:							
cheese	560	23.5	63.2	23.8	32	1184	3.2
ham	577	25.9	63.5	24.5	38	1347	3.2
pepperoni	622	26.2	63.4	29.4	46	1383	3.2
sausage and mush-							
room.	618	26.2	65.5	28.2	43	1356	3.7
veggie	576	24.0	65.0	24.7	32	1233	3.7
X-tra cheese and							
pepperoni	671	29.6	63.7	33.1	54	1508	3.2
hand-tossed:							
cheese	344	14.8	50.0	9.5	19	981	2.4
ham	362	17.2	50.3	10.2	26	1143	2.4
pepperoni	406	17.5	50.2	15.1	32	1179	2.5
sausage and mush-							
room.	402	17.5	52.2	13.9	31	1151	2.9
veggie	360	15.2	51.7	10.4	19	1028	3.0
X-tra cheese and							
pepperoni	455	20.9	50.5	18.8	42	1304	2.5
thin crust, ⅓ pie:							
cheese	364	16.1	40.1	15.5	26	1012	1.9
ham	388	19.3	40.5	16.5	35	1229	1.9
pepperoni	447	19.7	40.4	23.0	43	1277	2.0
sausage and mush-							
room.	442	19.8	43.1	21.4	41	1240	2.5
veggie	386	16.7	42.5	16.7	26	1076	2.6
X-tra cheese and							
pepperoni	512	24.2	40.8	28.0	56	1443	2.0
Donut, 1 pc., except as noted:							
plain:							
(*Awrey's*), 1.5 oz.	170	2.0	19.0	10.0	15	320	0
(*Awrey's*), 2 oz. . .	240	3.0	21.0	16.0	15	290	<1.0
(*Hostess*), 1 oz. . .	120	2.0	13.0	6.0	5	160	<1.0
(*Hostess* Jumbo),							
1.2 oz.	140	2.0	16.0	7.0	10	190	<1.0

Food and Measure	cal.	prot. (gms)	carbo. (gms)	fat (gms)	chol. (mgs)	sod. (mgs)	fiber (gms)
Donut, plain *(cont.)*							
(*Hostess* Old Fashion)	170	3.0	21.0	9.0	10	230	<1.0
(*Tastykake* Assorted)	180	3.0	19.0	11.0	15	210	1.0
assorted (*Hostess*)	200	3.0	23.0	11.0	10	230	<1.0
cinnamon:							
(*Hostess*)	110	2.0	15.0	5.0	5	140	<1.0
(*Hostess Gems*),							
6 pcs.	340	5.0	48.0	14.0	15	410	2.0
(*Tastykake* Assorted)	210	3.0	24.0	12.0	15	240	1.0
sugar (*Entenmann's*							
Variety Pack) . .	310	3.0	32.0	19.0	20	300	<1.0
coconut top (*Awrey's*)	210	2.0	25.0	12.0	10	190	0
crumb:							
(*Entenmann's*) . . .	260	3.0	34.0	13.0	15	230	<1.0
(*Entenmann's* Variety Pack)	420	4.0	52.0	22.0	20	360	1.0
(*Hostess*)	130	1.0	14.0	8.0	5	115	<1.0
crunch:							
(*Awrey's*)	280	3.0	35.0	15.0	15	320	<1.0
top (*Awrey's*) . . .	160	2.0	19.0	8.0	10	190	0
devil's food crumb							
(*Entenmann's*) . . .	250	3.0	33.0	12.0	15	240	1.0
frosted/iced, chocolate:							
(*Awrey's*), 1.75 oz.	200	2.0	23.0	11.0	15	240	<1.0
(*Awrey's*), 2.5 oz.	300	3.	31.0	18.0	20	340	<1.0
(*Hostess*), 1.4 oz.	180	2.0	20.0	11.0	5	170	1.0
(*Hostess Gems*),							
6 pcs.	390	5.0	42.0	23.0	10	360	2.0
(*Hostess* Jumbo),							
2 oz.	260	3.0	28.0	16.0	10	240	1.0
chocolate (*Awrey's*),							
1.75 oz.	190	2.0	25.0	10.0	5	150	<1.0
chocolate (*Awrey's*),							
2.5 oz.	280	3.0	34.0	16.0	5	200	1.0
chocolate, mini							
(*Hostess*), 5 pcs.	220	4.0	33.0	9.0	35	220	1.0

Food and Measure	cal.	prot. (gms)	carbo. (gms)	fat (gms)	chol. (mgs)	sod. (mgs)	fiber (gms)
custard Bismark							
(*Awrey's*)	350	5.0	36.0	20.0	0	370	1.0
mini (*Entenmann's*),							
2 pcs.	270	2.0	23.0	20.0	10	180	1.0
rich (*Entenmann's*)	280	3.0	27.0	19.0	10	240	1.0
rich (*Entenmann's*							
Variety Pack) . .	400	4.0	37.0	27.0	15	310	1.0
rich (*Tastykake*) . .	270	3.0	30.0	16.0	5	180	2.0
rich, mini (*Tas-*							
tykake), 4 pcs.	270	3.0	29.0	15.0	15	240	2.0
rich, w/raspberry							
(*Entenmann's*) . .	260	3.0	31.0	15.0	10	200	1.0
ring (*Awrey's*) . . .	350	5.0	33.0	21.0	0	370	1.0
sour creme (*Aw-*							
rey's)	430	4.0	52.0	23.0	0	360	<1.0
glazed:							
(*Entenmann's*							
Popems), 6 pcs.	240	2.0	33.0	11.0	15	210	0
(*Hostess* Old Fash-							
ion)	250	3.0	33.0	12.0	15	230	<1.0
(*Hostess* Party) . .	260	4.0	39.0	10.0	5	310	1.0
(*Hostess* Whirl) . .	180	3.0	28.0	7.0	<5	220	<1.0
buttermilk (*Enten-*							
mann's)	270	3.0	36.0	13.0	10	280	0
chocolate (*Enten-*							
mann's Popems),							
4 pcs.	200	2.0	29.0	10.0	15	190	<1.0
honey, devil's food							
(*Awrey's*)	310	4.0	43.0	14.0	15	530	2.0
honey, ring (*Aw-*							
rey's)	310	5.0	30.0	19.0	0	330	1.0
honey wheat (*Host-*							
ess Old Fashion)	250	3.0	33.0	12.0	25	270	1.0
orange (*Tastykake*)	220	2.0	33.0	9.0	5	200	1.0
sour creme (*Aw-*							
rey's)	420	4.0	52.0	23.0	0	340	0
honey wheat:							
(*Tastykake*)	230	1.0	33.0	10.0	5	180	1.0

Food and Measure	cal.	prot. (gms)	carbo. (gms)	fat (gms)	chol. (mgs)	sod. (mgs)	fiber (gms)
Donut, honey wheat *(cont.)*							
mini (*Tastykake*),							
6 pcs.	280	4.0	39.0	13.0	20	300	1.0
powdered sugar:							
(*Awrey's*), 1.5 oz.	170	2.0	19.0	10.0	15	220	0
(*Awrey's*), 2.5 oz.	390	5.0	44.0	22.0	25	470	1.0
(*Hostess*), 1 oz. . .	110	1.0	15.0	6.0	5	135	0
(*Hostess* Jumbo),							
1.3 oz.	160	2.0	19.0	9.0	5	170	<1.0
(*Hostess Gems*),							
6 pcs.	350	4.0	47.0	16.0	10	380	1.0
(*Tastykake* Assorted)	210	3.0	24.0	11.0	15	210	1.0
jelly Bismark (*Awrey's*)	320	18.0	35.0	18.0	0	310	1.0
mini (*Tastykake*),							
6 pcs.	290	4.0	40.0	12.0	25	350	1.0
raspberry fill (*Hostess O's*)	230	3.0	35.0	10.0	5	230	<1.0
sour creme, plain (*Awrey's*)	370	4.0	41.0	22.0	0	340	0
sprinkle topped (*Awrey's*)	160	2.0	19.0	8.0	10	190	0
stick, see "Cake, snack"							
strawberry filled:							
frosted (*Hostess Gems*), 3 pcs. . .	240	3.0	29.0	13.0	<5	210	1.0
powdered (*Hostess Gems*), 3 pcs. . .	210	3.0	31.0	9.0	<5	210	<1.0
vanilla iced:							
(*Awrey's* Long John)	380	5.0	33.0	21.0	0	370	1.0
jelly Bismark (*Awrey's*)	320	4.0	35.0	18.0	0	320	1.0
white, iced (*Awrey's*)	200	2.0	24.0	10.0	15	240	0
Donut, frozen, glazed							
(*Rich's*), 1 pc. . . .	130	2.0	16.0	7.0	0	55	0

Food and Measure	cal.	prot. (gms)	carbo. (gms)	fat (gms)	chol. (mgs)	sod. (mgs)	fiber (gms)
Dressing, see "Salad dressing" and specific listings							
Drum, freshwater, meat only:							
raw, 4 oz.	135	19.9	0	5.6	73	85	0
baked, broiled, or microwaved, 4 oz. . .	173	25.5	0	7.2	93	109	0
Duck, domesticated, roasted:							
meat w/skin, 4 oz. . .	382	21.5	0	32.1	95	67	0
meat only, 4 oz. . . .	228	26.6	0	12.7	101	74	0
Duck, wild, raw:							
meat w/skin, 4 oz. . .	239	19.8	0	17.2	91	64	0
breast meat, 4 oz. . .	139	22.5	0	4.8	n.a.	65	0
Duck sauce, see "Sweet and sour sauce"							

E

Food and Measure	cal.	prot. (gms)	carbo. (gms)	fat (gms)	chol. (mgs)	sod. (mgs)	fiber (gms)
Eclair, chocolate, frozen (*Rich's*), 1 pc.	190	2.0	24.0	9.0	40	115	0
Eel, meat only:							
raw, 4 oz.	209	20.9	0	3.2	143	58	0
baked, broiled, or microwaved, 4 oz. . .	268	26.8	0	17.0	183	74	0
Egg, chicken:							
raw, 1 large egg:							
whole	75	6.3	.6	5.0	213	63	0
white only	17	3.5	.3	0	0	55	0
yolk only[1]	59	2.8	.3	5.1	213	7	0
cooked:							
hard-boiled, chopped, 1 cup	210	17.1	1.5	14.4	578	169	0
poached, 1 large . .	74	6.2	.6	5.0	212	140	0
dried, 1 oz.:							
whole	168	13.0	1.4	11.9	544	148	0
whole, stabilized . .	174	13.7	.7	12.5	572	155	0
white, stabilized, flakes	100	21.8	1.2	<.1	0	328	0
yolk	195	8.7	.1	17.4	830	26	0
Egg, duck, 1 egg . .	130	9.0	1.0	9.6	619	102	0
Egg, goose, 1 egg	267	20.0	1.9	19.1	n.a.	n.a.	0
Egg, quail, 1 egg . .	14	1.2	<.1	1.0	76	n.a.	0
Egg, turkey, 1 egg	135	10.8	.9	9.4	737	n.a.	0
Egg, substitute or imitation, ¼ cup, except as noted:							
(*Egg Beaters*)	30	6.0	1.0	0	0	100	0

[1] *Includes a small portion of white.*

Food and Measure	cal.	prot. (gms)	carbo. (gms)	fat (gms)	chol. (mgs)	sod. (mgs)	fiber (gms)
(*Egg Watchers*) . . .	30	6.0	1.0	0	0	80	0
(*Morningstar Farms Better'n Eggs*) . . .	20	5.0	0	0	0	90	0
(*Morningstar Farms Scramblers*)	35	6.0	2.0	0	0	95	0
(*Second Nature*) . . .	40	6.0	3.0	0	0	115	0
Egg breakfast, freeze-dried, ½ cup:							
w/bacon:							
(*Mountain House*)	150	11.0	5.0	9.0	345	460	0
precooked (*Mountain House*) . . .	120	10.0	5.0	7.0	190	550	0
omelet, cheese (*Mountain House*)	180	13.0	7.0	11.0	335	530	0
Egg breakfast, frozen (see also specific listings), 1 pkg.:							
omelet, ham-cheese (*Weight Watchers*)	220	13.0	30.0	5.0	30	440	2.0
patty, egg:							
w/Canadian bacon (*Swanson Great Starts*)	240	9.0	33.0	6.0	25	720	2.0
w/pork and turkey (*Swanson Great Starts*)	280	14.0	32.0	9.0	45	800	3.0
scrambled:							
(*Swanson Great Starts* Egg Product)	240	20.0	22.0	13.0	40	510	1.0
(*Swanson Great Starts* Low Fat)	240	20.0	18.0	13.0	40	620	2.0
and bacon (*Swanson Great Starts*)	290	29.0	17.0	19.0	240	700	1.0
w/homefries (*Swanson Great Starts*)	200	18.0	15.0	12.0	190	390	2.0
and sausage (*Swanson Great Starts*)	360	40.0	21.0	26.0	280	800	3.0

Food and Measure	cal.	prot. (gms)	carbo. (gms)	fat (gms)	chol. (mgs)	sod. (mgs)	fiber (gms)
Egg breakfast sand-wich, frozen, 1 pkg.:							
biscuit, see "Sausage biscuit"							
w/cheese (*Swanson Great Starts*)	360	29.0	35.0	19.0	170	950	1.0
muffin:							
(*Weight Watchers*)	210	13.0	28.0	5.0	20	420	2.0
w/bacon and cheese (*Swanson Great Starts*)	290	23.0	25.0	15.0	95	750	2.0
w/Canadian bacon, cheese (*Hormel Quick Meal*) . . .	260	16.0	29.0	9.0	110	750	2.0
w/sausage, cheese (*Hormel Quick Meal*)	390	17.0	28.0	23.0	130	730	2.0
omelet (*Weight Watchers* Classic)	220	15.0	26.0	6.0	20	410	2.0
Egg roll, frozen, 3-oz. roll, except as noted:							
(*Empire* Kosher) . . .	190	6.0	28.0	6.0	2	350	2.0
(*Empire* Kosher Mini), 6 rolls	280	9.0	43.0	8.0	0	740	3.0
chicken:							
(*Chun King*)	170	7.0	25.0	5.0	10	450	4.0
(*La Choy*)	170	7.0	25.0	5.0	10	450	4.0
sweet and sour (*La Choy*)	180	6.0	29.0	4.0	5	30	3.0
chicken, mini:							
(*Chun King*), 12 rolls	400	11.0	58.0	14.0	15	510	6.0
(*La Choy*), 14 rolls	430	15.0	67.0	11.0	15	900	6.0
pork:							
(*Chun King*)	170	6.0	23.0	6.0	5	390	3.0
(*La Choy*)	170	6.0	23.0	6.0	5	390	3.0
moo shu (*La Choy*)	190	6.0	25.0	7.0	15	330	2.0

Food and Measure	cal.	prot. (gms)	carbo. (gms)	fat (gms)	chol. (mgs)	sod. (mgs)	fiber (gms)
pork and shrimp, mini:							
(*Chun King*),							
12 rolls	420	11.0	56.0	16.0	25	500	6.0
(*La Choy*), 14 rolls	430	15.0	65.0	12.0	15	890	7.0
bite size (*La Choy*),							
15 rolls	240	8.0	31.0	9.0	10	350	3.0
shrimp:							
(*Chun King*)	150	6.0	24.0	4.0	10	420	3.0
(*La Choy*)	150	6.0	24.0	4.0	10	420	3.0
shrimp, mini:							
(*Chun King*),							
12 rolls	370	10.0	57.0	11.0	15	700	7.0
(*La Choy*), 14 rolls	410	14.0	68.0	9.0	10	990	7.0
vegetables, w/lobster, mini (*La Choy*),							
14 rolls, 7.25 oz.	410	13.0	65.0	11.0	0	690	9.0
"Egg" roll, vegetarian, frozen (*Worthington*), 1 roll . .	180	6.0	20.0	8.0	0	380	2.0
Egg roll wrapper:							
(*Frieda's*), 2 pcs.,							
1.7 oz.	132	5.0	28.0	.5	0	252	1.0
(*Nasoya*), 1.5 oz. . .	117	4.5	23.7	.5	14	290	1.0
Eggnog, dairy, ½ cup:							
(*Borden*)	160	3.0	17.0	9.0	80	80	0
(*Borden* Light)	150	5.0	23.0	4.0	20	65	0
(*Crowley*)	190	4.0	23.0	9.0	65	130	0
(*Crowley* Light) . . .	120	4.0	22.0	2.0	45	95	0
(*Crowley* Nonfat) . .	130	5.0	25.0	0	20	75	0
Eggplant, fresh:							
raw, 1″ pcs., ½ cup	11	.4	2.5	.1	0	1	1.0
boiled, drained,							
1″ cubes, ½ cup	13	.4	3.2	.1	0	2	1.2
Japanese, raw, w/peel,							
(*Frieda's*), 3½ oz.	25	1.2	5.6	.2	0	2	n.a.
Eggplant appetizer:							
(*Progresso* Caponata),							
2 tbsp.	30	0	2.0	2.0	0	130	2.0

Food and Measure	cal.	prot. (gms)	carbo. (gms)	fat (gms)	chol. (mgs)	sod. (mgs)	fiber (gms)
Eggplant appetizer (cont.)							
roasted (Pelopon-							
nese), 2 tbsp. . . .	25	1.0	11.0	1.5	0	180	0
stuffed:							
baby (Krinos),							
1.1 oz., about							
2 pcs.	20	0	0	2.0	0	550	1.0
rolettes (Paesana),							
3¾ oz.	260	2.0	9.0	24.0	0	510	1.0
Eggplant entree, fro-							
zen:							
cutlets (Celentano),							
5 oz.	210	7.0	23.0	23.0	45	170	7.0
parmigiana:							
(Celentano),							
10-oz. pkg. . . .	420	14.0	30.0	27.0	45	800	23.0
(Celentano 14 oz.),							
½ pkg.	320	12.0	22.0	21.0	25	560	16.0
(Celentano Value							
Pack), 1 cup,							
8 oz.	360	9.0	25.0	25.0	25	640	15.0
(Mrs. Paul's),							
½ cup	220	22.0	19.0	14.0	10	530	3.0
rollettes, 10 oz.:							
(Celentano)	350	10.0	27.0	22.0	0	480.	6.0
(Celentano Great							
Choice)	330	11.0	39.0	15.0	55	660	7.0
Eggplant pickle relish							
(Patak's Brinjal),							
1 tbsp.	60	0	10.0	2.0	0	180	<1.0
Elderberry, ½ cup	53	.5	13.3	.4	0	n.a.	5.1
Empanadilla, frozen							
(Goya):							
plain, 2 pcs.	380	11.0	58.0	12.0	15	800	2.0
plain, cocktail size,							
7 pcs.	370	11.0	56.0	11.0	15	770	2.0
pizza flavor, 2 pcs.	370	11.0	56.0	12.0	15	930	4.0
Enchilada, canned							
(Gebhardt), 2 pcs.	260	4.5	20.5	19.0	25	685	3.0

Food and Measure	cal.	prot. (gms)	carbo. (gms)	fat (gms)	chol. (mgs)	sod. (mgs)	fiber (gms)
Enchilada dinner, frozen, 1 pkg., except as noted:							
(*Amy's*)	250	7.0	41.0	8.0	0	680	5.0
(*Chi-Chi's* Baja) . . .	580	25.0	82.0	17.0	50	2050	10.0
beef:							
(*Healthy Choice* Rio Grande)	410	14.0	70	8.0	15	480	9.0
(*Patio*)	350	12.0	52.0	10.0	15	1700	9.0
(*Patio* Chili 'n Beans Large), 2 pcs. . . .	250	12.0	35.0	7.0	15	1350	8.0
(*Swanson*)	470	26.0	60.0	17.0	20	1790	10.0
chili sauce w/ (*Banquet* Family), 1 pc.	130	4.0	19.0	14.0	25	610	2.0
beef and cheese (*Patio* Chili 'n Beans), 2 pcs.	250	12.0	35.0	6.0	20	1130	9.0
cheese (*Patio*)	330	13.0	52.0	8.0	15	1570	10.0
chicken:							
(*Chi-Chi's* Suprema)	580	24.0	71.0	23.0	80	2450	8.0
(*Healthy Choice* Suprema)	390	17.0	60.0	9.0	30	390	5.0
(*Patio*)	380	14.0	58.0	9.0	25	1470	9.0
Enchilada entree, frozen, 1 pkg., except as noted:							
beef:							
(*Banquet*)	380	15.0	54.0	12.0	15	1330	10.0
(*Patio* Family), 2 pcs.	200	5.0	31.0	6.0	10	740	5.0
and tamale, chili gravy w/ (*Morton*)	260	8.0	40.0	7.0	5	1000	8.0
black bean:							
(*Amy's* Family), 4.38 oz.	120	4.0	18.0	4.0	0	360	2.0
and vegetable (*Amy's* Family), 4.75 oz.	130	4.0	20.0	4.0	0	390	2.0

Food and Measure	cal.	prot. (gms)	carbo. (gms)	fat (gms)	chol. (mgs)	sod. (mgs)	fiber (gms)
Enchilada entree *(cont.)*							
cheese:							
(*Amy's*)	210	11.0	16.0	9.0	20	390	2.0
(*Amy's* Family),							
4.38 oz.	200	10.0	15.0	8.0	18	360	2.0
(*Banquet*)	340	15.0	56.0	6.0	15	1500	9.0
(*Patio* Family),							
2 pcs.	170	6.0	26.0	4.0	10	880	4.0
and rice (*Stouffer's*)	370	12.0	48.0	14.0	25.0	890	5.0
chicken:							
(*Banquet*)	360	15.0	54.0	10.0	20	1580	9.0
nacho grande							
(*Weight Watchers*)	290	15.0	42.0	8.0	20	560	4.0
and rice (*Stouffer's*)	370	16.0	45.0	14.0	30	970	3.0
chicken Suiza:							
(*Healthy Choice*) . .	270	14.0	43.0	4.0	20	290	6.0
(*Weight Watchers*)	270	14.0	33.0	9.0	40	540	4.0
w/rice (*Lean Cui-*							
sine)	290	12.0	48.0	5.0	25	530	5.0
Enchilada sauce,							
¼ cup:							
(*Chi-Chi's*)	30	0	3.0	1.5	0	210	0
(*La Victoria*)	20	0	3.0	1.0	0	400	0
(*Las Palmas*)	15	0	2.0	.5	0	310	1.0
(*Rosarita*)	25	0	3.0	1.0	0	410	0
green chili:							
(*Las Palmas*) . . .	25	0	3.0	1.5	0	260	0
(*Old El Paso*) . . .	30	<1.0	3.0	1.5	0	330	<1.0
hot:							
(*Las Palmas*) . . .	20	0	3.0	.5	0	330	1.0
(*Old El Paso*) . . .	30	0	4.0	1.5	0	190	<1.0
mild (*Old El Paso*) . .	25	0	4.0	1.0	0	160	<1.0
Enchilada seasoning							
mix:							
(*Durkee*), 1½ tsp. . .	10	0	2.0	0	0	260	0
(*Lawry's*), 2 tsp. . . .	20	0	4.0	0	0	260	0
(*Old El Paso*), 2 tsp.	10	0	2.0	0	0	540	<1.0
Endive, chopped,							
½ cup	4	.3	.8	.1	0	6	.8

Food and Measure	cal.	prot. (gms)	carbo. (gms)	fat (gms)	chol. (mgs)	sod. (mgs)	fiber (gms)
Endive, Belgian, see "Chicory, witloof"							
Eppaw, ½ cup	75	2.3	15.8	.9	0	6	n.a.
Escarole, see "Endive"							
Etouffee dinner mix (*Luzianne*), ¼ pkg.	200	5.0	42.0	1.0	0	1030	<1.0

F

Food and Measure	cal.	prot. (gms)	carbo. (gms)	fat (gms)	chol. (mgs)	sod. (mgs)	fiber (gms)
Fajita, canned (*Nalley* Superba), 1 cup:							
beef	230	15.0	30.0	6.0	15	720	12.0
chicken	230	13.0	30.0	6.0	15	810	13.0
Fajita entree, frozen:							
beef (*Tyson* Kit),							
3.6-oz. fajita	130	9.0	18.0	2.0	15	300	2.0
chicken:							
(*Healthy Choice* Fiesta), 7 oz. . . .	260	21.0	36.0	4.0	30	410	5.0
(*Tyson* Kit), 3.6-oz. fajita	120	8.0	18.0	1.5	15	410	2.0
Fajita sauce:							
(*S&W* Southwestern), 1 tbsp.	10	0	2.0	0	0	230	1.0
and marinade (*World Harbors* Guadalupe), 2 tbsp.	45	0	10.0	0	0	600	0
skillet (*Lawry's*), 2 tbsp.	15	0	2.0	0	0	600	0
Fajita seasoning mix:							
(*Lawry's*), 2 tsp. . . .	15	0	3.0	0	0	400	0
beef (*Durkee* Easy), ⅙ pkg.	15	0	4.0	0	0	550	0
Falafel mix:							
(*Casbah*), ⅛ pkg. . .	130	6.0	20.0	3.0	0	530	2.0
(*Fantastic Falafil*), ½ cup	250	15.0	42.0	4.0	0	610	11.0
(*Near East*), 2½ fried patties*	230	10.0	18.0	15.0	0	560	5.0

Food and Measure	cal.	prot. (gms)	carbo. (gms)	fat (gms)	chol. (mgs)	sod. (mgs)	fiber (gms)
Farina, whole grain							
(see also "Cereal"):							
dry, 1 oz.	105	3.0	22.1	.1	0	1	.8
cooked, 1 cup	116	3.4	24.6	.2	0	1	3.3
Fat, see specific list-							
ings							
Fat, imitation							
(*Rokeach Nyafat*),							
1 tbsp.	99	0	0	11.0	0	0	0
Fava beans, see							
"Broad beans"							
Feijoa, raw:							
(*Frieda's*), 1 oz. . . .	17	.3	4.0	.3	0	1	n.a.
w/skin, 1 medium,							
2.3 oz.	25	.6	5.3	.4	0	2	n.a.
pureed, ½ cup	60	1.5	12.9	1.0	0	4	n.a.
Fennel, bulb, raw,							
trimmed:							
1 oz.	9	.4	2.1	.1	0	15	n.a.
8.3-oz. bulb	72	2.9	17.1	.5	0	122	n.a.
sliced, ½ cup	27	1.1	6.3	.2	0	45	n.a.
Fennel seed:							
1 tsp.	7	.3	1.1	.3	0	2	<1.0
(*McCormick*), ¼ tsp.	3	.2	.4	.2	0	1	.3
Fenugreek seed,							
1 tsp.	12	.9	2.2	.2	0	2	<1.0
Fettuccine, plain:							
dry, see "Pasta"							
refrigerated (*Con-*							
tadina), 1¼ cup . .	250	10.0	45.0	3.5	85	30	2.0
Fettuccine entree,							
frozen, 1 pkg., ex-							
cept as noted:							
Alfredo:							
(*Banquet*)	370	12.0	39.0	18.0	30	940	4.0
(*Healthy Choice*) . .	250	11.0	39.0	5.0	15	480	3.0
(*Lean Cuisine*) . . .	270	13.0	38.0	7.0	15	590	2.0
(*Marie Callender's*),							
1 cup	350	10.0	29.0	21.0	45	400	2.0

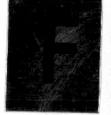

Food and Measure	cal.	prot. (gms)	carbo. (gms)	fat (gms)	chol. (mgs)	sod. (mgs)	fiber (gms)
Fettuccine entree, frozen, Alfredo *(cont.)*							
(*Stouffer's*)	580	14.0	42.0	39.0	120	810	4.0
w/broccoli (*Weight Watchers*)	230	10.0	34.0	6.0	20	450	3.0
w/four cheeses (*The Budget Gourmet*)	480	20.0	48.0	24.0	55	1120	3.0
w/broccoli and chicken (*Marie Callender's*), 1 cup . .	420	18.0	30.0	26.0	55	530	3.0
chicken, see "Chicken entree"							
primavera:							
(*Lean Cuisine*) . . .	260	15.0	33.0	8.0	15	580	4.0
(*Marie Callender's*), 1 cup	310	10.0	25.0	19.0	50	380	2.0
(*Stouffer's Lunch Express*)	420	15.0	33.0	25.0	95	690	6.0
Fettuccine entree mix:							
(*Noodle Roni*), 1 cup*	470	13.0	48.0	26.0	10	1110	2.0
w/creamy basil sauce (*Knorr* Cup), 1 pkg.	220	6.0	41.0	4.0	5	810	2.0
Fig:							
fresh:							
1 large, 2.3 oz. . .	47	.5	12.3	.2	0	1	2.1
1 medium, 1.8 oz.	37	.4	9.6	.2	0	1	1.7
Calimyrna (*Frieda's*), 1 oz.	23	.3	5.8	.1	0	<1	n.a.
canned, in syrup:							
½ cup	114	.5	29.7	.1	0	2	2.8
Kadota (*S&W*), 5 figs	140	0	32.0	1.0	0	5	3.0
dried:							
10 figs, 6.6 oz. . .	477	5.7	122.2	2.2	0	20	17.4
California, 4 figs, 2 oz.	143	2.4	38.8	.7	0	6	9.5
Calamata string (*Agora*), ½ cup . . .	250	3.0	58.0	2.0	0	<10	17.0

Food and Measure	cal.	prot. (gms)	carbo. (gms)	fat (gms)	chol. (mgs)	sod. (mgs)	fiber (gms)
Calimyrna or Mission (*Blue Ribbon/Sun-Maid*), 4 figs, 1½ oz. . . .	120	1.0	28.0	0	0	5	5.0
white/Mission (*Sonoma*), 3-4 figs, 1.4 oz.	110	1.0	26.0	0	0	0	5.0
Filberts:							
dried:							
1 oz.	179	3.7	4.4	17.8	0	1	1.7
chopped, 1 cup . .	727	15.0	17.6	72.0	0	3	7.0
blanched, 1 oz. . .	191	3.6	4.5	19.1	0	1	<2.0
dry-roasted:							
1 oz.	188	2.8	5.1	18.8	0	1	<2.0
salted, 1 oz.	188	2.8	5.1	18.8	0	221	<2.0
oil-roasted:							
1 oz.	187	4.1	5.4	18.1	0	1	1.8
salted, 1 oz.	187	4.1	5.4	18.1	0	223	1.8
Fillo pastry, frozen (*Apollo*), ⅛ pkg. . .	180	5.0	35.0	0	0	300	1.0
Fish, see specific listings							
"Fish," vegetarian:							
frozen (*Worthington*), 2 fillets	180	16.0	8.0	10.0	0	750	4.0
mix (*Loma Linda* Ocean Platter), ⅓ cup	90	14.0	8.0	1.0	0	450	4.0
Fish dinner, frozen (see also specific fish listings), 1 pkg.:							
battered portions, w/chips (*Swanson*)	480	31.0	55.0	20.0	45	1050	5.0
breaded sticks (*Swanson* Budget)	340	17.0	51.0	11.0	25	710	3.0

Food and Measure	cal.	prot. (gms)	carbo. (gms)	fat (gms)	chol. (mgs)	sod. (mgs)	fiber (gms)
Fish entree, frozen (see also specific fish listings):							
(*Van de Kamp's* Fish 'n Fries), 6.5 oz. . . .	380	13.0	41.0	18.0	25	370	2.0
baked, w/shells (*Lean Cuisine*), 9 oz.	260	19.0	28.0	8.0	50	580	3.0
cakes (*Mrs. Paul's*), 2 pcs.	200	12.0	23.0	8.0	15	680	2.0
and chips (*Swanson*), 1 pkg.	310	18.0	38.0	12.0	35	620	4.0
fillets, battered:							
(*Gorton's*), 2 pcs.	280	10.0	16.0	19.0	20	630	n.a.
(*Mrs. Paul's*), 1 pc.	170	17.0	13.0	11.0	15	460	1.0
(*Mrs. Paul's Crunchy*), 2 pcs.	250	20.0	23.0	13.0	25	680	2.0
(*Van de Kamp's*), 1 pc.	180	8.0	12.0	11.0	20	340	n.a.
lemon pepper (*Gorton's*), 2 pcs. . .	250	9.0	18.0	16.0	35	630	n.a.
fillets, breaded:							
(*Gorton's* Crunchy), 2 pcs.	270	12.0	17.0	17.0	25	480	n.a.
(*Mrs. Paul's*), 2 pcs.	240	18.0	20.0	12.0	25	390	1.0
(*Mrs. Paul's Healthy Treasures*), 1 pc.	170	5.0	21.0	3.0	30	290	2.0
(*Van de Kamp's*), 2 pcs.	280	11.0	17.0	19.0	35	270	n.a.
(*Van de Kamp's Crisp & Healthy*), 2 pcs.	150	12.0	20.0	2.5	30	380	n.a.
garlic and herb (*Gorton's Crunchy*), 2 pcs.	250	10.0	20.0	14.0	35	720	n.a.
hot and spicy (*Gorton's* Crunchy), 2 pcs.	250	10.0	19.0	14.0	30	620	n.a.
potato (*Gorton's*), 2 pcs.	290	11.0	17.0	20	25	270	n.a.

Food and Measure	cal.	prot. (gms)	carbo. (gms)	fat (gms)	chol. (mgs)	sod. (mgs)	fiber (gms)
Southern fried (*Gorton's* Crunchy), 2 pcs.	270	11.0	20.0	16.0	30	560	n.a.
fillets, grilled, 1 pc.:							
Italian herb (*Gorton's*)	130	18.0	2.0	6.0	60	250	0
lemon pepper (*Gorton's*)	120	17.0	1.0	6.0	60	170	0
fillets, in sauce:							
(*Mrs. Paul's* Kitchen), 1 pc.	120	8.0	4.0	5.0	25	450	1.0
lemon pepper (*Healthy Choice*), 10.7 oz.	290	14.0	47.0	5.0	25	360	7.0
grilled, w/vegetables (*Lean Cuisine* Cafe Classics), 8⅞ oz.	170 .	16.0	14.0	5.0	45	520	3.0
w/macaroni and cheese:							
(*Stouffer's* Home-style), 9 oz. . . .	430	24.0	37.0	21.0	70	930	2.0
(*Swanson*), 1 pkg.	350	23.0	38.0	15.0	30	930	4.0
nuggets (*Van de Kamp's*), 8 pcs. . .	280	11.0	20.0	18.0	25	600	n.a.
portions, battered:							
(*Gorton's*), 1 pc. . .	160	6.0	12.0	10.0	20	400	n.a.
(*Mrs. Paul's*), 2 pcs.	280	26.0	22.0	17.0	30	760	2.0
(*Van de Kamp's*), 2 pcs.	350	13.0	26.0	22.0	35	710	n.a.
portions, breaded:							
(*Mrs. Paul's*), 2 pcs.	190	15.0	16.0	10.0	15	280	1.0
(*Van de Kamp's*), 3 pcs.	330	14.0	23.0	21.0	35	410	n.a.
shapes, breaded (*Mrs. Paul's* Sea Pals), 5 pcs.	190	14.0	18.0	9.0	20	310	1.0
sticks, 1 pkg.:							
(*Kid Cuisine* Funtastic)	370	11.0	55.0	12.0	15	550	4.0

Food and Measure	cal.	prot. (gms)	carbo. (gms)	fat (gms)	chol. (mgs)	sod. (mgs)	fiber (gms)
Fish entree, sticks *(cont.)*							
(Swanson Fun Feast							
Frenzied)	360	22.0	47.0	14.0	25	640	4.0
sticks, battered:							
(Gorton's), 5 pcs.	290	10.0	18.0	20.0	20	600	n.a.
(Mrs. Paul's), 6 pcs.	240	23.0	13.0	11.0	15	460	1.0
(Van de Kamp's),							
6 pcs.	260	11.0	18.0	16.0	30	540	n.a.
sticks, breaded:							
(Gorton's Crunchy),							
6 pcs.	250	11.0	16.0	16.0	25	410	n.a.
(Mrs. Paul's), 6 pcs.	220	17.0	20.0	11.0	20	430	1.0
(Mrs. Paul's Crispy							
Crunchy), 5 pcs.	200	14.0	20.0	14.0	20	510	2.0
(Gorton's Value							
Pack), 6 pcs. . .	220	9.0	18.0	12.0	25	380	n.a.
(Van de Kamp's),							
6 pcs.	290	13.0	23.0	17.0	35	390	n.a.
(Van de Kamp's							
Snack/Value							
Pack), 6 pcs. . .	260	11.0	21.0	14.0	25	350	n.a.
(Van de Kamp's							
Crisp & Healthy),							
6 pcs.	180	13.0	26.0	3.0	25	440	n.a.
mini *(Mrs. Paul's)*,							
12 pcs.	220	17.0	20.0	11.0	30	330	2.0
mini *(Van de*							
Kamp's), 13 pcs.	250	11.0	19.0	14.0	30	330	n.a.
potato *(Gorton's)*,							
6 pcs.	220	10.0	22.0	16.0	25	270	n.a.
Fish sandwich, fillet,							
frozen, 1 pc.:							
(Hormel Quick Meal)	400	15.0	48.0	16.0	75	850	2.0
w/cheese *(Mrs.*							
Paul's)	330	23.0	38.0	15.0	25	630	3.0
Fish sauce mix,							
lemon butter							
(Weight Watcher's),							
¼ cup*	5	0	1.0	0	0	410	0

Food and Measure	cal.	prot. (gms)	carbo. (gms)	fat (gms)	chol. (mgs)	sod. (mgs)	fiber (gms)
Fish seasoning:							
batter seasoning, Cajun (*Tone's*), 1 tsp.	12	.3	2.6	.1	0	49	.1
seafood:							
(*Old Bay*), ½ tsp.	0	0	0	0	0	330	0
(*Tone's*), 1 tsp. . .	10	.5	.9	.7	0	1	.3
Fish seasoning and coating mix:							
(*Shake'n Bake*), ¼ pkt.	70	1.0	14.0	1.5	0	420	1.0
lemon butter (*Durkee/ French's* Roasting Bag), ¼ pkg. . . .	30	0	6.0	.5	0	380	0
lemon pepper–dill (*Durkee Easy*), ⅙ pkg.	20	0	4.0	.5	0	160	0
tomato basil (*Durkee Easy*), ⅐ pkg. . . .	15	0	4.0	0	0	170	0
Flatbread, see "Cracker"							
Flatfish, meat only:							
raw, 4 oz.	104	21.4	0	1.4	54	92	0
baked, broiled, or microwaved, 4 oz. . .	133	27.4	0	1.7	77	119	0
Flavor enhancer (*Ac'cent*), ½ tsp.	5	0	0	0	0	300	0
Flax seeds (*Arrowhead Mills*), 3 tbsp.	140	5.0	11.0	10.0	0	0	6.0
Flounder:							
fresh, see "Flatfish"							
frozen (*Van de Kamp's*), 4 oz. . . .	110	22.0	0	2.0	45	105	0
Flounder entree, fillets, frozen:							
battered (*Mrs. Paul's* Crunchy), 2 pcs. . .	260	22.0	24.0	14.0	30	540	2.0
breaded, 1 pc.:							
(*Mrs. Paul's* Premium)	240	18.0	23.0	12.0	35	530	2.0

Food and Measure	cal.	prot. (gms)	carbo. (gms)	fat (gms)	chol. (mgs)	sod. (mgs)	fiber (gms)
Flounder entree, breaded *(cont.)*							
(*Van de Kamp's* Light)	100	15.0	19.0	11.0	40	400	n.a.
Flour, see "Wheat flour" and specific listings							
Fra diavolo sauce, see "Pasta sauce"							
Frankfurter, 1 link, except as noted:							
(*Boar's Head*)	150	7.0	0	14.0	25	460	0
(*Hormel* 10), 1.6 oz.	140	5.0	2.0	13.0	40	450	0
(*Hormel* 8), 2 oz. . .	180	6.0	2.0	17.0	50	560	0
(*Hormel* Big 8), 2 oz.	180	6.0	1.0	17.0	40	540	0
(*Hormel Light & Lean 97*), 1.6 oz.	45	5.0	4.0	1.0	15	490	0
(*Hormel Light & Lean 97* Jumbo), 2 oz.	60	6.0	5.0	1.5	20	630	0
(*John Morrell* Fat Free), 1.4 oz. . . .	45	5.0	6.0	0	10	580	0
(*John Morrell* Lite)	90	4.0	5.0	6.0	30	570	0
(*Oscar Mayer* Wieners)	150	5.0	1.0	13.0	30	450	0
(*Oscar Mayer* Wieners Light)	110	7.0	1.0	9.0	35	590	0
(*Oscar Mayer* Wieners, Little), 6 links, 2 oz.	180	6.0	1.0	17.0	30	610	0
(*Oscar Mayer Big & Juicy* Wieners) . . .	240	9.0	1.0	22.0	45	690	0
(*Oscar Mayer Bun-Length* Wieners) . .	190	6.0	1.0	17.0	35	570	0
beef:							
(*Boar's Head* Lite)	90	7.0	0	6.0	25	270	0
(*Boar's Head* Giant)	160	7.0	1.0	14.0	30	440	0
(*Boar's Head* Skinless)	120	6.0	0	11.0	20	350	0
(*Hebrew National*), 1.7 oz.	150	6.0	1.0	14.0	30	370	0

Food and Measure	cal.	prot. (gms)	carbo. (gms)	fat (gms)	chol. (mgs)	sod. (mgs)	fiber (gms)
(*Hebrew National* 8 oz.)	140	6.0	1.0	13.0	30	360	0
(*Hebrew National* Bulk), 2.7 oz. . .	240	9.0	1.0	22.0	50	600	0
(*Hebrew National* Family Pack), 2 oz.	180	7.0	0	16.0	40	450	0
(*Hebrew National* Picnic Pack), 1.6 oz.	140	6.0	1.0	13.0	30	360	0
(*Hebrew National* Reduced Fat), 1.7 oz.	120	8.0	1.0	10.0	25	350	0
(*Hebrew National* Reduced Fat 3 lb.) 2.7 oz.	180	11.0	0	15.0	40	550	0
(*Hebrew National* Quarter Pound/ Jumbo)	350	14.0	1.0	34.0	75	890	0
(*Hormel* 8)	170	6.0	1.0	15.0	35	480	0
(*Hormel Light & Lean 97*)	45	5.0	4.0	1.0	15	490	0
(*Oscar Mayer*) . . .	140	5.0	1.0	13.0	25	450	0
(*Oscar Mayer* Light)	110	6.0	2.0	9.0	25	620	0
(*Oscar Mayer Big & Juicy*), 2.7 oz. . .	240	9.0	1.0	22.0	45	700	0
(*Oscar Mayer Big & Juicy* ¼ lb.) . . .	350	13.0	2.0	33.0	65	1050	0
(*Oscar Mayer Big & Juicy* Deli), 2.7 oz.	230	9.0	1.0	22.0	50	680	0
(*Oscar Mayer Bun-Length*)	190	6.0	2.0	17.0	35	570	0
(*Wranglers*)	170	7.0	1.0	15.0	40	530	0
cocktail:							
(*Hormel*), 5 links	160	7.0	1.0	14.0	40	550	0
beef (*Boar's Head*), 5 links	170	8.0	0	15.0	30	430	0

Food and Measure	cal.	prot. (gms)	carbo. (gms)	fat (gms)	chol. (mgs)	sod. (mgs)	fiber (gms)
Frankfurter, cocktail *(cont.)*							
beef (*Hebrew National*), 4 links	180	7.0	0	16.0	40	450	0
beef (*Hebrew National* 32 oz.), 6 links	160	6.0	0	15.0	35	410	0
smoked (*Hormel Smokies*), 5 links	180	8.0	1.0	16.0	40	530	0
cheese:							
(*Oscar Mayer*) . . .	140	5.0	1.0	13.0	35	520	0
(*Wranglers*)	170	7.0	1.0	15.0	40	550	0
hot and spicy (*Oscar Mayer Big & Juicy*)	220	10.0	1.0	20.0	45	750	0
smoked:							
(*Oscar Mayer Big & Juicy* Smokie) . .	220	10.0	1.0	19.0	50	770	0
(*Wranglers*)	170	7.0	1.0	15.0	40	530	0
turkey, see "Turkey frankfurter"							
"Frankfurter," vegetarian, 1 link:							
(*New Menu* VegiDog)	45	9.0	1.0	0	0	170	0
canned:							
(*Loma Linda* Big)	110	10.0	2.0	7.0	0	240	2.0
(*Loma Linda* Linketts)	70	7.0	1.0	4.5	0	160	1.0
(*Worthington* VejaLinks)	50	5.0	1.0	3.0	0	190	0
(*Worthington Super-Links*)	110	7.0	2.0	8.0	0	350	1.0
frozen:							
(*Morningstar Farms* Deli Franks) . . .	110	10.0	3.0	7.0	0	520	2.0
(*Natural Touch* Vege)	100	10.0	2.0	6.0	0	470	2.0
(*Worthington* Leanies)	110	7.0	2.0	8.0	0	430	1.0
corn battered (*Loma Linda* Corn Dog)	220	10.0	18.0	9.0	0	240	3.0

Food and Measure	cal.	prot. (gms)	carbo. (gms)	fat (gms)	chol. (mgs)	sod. (mgs)	fiber (gms)
refrigerated:							
chili (*Yves Veggie*							
Cuisine Dogs) . .	70	12.0	5.0	0	0	295	4.0
tofu (*Yves Veggie*							
Cuisine Weiners)	57	9.0	4.0	0	0	247	1.0
Frankfurter sandwich,							
frozen, 1 pc., except							
as noted:							
(*Hormel Quick Meal*							
Jumbo Dog)	350	13.0	28.0	21.0	55	920	3.0
bagel wrapped:							
(*Boar's Head* Bagel							
Dog	310	15.0	1.0	27.0	55	890	0
(*Hebrew National*							
Bagel Dog) . . .	400	14.0	47.0	17.0	35	710	2.0
on bun (*Swanson Fun*							
Feast)	350	18.0	47.0	12.0	35	800	3.0
w/cheese (*Hormel*							
Quick Meal Cheesey							
Dog)	310	10.0	29.0	17.0	45	860	1.0
chili w/cheese (*Hor-*							
mel Quick Meal) . .	350	12.0	30.0	20.0	60	850	2.0
corn dog:							
(*Hormel/Hormel*							
Quick Meal) . . .	220	6.0	25.0	11.0	45	520	1.0
mini (*Hormel Quick*							
Meal), 5 pcs. . .	250	6.0	23.0	15.0	50	570	1.0
Franks and beans,							
see "Beans and							
franks"							
French toast, frozen,							
2 pcs.:							
(*Aunt Jemima*)	240	9.0	38.0	6.0	80	360	1.0
(*Downyflake*)	260	9.0	43.0	6.0	50	640	2.0
cinnamon swirl:							
(*Aunt Jemima*) . . .	240	9.0	37.0	6.0	90	330	2.0
(*Downyflake*)	270	10.0	45.0	6.0	40	520	1.0

Food and Measure	cal.	prot. (gms)	carbo. (gms)	fat (gms)	chol. (mgs)	sod. (mgs)	fiber (gms)
French toast break-							
fast, frozen, 1 pkg.:							
cinnamon swirl							
(*Swanson Great*							
Starts)	440	43.0	34.0	28.0	150	580	2.0
w/sausage (*Swanson*							
Great Starts)	410	40.0	33.0	26.0	110	580	3.0
sticks, mini (*Swanson*							
Kids Breakfast							
Blast)	310	22.0	41.0	14.0	45	300	2.0
Frog's legs, meat							
only, raw, 4 oz. . . .	83	18.6	0	.3	n.a.	n.a.	0
Frosting, ready-to-							
spread, 2 tbsp.:							
caramel pecan (*Pills-*							
bury Supreme/							
Creamy Supreme)	150	0	19.0	8.0	0	65	0
chocolate:							
(*Betty Crocker*							
Creamy Deluxe)	150	0	24.0	6.0	0	75	0
(*Pillsbury Creamy*							
Supreme)	140	0	21.0	6.0	0	80	0
(*Pillsbury Supreme*)	140	0	21.0	6.0	0	75	0
(*Pillsbury Supreme/*							
Creamy Supreme							
Funfetti)	140	0	22.0	6.0	0	80	0
dark (*Pillsbury Su-*							
preme/Creamy							
Supreme)	130	0	20.0	6.0	0	45	0
fudge (*Pillsbury*							
Creamy Supreme)	140	0	21.0	6.0	0	80	0
fudge (*Pillsbury Su-*							
preme)	140	0	21.0	6.0	0	75	0
fudge (*Pillsbury Su-*							
preme/Creamy							
Supreme Reduced							
Fat)	140	0	26.0	3.5	0	85	0
milk (*Betty Crocker*							
Creamy Deluxe)	150	0	24.0	6.0	0	70	0

Food and Measure	cal.	prot. (gms)	carbo. (gms)	fat (gms)	chol. (mgs)	sod. (mgs)	fiber (gms)
milk (*Pillsbury Supreme/Creamy Supreme*)	140	0	21.0	6.0	0	60	<1.0
milk (*Pillsbury Supreme/Creamy Supreme Lovin' Lites*)	130	0	25.0	3.0	0	85	<1.0
milk, swirl w/fudge glaze (*Pillsbury Supreme/Creamy Supreme*)	140	0	22.0	6.0	0	60	<1.0
Swiss almond (*Betty Crocker Creamy Deluxe*)	150	0	25.0	5.0	0	45	0
coconut:							
almond (*Pillsbury Supreme*)	160	<1.0	18.0	9.0	0	60	<1.0
pecan (*Pillsbury Supreme/Creamy Supreme*)	160	0	17.0	10.0	0	60	<1.0
cookie (*Pillsbury Supreme/Creamy Supreme Oreo*)	150	0	23.0	6.0	0	75	0
cream cheese:							
(*Betty Crocker Creamy Deluxe*)	140	0	24.0	5.0	0	65	0
(*Pillsbury Supreme/ Creamy Supreme*)	150	0	24.0	6.0	0	70	0
creamy candy (*Pillsbury Supreme/ Creamy Supreme*)	150	0	22.0	7.0	0	95	0
lemon creme (*Pillsbury Supreme/ Creamy Supreme*)	150	0	24.0	6.0	0	75	0
rainbow chip (*Betty Crocker Creamy Deluxe*)	160	0	25.0	6.0	0	25	0

Food and Measure	cal.	prot. (gms)	carbo. (gms)	fat (gms)	chol. (mgs)	sod. (mgs)	fiber (gms)
Frosting *(cont.)*							
strawberry creme							
(*Pillsbury Supreme/*							
Creamy Supreme)	150	0	24.0	6.0	0	75	0
vanilla:							
(*Betty Crocker*							
Creamy Deluxe)	140	0	24.0	5.0	0	35	0
(*Pillsbury Supreme/*							
Creamy Supreme)	150	0	23.0	6.0	0	70	0
(*Pillsbury Creamy*							
Supreme Funfetti)	150	0	25.0	6.0	0	75	0
(*Pillsbury Supreme*							
Funfetti)	160	0	26.0	6.0	0	75	0
(*Pillsbury Supreme/*							
Creamy Supreme							
Lovin' Lites) . . .	140	0	29.0	3.0	0	70	0
French (*Betty*							
Crocker Creamy							
Deluxe)	140	0	24.0	5.0	0	20	0
French (*Pillsbury*							
Creamy Supreme)	150	0	20.0	8.0	0	45	0
French (*Pillsbury*							
Supreme)	160	0	26.0	6.0	0	75	0
pink (*Pillsbury Su-*							
preme/Creamy							
Supreme Funfetti)	150	0	24.0	6.0	0	70	0
swirl, w/fudge glaze							
(*Pillsbury Su-*							
preme/Creamy							
Supreme)	150	0	25.0	6.0	0	75	0
Frozen desserts, see							
"Ice cream and fro-							
zen desserts"							
Fructose (*Estee*),							
1 tsp.	16	0	4.0	0	0	0	0
Fruit, see specific list-							
ings							
Fruit, candied, see							
specific listings							

Food and Measure	cal.	prot. (gms)	carbo. (gms)	fat (gms)	chol. (mgs)	sod. (mgs)	fiber (gms)
Fruit, mixed, candied:							
(*S&W* Glace), 2 tbsp.	90	0	25.0	0	0	30	2.0
(*White Swan*),							
1 tbsp., .8 oz. . . .	70	0	18.0	0	0	15	1.0
(*White Swan* Deluxe),							
2 tbsp., 1.2 oz. . .	100	0	25.0	0	0	20	1.0
fruit and peel mix							
(*Paradise* Old En-							
glish), 1 tbsp., 8 oz.	70	0	18.0	0	0	15.0	1.0
cake mix (*Queen*							
Anne/Paradise Extra							
Fancy), 2 tbsp.,							
1.2 oz.	100	0	25.0	0	0	20	1.0
Fruit, mixed, canned							
(see also "Fruit							
cocktail"), ½ cup,							
except as noted:							
in juice, chunky:							
(*Del Monte*							
Naturals)	60	0	15.0	0	0	10	1.0
(*Libby's* Lite) . . .	60	0	4.0	0	0	5	1.0
(*S&W* Natural) . . .	70	1.0	19.0	0	0	20	3.0
in juice or extra light							
syrup (*Del Monte*							
Lite/Snack Cup) . .	60	0	15.0	0	0	10	1.0
in light syrup (*Del*							
Monte Snack Cup),							
3½ oz.	70	0	17.0	0	0	10	<1.0
in heavy syrup:							
(*Del Monte* Snack							
Cup), 4¼ oz. . .	90	0	23.0	0	0	10	1.0
chunky (*Del Monte*)	100	0	24.0	0	0	10	1.0
tropical salad:							
in light syrup (*Del*							
Monte)	80	0	21.0	0	0	10	1.0
in light syrup (*Dole*)	80	1.0	20.0	0	0	10	1.0
in heavy syrup . . .	110	.5	28.6	.1	0	3	1.7

Food and Measure	cal.	prot. (gms)	carbo. (gms)	fat (gms)	chol. (mgs)	sod. (mgs)	fiber (gms)
Fruit, mixed, dried:							
(*Del Monte*), ⅓ cup,							
1.4 oz.	110	<1.0	30.0	0	0	50	5.0
(*Dole Sun Giant*),							
1.5 oz.	100	1.0	24.0	0	0	35	3.0
(*Sonoma*), 1.4 oz. . . .	120	1.0	30.0	0	0	0	3.0
diced (*Sonoma*),							
⅓ cup	120	1.0	31.0	0	0	0	3.0
and nuts, see "Trail mix"							
Fruit, mixed, frozen:							
(*Big Valley*), ⅔ cup	60	1.0	14.0	0	0	0	2.0
(*Stilwell*), 1 cup . . .	50	1.0	20.0	0	0	10	2.0
Fruit bar, frozen (see also "Yogurt bar"), 1 pc.:							
all flavors:							
(*Dole*), 1.75 oz. . . .	45	0	11.0	0	0	5	0
(*Dole* 'n Sugar),							
1.75 oz.	25	0	6.0	0	0	5	0
except coconut							
(*Edy's*)	90	0	23.0	0	0	0	0
all flavors (*Starburst*)	50	0	12.0	0	0	0	0
banana cream (*Frozfruit*)	150	1.0	20.0	7.0	25	20	1.0
cantaloupe (*Frozfruit*)	60	0	15.0	0	0	5	0
cherry (*Frozfruit*) . .	70	1.0	18.0	0	0	0	1.0
coconut:							
(*Dole* Fruit 'n Juice)	210	3.0	33.0	7.0	10	50	0
(*Edy's* Calypso) . .	190	4.0	26.0	8.0	15	75	0
cream (*Frozfruit*)	170	2.0	17.0	11.0	20	25	2.0
cranberry-apple (*Frozfruit*)	80	0	20.0	0	0	0	<1.0
guava-pineapple (*Frozfruit*)	80	0	20.0	0	0	0	2.0
kiwi-strawberry (*Frozfruit*)	90	0	23.0	0	0	0	2.0
lemon:							
(*Frozfruit*)	90	0	22.0	0	0	10	0

Food and Measure	cal.	prot. (gms)	carbo. (gms)	fat (gms)	chol. (mgs)	sod. (mgs)	fiber (gms)
iced tea (*Frozfruit*)	80	0	19.0	0	0	10	0
lemonade (*Dole* Fruit 'n Juice)	120	1.0	28.0	0	0	55	0
lime (*Frozfruit*) . . .	90	0	21.0	0	0	10	0
orange (*Frozfruit*) . .	90	0	21.0	0	0	15	0
peach passion (*Dole* Fruit 'n Juice) . . .	70	0	17.0	0	0	5	0
piña colada, cream (*Frozfruit*)	170	2.0	23.0	8.0	20	20	1.0
pine-coconut (*Dole* Fruit 'n Juice) . . .	150	1.0	27.0	4.0	0	5	0
pine-orange-banana: (*Dole* Fruit 'n Juice), 2.5 oz.	70	0	16.0	0	0	5	0
(*Dole* Fruit 'n Juice), 4 oz.	150	0	27.0	4.0	0	5	0
pineapple (*Frozfruit*)	80	0	19.0	0	0	0	0
raspberry: (*Dole* Fruit 'n Juice)	70	0	16.0	0	0	5	0
(*Frozfruit*)	80	0	20.0	0	0	5	1.0
strawberry: (*Dole* Fruit 'n Juice), 2.5 oz.	70	0	17.0	0	0	5	0
(*Dole* Fruit 'n Juice), 4 oz.	110	0	26.0	0	0	5	0
(*Frozfruit*)	80	0	20.0	0	0	20	1.0
cream (*Frozfruit*)	130	1.0	21.0	5.0	20	20	1.0
strawberry-banana cream (*Frozfruit*)	140	1.0	21.0	6.0	20	20	1.0
tropical (*Frozfruit*) . .	90	0	23.0	0	0	0	1.0
watermelon (*Frozfruit*)	50	0	13.0	0	0	0	2.0
Fruit cocktail, canned, ½ cup: (*Del Monte* Very Cherry)	90	<1.0	22.0	0	0	10	<1.0
(*Hunt's*)	90	0	23.0	0	0	15	1.0
in extra light syrup (*Del Monte* Lite) . .	60	0	15.0	0	0	10	1.0

Food and Measure	cal.	prot. (gms)	carbo. (gms)	fat (gms)	chol. (mgs)	sod. (mgs)	fiber (gms)
Fruit cocktail *(cont.)*							
in juice:							
(*Del Monte*							
Naturals)	60	0	15.0	0	0	10	1.0
(*Libby's* Lite) . . .	60	0	15.0	0	0	10	1.0
(*S&W* Natural) . . .	80	1.0	20.0	0	0	20	2.0
in heavy syrup:							
(*Del Monte*)	100	0	24.0	0	0	10	1.0
(*S&W*)	90	0	23.0	0	0	15	1.0
honey flavor (*Del*							
Monte Natural) . .	80	<1.0	20.0	0	0	10	<1.0
in light syrup	72	.5	18.8	.1	0	7	1.4
Fruit dip, 2 tbsp.:							
caramel (*Smucker's*							
Fat Free)	130	1.0	30.0	0	0	85	0
chocolate (*Smucker's*							
Fat Free)	130	2.0	31.0	0	0	75	<1.0
Fruit drink blends							
(see also "Citrus							
drinks," "Soft							
drinks" and specific							
listings), 8 fl. oz.,							
except as noted:							
(*Capri Sun Mountain*							
Cooler), 6.75 fl. oz.	100	0	26.0	0	0	20	0
(*Capri Sun Pacific*							
Cooler), 6.75 fl. oz.	100	0	29.0	0	0	20	0
(*Capri Sun Surfer*							
Cooler), 6.75 fl. oz.	100	0	27.0	0	0	20	0
(*Dole* Fruit Fiesta),							
16 fl. oz.	270	0	40.0	0	0	40	0
(*Dole* Lanai/Tropical							
Breeze), 16 fl. oz.	240	1.0	59.0	0	0	40	0
(*Hi-C* Ecto Cooler) . .	120	0	33.0	0	0	25	0
(*Lincoln* Party)	140	0	34.0	0	0	45	0
(*Snapple* Bali Blast)	120	0	30.0	0	0	10	0
(*Snapple* Samoan							
Splash)	120	0	29.0	0	0	10	0
(*Tropicana*)	130	0	32.0	0	0	15	0

Food and Measure	cal.	prot. (gms)	carbo. (gms)	fat (gms)	chol. (mgs)	sod. (mgs)	fiber (gms)
(*Veryfine* Avalanche)	110	0	26.0	0	0	20	0
(*Veryfine* Tropical Breeze)	120	0	30.0	0	0	10	0
nectar (*Kern's* Tropical), 11.5 fl. oz. . . .	210	3.0	48.0	0	0	10	0
punch:							
(*Capri Sun*), 6.75 fl. oz.	100	0	26.0	0	0	20	0
(*Capri Sun Maui*), 6.75 fl. oz.	100	0	28.0	0	0	20	0
(*Capri Sun Safari*), 6.75 fl. oz.	100	0	25.0	0	0	20	0
(*Dole* Paradise), 10 fl. oz.	150	0	38.0	0	0	25	0
(*Dole* Tropical), 10 fl. oz.	130	1.0	33.0	0	0	25	0
(*Farmer's Market* Tropical)	120	0	29.0	0	0	0	0
(*Heinke's* California/ Paradise)	110	0	28.0	0	0	20	0
(*Heinke's* Macchu Pichu)	120	0	30.0	0	0	25	0
(*Hi-C*)	120	0	33.0	0	0	30	0
(*Hi-C* Hula)	110	0	30.0	0	0	30	0
(*Minute Maid*) . . .	120	0	31.0	0	0	25	0
(*Minute Maid* Box)	120	0	33.0	0	0	30	0
(*R.W. Knudsen* Rain Forest/Tropical)	120	0	29.0	0	0	20	0
(*Snapple*)	110	0	28.0	0	0	10	0
(*Tree Top*)	130	0	32.0	0	0	50	0
frozen*, 8 fl. oz.:							
(*Dole* Fruit Fiesta)	140	0	34.0	0	0	20	0
(*Dole* Lanai/Tropical Breeze)	120	0	30.0	0	0	20	0
(*R.W. Knudsen* Tropical)	120	0	29.0	0	0	20	0
punch (*Minute Maid*)	120	0	31.0	0	0	5	0

Food and Measure	cal.	prot. (gms)	carbo. (gms)	fat (gms)	chol. (mgs)	sod. (mgs)	fiber (gms)
Fruit glace, see "Fruit, mixed, candied" and specific listings							
Fruit glaze, see "Glaze, fruit"							
Fruit juice blends, (see also specific listings), 8 fl. oz., except as noted:							
(*R.W. Knudsen* Morning Blend)	120	1.0	31.0	0	0	15	0
(*R.W. Knudsen* Natural Breakfast) . . .	110	1.0	27.0	0	0	35	0
(*R.W. Knudsen* Vita)	120	2.0	29.0	0	0	35	0
(*Season's Best* Medley)	130	<1.0	32.0	0	0	25	0
(*Snapple* Vitamin Supreme), 10 fl. oz.	150	0	38.0	0	0	20	0
punch:							
(*After the Fall* Maui)	90	1.0	23.0	0	0	15	0
(*After the Fall* Sangria de la Noche)	125	1.0	30.0	0	0	10	0
(*Apple & Eve* Nothin' But Juice)	120	1.0	29.0	0	0	30	0
(*Juicy Juice*)	130	1.0	32.0	0	0	10	0
(*Tree Top*), 10 fl. oz.	150	0	37.0	0	0	30	0
(*Veryfine* Juice-Ups)	140	0	36.0	0	0	15	0
tropical fruit:							
(*Dole*)	140	1.0	35.0	0	0	30	0
(*Dole*), 10 fl. oz. . . .	180	1.0	44.0	0	0	45	0
(*Juicy Juice*)	130	1.0	29.0	0	0	10	0
frozen* (*Dole*) . . .	140	1.0	34.0	0	0	30	0
Fruit and nut mix, see "Trail mix"							
Fruit pectin (*Sure•Jell*), ¼ tsp.	5	0	1.0	0	0	0	0
Fruit protector (*Ever-Fresh*), ¼ tsp.	5	0	1.0	0	0	0	0

Food and Measure	cal.	prot. (gms)	carbo. (gms)	fat (gms)	chol. (mgs)	sod. (mgs)	fiber (gms)
Fruit snack (see also specific listings), 1 oz., except as noted:							
all varieties:							
(*Fruit Roll Ups*) . .	110	0	24.0	1.0	0	105	0
(*Roller Blade*), .9 oz.	90	0	21.0	1.0	0	30	0
(*Smart Snackers*), .5 oz.	50	0	13.0	0	0	125	2.0
(*String Thing*), .7 oz.	80	0	17.0	1.0	0	45	0
apple:							
(*Stretch Island*) . .	90	0	25.0	0	0	0	3.0
organic (*Stretch Island*)	90	0	24.0	0	0	10	2.0
apricot (*Stretch Island*)	90	1.0	23.0	0	0	0	2.0
blackberry, cherry, grape, or raspberry (*Stretch Island*) . .	90	0	24.0	0	0	0	2.0
grape, organic (*Stretch Island*) . .	90	0	24.0	0	0	5	2.0
raspberry, organic (*Stretch Island*) . .	90	1.0	25.0	0	0	10	2.0
tropical (*Stretch Island*)	90	<1.0	22.0	0	0	0	1.0
Fruit spreads (see also "Jam and preserves"), 1 tbsp.:							
all varieties:							
(*Kraft* Reduced Calorie)	20	0	5.0	0	0	20	0
(*Polaner*)	40	0	10.0	0	0	0	0
(*R.W. Knudsen*) . .	50	0	13.0	0	0	0	0
(*Simply Fruit*) . . .	40	0	10.0	0	0	0	0
(*Slenderella* Reduced Calorie) . .	20	0	5.0	0	0	10	0
(*Smucker's Bagel Toppers*)	40	0	10.0	0	0	15	0

Food and Measure	cal.	prot. (gms)	carbo. (gms)	fat (gms)	chol. (mgs)	sod. (mgs)	fiber (gms)
Fruit spreads *(cont.)*							
and peanuts							
(*Smucker's* Super							
Spreaders)	40	0	10.0	0	0	10	0
Fruit syrup (see also							
specific listings),							
¼ cup:							
(*Smucker's*)	210	0	52.0	0	0	0	0
light (*Smucker's*) . .	130	0	33.0	0	0	0	0
and maple							
(*R.W. Knudsen*) . .	150	0	38.0	0	0	0	0
Fudge, see "Candy"							
Fudge topping, see							
"Chocolate topping"							
Fusilli pasta mix,							
w/creamy pesto							
(*Knorr*), ⅔ cup . .	250	9.0	47.0	3.0	<5	790	3.0

G

Food and Measure	cal.	prot. (gms)	carbo. (gms)	fat (gms)	chol. (mgs)	sod. (mgs)	fiber (gms)
Garbanzo beans, see "Chickpeas"							
Garbanzo flour (*Arrowhead Mills*), ¼ cup	90	5.0	15.0	1.0	0	0	3.0
Garden salad, ½ cup:							
dill (*S&W*)	50	2.0	14.0	0	0	560	3.0
marinated (*S&W*) . .	50	2.0	13.0	0	0	880	3.0
Garlic:							
trimmed, 1 oz.	42	1.8	9.4	.1	0	5	.6
1 clove, .1 oz.	4	.2	1.0	<.1	0	1	.1
crushed:							
(*Christopher Ranch*), 1 tsp.	10	0	1.0	0	0	0	0
(*Frieda's*), 1 oz. . . .	39	1.8	8.7	.1	0	5	0
granulated/minced:							
1 tsp.	13	.7	2.9	0	0	1	0
(*Tone's*), ¼ tsp. . . .	5	0	1.0	0	0	0	0
Garlic, pickled (*Christopher Ranch*), 3 pcs., ¼ oz.	5	0	0	0	0	80	0
Garlic dip, 2 tbsp.:							
(*Nalley*)	130	1.0	2.0	13.0	10	190	0
Italian, creamy (*Marie's*)	180	1.0	3.0	19.0	15	220	0
roasted, and onion (*Marie's* Fat Free)	35	0	7.0	0	0	350	1.0
Garlic dressing (*Christopher Ranch*), 1 tbsp.	53	0	1.0	5.0	10	133	2.0

Food and Measure	cal.	prot. (gms)	carbo. (gms)	fat (gms)	chol. (mgs)	sod. (mgs)	fiber (gms)
Garlic pepper:							
1 tsp.	8	.3	1.8	0	0	360	.3
(*Tone's*), ¼ tsp. . . .	0	0	0	0	0	90	0
(*Lawry's*), ¼ tsp. . .	0	0	0	0	0	70	0
Garlic pickle relish							
(*Patak's*), 1 tbsp.	45	<1.0	4.0	3.0	0	430	<1.0
Garlic powder:							
1 tsp.	10	.5	2.3	0	0	1	0
(*McCormick*), ¼ tsp.	3	.1	.5	0	0	<1	.2
(*Tone's*), ¼ tsp. . . .	5	0	1.0	0	0	0	0
Garlic salt:							
1 tsp.	3	.1	.5	0	0	2233	0
(*Tone's*), ¼ tsp. . . .	0	0	0	0	0	560	0
(*Durkee* California),							
½ tsp.	0	0	0	0	0	240	0
(*Lawry's*), ¼ tsp. . .	0	0	0	0	0	240	0
(*Morton*), ½ tsp. . .	2	<1.0	<1.0	0	0	650	0
Garlic spread:							
(*Lawry's* Concentrate),							
2 tsp.	50	0	1.0	6.0	0	80	0
(*Lawry's* Ready-to-							
Spread), 1 tbsp. . .	100	0	2.0	10.0	0	190	0
Garlic sprouts (*Jona-*							
than's), 1 cup, 4 oz.	70	5.0	14.0	.5	0	10	3.0
Garlic-basil, chopped							
(*Paesana*), 1 tsp.	6	0	0	0	0	0	0
Gefilte fish, drained:							
(*Manischewitz* Gold/							
Jelled Broth), 1 ball,							
w/jell	110	5.0	10.0	5.0	10	460	1.0
(*Manischewitz* Gold							
Vegetable Medley),							
1 ball, ⅙ carrot . .	80	5.0	5.0	4.0	20	250	1.0
(*Manischewitz* Gold							
w/Olives/Carrots),							
1 ball, ¼ carrot . .	60	5.0	3.0	3.0	15	270	1.0
zesty (*Manischewitz*							
Gold/Brine), 1 ball	70	5.0	4.0	4.0	15	310	1.0

Food and Measure	cal.	prot. (gms)	carbo. (gms)	fat (gms)	chol. (mgs)	sod. (mgs)	fiber (gms)
Gelatin, unflavored							
(*Knox*), 1 pkt. . . .	25	6.0	0	0	0	10	0
Gelatin dessert,							
½ cup, except as							
noted:							
all flavors:							
(*Del Monte* Snack)	70	0	19.0	0	0	40	<1.0
(*Hunt's Snack Pack*)	100	0	25.0	0	0	40	0
(*Jell-O* Snacks) . .	80	1.0	18.0	0	0	45	0
(*Jell-O* Sugar Free							
Snacks), 3.2 oz.	10	1.0	0	0	0	50	0
except strawberry							
(*Kraft Handi-*							
Snacks)	80	0	20.0	0	0	40	0
strawberry (*Kraft*							
Handi-Snacks) . . .	80	0	20.0	0	0	45	0
Gelatin dessert mix*:							
all flavors, ½ cup:							
(*Jell-O* Sugar Free)	10	1.0	0	0	0	—[1]	0
except black rasp-							
berry (*Jell-O*) . .	80	2.0	19.0	0	0	—[2]	0
black raspberry							
(*Jell-O*), ½ cup . .	80	2.0	20.0	0	0	35	0
strawberry, ½ cup:							
(*D-Zerta*)	10	2.0	0	0	0	5	0
(*Jell-O 1-2-3*),							
⅔ cup	130	2.0	26.0	1.5	0	45	0
Gelatin drink mix, or-							
ange (*Knox*), 1 pkt.	40	6.0	4.0	0	0	15	0
Giardiniera, see							
"Vegetables, mixed,							
pickled"							
Ginger, trimmed root:							
1 oz.	20	.5	4.3	.2	0	4	.6
sliced, ¼ cup	17	.4	3.6	.2	0	3	.5

[1] *Sodium values vary between 50 mgs. and 70 mgs. according to flavor.*
[2] *Sodium values vary between 35 mgs. and 75 mgs. according to flavor.*

Food and Measure	cal.	prot. (gms)	carbo. (gms)	fat (gms)	chol. (mgs)	sod. (mgs)	fiber (gms)
Ginger, candied or crystallized:							
(*Frieda's*), 1 oz. . . .	96	.1	24.7	.1	0	n.a.	1.0
(*Paradise/White Swan*), 3 pcs., 1 oz.	100	0	26.0	0	0	10	1.0
Ginger, ground:							
1 tsp.	6	.2	1.3	.1	0	1	.2
(*McCormick*), ¼ tsp.	2	0	.4	0	0	<1	.1
Ginger, pickled, Japanese, 1 oz.	10	.1	2.1	<.1	0	105	n.a.
Ginger drink (*Santa Cruz* Hawaiian), 8 fl. oz.	110	0	27.0	0	0	35	0
Ginkgo nut, shelled:							
raw, 1 oz.	52	1.2	10.7	.5	0	2	<1.0
canned, drained, 1 oz.	32	.6	6.3	.5	0	87	2.6
dried, 1 oz.	99	2.9	20.6	.8	0	4	n.a.
Glace, cake, see "Fruit, mixed, candied"							
Glaze, fruit, 2 tbsp., except as noted:							
for banana, creamy (*Marie's*)	60	.5	8.0	2.5	0	50	0
for blueberries (*Marie's*)	40	0	10.0	0	0	30	0
for peaches (*Marie's*)	40	0	10.0	0	0	50	0
for strawberries (*Marie's*)	40	0	9.0	0	0	30	0
pie, strawberry (*Smucker's*), 2 oz.	80	0	21.0	0	0	0	0
Glaze, ham, see "Ham glaze"							
Glaze mix, see "Seasoning and coating mix"							
Gluten, see "Wheat flour"							

Food and Measure	cal.	prot. (gms)	carbo. (gms)	fat (gms)	chol. (mgs)	sod. (mgs)	fiber (gms)
Goat, meat only,							
roasted, 4 oz. . . .	162	30.7	0	3.4	85	98	0
Godfather's Pizza,							
1 slice:							
cheese, original crust:							
mini, ¼ pie	138	6.0	20.0	4.0	13	159	n.a.
small, ⅙ pie	239	10.0	32.0	7.0	25	289	n.a.
medium, ⅛ pie . .	242	10.0	35.0	7.0	22	285	n.a.
large, ¹⁄₁₀ pie	271	12.0	37.0	8.0	28	329	n.a.
cheese, golden crust:							
small, ⅙ pie	213	8.0	27.0	8.0	19	258	n.a.
medium, ⅛ pie . .	229	8.0	28.0	9.0	19	272	n.a.
large, ¹⁄₁₀ pie	261	8.0	31.0	11.0	23	314	n.a.
combo, original crust:							
mini, ¼ pie	164	8.0	21.0	5.0	17	287	n.a.
small, ⅙ pie	299	15.0	34.0	11.0	37	573	n.a.
medium, ⅛ pie . .	318	16.0	37.0	12.0	38	569	n.a.
large, ¹⁄₁₀ pie	332	16.0	39.0	12.0	39	617	n.a.
combo, golden crust:							
small, ⅙ pie	273	13.0	29.0	12.0	31	542	n.a.
medium, ⅛ pie . .	283	13.0	30.0	13.0	29	526	n.a.
large, ¹⁄₁₀ pie	322	14.0	33.0	15.0	34	602	n.a.
Goose, roasted:							
meat w/skin, 4 oz. . .	346	28.5	0	24.9	103	79	0
meat only, 4 oz. . . .	270	32.9	0	14.4	109	86	0
Goose fat, 1 oz. . . .	255	0	0	28.3	28	0	0
Goose liver, see							
"Liver" and "Pâté"							
Gooseberry, ½ cup:							
fresh	34	.7	7.6	.4	0	1	3.2
canned, light syrup	93	.8	23.6	.3	0	3	3.0
Gorgonzola sauce,							
refrigerated (*Monte-*							
rey Pasta Com-							
pany), 4 oz.	400	8.0	3.0	40.0	145	390	0
Goulash seasoning							
mix (*Knorr* Recipe),							
1⅓ tbsp.	35	1.0	6.0	1.0	0	450	0

Food and Measure	cal.	prot. (gms)	carbo. (gms)	fat (gms)	chol. (mgs)	sod. (mgs)	fiber (gms)
Gourd, boiled, ½ cup:							
dishcloth, 1″ slices	50	.6	12.8	.3	0	18	<1.0
white-flower, 1″ cubes	11	.4	2.7	<.1	0	1	<1.0
Grains, see specific listings							
Granadilla, see "Passion fruit"							
Granola, see "Cereal"							
Granola and cereal bar (see also "Snack bar"), 1 bar, except as noted:							
(*Rice Krispies Treats*)	90	1.0	18.0	2.0	0	75	0
all varieties:							
(*Health Valley* Fat Free Granola) . .	140	2.0	35.0	0	0	5	3.0
(*Health Valley Healthy Breakfast Bakes* Fat Free)	110	2.0	26.0	0	0	25	3.0
(*Health Valley Healthy Cereal Bars* No Fat) . . .	100	2.0	26.0	0	0	0	3.0
(*Health Valley Healthy Energy Bars*)	180	3.0	40.0	1.5	0	10	4.0
(*Kellogg's* Low Fat)	80	2.0	16.0	1.5	0	60	1.0
(*Nature's Choice* Fat Free Granola) . .	90	1.0	23.0	0	0	10	2.0
(*Nature's Choice Real Fruit*), 2 bars	100	<1.0	26.0	0	0	20	0
(*Nutri-Grain*)	140	2.0	27.0	3.0	0	60	1.0
except apple berry and oatmeal cookie (*Quaker Chewy* Lowfat)	110	2.0	22.0	2.0	0	105	1.0
scones (*Health Valley*)	180	4.0	43.0	0	0	160	5.0
w/almonds, chewy (*Little Debbie*) . . .	200	3.0	25.0	10.0	0	95	2.0

Food and Measure	cal.	prot. (gms)	carbo. (gms)	fat (gms)	chol. (mgs)	sod. (mgs)	fiber (gms)
apple, blueberry, or peach filled (*Na--ture's Choice* Fat Free Cereal)	110	2.0	27.0	0	0	90	2.0
apple berry (*Quaker Chewy* Lowfat) . . .	110	2.0	22.0	2.0	0	100	1.0
blueberry (*Kudos* Low Fat)	90	1.0	15.0	1.5	0	90	1.0
carob chip (*Nature's Choice* Granola) . .	80	2.0	16.0	2.0	0	5	2.0
chocolate chip:							
(*Kudos*)	90	1.0	13.0	3.0	0	60	1.0
(*Kudos* Enrobed)	120	2.0	18.0	5.0	5	75	1.0
(*Carnation* Chewy)	150	2.0	22.0	6.0	0	80	1.0
(*Little Debbie*) . . .	220	3.0	33.0	10.0	0	95	2.0
(*Nature's Choice* Grrr-Nola Treats)	80	1.0	15.0	2.0	0	5	1.0
(*Quaker Chewy*) . .	120	2.0	21.0	3.5	0	70	1.0
(*Rice Krispies*) . . .	120	1.0	20.0	4.0	0	60	1.0
chunk (*Carnation* Granola)	140	2.0	22.0	2.0	0	55	1.0
cinnamon:							
and oats (*Barbara's* Granola)	260	6.0	31.0	15.0	0	105	2.0
raisin (*Nature's Choice* Granola)	80	2.0	16.0	2.0	0	5	3.0
coconut almond (*Barbara's* Granola) . .	290	6.0	23.0	20.0	0	20	3.0
cranberry, raspberry, or strawberry filled (*Nature's Choice* Fat Free Cereal)	110	2.0	27.0	0	0	110	2.0
fudge:							
nutty (*Kudos*) . . .	130	2.0	18.0	5.0	5	65	1.0
dipped, macaroon (*Little Debbie*) . .	280	3.0	34.0	16.0	0	100	3.0
dipped, w/peanuts (*Little Debbie*) . .	270	4.0	33.0	15.0	0	95	2.0

Food and Measure	cal.	prot. (gms)	carbo. (gms)	fat (gms)	chol. (mgs)	sod. (mgs)	fiber (gms)
Granola and cereal bar *(cont.)*							
milk and cookies (*Kudos*)	130	2.0	18.0	5.0	5	70	1.0
oats and honey:							
(*Carnation* Granola)	130	2.0	23.0	4.0	0	55	1.0
(*Little Debbie*) . . .	210	3.0	32.0	9.0	0	105	2.0
(*Nature's Choice* Granola)	80	2.0	15.0	2.0	0	5	2.0
oatmeal cookie (*Quaker Chewy* Lowfat)	110	1.0	22.0	2.0	0	105	1.0
oatmeal raisin:							
(*Little Debbie*) . . .	160	2.0	33.0	3.0	0	120	2.0
(*Sweet Success*) . .	120	2.0	23.0	4.0	<5	30	3.0
peanut butter:							
(*Barbara's* Granola)	260	9.0	28.0	15.0	0	75	3.0
(*Kudos*)	130	2.0	18.0	5.0	5	85	1.0
(*Nature's Choice* Granola)	80	2.0	14.0	3.0	0	5	2.0
chocolate chip (*Carnation* Chewy) . .	150	3.0	21.0	2.0	0	90	1.0
chocolate chip (*Quaker Chewy*)	120	3.0	19.0	4.5	0	85	1.0
and jelly (*Nature's Choice Grrr-Nola*)	80	1.0	14.0	3.0	0	5	2.0
strawberry (*Kudos* Low Fat)	80	1.0	15.0	1.5	0	90	1.0
Grape, ½ cup, except as noted:							
fresh, American type (slipskin):							
10 medium	15	.2	4.1	.1	0	tr.	.3
peeled and seeded	29	.3	7.9	.2	0	1	.6
fresh, European type (adherent skin):							
seeded, 1 lb.	287	2.7	72.0	2.3	0	7	2.7
seedless, 10 medium	36	.3	8.9	.3	0	1	.3
seedless or seeded	57	.5	14.2	.5	0	2	.5

Food and Measure	cal.	prot. (gms)	carbo. (gms)	fat (gms)	chol. (mgs)	sod. (mgs)	fiber (gms)
canned, seedless:							
heavy syrup	94	.6	25.2	.1	0	7	.5
heavy syrup (*S&W*)	100	<1.0	23.0	0	0	20	<1.0
heavy syrup (*S&W* Fancy Jubilee) . .	130	<1.0	33.0	0	0	35	<1.0
Grape drink, 8 fl. oz., except as noted:							
(*Capri Sun*), 6.75 fl. oz.	110	0	28.0	0	0	20	0
(*Dole*), 10 fl. oz. . . .	150	0	38.0	0	0	25	0
(*Hi-C*)	120	0	33.0	0	0	30	0
(*Lincoln*)	130	0	32.0	0	0	45	0
(*Veryfine* Glacial) . .	110	0	28.0	0	0	5	0
grapeade (*Snapple*)	110	0	28.0	0	0	10	0
frozen* (*Minute Maid*)	120	0	33.0	0	0	5	0
Grape drink blends:							
apple (*Tree Top*), 11.5 fl. oz.	190	0	49.0	0	0	35	0
punch:							
(*Minute Maid*), 8 fl. oz.	120	0	32.0	0	0	25	0
frozen* (*Minute Maid*), 8 fl. oz.	120	0	32.0	0	0	5	0
Grape drink mix, 8 fl. oz.*:							
(*Kool-Aid*)	100	0	25.0	0	0	15	0
(*Kool-Aid* w/sugar)	60	0	16.0	0	0	0	0
Grape juice, 8 fl. oz.:							
(*After the Fall* Concord)	130	1.0	31.0	0	0	10	0
(*Goya*)	140	1.0	36.0	0	0	10	1.0
(*Juicy Juice*)	130	1.0	32.0	0	0	10	0
(*Lucky Leaf*)	140	0	34.0	0	0	35	0
(*R.W. Knudsen*) . . .	150	1.0	37.0	0	0	30	0
(*R.W. Knudsen* Concord)	160	0	40.0	0	0	15	0
(*Season's Best*) . . .	160	<1.0	39.0	0	0	25	0
(*Veryfine*)	150	0	37.0	0	0	30	0
(*Veryfine* Juice-Ups)	130	0	32.0	0	0	10	0

Food and Measure	cal.	prot. (gms)	carbo. (gms)	fat (gms)	chol. (mgs)	sod. (mgs)	fiber (gms)
Grape leaves, in jars, (*Krinos*), 1 leaf . .	5	0	0	0	0	200	1.0
Grape leaves, stuffed, in jars (*Perfecta* Dolma-dakia), 4.35 oz. . .	220	3.0	19.0	15.0	0	780	4.0
Grapefruit, fresh:							
pink or red, California or Arizona:							
½ medium, 3¾″ . .	46	.6	11.9	.1	0	<1	1.4
sections w/juice, ½ cup	43	.6	11.1	.1	0	<1	1.3
pink or red, Florida:							
½ medium, 3¾″ . .	37	.7	9.2	.1	0	<1	1.4
sections w/juice, ½ cup	34	.6	8.6	.1	0	<1	1.3
white, California:							
½ medium, 3¾″ . .	43	1.0	10.7	.1	0	<1	1.3
sections w/juice, ½ cup	42	1.0	10.5	.1	0	<1	1.3
white, Florida:							
½ medium, 3¾″ . .	38	.7	9.7	.1	0	<1	.2
sections w/juice, ½ cup	38	.7	9.4	.1	0	<1	.2
Grapefruit, canned							
in juice, ½ cup . . .	46	.9	11.4	.1	0	9	.5
(*S&W* Natural Style), ⅔ cup	50	0	14.0	0	0	25	0
Grapefruit, Chinese, see "Pummelo"							
Grapefruit drink, 8 fl. oz., except as noted:							
pink:							
(*Ocean Spray*) . . .	110	<1.0	28.0	0	0	35	0
(*Tree Top* Desert Ice)	120	0	29.0	0	0	25	0
(*Tropicana Twister*)	120	0	29.0	0	0	20	0

Food and Measure	cal.	prot. (gms)	carbo. (gms)	fat (gms)	chol. (mgs)	sod. (mgs)	fiber (gms)
(*Tropicana Twister*), 11.5 fl. oz.	160	0	40.0	0	0	30	0
(*Tropicana Twister* Light)	35	0	10.0	0	0	20	0
ruby red:							
(*Ocean Spray*) . . .	130	0	33.0	0	0	35	0
and tangerine							
(*Ocean Spray*) . .	130	0	32.0	0	0	35	0
Grapefruit juice,							
8 fl. oz., except as noted:							
fresh, 6 fl. oz.	72	.9	17.0	.2	0	2	.2
(*Dole*), 10 fl. oz. . . .	120	2.0	29.0	0	0	25	0
(*Goya*)	160	2.0	36.0	0	0	0	1.0
(*Ocean Spray*)	100	1.0	24.0	0	0	35	<1.0
(*S&W*), 6 fl. oz. . . .	80	1.0	18.0	0	0	0	0
(*S&W*)	100	1.0	25.0	0	0	0	0
(*Tree Top*)	100	0	25.0	0	0	30	0
(*Veryfine*)	90	2.0	20.0	0	0	15	0
blend:							
(*Dole* Sunripe) . . .	130	1.0	31.0	0	0	30	0
cranberry (*Apple & Eve* Ruby Red)	120	1.0	30	0	0	10	0
golden (*Tropicana*) . .	90	<1.0	23.0	0	0	0	0
pink or white							
(*R.W. Knudsen*) . .	100	2.0	23.0	0	0	35	0
red (*R.W. Knudsen* Rio)	140	2.0	35.0	0	0	10	0
ruby red:							
(*Tropicana* Carton)	100	<1.0	23.0	0	0	0	0
(*Tropicana* Plastic)	100	<1.0	25.0	0	0	0	0
frozen* (*Minute Maid*)	100	0	24.0	0	0	0	0
Gravy, see specific listings							
Great northern beans:							
dried:							
boiled, ½ cup	104	7.3	18.6	.4	0	2	6.2
(*Goya*), ¼ cup . . .	70	8.0	22.0	0	0	20	13.0

Food and Measure	cal.	prot. (gms)	carbo. (gms)	fat (gms)	chol. (mgs)	sod. (mgs)	fiber (gms)
Great northern beans *(cont.)*							
canned, ½ cup:							
w/liquid	150	9.7	27.6	.5	0	6	6.4
(*Allens*)	100	6.0	19.0	.5	0	310	7.0
(*Eden* Organic) . .	120	7.0	23.0	0	0	15	7.0
(*Goya*)	80	6.0	18.0	4.0	0	370	6.5
(*Green Giant/Joan of Arc*)	100	6.0	18.0	.5	0	290	6.0
(*Stokely*)	110	6.0	19.0	.5	0	350	3.0
(*Sun-Vista*)	70	6.0	17.0	0	0	490	6.0
w/sausage (*Trappey's*)	100	6.0	18.0	1.0	0	460	7.0
Green beans, fresh:							
raw, ½ cup	17	1.0	3.9	.1	0	3	1.9
boiled, drained, ½ cup	22	1.2	4.9	.2	0	2	2.0
Green beans, canned, ½ cup:							
(*Allens* Shells Out)	30	2.0	6.0	0	0	460	2.0
(*Goya*)	20	1.0	4.0	0	0	300	2.0
(*Green Giant Kitchen Sliced*)	20	<1.0	4.0	0	0	400	1.0
(*Green Giant Kitchen Sliced* Less Sodium)	20	2.0	3.0	0	0	200	1.0
(*Stokely*)	20	1.0	4.0	0	0	350	1.0
(*Stokely* No Salt) . .	20	1.0	4.0	0	0	25	1.0
all varieties:							
(*Del Monte*)	20	1.0	4.0	0	0	360	2.0
(*Del Monte* No Salt)	20	1.0	4.0	0	0	10	2.0
whole, cut, or French (*S&W*)	20	1.0	4.0	0	0	340	2.0
cut:							
(*Allens* No Salt) . .	15	0	3.0	0	0	10	2.0
(*Allens/Sunshine/ Alma/Crest Top*)	30	0	6.0	.5	0	320	3.0
(*Green Giant*) . . .	20	2.0	3.0	0	0	400	1.0
(*Green Giant* Less Sodium)	20	2.0	3.0	0	0	200	1.0
w/wax beans (*S&W*)	20	1.0	3.0	0	0	135	2.0

Food and Measure	cal.	prot. (gms)	carbo. (gms)	fat (gms)	chol. (mgs)	sod. (mgs)	fiber (gms)
French style:							
(*Allens*)	25	<1.0	4.0	0	0	300	2.0
(*Green Giant*) . . .	20	2.0	3.0	0	0	390	1.0
Italian cut:							
(*Allens/Sunshine*)	35	1.0	7.0	.5	0	320	3.0
(*Del Monte*)	30	1.0	6.0	0	0	360	3.0
w/potatoes (*Allen/Sunshine*)	35	1.0	7.0	0	0	220	2.0
Green beans, dilled (*S&W*), 1 oz. . . .	20	0	5.0	0	0	125	1.0
Green beans, freeze-dried (*Mountain House*), ⅔ cup . .	25	1.0	5.0	0	0	0	2.0
Green beans, frozen:							
(*Seabrook*), 1 cup . .	25	1.0	4.0	0	0	10	2.0
cut, ⅔ cup:							
(*Green Giant*) . . .	25	1.0	5.0	0	0	0	2.0
(*Green Giant Harvest Fresh*) . . .	25	<1.0	5.0	0	0	95	2.0
sliced (*Stilwell*), ⅔ cup	25	1.0	4.0	0	0	10	2.0
Green bean combinations, frozen:							
and almonds (*Green Giant Harvest Fresh*), ⅔ cup . . .	60	2.0	5.0	3.0	0	95	2.0
mushroom casserole (*Stouffer's*), 3.8 oz.	140	3.0	13.0	8.0	10	530	2.0
Green peas, see "Peas, green"							
Greens (see also specific listings), mixed, canned (*Allens/Sunshine*), ½ cup . . .	30	1.0	8.0	.5	0	10	4.0
Grenadine syrup, 2 tbsp.:							
(*Mr. & Mrs. "T"*) . .	80	0	18.0	0	0	5	0
(*Rose's*)	90	0	22.0	0	0	10	0

Food and Measure	cal.	prot. (gms)	carbo. (gms)	fat (gms)	chol. (mgs)	sod. (mgs)	fiber (gms)
Grilling sauce (see also specific listings), 2 tbsp., except as noted:							
Chardonnay (*Knorr*)	35	0	2.0	2.5	0	380	0
herb, Tuscan (*Knorr*)	35	0	2.0	2.5	0	450	0
mandarin ginger (*Knorr* Microwave)	45	<1.0	3.0	3.5	0	350	0
Parmesano (*Knorr* Microwave), 3 tbsp.	50	1.0	3.0	3.5	<5	680	0
plum, spicy (*Knorr*)	50	<1.0	9.0	1.5	0	490	0
tequila lime (*Knorr*)	40	<1.0	5.0	2.0	0	510	0
Grits, see "Corn grits"							
Ground cherry, ½ cup	37	1.3	7.8	.5	0	n.a.	2.0
Grouper, meat only:							
raw, 4 oz.	104	22.0	0	1.2	42	60	0
baked, broiled, or microwaved, 4 oz. . .	134	28.2	0	1.5	53	60	0
Guacamole dip (see also "Avocado dip") (*Nalley*), 2 tbsp. . .	120	1.0	2.0	12.0	10	170	0
Guacamole seasoning (*Lawry's*), ½ tsp.	5	0	1.0	0	0	130	0
Guanabana, frozen chunks (*Goya*), ⅓ pkg.	60	1.0	13.0	0	0	20	2.0
Guanabana nectar, canned (*Goya*), 12 fl. oz.	230	1.0	57.0	0	0	20	1.0
Guava:							
1 medium, 4 oz. . . .	45	.7	10.7	.5	0	2	4.9
½ cup	42	.7	9.8	.5	0	2	4.5
strawberry, ½ cup . .	85	.7	21.2	.7	0	45	7.8
Guava drink, 8 fl. oz.:							
(*Mauna La'l*)	130	0	32.0	0	0	35	0
(*Snapple* Guava Mania)	110	0	29.0	0	0	10	0

Food and Measure	cal.	prot. (gms)	carbo. (gms)	fat (gms)	chol. (mgs)	sod. (mgs)	fiber (gms)
Guava juice (*After the Fall* Maya), 8 fl. oz.	110	1.0	26.0	0	0	20	0
Guava nectar:							
(*Goya*), 12 fl. oz. . .	240	1.0	59.0	0	0	25	2.0
(*Kern's*), 8 fl. oz. . .	150	0	38.0	0	0	5	0
(*Libby's/Kern's*),							
11.5 fl. oz.	220	0	54.0	0	0	10	0
Guava paste (*Goya*),							
³/₄-in. slice	100	0	24.0	0	0	10	1.0
Guava sauce, ½ cup	43	.4	11.3	.2	0	4	4.3
Guavadilla, see "Passion fruit"							
Guinea hen, raw:							
meat w/skin, 4 oz. . .	179	26.5	0	7.3	n.a.	n.a.	0
meat only, 4 oz. . . .	125	23.4	0	2.8	71	n.a.	0
Gumbo dinner mix							
(*Luzianne*), ⅕ pkg.	160	4.0	33.0	1.0	0	760	1.0
Gyro mix (*Casbah*),							
¹/₁₀ pkg.	64	2.0	12.0	0	0	470	0

H

Food and Measure	cal.	prot. (gms)	carbo. (gms)	fat (gms)	chol. (mgs)	sod. (mgs)	fiber (gms)
Häagen-Dazs Ice Cream Shop, ½ cup:							
ice cream:							
cappuccino	270	5.0	22.0	18.0	120	85	0
cherry, brandied . .	250	4.0	24.0	15.0	100	80	0
chocolate, Belgian	330	5.0	29.0	18.0	90	80	0
chocolate Swiss al- mond	300	6.0	24.0	21.0	105	75	0
coffee chip	300	5.0	26.0	20.0	105	80	0
macadamia nut . .	330	5.0	24.0	24.0	n.a.	n.a.	0
maple walnut . . .	330	6.0	18.0	26.0	125	75	0
pralines & cream	290	5.0	27.0	18.0	100	180	0
vanilla chip	300	5.0	26.0	20.0	105	80	0
sorbet:							
lemon	140	0	35.0	0	0	20	0
orange	140	0	36.0	0	0	20	0
raspberry	110	0	27.0	0	0	15	0
yogurt, soft-serve:							
chocolate	120	4.0	26.0	0	0	65	0
coffee	140	5.0	22.0	4.0	35	75	0
raspberry	140	4.0	21.0	4.0	35	70	0
strawberry	120	4.0	26.0	0	5	70	0
vanilla	110	5.0	22.0	0	5	75	0
Haddock, meat only:							
raw, 4 oz.	99	21.5	0	.8	65	78	0
baked, broiled, or mi- crowaved, 4 oz. . .	127	27.5	0	1.1	84	99	0
smoked, 4 oz.	132	28.6	0	1.1	87	865	0

Food and Measure	cal.	prot. (gms)	carbo. (gms)	fat (gms)	chol. (mgs)	sod. (mgs)	fiber (gms)
Haddock entree, frozen:							
battered, 2 pcs.:							
(*Mrs. Paul's* Crunchy)	250	18.0	25.0	12.0	25	630	2.0
(*Van de Kamp's*) . .	260	13.0	18.0	16.0	30	530	n.a.
breaded:							
(*Mrs. Paul's*), 1 pc.	230	17.0	17.0	11.0	35	390	2.0
(*Van de Kamp's*), 2 pcs.	280	12.0	19.0	17.0	25	310	n.a.
(*Van de Kamp's Light*), 1 pc. . . .	90	14.0	19.0	10.0	30	410	n.a.
Hake, see "Whiting"							
Halibut, meat only:							
Atlantic and Pacific:							
raw, 4 oz.	124	23.6	0	2.6	37	61	0
baked, broiled, or microwaved, 4 oz.	159	30.3	0	3.3	46	78	0
Greenland:							
raw, 4 oz.	211	16.3	0	15.7	52	91	0
baked, broiled, or microwaved, 4 oz.	271	20.9	0	20.1	67	117	0
Halibut, frozen, fillet or steaks (*Peter Pan*), 4 oz.	110	20.0	0	3.0	45	55	0
Halibut entree, frozen, battered (*Van de Kamp's*), 3 pcs.	300	13.0	16.0	21.0	20	520	n.a.
Halvah, chocolate (*Joyva*), 1.75 oz.	340	4.0	16.0	22.0	0	105	2.0
Ham, fresh, meat only:							
whole leg, roasted:							
lean w/fat, 4 oz. . .	333	28.4	0	23.5	105	67	0
lean w/fat, chopped or diced, 1 cup	411	35.0	0	29.0	131	83	0
lean only, 4 oz. . .	249	32.1	0	12.5	107	73	0
lean only, chopped or diced, 1 cup	309	39.7	0	15.4	131	90	0

Food and Measure	cal.	prot. (gms)	carbo. (gms)	fat (gms)	chol. (mgs)	sod. (mgs)	fiber (gms)
Ham *(cont.)*							
rump half, roasted:							
lean w/fat, 4 oz. . . .	311	30.2	0	20.2	108	69	0
lean only, 4 oz. . . .	251	33.0	0	12.1	109	74	0
shank half, roasted:							
lean w/fat, 4 oz. . . .	344	27.6	0	25.1	104	66	0
lean only, 4 oz. . . .	244	32.0	0	11.9	104	73	0
Ham, cured:							
whole leg, lean w/fat:							
unheated, 4 oz. . . .	279	21.0	.1	21.0	64	1456	0
roasted, 4 oz.	276	24.5	0	19.0	70	1346	0
roasted, chopped or							
diced, 1 cup . . .	341	30.2	0	23.5	86	1661	0
whole leg, lean only:							
unheated, 4 oz. . .	167	25.3	.1	6.5	59	1719	0
roasted, 4 oz.	178	28.4	0	6.2	62	1505	0
roasted, chopped or							
diced, 1 cup . . .	219	35.1	0	7.7	78	1858	0
boneless (11% fat):							
unheated, 4 oz. . .	206	19.9	3.5	12.0	65	1493	0
roasted, 4 oz.	202	25.7	0	10.2	67	1701	0
roasted, chopped or							
diced, 1 cup . . .	249	31.7	0	12.6	83	2100	0
boneless, extra lean							
(5% fat):							
unheated, 4 oz. . .	149	21.9	1.1	5.6	53	1620	0
roasted, 4 oz.	164	23.7	1.7	6.3	60	1364	0
roasted, chopped or							
diced, 1 cup . . .	203	29.3	2.1	7.7	74	1684	0
Ham, canned or re-							
frigerated, 3 oz.,							
except as noted:							
(*Black Label* Refriger-							
ated)	100	14.0	0	5.0	40	960	0
(*Black Label* Shelf)	110	14.0	0	5.0	45	900	0
(*Curemaster* Half) . .	80	14.0	0	3.0	40	940	0
(*Hormel Light &*							
Lean)	90	14.0	2.0	2.5	35	950	0

Food and Measure	cal.	prot. (gms)	carbo. (gms)	fat (gms)	chol. (mgs)	sod. (mgs)	fiber (gms)
(*John Morrell* Boneless)	140	13.0	2.0	9.0	45	840	0
(*Jones Dairy Farm Country Carved Family/Dainty*) . . .	100	0	17.0	4.0	50	930	0
(*Jones Dairy Farm Country Club*) . . .	100	17.0	0	4.0	50	930	0
(*Jones Dairy Farm Family/Dainty*) . . .	100	17.0	0	4.0	50	930	0
(*Jones Dairy Farm Homestead*)	140	16.0	0	8.0	55	750	0
(*Jones Dairy Farm* Old Fashioned)	220	15.0	0	18.0	65	1200	0
baked (*Louis Rich Dinner*), 3.3-oz. slice	80	16.0	1.0	1.5	40	1150	0
Black Forest (*Boar's Head* Baby)	90	16.0	3.0	1.5	45	900	0
chunk (*Hormel*), 2 oz.	90	9.0	0	6.0	30	600	0
fully cooked (*Jones Dairy Farm*)	240	13.0	0	21.0	65	740	0
honey:							
(*Jones Dairy Farm Country Carved Family*)	100	16.0	0	4.0	45	950	0
(*Patrick Cudahy ReaLean*)	90	11.0	5.0	2.5	30	1050	0
maple:							
(*Boar's Head Baby Honey Coat*) . . .	90	16.0	4.0	1.5	35	870	0
(*Jones Dairy Farm Country Carved Family*)	100	15.0	1.0	4.0	45	810	0
semi-boneless (*Jones Dairy Farm*)	180	16.0	0	13.0	60	800	0
skinless, shankless (*Jones Dairy Farm*)	160	16.0	0	11.0	60	680	0
slice:							
(*Oscar Mayer*) . . .	80	14.0	0	3.0	40	1010	0

Food and Measure	cal.	prot. (gms)	carbo. (gms)	fat (gms)	chol. (mgs)	sod. (mgs)	fiber (gms)
Ham, canned or refrigerated, slice *(cont.)*							
smoke flavor (*Patrick Cudahy ReaLean*)	80	11.0	4.0	2.5	30	1010	0
smoked or maple glaze (*Boar's Head Sweet Slice*)	110	15.0	<1.0	5.0	40	780	0
smoked, semi-boneless (*Boar's Head*)	130	15.0	1.0	7.0	50	800	0
spiral sliced:							
(*Jones Dairy Farm*)	180	16.0	0	11.0	60	680	0
(*Spiral Cure 81 Half*)	150	15.0	1.0	9.0	50	1090	0
steak:							
(*Jones Dairy Farm Lean Choice/Rock River*)	100	17.0	0	4.0	50	930	0
(*Oscar Mayer*), 2 oz.	60	10.0	0	2.0	30	750	0
honey (*Patrick Cudahy*)	100	14.0	4.0	3.5	45	920	0
smoke flavor (*Patrick Cudahy*) . . .	90	14.0	1.0	3.0	40	1000	0
Virginia:							
(*Boar's Head* Ready-to-Eat)	100	14.0	3.0	3.0	40	1010	0
smoked (*Boar's Head* Baby Gourmet)	90	16.0	1.0	4.0	45	900	0
"Ham," vegetarian, frozen:							
roll (*Worthington Wham*), ⅜" slice	100	9.0	2.0	6.0	0	520	0
sliced (*Worthington Wham*), 2 slices . .	80	7.0	1.0	5.0	0	430	0
Ham and asparagus, frozen, bake (*Stouffer's*), 9½ oz.	520	16.0	32.0	36.0	75	1040	2.0
Ham bologna (*Boar's Head*), 2 oz.	80	9.0	2.0	4.0	30	660	0

Food and Measure	cal.	prot. (gms)	carbo. (gms)	fat (gms)	chol. (mgs)	sod. (mgs)	fiber (gms)
Ham glaze:							
(*Crosse & Blackwell*), 1 tbsp.	30	0	8.0	0	0	25	0
(*Marzetti*), 2 tbsp. . . .	35	0	9.0	0	0	105	0
Ham lunch meat (see also "Prosciutto"), 2 oz., except as noted:							
(*Boar's Head* Deluxe)	60	9.0	2.0	1.0	25	590	0
(*Boar's Head* Lower Sodium Extra Lean)	50	10.0	<1.0	1.0	20	460	0
(*Healthy Deli* Cinnamon Apple Grove)	70	9.0	4.0	1.5	20	480	0
(*Healthy Deli* Deluxe)	60	9.0	1.0	1.5	20	480	0
(*Healthy Deli* Less Sodium)	60	9.0	2.0	1.5	20	330	0
(*Healthy Deli* Old Tyme Taverne) . . .	60	10.0	1.0	1.5	20	470	0
(*Hormel Light & Lean* 97), 1-oz. slice . .	25	4.0	0	1.0	15	340	0
(*Hormel Light & Lean* 97 Deli)	50	9.0	0	2.0	25	720	0
(*Jones Dairy Farm Lean Choice*), 2 slices	50	9.0	0	1.5	30	420	0
(*Menumaster*), 1 oz.	30	4.0	1.0	1.0	10	320	0
(*Old Tyme*), 1 oz. . .	35	5.0	0	1.5	15	280	0
(*Oscar Mayer* Lower Sodium), 3 slices	70	10.0	2.0	2.5	30	520	0
baked:							
(*Louis Rich Carving Board*), 2 slices	50	8.0	1.0	1.5	25	550	0
(*Oscar Mayer*), 3 slices, 2.2 oz.	60	11.0	2.0	1.0	30	720	0
(*Oscar Mayer Healthy Favorites*), 4 slices	50	9.0	0	1.0	25	600	0
baked, Virginia:							
(*Healthy Deli*) . . .	60	9.0	3.0	1.5	20	480	0

Food and Measure	cal.	prot. (gms)	carbo. (gms)	fat (gms)	chol. (mgs)	sod. (mgs)	fiber (gms)
Ham lunch meat, baked, Virginia *(cont.)*							
(*Healthy Deli* Less Sodium)	70	9.0	3.0	1.5	20	330	0
Black Forest:							
(*Boar's Head*) . . .	60	10.0	2.0	.5	30	580	0
(*Healthy Deli*) . . .	60	10.0	1.0	1.5	20	480	0
boiled:							
(*Oscar Mayer*), 3 slices, 2.2 oz.	60	10.0	0	2.5	30	820	0
(*Oscar Mayer Deli-Thin*), 4 slices . .	50	9.0	0	2.0	25	680	0
(*Patrick Cudahy*), 1-oz. slice	30	5.0	<1.0	1.0	15	360	0
cappacola:							
(*Boar's Head* Cappy)	60	10.0	3.0	1.5	15	530	0
(*Healthy Deli* Cappi)	60	9.0	2.0	1.5	20	480	0
chopped:							
(*Black Label*) . . .	140	7.0	3.0	11.0	30	650	0
(*Oscar Mayer*), 1-oz. slice	45	4.0	1.0	3.0	15	340	0
cooked:							
(*Alpine Lace*) . . .	60	9.0	1.0	2.0	25	440	0
(*Hormel* Deli) . . .	60	8.0	2.0	2.5	20	680	0
(*Hormel* Low Salt)	60	8.0	1.0	2.5	25	510	0
(*Patrick Cudahy* Less Sodium), 1-oz. slice	30	5.0	0	1.0	15	180	0
honey:							
(*Healthy Deli* Honey Valley Farms) . .	60	9.0	2.0	1.5	20	480	0
(*Louis Rich Carving Board* Thin), 6 slices	70	11.0	2.0	1.5	30	710	0
(*Louis Rich Carving Board* Traditional)	50	8.0	2.0	1.5	25	530	0
(*Oscar Mayer*), 3 slices, 2.2 oz.	70	10.0	2.0	2.5	30	760	0
(*Oscar Mayer Deli-Thin*), 4 slices . .	60	9.0	2.0	2.0	25	630	0

Food and Measure	cal.	prot. (gms)	carbo. (gms)	fat (gms)	chol. (mgs)	sod. (mgs)	fiber (gms)
(*Oscar Mayer Healthy Favorites*), 4 slices	50	9.0	2.0	1.5	25	630	0
(*Patrick Cudahy*), 1-oz. slice	35	5.0	1.0	1.0	15	310	0
hot (*Healthy Deli* Rodeo)	60	9.0	1.0	1.5	20	480	0
jalapeño (*Healthy Deli*)	60	8.0	3.0	1.5	15	480	0
maple:							
(*Boar's Head Honey Coat*)	60	10.0	3.0	1.0	20	570	0
(*Healthy Deli* Vermont)	60	9.0	3.0	1.5	20	460	0
(*Patrick Cudahy*), 1-oz. slice	35	5.0	2.0	1.0	15	290	0
minced, 1 oz.	75	4.6	.5	5.9	20	353	0
pepper:							
(*Boar's Head*) . . .	70	9.0	3.0	2.0	30	590	0
(*Healthy Deli*) . . .	60	9.0	2.0	1.5	20	470	0
smoked:							
(*Boar's Head* Gourmet)	60	10.0	2.0	.5	30	580	0
(*Hormel Light & Lean* 97 Deli) . .	50	8.0	2.0	1.5	20	700	0
(*Louis Rich Carving Board*), 2 slices	45	8.0	0	1.5	20	570	0
(*Oscar Mayer*), 3 slices, 2.2 oz.	60	10.0	0	2.5	30	750	0
(*Oscar Mayer Deli-Thin*), 4 slices . .	50	9.0	0	2.0	25	620	0
(*Oscar Mayer Healthy Favorites*), 4 slices	59	9.0	0	1.5	25	620	0
double (*Healthy Deli*)	60	10.0	1.0	1.5	20	470	0
spiced (*Boar's Head*)	120	7.0	1.0	10.0	30	570	0
Virginia:							
(*Boar's Head*) . . .	60	9.0	3.0	1.0	25	590	0
(*Healthy Deli*) . . .	60	9.0	2.0	1.5	20	480	0

Food and Measure	cal.	prot. (gms)	carbo. (gms)	fat (gms)	chol. (mgs)	sod. (mgs)	fiber (gms)
Ham patty (*Hormel*), 2-oz. patty	180	7.0	1.0	17.0	35	550	0
Ham salad spread (*Libby's Spreadables*), ⅓ cup . . .	110	8.0	8.0	4.5	20	620	4.0
Ham spread:							
deviled:							
(*Cure 81*), 2 oz. . .	150	9.0	1.0	12.0	40	430	0
(*Underwood*), ¼ cup	160	8.0	0	14.0	45	440	0
w/crackers (*Red Devil* Snackers), 1 pkg.	310	11.0	18.0	22.0	50	680	1.0
honey:							
(*Underwood*), ¼ cup	180	8.0	3.0	16.0	45	330	0
w/crackers (*Red Devil* Snackers), 1 pkg.	340	11.0	20.0	24.0	50	560	1.0
Ham and asparagus au gratin, frozen (*The Budget Gourmet* Light & Healthy), 8.7 oz. . .	290	17.0	26.0	13.0	50	870	3.0
Ham and cheese loaf (*Oscar Mayer*), 1 oz.	70	4.0	1.0	5.0	20	350	0
Ham and cheese patty (*Hormel*), 2-oz. patty	190	7.0	0	17.0	45	470	0
Ham and cheese sandwich, frozen, 1 pc.:							
(*Croissant Pockets*)	360	13.0	39.0	17.0	45	710	5.0
(*Hormel Quick Meal*)	330	19.0	46.0	8.0	35	860	2.0
(*Hot Pockets*)	340	14.0	37.0	15.0	45	840	4.0
Hamburger, see "Beef entree, frozen"							

Food and Measure	cal.	prot. (gms)	carbo. (gms)	fat (gms)	chol. (mgs)	sod. (mgs)	fiber (gms)
"Hamburger," vegetarian:							
(*New Menu* VegiBurger), 3 oz.	110	13.0	12.0	1.0	0	320	1.0
canned:							
(*LaLoma Redi-Burger*), ⅝″ slice	170	16.0	5.0	10.0	0	460	4.0
(*Loma Linda Vege-Burger*), ¼ cup	70	11.0	2.0	1.5	0	115	2.0
(*Worthington*), ¼ cup	60	9.0	2.0	2.0	0	270	1.0
frozen, 1 patty:							
(*Amy's* California)	100	4.0	17.0	3.0	0	290	3.0
(*Amy's* Chicago) . .	160	9.0	20.0	5.0	5	390	4.0
(*Green Giant Harvest Burgers* Original)	140	18.0	8.0	4.0	0	380	5.0
(*Ken & Robert's* Veggie Burger)	130	5.0	26.0	1.0	0	260	3.0
(*Morningstar Farms* Better'n Burgers)	70	11.0	6.0	0	0	360	3.0
(*Morningstar Farms* Grillers)	140	14.0	5.0	7.0	0	260	3.0
(*Natural Touch* Vegan Burger) . .	70	11.0	6.0	0	0	370	3.0
(*Natural Touch* Vege Burger)	140	15.0	4.0	6.0	0	320	4.0
black bean, spicy (*Morningstar Farms*)	100	8.0	16.0	1.0	0	470	5.0
garden grain (*Morningstar Farms*)	120	6.0	18.0	2.5	<5	280	4.0
garden vegetable (*Morningstar Farms*)	100	10.0	9.0	2.5	0	350	4.0
garden vegetable (*Natural Touch*)	100	10.0	8.0	2.5	0	280	3.0

Food and Measure	cal.	prot. (gms)	carbo. (gms)	fat (gms)	chol. (mgs)	sod. (mgs)	fiber (gms)
"Hamburger," vegetarian, frozen *(cont.)*							
Italian (*Green Giant Harvest Burgers*)	140	17.0	8.0	4.5	0	370	5.0
Southwestern (*Green Giant Harvest Burgers*) . .	140	16.0	9.0	4.0	0	370	5.0
tofu (*Natural Touch Okara*)	110	11.0	4.0	5.0	0	360	3.0
frozen, ground (*Worthington*), ½ cup	80	11.0	3.0	2.5	0	270	3.0
refrigerated, 1 patty:							
(*Hempeh Burger*)	140	10.0	12.0	6.0	0	110	5.0
(*Yves Veggie Cuisine*)	83	11.0	9.0	0	0	380	4.0
mix, dry:							
(*Worthington Granburger*), 3 tbsp.	60	10.0	3.0	.5	0	410	2.0
chunks (*Loma Linda Vita-Burger*), ¼ cup	70	10.0	6.0	1.0	0	350	3.0
granules (*LaLoma Vita-Burger*), 3 tbsp.	70	10.0	6.0	1.0	0	350	3.0
mix, 1 patty*:							
(*Fantastic Nature's Burger* Original)	170	8.0	30.0	3.0	0	320	5.0
(*Fantastic Nature's Burger* BBQ) . . .	170	7.0	34.0	1.5	0	580	5.0
Hamburger entree mix, dry:							
beef pasta (*Hamburger Helper*), ⅔ cup	120	4.0	23.0	1.0	0	860	<1.0
beef taco (*Hamburger Helper*), ½ cup . .	160	5.0	30.0	2.0	0	870	1.0
w/cheese (*Hamburger Mate*), ⅕ pkg. . . .	160	6.0	30.0	2.5	5	1120	1.0

Food and Measure	cal.	prot. (gms)	carbo. (gms)	fat (gms)	chol. (mgs)	sod. (mgs)	fiber (gms)
cheeseburger maca-roni (*Hamburger Helper*), ⅓ cup . .	180	5.0	28.0	5.0	5	930	<1.0
chili (*Hamburger Mate*), ⅕ pkg. . . .	160	6.0	31.0	1.0	0	1410	1.0
fettuccine alfredo (*Hamburger Helper*), ½ cup	140	5.0	24.0	3.0	0	820	<1.0
Italian, zesty (*Hamburger Helper*), ½ cup	160	5.0	34.0	1.0	0	840	<1.0
lasagna (*Hamburger Helper*), ⅔ cup . .	140	4.0	30.0	1.0	0	910	0
w/noodles (*Hamburger Mate*), ⅕ pkg.	150	6.0	27.0	1.5	25	920	<1.0
w/pasta and tomato sauce (*Hamburger Mate*), ⅕ pkg. . . .	160	6.0	32.0	1.0	0	1100	1.0
pizza pasta (*Hamburger Helper*), ½ cup	150	4.0	30.0	1.5	0	620	1.0
stroganoff (*Hamburger Helper*), ⅔ cup	170	4.0	30.0	3.0	<5	880	<1.0
Hardee's, 1 serving:							
breakfast items:							
apple cinnamon rai-sin biscuit	200	2.0	30.0	8.0	0	350	n.a.
Big Country:							
bacon	820	33.0	62.0	49.0	535	1870	n.a.
sausage	1000	41.0	62.0	66.0	570	2310	n.a.
biscuit:							
bacon and egg	530	19.0	45.0	30.0	270	1280	n.a.
bacon, egg, cheese	610	24.0	45.0	37.0	280	1630	n.a.
country ham . .	430	15.0	45.0	22.0	25	1930	n.a.
ham	400	9.0	47.0	20.0	15	1340	n.a.
ham, egg, cheese	540	20.0	48.0	30.0	285	1660	n.a.

Food and Measure	cal.	prot. (gms)	carbo. (gms)	fat (gms)	chol. (mgs)	sod. (mgs)	fiber (gms)
Hardee's, breakfast items *(cont.)*							
Rise 'n' Shine	190	6.0	44.0	21.0	0	1000	n.a.
sausage	510	14.0	44.0	31.0	25	1360	n.a.
sausage and egg	600	22.0	45.0	37.0	285	1440	n.a.
ultimate omelet	530	18.0	45.0	30.0	175	1330	n.a.
Biscuit 'n' Gravy . .	510	10.0	55.0	28.0	15	1500	n.a.
Frisco sandwich,							
ham	500	24.0	46.0	25.0	290	1370	n.a.
hash rounds, regu-							
lar	230	3.0	24.0	14.0	0	560	n.a.
pancakes, 3	280	8.0	56.0	2.0	15	890	n.a.
burgers:							
bacon cheeseburger	530	29.0	29.0	34.0	85	970	n.a.
cheeseburger . . .	390	22.0	31.0	20	65	990	n.a.
cheeseburger, ¼ lb.	420	24.0	31.0	22.0	75	870	n.a.
cheeseburger, big							
double	630	40.0	32.0	38.0	130	1520	n.a.
Big Hardee	590	36.0	33.0	35.0	120	1150	n.a.
Big Hardee							
w/cheese	690	41.0	34.0	43.0	130	1600	n.a.
Frisco burger . . .	740	33.0	43.0	49.0	105	1370	n.a.
hamburger	340	20.0	30.0	16.0	60	770	n.a.
Hardee Jr.	400	21.0	32.0	21.0	60	850	n.a.
Hardee Jr. w/cheese	450	23.0	33.0	25.0	65	1070	n.a.
Mushroom 'n' Swiss	610	41.0	31.0	36.0	130	1420	n.a.
sandwiches:							
chicken, grilled . .	290	23.0	30.0	9.0	65	860	n.a.
chicken fillet	420	24.0	46.0	15.0	50	1190	n.a.
Fisherman's Fillet	450	23.0	45.0	20.0	60	1100	n.a.
Hot Ham 'n' Cheese	300	16.0	35.0	11.0	50	1390	n.a.
roast beef, big . . .	410	24.0	28.0	23.0	70	1140	n.a.
roast beef, regular	270	15.0	28.0	11.0	30	770	n.a.
chicken:							
breast	370	29.0	29.0	15.0	75	1190	n.a.
leg	170	13.0	15.0	7.0	45	570	n.a.
thigh	330	19.0	30.0	15.0	60	1000	n.a.
wing	200	10.0	23.0	8.0	30	740	n.a.
salads:							
garden	220	12.0	11.0	13.0	40	350	n.a.

Food and Measure	cal.	prot. (gms)	carbo. (gms)	fat (gms)	chol. (mgs)	sod. (mgs)	fiber (gms)
grilled chicken . . .	150	20.0	11.0	3.0	60	610	n.a.
side salad	25	1.0	4.0	<1.0	0	45	n.a.
dressings:							
French, fat free . .	70	0	17.0	0	0	580	0
ranch	290	1.0	6.0	29.0	25	510	0
Thousand Island . .	250	1.0	9.0	23.0	35	540	0
side dishes:							
baked beans, 5 oz.	170	8.0	32.0	1.0	0	600	n.a.
coleslaw, 4 oz. . . .	240	2.0	13.0	20.0	10	340	n.a.
fries, small	240	4.0	33.0	10.0	0	100	n.a.
fries, medium . . .	350	5.0	49.0	15.0	0	150	n.a.
fries, large	430	6.0	59.0	18.0	0	190	n.a.
gravy, 1.5 oz. . . .	20	<1.0	3.0	<1.0	0	260	n.a.
mashed potato,							
4 oz.	70	2.0	14.0	<1.0	0	330	n.a.
desserts/shakes:							
Big Cookie	280	4.0	41.0	12.0	15	150	n.a.
Cool Twist cone:							
chocolate	180	5.0	34.0	2.0	15	110	n.a.
vanilla	170	4.0	34.0	2.0	10	130	n.a.
vanilla/chocolate	180	4.0	34.0	2.0	10	120	n.a.
Cool Twist sundae:							
hot fudge	290	7.0	51.0	6.0	20	310	n.a.
strawberry . . .	210	5.0	43.0	2.0	10	140	n.a.
peach cobbler, 6 oz.	310	2.0	60.0	7.0	0	360	n.a.
shake:							
chocolate	370	13.0	67.0	5.0	30	270	0
peach	390	10.0	77.0	4.0	25	290	0
strawberry . . .	420	11.0	83.0	4.0	20	270	0
vanilla	350	12.0	65.0	5.0	20	300	0
Hash (see also specific hash listings), canned (Mary Kitchen Fiesta),							
1 cup	210	21.0	29.0	23.0	75	1060	4.0
Hazelnut, see "Filberts"							

Food and Measure	cal.	prot. (gms)	carbo. (gms)	fat (gms)	chol. (mgs)	sod. (mgs)	fiber (gms)
Hazelnut butter (*Roaster Fresh*), 1 oz.	188	4.0	5.0	19.0	0	1	0
Head cheese (*Oscar Mayer*), 1-oz. slice	50	5.0	0	4.0	25	360	0
Heart, braised or simmered, 4 oz.:							
beef	199	32.6	.5	6.4	219	71	0
chicken, broiler-fryer	210	30.0	.1	9.0	274	54	0
lamb	210	28.3	2.2	9.0	282	71	0
pork	168	26.8	.5	5.7	251	40	0
turkey	201	30.3	2.3	6.9	256	62	0
veal . . . . ´.	211	33.0	.1	7.7	200	66	0
Hearts of palm, see "Palm"							
Herbs, see specific listings							
Herbs, mixed (*Lawry's* Pinch of Herbs), ¼ tsp. . . .	0	0	0	0	0	80	0
Herring, fresh:							
Atlantic, meat only:							
raw, 4 oz.	180	20.4	0	10.3	68	102	0
baked, broiled, or microwaved, 4 oz.	230	26.1	0	13.1	87	130	0
kippered, 4 oz. . . .	246	27.9	0	14.0	93	1041	0
pickled, 4 oz. . . .	297	16.1	10.9	20.4	15	987	0
lake, see "Cisco"							
Pacific, meat only:							
raw, 4 oz.	224	18.6	0	15.8	87	84	0
baked, broiled, or microwaved, 4 oz.	284	23.8	0	20.2	112	108	0
Herring, canned, see "Sardine"							
Herring, in jars, drained, 2 oz., except as noted:							
(*Vita* Homestyle) . . .	130	9.0	5.0	8.0	40	600	0
(*Vita* Party Snacks)	120	9.0	10.0	5.0	30	480	0

Food and Measure	cal.	prot. (gms)	carbo. (gms)	fat (gms)	chol. (mgs)	sod. (mgs)	fiber (gms)
lunch, sliced (*Vita*)	130	9.0	5.0	8.0	40	600	0
in sour cream (*Vita*),							
¼ cup, 2¼ oz. . . .	120	7.0	8.0	7.0	35	600	0
roll mops (*Vita*),							
2½ oz., about 1 pc.	140	11.0	9.0	7.0	50	1250	0
Herring salad (*Vita*),							
¼ cup	110	4.0	15.0	4.0	20	600	0
Hickory nut, dried,							
shelled, 1 oz. . . .	187	3.6	5.2	18.3	0	tr.	1.8
Hoisin sauce:							
(*House of Tsang*),							
1 tsp.	15	0	3.0	0	0	105	0
(*Lee Kum Kee*),							
2 tbsp.	100	<1.0	25.0	0	0	1060	0
Hollandaise grilling							
sauce (*Knorr* Micro-							
wave), 2 tbsp. . . .	45	0	1.0	4.5	15	200	0
Hollandaise sauce							
mix:							
(*Durkee*), ¹⁄₁₀ pkg. . .	10	0	2.0	0	5	70	0
(*French's*), 2 tbsp. . .	10	0	2.0	0	5	75	0
(*Knorr*), ¹⁄₁₀ pkg. . . .	10	0	2.0	0	0	85	0
Homestyle gravy mix:							
(*Durkee*), ¼ cup* . .	15	.5	3.0	.5	0	240	0
(*French's*), ¼ cup*	10	0	3.0	.5	0	230	0
(*Pillsbury*), ¼ cup*	10	0	3.0	0	0	270	0
Hominy, canned:							
golden, ½ cup:							
(*Allens/Uncle Wil-*							
liam)	120	2.0	27.0	.5	0	340	4.0
(*Goya*)	120	2.0	27.0	0	0	340	4.0
(*Sun-Vista*)	70	2.0	19.0	0	0	540	3.0
(*Van Camp's*) . . .	80	1.0	17.0	1.0	0	540	1.0
Mexican (*Allens/Uncle*							
William), ½ cup . .	120	2.0	25.0	1.0	0	340	3.0
white, ½ cup:							
(*Allens/Uncle Wil-*							
liam)	100	2.0	22.0	.5	0	340	4.0
(*Goya*)	100	2.0	22.0	.5	0	340	4.0

Food and Measure	cal.	prot. (gms)	carbo. (gms)	fat (gms)	chol. (mgs)	sod. (mgs)	fiber (gms)
Hominy, white *(cont.)*							
(*Sun-Vista*)	65	2.0	18.0	.5	0	530	3.0
(*Van Camp's*) . . .	80	1.0	16.0	1.0	0	530	1.0
Hominy grits, dry, see "Corn grits"							
Honey (*Aunt Sue's/ Grandma's/Sue Bee*), 1 tbsp.	60	0	17.0	0	0	0	0
Honey bun, see "Bun, sweet"							
Honey butter (*Downey's*), .5 oz.	60	0	8.0	1.0	<5	10	0
Honey loaf (*Oscar Mayer*), 1-oz. slice	35	5.0	1.0	1.0	15	380	0
Honey mustard sauce, California style (*Rice Road*), 1 tbsp.	20	0	4.0	0	0	270	0
Honey roll sausage, beef, 1 oz.	52	5.3	.6	3.0	14	375	0
Honeycomb, strained (*Frieda's*), 1 oz. . .	86	.1	23.3	0	0	1	0
Honeydew:							
1/10 melon, 7" × 2" . .	46	.6	11.8	.1	0	13	.8
pulp, cubed, 1/2 cup	30	.4	7.8	.1	0	9	.5
Hors d'oeuvre kit, frozen, 1 filled sheet, except as noted:							
(*Pepperidge Farm*), 7 sheets	470	11.0	41.0	28.0	15	520	7.0
beef Stroganoff (*Pepperidge Farm*) . . .	420	13.0	27.0	29.0	40	500	5.0
chicken à la king (*Pepperidge Farm*)	400	11.0	28.0	26.0	35	590	5.0
shrimp Newburg (*Pepperidge Farm*)	340	8.0	31.0	20.0	60	670	4.0

Food and Measure	cal.	prot. (gms)	carbo. (gms)	fat (gms)	chol. (mgs)	sod. (mgs)	fiber (gms)
Horseradish, fresh:							
leafy tips, ½ cup:							
raw, chopped . . .	6	.9	.8	.1	0	1	.2
boiled, drained,							
chopped	13	1.1	2.3	.2	0	2	.4
pods, ½ cup:							
raw, sliced	19	1.1	4.3	.1	0	21	1.6
boiled, drained,							
sliced	21	1.2	4.8	.1	0	25	2.5
Horseradish, prepared, 1 tsp., except as noted:							
(*Boar's Head*)	0	0	0	0	0	30	0
(*Heluva* Good)	0	0	0	0	0	6	0
(*Kraft*)	0	0	0	0	0	50	0
cream style (*Kraft*)	0	0	0	0	0	50	0
red (w/beets):							
(*Gold's*)	0	0	0	0	0	30	0
(*Hebrew National*),							
½ cup	25	0	4.0	0	0	800	0
(*Rosoff*), 1 tbsp. . .	8	0	2.0	0	0	160	0
white (*Rosoff*),							
1 tbsp.	7	0	1.0	0	0	160	0
Horseradish sauce:							
(*Heinz*), 1 tsp.	25	0	1.0	2.5	0	35	0
(*Reese's*), 2 tbsp. . .	100	0	4.0	9.0	15	260	0
(*Sauceworks*), 2 tbsp.	20	0	<1.0	1.5	<5	35	0
Hot dog, see "Frankfurter"							
Hot dog sauce, see "Chili sauce"							
Hot fudge sauce, see "Chocolate topping"							
Hot sauce, see "Pepper sauce" and specific listings							
Hubbard squash:							
raw (*Frieda's*), 1 oz.	14	.5	3.3	.1	0	<1	n.a.
baked, cubed, ½ cup	51	2.5	11.0	.6	0	8	2.9

Food and Measure	cal.	prot. (gms)	carbo. (gms)	fat (gms)	chol. (mgs)	sod. (mgs)	fiber (gms)
Hubbard squash *(cont.)*							
boiled, drained,							
mashed, ½ cup . .	35	1.8	7.6	.4	0	6	3.4
Hummus *(Casbah)*,							
1 oz.	85	3.5	7.5	4.5	0	130	1.0
Hummus mix:							
(Casbah), 1 oz. . . .	120	5.0	14.0	5.0	0	180	1.0
dip *(Fantastic Foods)*,							
2 tbsp.*	60	3.0	9.0	2.0	0	220	2.0
Hushpuppies, frozen							
(Stilwell), 3 pcs. . .	140	2.0	19.0	6.0	0	310	2.0
Hyacinth beans,							
½ cup:							
fresh, boiled, drained	22	1.3	4.1	.1	0	1	n.a.
dried, boiled	114	7.9	20.1	.6	0	7	n.a.

I

Food and Measure	cal.	prot. (gms)	carbo. (gms)	fat (gms)	chol. (mgs)	sod. (mgs)	fiber (gms)
Ice, Italian (*Luigi's*), 6 fl. oz.:							
cherry	120	<1.0	28.0	0	0	10	0
chocolate fudge . . .	150	<1.0	38.0	0	0	10	0
grape	110	0	26.0	0	0	10	0
lemon	110	<1.0	25.0	0	0	10	0
strawberry	110	<1.0	26.0	0	0	10	0
Ice bar, see "Fruit bar, frozen"							
Ice cream, ½ cup:							
almond praline (*Edys Grand*)	160	3.0	20.0	8.0	25	85	0
amaretto (*Häagen-Dazs DiSaronno*) . .	260	4.0	26.0	15.0	95	80	0
banana split (*Edy's Grand*)	170	3.0	19.0	10.0	20	50	0
(*Ben & Jerry's Chubby Hubby*) . .	350	8.0	31.0	23.0	75	160	2.0
(*Ben & Jerry's Chunky Monkey*) . .	280	4.0	29.0	18.0	70	50	1.0
(*Ben & Jerry's Rainforest Crunch*)	300	5.0	24.0	23.0	85	140	0
(*Ben & Jerry's Wavy Gravy*)	330	6.0	29.0	24.0	80	95	2.0
brownie:							
batter (*Edy's Grand*)	150	3.0	18.0	8.0	25	55	0
fudge (*Healthy Choice*)	120	3.0	22.0	2.0	5	55	<2.0
fudge, double (*Edy's Grand*)	160	2.0	19.0	9.0	25	40	0

Food and Measure	cal.	prot. (gms)	carbo. (gms)	fat (gms)	chol. (mgs)	sod. (mgs)	fiber (gms)
Ice cream, brownie *(cont.)*							
'n fudge (*Edy's* Grand Light) . . .	110	3.0	18.0	4.0	20	45	0
Brownies à la Mode (*Häagen-Dazs Ex-träas*)	280	5.0	25.0	18.0	100	130	0
butter pecan:							
(*Ben & Jerry's*) . .	310	5.0	20.0	25.0	85	125	1.0
(*Edy's Grand*) . . .	160	3.0	16.0	9.0	25	50	0
(*Edy's Grand* Light)	120	3.0	16.0	5.0	20	45	0
(*Häagen-Dazs*) . . .	320	5.0	20.0	24.0	105	140	<1.0
crunch (*Healthy* Choice)	120	3.0	22.0	2.0	<5	60	1.0
cappuccino chocolate chunk (*Healthy* Choice)	120	3.0	60.0	2.0	10	60	1.0
Cappuccino Commo-tion (*Häagen-Dazs* Exträas)	310	5.0	25.0	21.0	100	105	1.0
Caramel Cone Explo-sion (*Häagen-Dazs* Exträas)	310	5.0	27.0	20.0	95	130	<1.0
caramel cream, dreamy (*Edy's* Grand Light)	110	3.0	16.0	4.0	25	50	0
caramel praline crunch (*Edy's* Fat Free)	110	3.0	24.0	0	0	85	0
cheesecake chunk (*Edy's Grand* Light)	120	3.0	16.0	5.0	25	35	0
cherry chocolate chip:							
(*Ben & Jerry's* Cherry Garcia) . .	240	3.0	25.0	16.0	75	55	0
(*Edy's Grand*) . . .	150	3.0	18.0	8.0	25	35	0
cherry vanilla:							
black (*Edy's Grand* No Sugar)	100	3.0	14.0	4.0	15	45	0
black, swirl (*Edy's* Fat Free)	100	4.0	21.0	0	0	70	0

Food and Measure	cal.	prot. (gms)	carbo. (gms)	fat (gms)	chol. (mgs)	sod. (mgs)	fiber (gms)
chocolate:							
(*Edy's Grand*) . . .	140	3.0	15.0	9.0	30	30	0
(*Edy's Grand* No Sugar)	100	3.0	13.0	4.0	15	45	0
(*Häagen-Dazs*) . . .	270	5.0	22.0	18.0	115	75	1.0
triple (*Edy's Grand* No Sugar)	100	3.0	15.0	5.0	10	55	0
triple (*Weight Watchers Tor-nado*)	150	4.0	26.0	3.5	5	80	1.0
chocolate almond fudge (*Edy's Grand* Light)	120	4.0	15.0	5.0	25	35	0
chocolate chip:							
(*Edy's Grand* Chips!)	160	3.0	17.0	8.0	25	35	0
(*Edy's Grand* No Sugar)	100	3.0	14.0	5.0	15	50	0
cookie dough (*Ben & Jerry's*)	270	3.0	30.0	15.0	75	85	0
chocolate (*Edy's Grand*)	160	2.0	17.0	10.0	30	25	0
chocolate (*Häagen-Dazs*)	300	5.0	26.0	20.0	100	70	2.0
chunk (*Healthy Choice*)	110	3.0	21.0	2.0	<5	60	1.0
mint (*Healthy Choice*)	120	3.0	21.0	2.0	<5	50	<1.0
mint (*Edy's Grand* Chips!)	160	3.0	17.0	9.0	25	35	0
chocolate cookie, mint (*Ben & Jerry's*) . .	260	4.0	27.0	17.0	80	120	1.0
chocolate fudge:							
(*Edy's* Fat Free) . .	100	4.0	24.0	0	0	75	0
(*Edy's* No Fat/Sugar)	80	4.0	21.0	0	0	55	0
chunk (*Edy's* Low Fat)	110	3.0	22.0	2.0	5	50	0
mousse (*Edy's Grand* Light) . . .	110	3.0	17.0	4.0	25	40	0

Food and Measure	cal.	prot. (gms)	carbo. (gms)	fat (gms)	chol. (mgs)	sod. (mgs)	fiber (gms)
Ice cream, chocolate fudge *(cont.)*							
mousse (*Healthy* Choice)	120	3.0	21.0	2.0	<5	50	1.0
sundae (*Edy's* Grand)	170	3.0	18.0	10.0	20	55	0
coffee:							
(*Ben & Jerry's Cafe* Ole)	230	4.0	22.0	16.0	90	55	0
(*Edy's Grand*) . . .	140	3.0	15.0	8.0	25	35	0
(*Häagen-Dazs*) . . .	270	5.0	21.0	18.0	120	85	0
coffee fudge:							
(*Edy's* Fat Free) . .	100	3.0	23.0	0	0	75	0
(*Edy's* No Fat/Sugar)	80	3.0	20.0	0	0	55	0
almond (*Ben &* Jerry's)	290	6.0	24.0	20.0	75	85	2.0
coffee toffee crunch (*Ben & Jerry's*) . .	280	4.0	28.0	19.0	80	120	0
cookie chunk (*Edy's* Fat Free)	110	4.0	23.0	0	0	105	0
cookies and cream:							
(*Edy's Grand*) . . .	150	3.0	18.0	8.0	25	75	0
(*Edy's Grand* Light)	110	3.0	15.0	4.0	25	55	0
(*Edy's* Low Fat) . .	110	3.0	21.0	2.0	5	55	0
(*Häagen-Dazs*) . . .	270	5.0	23.0	17.0	110	115	0
(*Healthy Choice*) . .	120	3.0	21.0	2.0	<5	90	<1.0
mint (*Edy's Grand* Light)	110	3.0	15.0	4.0	25	55	0
cookie dough:							
(*Edy's Grand*) . . .	170	3.0	20.0	9.0	25	65	0
(*Edy's Grand* Light)	120	3.0	18.0	5.0	20	60	0
(*Weight Watchers* Craze)	140	3.0	24.0	3.5	5	85	1.0
Cookie Dough Dynamo (*Häagen-Dazs Exträas*) . . .	300	4.0	29.0	19.0	95	140	0
espresso chip:							
(*Edy's Grand*) . . .	150	3.0	16.0	8.0	25	30	0
(*Edy's* Low Fat) . .	100	3.0	20.0	2.0	5	40	0

Food and Measure	cal.	prot. (gms)	carbo. (gms)	fat (gms)	chol. (mgs)	sod. (mgs)	fiber (gms)
fudge (*Edy's Grand Light*)	110	3.0	18.0	4.0	15	40	0
French silk (*Edy's Grand* Light)	120	3.0	18.0	5.0	20	40	0
fudge chunk (*Ben & Jerry's* New York)	290	4.0	28.0	20.0	45	45	2.0
ice cream sandwich (*Edy's Grand*) . . .	150	3.0	13.0	8.0	25	75	0
Irish cream (*Häagen-Dazs Baileys*) . . .	280	4.0	23.0	18.0	110	100	0
macadamia brittle (*Häagen-Dazs*) . . .	300	4.0	25.0	20.0	110	120	0
marble fudge:							
(*Edy's* Fat Free) . .	100	3.0	23.0	0	0	75	0
(*Edy's Grand* No Sugar)	100	3.0	15.0	4.0	15	55	0
mint fudge:							
(*Edy's* Fat Free) . .	100	3.0	23.0	0	0	75	0
(*Edy's Grand* No Sugar)	100	3.0	15.0	4.0	15	55	0
mocha fudge:							
(*Ben & Jerry's*) . .	270	5.0	30.0	18.0	85	65	1.0
(*Edy's Grand* No Sugar)	100	3.0	15.0	4.0	15	55	0
almond (*Edy's Grand* Light) . . .	110	3.0	16.0	4.0	15	35	0
Peanut Butter Burst (*Häagen-Dazs Ex-träas*)	330	6.0	26.0	22.0	95	150	1.0
peanut butter cup:							
(*Ben & Jerry's*) . .	370	8.0	30.0	26.0	75	140	2.0
(*Edy's Grand* Light)	120	3.0	17.0	5.0	15	45	0
praline (*Weight Watchers Positively Crunch*)	140	3.0	25.0	3.0	5	105	0
praline caramel:							
(*Edy's Grand* Light)	120	3.0	18.0	4.0	20	60	0
(*Healthy Choice*) . .	120	3.0	25.0	2.0	<5	70	<1.0

Food and Measure	cal.	prot. (gms)	carbo. (gms)	fat (gms)	chol. (mgs)	sod. (mgs)	fiber (gms)
Ice cream *(cont.)*							
raspberry vanilla swirl							
(*Edy's* No Fat/Sugar)	70	4.0	18.0	0	0	45	0
rocky road:							
(*Edy's Grand*) . . .	170	3.0	17.0	10.0	25	30	0
(*Edy's Grand* Light)	120	3.0	16.0	4.0	20	35	0
(*Edy's* Low Fat) . .	110	3.0	21.0	2.0	5	35	0
(*Healthy Choice*) . .	140	3.0	28.0	2.0	<5	60	2.0
(*Weight Watchers*							
Reckless)	140	4.0	23.0	3.0	5	75	1.0
rum raisin (*Häagen-*							
Dazs)	270	4.0	22.0	17.0	110	75	0
strawberry:							
(*Edy's Grand*) . . .	130	2.0	17.0	6.0	20	25	0
(*Edy's Grand* No							
Sugar)	90	3.0	13.0	4.0	15	45	0
(*Häagen-Dazs*) . . .	250	4.0	23.0	16.0	95	80	<1.0
strawberry cheesecake							
chunk (*Edy's Grand*)	150	3.0	18.0	8.0	30	30	0
Strawberry Cheese-							
cake Craze (*Häagen-*							
Dazs Exträas) . . .	290	4.0	28.0	18.0	100	160	<1.0
strawberry shortcake							
(*Edy's* Fat Free) . .	100	3.0	22.0	0	0	85	0
toffee n' caramel							
(*Edy's Heath* Low							
Fat)	120	2.0	23.0	2.0	5	40	0
toffee crunch, English							
(*Ben & Jerry's*) . .	280	3.0	28.0	19.0	80	115	0
Triple Brownie Over-							
load (*Häagen-Dazs*							
Exträas)	300	5.0	26.0	20.0	90	100	1.0
vanilla:							
(*Ben & Jerry's*) . .	230	4.0	21.0	17.0	95	55	0
(*Edy's* Fat Free) . .	90	4.0	20.0	0	0	70	0
(*Edy's* No Fat/Sugar)	80	4.0	18.0	0	0	45	0
(*Edy's Grand*) . . .	150	2.0	14.0	10.0	35	30	0
(*Edy's Grand* Light)	100	3.0	14.0	4.0	25	35	0

Food and Measure	cal.	prot. (gms)	carbo. (gms)	fat (gms)	chol. (mgs)	sod. (mgs)	fiber (gms)
(*Edy's Grand* No Sugar)	100	3.0	13.0	4.0	15	50	0
(*Edy's* Low Fat) . .	100	3.0	19.0	2.0	10	40	0
(*Häagen-Dazs*) . . .	270	5.0	21.0	18.0	120	85	0
(*Healthy Choice*) . .	100	3.0	18.0	2.0	5	50	1.0
(*Weight Watchers* Oh So Very) . . .	120	4.0	20.0	2.5	5	65	1.0
French (*Edy's* Grand)	160	2.0	16.0	10.0	55	30	0
bean (*Edy's Grand*)	150	2.0	15.0	9.0	30	30	0
vanilla caramel:							
(*Edy's* No Fat/Sugar)	80	3.0	20.0	0	0	55	0
(*Edy's Grand* No Sugar)	100	3.0	15.0	4.0	15	55	0
fudge swirl (*Ben & Jerry's*)	280	4.0	33.0	17.0	95	75	1.0
vanilla chocolate strawberry (*Edy's* Grand)	130	3.0	15.0	7.0	25	30	0
vanilla chocolate swirl (*Edy's* No Fat/Sugar)	80	4.0	19.0	0	0	45	0
vanilla fudge (*Häagen-Dazs*)	280	5.0	25.0	18.0	105	105	0
vanilla Swiss almond (*Häagen-Dazs*) . . .	310	6.0	23.0	21.0	105	80	1.0
"Ice cream," imitation, (see also "Ice cream, tofu" and "Ice cream and frozen desserts"), ½ cup, except as noted:							
bar, 1 bar:							
chocolate (*Rice Dream*)	270	2.0	32.0	15.0	0	95	2.0
nutty, chocolate or vanilla (*Rice Dream*)	260	4.0	23.0	18.0	0	55	2.0

Food and Measure	cal.	prot. (gms)	carbo. (gms)	fat (gms)	chol. (mgs)	sod. (mgs)	fiber (gms)
"Ice cream," imitation, bar *(cont.)*							
strawberry *(Rice Dream)*	250	1.0	31.0	13.0	0	80	1.0
cappuccino *(Rice Dream)*	130	1.0	19.0	5.0	0	70	1.0
carob:							
(Rice Dream) . . .	130	1.0	20.0	5.0	0	70	1.0
almond *(Rice Dream)*	140	1.0	20.0	6.0	0	85	2.0
chip *(Rice Dream)*	130	1.0	20.0	6.0	0	70	1.0
cocoa marble fudge *(Rice Dream)* . . .	130	1.0	21.0	6.0	0	75	1.0
cookies 'n dream *(Rice Dream)* . . .	140	1.0	21.0	6.0	0	70	1.0
lemon *(Rice Dream)*	130	1.0	19.0	5.0	0	70	1.0
mint carob chip *(Rice Dream)*	130	1.0	20.0	6.0	0	70	1.0
Neapolitan *(Rice Dream)*	120	1.0	19.0	5.0	0	70	1.0
peanut butter fudge *(Rice Dream)* . . .	130	2.0	21.0	6.0	0	75	1.0
pie, cookie, 1 pie:							
chocolate or mint *(Rice Dream)* . .	320	3.0	39.0	18.0	0	80	2.0
mocha *(Rice Dream)*	320	3.0	40.0	17.0	0	80	1.0
vanilla *(Rice Dream)*	290	3.0	37.0	15.0	0	70	2.0
strawberry *(Rice Dream)*	110	1.0	18.0	5.0	0	65	1.0
vanilla or vanilla fudge *(Rice Dream)* . . .	130	1.0	19.0	5.0	0	70	1.0
vanilla Swiss almond *(Rice Dream)* . . .	130	1.0	20.0	6.0	0	70	1.0
wildberry *(Rice Dream)*	110	0	18.0	5.0	0	65	1.0

Food and Measure	cal.	prot. (gms)	carbo. (gms)	fat (gms)	chol. (mgs)	sod. (mgs)	fiber (gms)
"Ice cream," tofu							
(see also "Sorbet"),							
½ cup, except as							
noted:							
all fruit flavors (*Tofutti*							
Fruitti)	100	2.0	20.0	0	0	90	0
better pecan (*Tofutti*)	220	1.0	22.0	13.0	0	200	0
chocolate:							
(*Tofutti*)	180	3.0	18.0	11.0	0	180	0
cake (*Tofutti*) . . .	210	3.0	26.0	11.0	0	100	1.0
fudge (*Tofutti* Low							
Fat)	120	2.0	25.0	2.0	0	98	0
coffee marshmallow							
(*Tofutti* Low Fat) . .	100	1.0	24.0	1.0	0	77	0
passion island fruit							
(*Tofutti* Low Fat) . .	100	1.0	21.0	1.0	0	100	0
peach mango (*Tofutti*							
Low Fat)	100	1.0	23.0	1.0	0	102	0
sandwich, 1 pc.:							
chocolate (*Tofutti*							
Cuties)	130	2.0	16.0	5.0	0	110	0
vanilla or wildberry							
(*Tofutti Cuties*)	121	2.0	17.0	5.0	0	121	0
soft serve, all flavors:							
(*Tofutti*)	190	2.0	20.0	4.0	0	95	0
(*Tofutti* Lite)	90	2.0	20.0	1.0	0	80	0
sticks, 1 bar:							
chocolate (*Tofutti*							
Fruitti)	120	1.0	15.0	5.0	0	20	0
fudge (*Tofutti*							
Teddy)	70	1.0	19.0	1.0	0	53	0
fudge (*Tofutti*							
Treats)	30	1.0	6.0	0	0	86	0
strawberry banana							
(*Tofutti* Low Fat) . .	100	1.0	23.0	1.0	0	92	0
vanilla:							
(*Tofutti*)	190	2.0	20.0	11.0	0	210	0
(*Tofutti Cutie* Slice),							
1 slice	140	1.0	15.0	8.0	0	150	0

Food and Measure	cal.	prot. (gms)	carbo. (gms)	fat (gms)	chol. (mgs)	sod. (mgs)	fiber (gms)
"Ice cream," tofu, vanilla *(cont.)*							
almond bark							
(*Tofutti*)	210	3.0	21.0	13.0	0	130	0
chocolate covered							
(*Tofutti Cutie*),							
1 pie	250	1.0	18.0	19.0	0	130	0
fudge (*Tofutti*) . . .	190	2.0	25.0	9.0	0	130	0
fudge (*Tofutti* Low							
Fat)	120	2.0	24.0	2.0	0	90	0
wildberry:							
(*Tofutti*)	190	2.0	24.0	9.0	0	190	0
(*Tofutti* Slice),							
1 slice	80	1.0	18.0	2.0	0	25	0
chocolate covered							
(*Tofutti* Slice),							
1 slice	180	1.0	18.0	10.0	0	75	0
Ice cream bar, 1 bar,							
except as noted:							
almond:							
(*DoveBar*)	280	5.0	23.0	19.0	30	110	1.0
(*DoveBar* Single)	350	6.0	29.0	24.0	40	140	1.0
praline (*Edy's*							
Grand)	270	4.0	27.0	17.0	25	75	0
(*Butterfinger*)	190	2.0	16.0	13.0	15	35	0
(*Klondike* Original) . .	290	3.0	24.0	20.0	15	65	0
Caramel Cone Explo-							
sion:							
(*Häagen-Dazs Ex-*							
träas)	330	4.0	30.0	22.0	60	150	<1.0
(*Häagen-Dazs Ex-*							
träas Single) . . .	350	4.0	32.0	23.0	65	160	<1.0
caramel creme							
w/toffee chips							
(*DoveBar*)	280	3.0	31.0	16.0	30	100	0
caramel nut (*Weight*							
Watchers)	130	2.0	14.0	8.0	5	25	0
chocolate:							
(*Nestlé Crunch*) . .	200	2.0	17.0	14.0	15	40	0
(*3 Musketeers*) . .	140	2.0	16.0	8.0	10	30	0

Food and Measure	cal.	prot. (gms)	carbo. (gms)	fat (gms)	chol. (mgs)	sod. (mgs)	fiber (gms)
(*3 Musketeers* Single)	190	2.0	22.0	11.0	20	40	0
(*Weight Watchers* Treat)	100	3.0	21.0	1.0	10	150	1.0
dark (*Häagen-Dazs*)	320	4.0	27.0	22.0	70	70	3.0
dark (*Häagen-Dazs* Single)	400	5.0	33.0	27.0	85	90	4.0
double (*Dove* Bite Size), 5 bars . . .	360	4.0	37.0	23.0	30	40	1.0
chocolate cookie dough (*Ben & Jerry's*)	420	5.0	44.0	25.0	55	145	<1.0
chocolate dip (*Weight Watchers*)	100	2.0	11.0	6.0	5	15	0
cookies 'n cream (*Edy's Grand*) . . .	260	4.0	27.0	17.0	25	90	0
Cookie Dough Dynamo (*Häagen-Dazs Exträas*) . . .	380	4.0	34.0	25.0	65	125	1.0
coffee w/almond crunch: (*Häagen-Dazs*) . . .	290	4.0	22.0	21.0	80	70	<1.0
(*Häagen-Dazs* Single)	360	5.0	27.0	26.0	100	85	1.0
eggnog, dark chocolate (*Dove* Bite Size), 5 bars	350	3.0	35.0	22.0	35	35	0
fudge chunk (*Ben & Jerry's* New York)	390	6.0	27.0	31.0	30	55	4.0
Iced Cappuccino: (*Häagen-Dazs Exträas*)	290	4.0	21.0	21.0	70	60	<1.0
(*Häagen-Dazs Exträas* Single) . . .	330	5.0	24.0	24.0	80	70	<1.0
(*Milky Way*)	140	2.0	19.0	7.0	5	50	0
mocha cashew crunch (*DoveBar*)	260	3.0	25.0	17.0	30	55	0
(*Nestlé Crunch* Crunch King) . . .	270	3.0	21.0	19.0	20	45	0

Food and Measure	cal.	prot. (gms)	carbo. (gms)	fat (gms)	chol. (mgs)	sod. (mgs)	fiber (gms)
Ice cream bar *(cont.)*							
(*Nestlé Crunch* Re-duced Fat)	130	3.0	14.0	7.0	5	40	0
rocky road (*Edy's Grand*)	270	4.0	23.0	19.0	25	40	0
toffee crunch, English (*Ben & Jerry's*) . .	330	4.0	33.0	22.0	65	105	<1.0
mousse, 2 bars:							
chocolate (*Weight Watchers*)	70	4.0	18.0	1.0	5	80	4.0
berries 'n cream (*Weight Watchers*)	70	3.0	17.0	1.5	0	75	1.0
orange vanilla (*Weight Watchers Treat*), 2 bars	70	4.0	17.0	1.0	5	80	3.0
peppermint w/dark chocolate (*DoveBar*)	290	3.0	31.0	17.0	30	40	0
peppermint w/dark chocolate (*Dove* Bite Size), 5 bars	360	3.0	39.0	22.0	30	35	0
pralines 'n creme, crispy (*Weight Watchers*)	130	2.0	15.0	7.0	5	40	0
(*Snickers*)	190	3.0	18.0	12.0	15	50	0
(*Snickers* Snack), 4 bars	390	7.0	38.0	25.0	25	105	7.0
toffee crunch (*Weight Watchers*)	120	2.0	12.0	7.0	5	25	0
Triple Brownie Over-load:							
(*Häagen-Dazs Ex-träas*)	320	4.0	23.0	23.0	80	95	1.0
(*Häagen-Dazs Ex-träas Single*) . . .	380	5.0	28.0	27.0	95	110	1.0
vanilla:							
(*Ben & Jerry's*) . .	330	4.0	29.0	23.0	75	55	<1.0
(*Dove* Bite Size), 5 bars	360	4.0	34.0	24.0	40	60	0
(*Nestlé Crunch*) . .	200	2.0	16.0	14.0	15	40	0

Food and Measure	cal.	prot. (gms)	carbo. (gms)	fat (gms)	chol. (mgs)	sod. (mgs)	fiber (gms)
(3 Musketeers) . .	190	2.0	21.0	10.0	20	40	0
brownie (Ben & Jerry's)	330	4.0	43.0	17.0	60	170	2.0
French (Dove Bite Size), 5 bars . . .	370	4.0	37.0	23.0	60	45	0
white coated (DoveBar)	270	3.0	26.0	17.0	30	50	0
vanilla, w/almonds:							
(Edy's Grand) . . .	270	5.0	23.0	20.0	30	45	0
(Häagen-Dazs) . . .	300	5.0	21.0	22.0	70	65	1.0
(Häagen-Dazs Single)	370	6.0	26.0	27.0	90	80	1.0
vanilla, dark chocolate:							
(DoveBar)	260	3.0	27.0	17.0	25	30	1.0
(DoveBar Single)	330	4.0	34.0	21.0	30	40	1.0
(Häagen-Dazs) . . .	320	4.0	27.0	22.0	70	50	4.0
(Häagen-Dazs Single)	400	5.0	33.0	27.0	85	65	4.0
vanilla, milk chocolate:							
(DoveBar)	260	3.0	25.0	17.0	30	45	0
(DoveBar Single)	330	4.0	31.0	21.0	40	55	0
(Häagen-Dazs) . . .	280	4.0	20.0	20.0	75	65	0
(Häagen-Dazs Single)	330	5.0	24.0	24.0	90	75	<1.0
(Weight Watchers Arctic D'Lites) . . .	130	3.0	14.0	7.0	5	20	0
Ice cream cone or cup, plain, 1 pc.:							
cone:							
(Oreo)	50	1.0	10.0	1.0	0	110	<1.0
cinnamon (Teddy Grahams)	60	1.0	13.0	.5	0	55	<1.0
sugar (Comet) . . .	50	<1.0	11.0	0	0	40	<1.0
waffle (Comet) . .	70	1.0	14.0	.5	0	30	1.0
cup (Comet)	20	0	40	0	0	20	0

Food and Measure	cal.	prot. (gms)	carbo. (gms)	fat (gms)	chol. (mgs)	sod. (mgs)	fiber (gms)
Ice cream cone, filled, 1 cone:							
caramel almond crunch (*Edy's Grand*)	350	6.0	40.0	20.0	30	110	0
chocolate (*Drumstick*)	320	6.0	36.0	17.0	25	90	2.0
chocolate dipped (*Drumstick*)	320	5.0	40.0	16.0	25	90	1.0
chocolate fudge, double (*Edy's Grand*)	390	7.0	30.0	27.0	20	130	0
cookies 'n cream (*Edy's Grand*) . . .	340	5.0	29.0	20.0	30	110	0
vanilla:							
(*Drumstick*)	340	6.0	35.0	19.0	20	90	2.0
caramel (*Drumstick*)	360	6.0	38.0	20.0	25	100	2.0
fudge (*Drumstick*)	360	5.0	39.0	20.0	20	100	2.0
fudge sundae (*Edy's Grand*)	340	5.0	41.0	19.0	30	80	0
Ice cream cup, filled:							
chocolate:							
(*Carnation*), 3 fl. oz.	140	2.0	16.0	8.0	25	40	0
malt (*Carnation*), 12 fl. oz.	270	7.0	48.0	6.0	20	130	1.0
sundae (*Carnation*), 5 fl. oz.	210	2.0	30.0	9.0	30	55	1.0
vanilla:							
(*Carnation*), 3 fl. oz.	100	1.0	11.0	6.0	20	30	0
(*Carnation*), 5 fl. oz.	170	2.0	19.0	10.0	35	50	0
strawberry:							
(*Carnation*), 3 fl. oz.	100	2.0	29.0	8.0	30	55	0
sundae (*Carnation*), 5 fl. oz.	200	2.0	29.0	8.0	30	55	0
Ice cream and frozen desserts, ½ cup, except as noted:							
bananas Foster (*Healthy Choice*) . .	110	3.0	21.0	1.5	5	60	1.0

Food and Measure	cal.	prot. (gms)	carbo. (gms)	fat (gms)	chol. (mgs)	sod. (mgs)	fiber (gms)
Black Forest (*Healthy Choice*)	120	3.0	23.0	2.0	5	50	1.0
brownie, 1 pc.:							
à la mode (*Weight Watchers*)	190	5.0	34.0	4.0	5	170	2.0
chocolate frosted (*Weight Watchers*)	100	2.0	22.0	2.5	0	135	3.0
double fudge parfait (*Weight Watchers*)	190	6.0	39.0	2.5	5	170	2.0
fudge, a la mode (*Healthy Choice*)	120	3.0	22.0	2.0	5	55	<2.0
peanut butter fudge (*Weight Watchers*)	110	2.0	21.0	2.5	0	140	3.0
cappuccino mocha fudge (*Healthy Choice*)	120	3.0	23.0	2.0	<5	50	1.0
caramel fudge à la mode (*Weight Watchers*), 2.96 oz.	160	4.0	29.0	3.0	5	180	0
cheesecake, 1 pc.:							
brownie (*Weight Watchers*)	200	9.0	33.0	6.0	5	220	4.0
chocolate, triple (*Weight Watchers*)	200	7.0	32.0	5.0	10	200	1.0
French (*Weight Watchers*)	180	7.0	28.0	5.0	15	230	2.0
New York (*Weight Watchers*)	150	6.0	21.0	5.0	10	140	0
cherry chocolate chunk (*Healthy Choice*)	110	3.0	19.0	2.0	<5	55	<1.0
chocolate:							
caramel mousse (*Weight Watchers*), 1 pc.	200	5.0	34.0	4.0	5	120	2.0
chip cookie dough sundae (*Weight Watchers*), 1 pc.	180	3.0	33.0	4.0	5	115	2.0

Food and Measure	cal.	prot. (gms)	carbo. (gms)	fat (gms)	chol. (mgs)	sod. (mgs)	fiber (gms)
Ice cream and frozen desserts, chocolate *(cont.)*							
eclair (*Weight Watchers*), 1 pc.	150	2.0	25.0	4.0	30	160	2.0
eclair, triple (*Weight Watchers*), 1 pc.	160	3.0	25.0	5.0	30	190	1.0
malt (*Milky Way*), 1 cup	220	7.0	44.0	3.0	10	135	2.0
mocha pie (*Weight Watchers*), 1 pc.	170	6.0	31.0	4.0	5	125	2.0
mousse (*Weight Watchers*), 1 pc.	190	6.0	31.0	5.0	5	150	3.0
raspberry royale (*Weight Watchers*), 1 pc.	190	5.0	39.0	3.0	15	190	2.0
fudge cake, double (*Weight Watchers*), 1 pc.	190	4.0	36.0	4.5	0	200	2.0
loaf, ⅕ of 12-oz. pkg.:							
cappuccino (*Viennetta*)	190	3.0	18.0	12.0	25	35	0
chocolate, mint, or vanilla (*Viennetta*)	190	3.0	18.0	12.0	25	40	0
mud pie, Mississippi (*Weight Watchers*), 1 pc.	160	4.0	24.0	5.0	5	120	0
nuggets, w/chocolate:							
(*Nestlé Crunch*), 8 pcs.	310	4.0	25.0	21.0	20	60	0
dark (*Bon-Bons*), 5 pcs.	190	2.0	16.0	13.0	15	35	0
dark (*Bon-Bons*), 8 pcs.	310	3.0	26.0	21.0	25	55	0
milk (*Bon-Bons*), 5 pcs.	200	2.0	17.0	14.0	10	35	0
milk (*Bon-Bons*), 8 pcs.	330	3.0	27.0	23.0	20	60	0
praline:							
caramel cluster (*Healthy Choice*)	130	3.0	25.0	2.0	<5	70	<1.0

Food and Measure	cal.	prot. (gms)	carbo. (gms)	fat (gms)	chol. (mgs)	sod. (mgs)	fiber (gms)
pecan mousse (*Weight Watchers*), 2.71 oz. . .	170	4.0	31.0	3.5	0	140	0
toffee crunch parfait (*Weight Watchers*), 5.1 fl. oz.	190	5.0	40.0	3.0	5	140	2.0
strawberry parfait royale (*Weight Watchers*), 5.24 fl. oz. . .	180	5.0	35.0	2.0	10	100	0
turtle fudge cake (*Healthy Choice*) . .	130	3.0	25.0	2.0	<5	60	2.0
Ice cream sandwich, 1 pc.:							
chocolate chip cookie (*Chipwich* Jr.) . . .	240	3.0	35.0	10.0	20	135	<1.0
cookies and cream (*Cool Creations*) . .	240	2.0	34.0	11.0	15	250	1.0
(*Klondike* Big Bear)	200	3.0	31.0	7.0	15	130	<1.0
(*Klondike* Krispy) . .	300	3.0	28.0	20.0	25	85	0
mini (*Cool Creations*)	110	1.0	16.0	5.0	10	70	0
Ice cream and sorbet, see "Sorbet"							
Icing, see "Frosting"							
Italian beans, in sauce, (*Green Giant/ Joan of Arc*), ½ cup	130	5.0	24.0	1.0	0	480	5.0
Italian cut beans, see "Green beans"							
Italian seasoning, 1 tsp.	3	.1	.6	.1	0	<1	.2

J

Food and Measure	cal.	prot. (gms)	carbo. (gms)	fat (gms)	chol. (mgs)	sod. (mgs)	fiber (gms)
Jack-in-the-Box,							
1 serving:							
breakfast:							
Breakfast Jack . . .	300	18.0	30.0	12.0	185	890	0
Country Crock							
Spread, .2 oz. . .	25	0	0	3.0	0	40	0
croissant, sausage	670	21.0	39.0	48.0	250	940	2.0
croissant, supreme	570	21.0	39.0	36.0	245	1240	2.0
hash browns	160	1.0	14.0	11.0	0	310	1.0
jelly, grape, .5 oz.	40	0	9.0	0	0	5	0
pancake platter . .	400	13.0	59.0	12.0	30	980	3.0
pancake syrup,							
1½ oz.	120	0	30.0	0	0	5	0
sandwich, breakfast:							
sourdough . . .	380	21.0	31.0	20.0	235	1120	0
ultimate	620	36.0	39.0	35.0	455	1800	<1
scrambled egg							
pocket	430	29.0	31.0	21.0	355	1060	0
sandwiches:							
beef, Monterey roast	540	30.0	40.0	30.0	75	1270	3.0
cheeseburger:							
regular	320	16.0	32.0	15.0	35	670	0
double	450	24.0	35.0	24.0	75	970	0
ultimate	1030	50.0	30.0	79.0	205	1200	0
bacon bacon . .	710	35.0	41.0	45.0	115	1280	0
Colossus	1100	54.0	30.0	84.0	220	1510	0
The Outlaw							
Burger	720	31.0	56.0	40.0	95	1510	0
chicken	400	20.0	38.0	18.0	45	1290	0
chicken, Caesar . .	520	27.0	44.0	26.0	55	1050	4.0

Food and Measure	cal.	prot. (gms)	carbo. (gms)	fat (gms)	chol. (mgs)	sod. (mgs)	fiber (gms)
chicken, spicy							
crispy	560	24.0	55.0	27.0	50	1020	0
chicken, supreme	620	25.0	48.0	36.0	75	1520	0
chicken fajita pita	290	24.0	29.0	8.0	35	700	3.0
chicken fillet, grilled	430	29.0	36.0	19.0	65	1070	0
The Really Big							
Chicken Sandwich	900	40.0	58.0	56.0	120	2150	1.0
fish supreme	590	22.0	49.0	34.0	70	1180	0
hamburger:							
regular	280	13.0	31.0	11.0	25	470	0
quarter-pounder	510	26.0	39.0	27.0	65	1080	0
sourdough,							
grilled	670	32.0	39.0	43.0	110	1180	0
Jumbo Jack	560	26.0	41.0	32.0	65	740	0
Jumbo Jack							
w/cheese	650	31.0	42.0	40.0	90	1150	0
entrees:							
chicken teriyaki							
bowl	580	28.0	115.0	1.5	30	1220	6.0
taco	190	7.0	15.0	11.0	20	410	2.0
taco, super	280	12.0	22.0	17.0	30	720	3.0
salads:							
chicken, garden . .	200	23.0	8.0	9.0	65	420	3.0
side	70	4.0	3.0	4.0	10	80	2.0
finger foods:							
chicken strips,							
4 pcs.	290	25.0	18.0	13.0	50	700	0
chicken strips,							
6 pcs.	450	39.0	28.0	20.0	80	1100	0
egg rolls, 3 pcs. . .	440	3.0	54.0	24.0	30	960	4.0
egg rolls, 5 pcs. . .	750	5.0	92.0	41.0	50	1640	7.0
jalapeños, stuffed,							
7 pcs.	420	15.0	29.0	27.0	55	1620	3.0
jalapeños, stuffed,							
10 pcs.	600	22.0	41.0	39.0	75	2320	4.0
potato wedges							
w/bacon, cheddar	800	20.0	49.0	58.0	55	1470	4.0

Food and Measure	cal.	prot. (gms)	carbo. (gms)	fat (gms)	chol. (mgs)	sod. (mgs)	fiber (gms)
Jack-in-the-Box *(cont.)*							
side dishes:							
fries:							
small	220	3.0	28.0	11.0	0	120	3.0
regular	350	4.0	45.0	17.0	0	190	4.0
jumbo	400	5.0	51.0	19.0	0	220	4.0
super scoop . .	590	8.0	76.0	29.0	0	330	6.0
seasoned, curly	360	5.0	39.0	20.0	0	1070	4.0
onion rings	380	5.0	38.0	23.0	0	450	0
sauces:							
barbeque, 1 oz. . .	45	1.0	11.0	0	0	300	0
buttermilk, .9 oz.	130	<1.0	3.0	13.0	10	240	<1
soy, .3 oz.	5	<1.0	<1.0	0	0	480	<1
sweet and sour,							
1 oz.	40	<1.0	11.0	0	0	160	0
tartar, 1 oz.	150	0	2.0	15.0	10	200	0
dressings, 2 oz.:							
blue cheese	210	1.0	11.0	18.0	15	750	0
buttermilk, house	290	1.0	6.0	30.0	20	560	0
Italian, low calorie	25	0	2.0	1.5	0	670	0
Thousand Island . .	250	1.0	10.0	24.0	20	570	0
condiments:							
cheese, 1 slice:							
American	45	2.0	0	3.5	10	200	0
Swiss style . . .	40	3.0	0	3.0	10	190	0
croutons, .4 oz. . .	50	1.0	8.0	2.0	0	105	0
guacamole, .9 oz.	50	<1.0	3.0	4.0	0	95	0
hot sauce pkt. . . .	5	<1.0	1.0	0	0	110	0
ketchup pkt.	10	0	3.0	0	0	100	0
mayonnaise pkt. . . .	150	0	0	17.0	15	120	0
mustard pkt.	5	0	0	0	0	55	0
mustard pkt., Chi-							
nese hot	10	0	1.0	0	0	50	0
salsa, 1 oz.	10	0	2.0	0	0	200	0
sour cream, 1.1. oz.	60	1.0	1.0	6.0	20	30	0
desserts:							
apple turnover . . .	350	3.0	48.0	19.0	0	460	0
cheesecake	310	8.0	29.0	18.0	65	210	2.0

Food and Measure	cal.	prot. (gms)	carbo. (gms)	fat (gms)	chol. (mgs)	sod. (mgs)	fiber (gms)
cheesecake, choco- late chip cookie dough	360	7.0	44.0	18.0	45	200	1.0
shakes:							
chocolate	390	9.0	74.0	6.0	25	210	<1
strawberry	330	9.0	60.0	7.0	30	180	0
vanilla	350	9.0	62.0	7.0	30	180	0
Jackfruit, trimmed,							
1 oz.	27	.4	6.8	.1	0	1	.5
Jalapeño, see "Pep- per, jalapeño"							
Jalapeño dip, 2 tbsp.:							
(*Kraft*)	60	1.0	3.0	4.0	15	260	0
(*Old El Paso*)	30	1.0	4.0	1.0	<5	125	2.0
and cheddar:							
(*Breakstone's*) . . .	60	1.0	2.0	4.0	15	170	0
(*Frito-Lay*)	50	2.0	3.0	3.0	5	280	0
cheese (*Kraft* Pre- mium)	60	2.0	1.0	5.0	15	250	0
Jam and preserves (see also "Fruit spreads"), 1 tbsp., except as noted:							
all varieties:							
(*Knott's Berry Farm*), 1 tsp. . .	18	0	4.0	0	0	0	0
(*Smucker's*)	50	0	13.0	0	0	0	0
(*Smucker's* Reduced Sugar)	25	0	6.0	0	0	0	0
(*Smucker's* Light)	10	0	5.0	0	0	0	0
apricot, raspberry or strawberry (*Kraft*)	50	0	13.0	0	0	10	0
blackberry (*Kraft*) . .	50	0	13.0	0	0	10	<1.0
grape (*Kraft*)	60	0	14.0	0	0	10	0
mango (*Goya*)	46	0	11.0	0	0	<1	0
orange marmalade:							
(*Crosse & Black- well*)	60	0	16.0	0	0	5	0
(*Kraft*)	50	0	14.0	0	0	10	0

Food and Measure	cal.	prot. (gms)	carbo. (gms)	fat (gms)	chol. (mgs)	sod. (mgs)	fiber (gms)
Jam and preserves, orange marmalade *(cont.)*							
(*Smucker's*)	50	0	13.0	0	0	0	0
papaya (*Goya*)	45	0	11.0	0	0	<1	0
passion fruit (*Goya*)	45	0	12.0	0	0	0	0
peach or pineapple							
(*Kraft*)	50	0	14.0	0	0	10	0
pineapple (*Goya*) . .	45	0	11.0	0	0	0	0
plum, red (*Kraft*) . .	60	0	13.0	0	0	10	0
strawberry (*Goya*) . .	45	0	11.0	0	0	0	0
strawberry (*Kraft*) . .	50	0	13.0	0	0	10	0
Jambalaya dinner							
mix (*Luzianne*),							
¼ pkg.	200	5.0	43.0	1.0	0	690	1.0
Java plum:							
3 medium, .4 oz. . .	5	.1	1.4	<.1	0	1	<1.0
seeded, ½ cup	41	.5	10.5	.2	0	9	<1.0
Jelly, 1 tbsp., except							
as noted:							
all fruit flavors:							
(*Knott's Berry*							
Farm), 1 tsp. . .	18	0	4.0	0	0	0	0
(*Smucker's*)	50	0	13.0	0	0	0	0
except apple, grape							
and strawberry							
(*Kraft*)	50	0	13.0	0	0	10	0
apple or strawberry							
(*Kraft*)	60	0	14.0	0	0	10	0
apple mint (*Crosse &*							
Blackwell)	50	0	13.0	0	0	0	0
currant, red (*Crosse*							
& Blackwell)	60	0	14.0	0	0	0	0
grape:							
(*Goya*)	45	0	11.0	0	0	0	0
(*Kraft*)	50	0	14.0	0	0	10	0
guava (*Goya*)	50	0	12.0	0	0	<1	0
pepper:							
mild (*Tabasco*) . . .	60	0	14.0	0	0	10	0
spicy (*Tabasco*) . .	50	0	12.0	0	0	40	0

Food and Measure	cal.	prot. (gms)	carbo. (gms)	fat (gms)	chol. (mgs)	sod. (mgs)	fiber (gms)
Jerk sauce (*World Harbors* Blue Mountain), 2 tbsp.	40	0	10.0	0	0	90	0
Jerusalem artichoke:							
sliced, ½ cup	57	1.5	13.1	<.1	0	n.a.	1.2
stored (*Frieda's Sunchoke*), 1 oz. . . .	75	2.3	16.7	.1	0	n.a.	n.a.
Jicama, see "Yam bean tuber"							
Jujube:							
raw, seeded, 1 oz. . . .	22	.3	5.7	.1	0	1	n.a.
dried, 1 oz.	81	1.0	20.1	.3	0	3	n.a.
Jute, potherb:							
raw, ½ cup	5	.7	.8	<.1	0	1	n.a.
boiled, drained, ½ cup	16	1.6	3.1	.1	0	5	.9

K

Food and Measure	cal.	prot. (gms)	carbo. (gms)	fat (gms)	chol. (mgs)	sod. (mgs)	fiber (gms)
Kale, ½ cup, except as noted:							
fresh:							
raw, chopped . . .	17	1.1	3.4	.2	0	15	.7
boiled, drained, chopped	21	1.2	3.7	.3	0	15	1.3
canned (*Allens/Sunshine*)	25	2.0	3.0	.5	0	20	2.0
frozen (*Seabrook*), 3 oz.	30	2.0	2.0	0	0	20	2.0
Kale, Scotch, ½ cup:							
raw, chopped	14	1.0	2.8	.2	0	24	<1.0
boiled, drained, chopped	18	1.2	3.7	.3	0	29	<2.0
Kamranga, see "Carambola"							
Kamut flakes, see "Cereal"							
Kamut flour (*Arrowhead Mills*), ¼ cup	110	4.0	25.0	.5	0	0	4.0
Kasha, see "Buckwheat groats"							
Kelp, see "Seaweed"							
Ketchup, 1 tbsp.:							
(*Del Monte*)	15	0	4.0	0	0	190	0
(*Healthy Choice*) . . .	10	0	2.0	0	0	100	0
(*Heinz*)	15	0	4.0	0	0	190	0
(*Hunt's*)	15	0	3.0	0	0	200	0
(*Hunt's* No Salt) . . .	15	0	3.0	0	0	<10	0
(*Smucker's*)	25	0	7.0	0	0	110	0

Food and Measure	cal.	prot. (gms)	carbo. (gms)	fat (gms)	chol. (mgs)	sod. (mgs)	fiber (gms)
KFC, 1 serving:							
Original Recipe:							
breast	360	33.0	12.0	20.0	115	870	1.0
drumstick	130	13.0	4.0	7.0	70	210	0
thigh	260	19.0	9.0	17.0	110	570	1.0
wing, whole	150	11.0	7.0	8.0	40	380	0
Colonel's Rotisserie Gold:							
breast/wing	335	40.0	1.0	18.7	157	1104	0
breast/wing, w/out skin/wing	199	37.0	0	5.9	97	667	0
thigh/leg	333	30.0	1.0	23.7	163	980	0
thigh/leg, w/out skin	217	27.0	0	12.2	128	772	0
Extra Tasty Crispy:							
breast	470	31.0	25.0	28.0	80	930	1.0
drumstick	190	13.0	8.0	11.0	60	260	<1.0
thigh	370	19.0	18.0	25.0	70	540	2.0
wing, whole	200	10.0	10.0	13.0	45	290	<1.0
Hot & Spicy:							
breast	530	32.0	23.0	35.0	110	1110	2.0
drumstick	190	13.0	10.0	11.0	50	300	<1.0
thigh	370	18.0	13.0	27.0	90	570	1.0
wing, whole	210	10.0	9.0	15.0	50	340	<1.0
chicken pot pie . . .	730	28.0	67.0	40.0	70	2050	5.0
Crispy Strips, 4 pcs.	323	24.6	12.0	19.6	50	815	n.a.
Hot Wings, 6 pcs. . .	471	27.0	18.0	33.0	150	1230	n.a.
Kentucky Nuggets, 6 pcs.	284	16.0	15.0	18.0	66	865	n.a.
sandwiches:							
chicken	497	28.6	45.5	22.3	52	1213	n.a.
Colonel's chicken	482	21.0	39.0	27.0	47	1060	n.a.
BBQ chicken	256	17.0	28.0	8.0	57	782	2.0
sides/specials:							
BBQ baked beans	132	5.0	24.0	2.0	3	535	4.0
beans, red, and rice	114	4.0	18.0	3.0	4	315	2.0
biscuit	200	3.0	20.0	12.0	2	564	1.0
coleslaw	114	1.0	13.0	6.0	<5	177	n.a.
corn-on-the-cob . .	222	4.0	27.0	12.0	0	76	8.0
corn bread	228	3.0	25.0	13.0	42	194	1.0

Food and Measure	cal.	prot. (gms)	carbo. (gms)	fat (gms)	chol. (mgs)	sod. (mgs)	fiber (gms)
KFC, sides/specials *(cont.)*							
garden rice	75	2.0	15.0	1.0	0	576	1.0
macaroni & cheese	162	7.0	15.0	8.0	16	531	0
mashed potatoes							
w/gravy	109	1.0	16.0	5.0	<1	386	2.0
Mean Greens . . .	52	3.0	8.0	2.0	6	477	3.0
potato salad	180	3.0	18.0	11.0	11	423	2.0
potato wedges . . .	192	3.0	25.0	9.0	3	428	3.0
Kidney beans:							
dry:							
boiled, ½ cup . . .	112	7.6	20.1	.4	0	2	6.5
uncooked (*Arrow-*							
head Mills),							
¼ cup	160	11.0	29.0	.5	0	0	10.0
canned, red, ½ cup:							
w/liquid	108	6.7	20.0	.4	0	437	8.2
(*Eden* Organic) . .	100	8.0	18.0	0	0	15	10.0
(*Hunt's*)	95	6.5	19.5	.5	0	485	5.0
(*Progresso*)	110	7.0	20.0	.5	0	280	8.0
baked (*B&M*) . . .	170	7.0	32.0	2.0	<5	440	6.0
baked (*Friends*) . .	160	7.0	32.0	1.0	<5	510	6.0
dark (*Allens/East*							
Texas Fair/Trap-							
pey's)	130	8.0	22.0	1.0	0	310	8.0
dark (*Goya*)	90	7.0	18.0	4.0	0	380	7.0
dark (*Van Camp's*)	90	6.0	20.0	0	0	760	6.0
dark or light (*Green*							
Giant/Joan of Arc)	110	8.0	20.0	0	0	340	6.0
dark or light							
(*Stokely*)	120	7.0	21.0	.5	0	380	5.0
dark or light							
(*Stokely* No							
Sugar)	110	7.0	19.0	.5	0	250	5.0
light (*Allens/Trap-*							
pey's)	120	6.0	22.0	1.0	0	340	8.0
light (*Van Camp's*)	90	6.0	20.0	0	0	390	6.0
w/bacon, light							
(*Trappey's* New							
Orleans)	110	6.0	20.0	1.0	0	410	6.0

Food and Measure	cal.	prot. (gms)	carbo. (gms)	fat (gms)	chol. (mgs)	sod. (mgs)	fiber (gms)
w/chili gravy (*Trappey's*)	110	6.0	20.0	1.0	0	510	7.0
w/jalapeños, light (*Trappey's*) . . .	110	6.0	19.0	1.0	0	420	6.0
in tomato sauce (*Goya* Guisadas)	110	6.0	18.0	1.0	0	620	5.0
canned, white (*Progresso* Cannellini), ½ cup	100	5.0	18.0	.5	0	270	5.0
Kidney beans, sprouted, raw, ½ cup	27	3.9	3.8	.5	0	n.a.	<1.0
Kidneys, braised:							
beef, 4 oz.	163	28.9	1.1	3.9	439	152	0
lamb, 4 oz.	155	26.8	1.1	4.1	641	171	0
pork, 4 oz.	171	28.8	0	5.3	544	91	0
pork, chopped, 1 cup	211	35.6	0	6.6	673	111	0
veal, 4 oz.	185	29.8	0	6.4	897	125	0
Kielbasa (see also "Polish sausage"):							
(*Boar's Head*), 2 oz.	120	9.0	0	10.0	50	440	0
(*Jones Dairy Farm* Dinner), 1 link . . .	190	10.0	1.0	16.0	40	560	0
Kishka (*Hebrew National*), 2 oz.	160	5.0	10.0	11.0	15	430	2.0
Kiwi:							
1 large, 3.7 oz. . . .	55	.9	13.5	.4	0	4	3.1
1 medium, 3.1 oz. . . .	46	.8	11.3	.3	0	4	2.6
fuzzless (*Frieda's*), 1 oz.	10	.2	2.1	<.1	0	n.a.	n.a.
Kiwi, dried (*Sonoma*), 7–8 pcs., 1 oz. . .	90	1.0	19.0	1.0	0	0	2.0
Kiwi punch (*After the Fall* Bear), 8 fl. oz.	100	1.0	24.0	0	0	15	0
Kiwi-strawberry drink, 8 fl. oz.:							
(*Snapple*)	120	0	29.0	0	0	10	0
(*Snapple* Diet)	20	0	5.0	0	0	10	0

Food and Measure	cal.	prot. (gms)	carbo. (gms)	fat (gms)	chol. (mgs)	sod. (mgs)	fiber (gms)
Knockwurst, beef:							
(*Boar's Head*), 4 oz.	310	15.0	1.0	27.0	50	950	0
beef (*Hebrew National*), 3-oz. link	260	10.0	1.0	25.0	55	670	0
Kohlrabi, ½ cup:							
raw, sliced	19	1.2	4.3	.1	0	14	2.5
boiled, drained, sliced	24	1.5	5.5	.1	0	17	.9
Kumquat:							
1 medium, .7 oz. . .	12	.2	3.1	<.1	0	1	1.3
seeded, 1 oz.	18	.3	4.7	<.1	0	2	1.9

L

Food and Measure	cal.	prot. (gms)	carbo. (gms)	fat (gms)	chol. (mgs)	sod. (mgs)	fiber (gms)
Lamb, choice grade, meat only, 4 oz., except as noted:							
cubed, leg/shoulder:							
braised or stewed	253	38.2	0	10.0	122	79	0
broiled	211	31.8	0	8.3	102	86	0
foreshank, braised:							
lean w/fat	276	32.2	0	15.3	120	82	0
lean only	212	35.2	0	6.8	118	84	0
ground:							
raw . . , ...	320	18.8	0	26.5	83	67	0
broiled	321	28.1	0	22.3	110	92	0
broiled, 1 cup . . .	328	28.7	0	23.1	113	94	0
leg, whole, roasted:							
lean w/fat	293	29.0	0	18.7	105	75	0
lean w/fat, 1 slice, 3″ diam. × ¼″ . .	73	7.2	0	4.7	26	19	0
lean only	217	32.1	0	8.8	101	77	0
lean only, 3″ slice	54	8.0	0	2.2	25	19	0
leg, shank, roasted:							
lean w/fat	255	29.9	0	14.1	102	74	0
lean w/fat, 1 slice, 3″ diam. × ¼″ . .	64	7.5	0	3.5	26	18	0
lean only	204	31.9	0	7.6	99	75	0
lean only, 3″ slice	51	8.0	0	1.9	25	19	0
leg, sirloin, roasted:							
lean w/fat	331	27.9	0	23.4	110	77	0
lean w/fat, 1 slice, 3″ diam. × ¼″ . .	83	7.0	0	5.9	27	19	0
lean only	231	32.1	0	10.4	104	81	0
lean only, 3″ slice	58	8.0	0	2.6	26	20	0

Food and Measure	cal.	prot. (gms)	carbo. (gms)	fat (gms)	chol. (mgs)	sod. (mgs)	fiber (gms)
Lamb *(cont.)*							
loin chop, broiled:							
lean w/fat, 2¼ oz.							
(4.2 oz. raw							
w/bone)	201	16.1	0	14.7	64	49	0
lean w/fat	358	28.5	0	26.2	113	87	0
lean only, 1.6 oz.							
(4.2 oz. raw							
w/bone and fat)	100	13.9	0	4.5	44	39	0
lean only	245	34.0	0	11.0	108	95	0
loin, roasted:							
lean w/fat	350	25.6	0	26.8	108	73	0
lean only	229	30.2	0	11.1	99	75	0
rib:							
broiled, lean w/fat	409	25.1	0	33.6	112	86	0
broiled, lean only	266	31.5	0	14.7	103	96	0
roasted, lean w/fat	407	24.0	0	33.8	110	83	0
roasted, lean only	263	29.7	0	15.1	100	92	0
shoulder, whole:							
braised, lean w/fat	390	32.5	0	27.8	132	85	0
braised, lean only	321	37.2	0	10.0	133	90	0
roasted, lean w/fat	313	25.5	0	22.6	104	75	0
roasted, lean only	231	28.3	0	12.2	99	77	0
Lamb, New Zealand,							
frozen, meat only,							
4 oz.:							
foreshank:							
braised, lean w/fat	293	30.6	0	18.0	116	53	0
braised, lean only	211	34.9	0	6.8	115	56	0
leg, whole:							
roasted, lean w/fat	279	28.1	0	17.6	115	49	0
roasted, lean only	205	31.4	0	7.9	113	51	0
loin chop:							
broiled, lean w/fat	357	26.6	0	27.1	127	56	0
broiled, lean only	226	33.2	0	9.3	129	62	0
rib:							
roasted, lean w/fat	386	21.5	0	32.6	113	49	0
roasted, lean only	222	27.7	0	11.5	107	54	0

Food and Measure	cal.	prot. (gms)	carbo. (gms)	fat (gms)	chol. (mgs)	sod. (mgs)	fiber (gms)
shoulder:							
braised, lean w/fat	405	32.0	0	29.8	139	58	0
braised, lean only	323	38.6	0	17.6	144	64	0
Lamb curry entree,							
frozen (*Curry Classics*), 10 oz.	480	37.0	16.0	29.0	n.a.	1210	6.0
Lamb's-quarters,							
boiled, drained,							
chopped, ½ cup . .	29	2.9	4.5	.6	0	n.a.	1.9
Lard, pork:							
1 tbsp.	115	0	0	12.8	12	<1	0
(*Goya*), 1 tbsp. . . .	130	0	0	14.0	15	0	0
Lasagna entree,							
canned:							
(*Hormel*), 7½-oz. can	250	8.0	24.0	14.0	25	940	1.0
(*Hormel* Micro Cup),							
7½ oz.	250	8.0	24.0	14.0	25	950	1.0
(*Libby's Diner*),							
7¾ oz.	200	9.0	25.0	7.0	15	860	3.0
(*Nalley*), 1 cup	250	15.0	33.0	6.0	45	1070	6.0
(*Nalley*), 7½-oz. can	200	10.0	26.0	6.0	25	990	5.0
and beef (*Hormel*							
Micro Cup),							
10½ oz.	359	12.0	34.0	19.0	34	1384	3.0
cheese, three (*Nalley*),							
7½-oz. can	180	11.0	21.0	6.0	35	840	5.0
Italian (*Top Shelf*),							
10 oz.	340	22.0	28.0	16.0	60	990	3.0
Lasagna entree,							
freeze-dried (*Mountain House*), 1 cup	240	14.0	24.0	9.0	35	570	3.0
Lasagna entree, frozen, 1 pkg., except							
as noted:							
(*Celentano*)	400	18.0	51.0	14.0	80	650	7.0
(*Celentano*),							
½ of 14-oz. pkg.	280	15.0	33.0	10.0	75	660	8.0
(*Celentano* 25 oz.),							
1 cup	360	20.0	31.0	17.0	95	820	11.0

Food and Measure	cal.	prot. (gms)	carbo. (gms)	fat (gms)	chol. (mgs)	sod. (mgs)	fiber (gms)
Lasagna entree, frozen *(cont.)*							
(*Celentano* Great Choice)	260	18.0	42.0	2.5	20	650	2.0
(*Celentano* Value Pack), 1 cup	320	14.0	41.0	11.0	65	520	6.0
(*Healthy Choice* Roma)	390	26.0	60.0	5.0	15	580	9.0
cheese:							
(*Lean Cuisine* Classic)	290	20.0	38.0	6.0	30	560	5.0
casserole (*Lean Cuisine Lunch Express*)	270	14.0	38.0	7.0	15	590	5.0
w/chicken scaloppini (*Lean Cuisine Cafe Classics*) . .	290	20.0	34.0	8.0	40	560	4.0
four (*Stouffer's*) . .	410	22.0	37.0	19.0	55	840	3.0
Italian (*Weight Watchers*)	300	20.0	38.0	8.0	30	550	5.0
three (*The Budget Gourmet*)	370	20.0	38.0	16.0	60	870	5.0
extra cheese (*Marie Callender's*), 1 cup	330	15.0	32.0	16.0	32	770	4.0
Florentine (*Smart Ones*)	200	10.0	34.0	2.0	10	590	6.0
garden (*Weight Watchers*)	270	14.0	36.0	7.0	30	540	5.0
w/meat sauce:							
(*Banquet*)	290	14.0	39.0	9.0	10	900	6.0
(*Banquet* Bake at Home), 8-oz. cup	240	12.0	32.0	7.0	15	650	5.0
(*Banquet* Family), 1 cup	230	12.0	3.0	8.0	35	530	3.0
(*The Budget Gourmet* Light & Healthy)	250	15.0	31.0	7.0	30	690	3.0
(*Lean Cuisine*) . . .	290	20.0	35.0	8.0	35	560	6.0
(*Marie Callender's*), 7 oz.	370	17.0	34.0	18.0	35	740	4.0

Food and Measure	cal.	prot. (gms)	carbo. (gms)	fat (gms)	chol. (mgs)	sod. (mgs)	fiber (gms)
(*Stouffer's*)	360	27.0	34.0	13.0	50	780	5.0
(*Stouffer's*),							
⅓ of 21-oz. pkg.	260	19.0	24.0	10.0	35	560	4.0
(*Stouffer's Lunch*							
Express)	330	18.0	42.0	10.0	40	910	5.0
(*Swanson*)	410	23.0	45.0	15.0	65	1080	5.0
(*Weight Watchers*)	270	14.0	38.0	7.0	35	570	6.0
casserole (*Swanson*)	330	14.0	41.0	9.0	25	1050	3.0
primavera:							
(*Celentano* Great							
Choice)	240	17.0	33.0	7.0	20	600	7.0
(*Celentano* Selects)	210	11.0	32.0	4.0	0	510	5.0
sausage, Italian (*The*							
Budget Gourmet)	430	20.0	40.0	21.0	60	730	4.0
vegetable:							
(*Amy's* Family),							
7 oz.	200	10.0	27.0	8.0	10	480	4.0
(*Banquet*)	260	11.0	41.0	6.0	10	850	7.0
(*The Budget Gour-*							
met Light &							
Healthy)	290	15.0	29.0	10.0	20	770	5.0
(*Lean Cuisine*) . . .	270	17.0	35.0	7.0	20	540	3.0
(*Stouffer's*)	450	20.0	41.0	23.0	40	980	5.0
(*Stouffer's*), 1/12 of							
96-oz. pkg. . . .	340	12.0	34.0	17.0	20	760	3.0
w/cheese (*Amy's*)	300	15.0	39.0	10.0	15	680	5.0
cheesy (*Swanson*)	350	20.0	40.0	13.0	20	1360	3.0
tofu (*Amy's*)	300	18.0	41.0	10.0	0	630	6.0
Lasagna entree mix, dry							
(*Master-A-Meal*),							
⅕ pkg.	150	5.0	30.0	1.0	0	1100	1.0
Leek:							
fresh:							
raw, 9.9-oz. leek . .	76	1.9	17.6	.4	0	25	2.2
raw, chopped,							
½ cup	32	.8	7.4	.2	0	10	.9
boiled, drained,							
chopped, ½ cup	16	.4	4.0	.1	0	6	<1.0
freeze-dried, 1 tbsp.	1	<.1	.2	tr.	0	<1	<1.0

Food and Measure	cal.	prot. (gms)	carbo. (gms)	fat (gms)	chol. (mgs)	sod. (mgs)	fiber (gms)
Lemon:							
2⅛″ lemon, 3.9 oz.	22	1.3	11.6	.3	0	3	n.a.
1 wedge, ¼ medium	5	.3	2.9	.1	0	1	n.a.
peeled, 2⅛″ lemon	17	.6	5.4	.2	0	1	1.6
Lemon herb sauce							
mix (*Knorr*), 1 tbsp.	30	1.0	4.0	1.0	0	240	0
Lemon juice:							
fresh, 1 tbsp.	4	.1	1.3	0	0	<1	.1
bottled (*ReaLemon*),							
1 tsp.	0	0	0	0	0	0	0
Lemon peel:							
fresh, 1 tbsp.	—[1]	.1	1.0	<.1	0	0	.6
candied:							
(*S&W*), 1.1 oz. . .	80	0	23.0	0	0	25	2.0
diced (*Paradise/*							
White Swan),							
2 tbsp., 1 oz. . .	80	0	21.0	0	0	15	2.0
Lemon pepper:							
1 tsp.	7	.2	1.5	0	0	425	.3
(*Lawry's*), ¼ tsp. . .	0	0	0	0	0	80	0
(*Tone's*), ¼ tsp. . . .	0	0	0	0	0	105	0
salt (*McCormick*),							
¼ tsp.	0	0	0	0	0	120	0
Lemon sauce (*House*							
of Tsang), 2 tbsp.	70	0	17.0	0	0	10	0
Lemonade, 8 fl. oz.,							
except as noted:							
(*After the Fall*)	90	1.0	23.0	0	0	10	0
(*Heinke's* Old Fashion)	120	0	29.0	0	0	35	0
(*Minute Maid*)	110	0	31.0	0	0	25	0
(*R.W. Knudsen*) . . .	120	0	29.0	0	0	35	0
(*Santa Cruz*)	120	0	29.0	0	0	35	0
(*Snapple*)	110	0	29.0	0	0	10	0
(*Tropicana*)	120	0	29.0	0	0	20	0
(*Tropicana*),							
11.5 fl. oz.	160	<1.0	39.0	0	0	20	0

[1] *Cannot be calculated; no digestibility value for fresh peel.*

Food and Measure	cal.	prot. (gms)	carbo. (gms)	fat (gms)	chol. (mgs)	sod. (mgs)	fiber (gms)
(*Veryfine* Chillers),							
11.5 fl. oz.	180	0	45.0	0	0	15	0
pink:							
(*Minute Maid*) . . .	110	0	31.0	0	0	25	0
(*Snapple*)	120	0	29.0	0	0	10	0
(*Snapple* Diet) . . .	20	0	4.0	0	0	10	0
(*Veryfine* Chillers),							
11.5 fl. oz.	180	0	45.0	0	0	15	0
frozen* (*Minute Maid*)	110	0	30.0	0	0	0	0
Lemonade fruit							
blends, 8 fl. oz.:							
all fruit flavors:							
(*R.W. Knudsen*) . .	120	0	29.0	0	0	35	0
(*Santa Cruz*)	120	0	29.0	0	0	35	0
cherry:							
(*Snapple*)	130	0	31.0	0	0	10	0
(*Veryfine* Chillers)	120	0	29.0	0	0	15	0
cranberry:							
(*Heinke's*)	120	0	29.0	0	0	35	0
(*Minute Maid*) . . .	120	0	32.0	0	0	25	0
frozen* (*Minute*							
Maid)	110	0	30.0	0	0	0	0
ginger (*R.W. Knudsen*							
Echinecea)	100	0	25.0	0	0	8	0
lime (*Veryfine* Chill-							
ers)	120	0	29.0	0	0	5	0
peach:							
(*Snapple*)	120	0	31.0	0	0	10	0
(*Veryfine* Chillers)	120	0	31.0	0	0	15	0
raspberry:							
(*Minute Maid*) . . .	120	0	32.0	0	0	25	0
frozen* (*Minute*							
Maid)	110	0	30.0	0	0	0	0
strawberry:							
(*Snapple*)	120	0	29.0	0	0	10	0
(*Veryfine* Chillers)	120	0	30.0	0	0	15	0
tangerine (*Veryfine*							
Chillers)	120	0	31.0	0	0	10	0
tropical (*Minute Maid*)	120	0	32.0	0	0	25	0

Food and Measure	cal.	prot. (gms)	carbo. (gms)	fat (gms)	chol. (mgs)	sod. (mgs)	fiber (gms)
Lemonade mix*,							
8 fl. oz.:							
(*Country Time*) . . .	70	0	17.0	0	0	15	0
(*Country Time* Punch)	70	0	16.0	0	0	10	0
(*Country Time/Kool-*							
Aid Sugar Free) . .	5	0	0	0	0	0	0
(*Crystal Light*)	5	0	0	0	0	0	0
(*Hi-C* Pink)	100	0	26.0	0	0	15	0
(*Kool-Aid*							
Presweetened) . . .	70	0	17.0	0	0	0	0
w/sugar (*Kool-Aid*)	100	0	25.0	0	0	15	0
Lentil:							
dry, green or red (*Ar-*							
rowhead Mills),							
¼ cup	150	11.0	27.0	0	0	15	9.0
dry, red (*Goya*),							
¼ cup	180	13.0	31.0	0	0	0	9.0
cooked, ½ cup . . .	115	8.9	19.9	.4	0	2	7.8
Lentil, sprouted, raw,							
½ cup	40	3.4	8.4	.2	0	4	n.a.
Lentil dishes, canned							
(*Patak's* Moong							
Dhal), ½ cup . . .	160	7.0	20.0	6.0	5	630	4.0
Lentil dishes, mix:							
hearty, and wild rice							
(*Spice Islands* Quick							
Meal), 1 pkg. . . .	190	10.0	37.0	1.5	0	500	3.0
and herb (*Eastern Tra-*							
ditions), 2 oz. . . .	160	5.0	35.0	.5	0	430	1.0
pilaf:							
(*Casbah*), 1 oz. . .	100	5.0	19.0	0	0	230	1.0
(*Near East*), 1 cup*	210	10.0	37.0	4.0	0	650	5.0
almond (*Spice Is-*							
lands Quick Meal),							
1 pkg.	190	6.0	37.0	2.0	0	490	2.0
Lentil rice loaf, fro-							
zen (*Natural Touch*),							
1" slice	170	8.0	14.0	9.0	0	370	4.0

Food and Measure	cal.	prot. (gms)	carbo. (gms)	fat (gms)	chol. (mgs)	sod. (mgs)	fiber (gms)
Lettuce (see also "Salad blend mix"):							
bibb or Boston:							
1 head, 5″ diam.	21	2.1	3.8	.4	0	8	1.6
2 inner leaves . . .	2	.2	.4	<.1	0	1	.5
butter (*Dole*), 1 head	21	2.0	4.0	.1	0	8	2.0
cos or romaine:							
1 inner leaf	2	.2	.2	<.1	0	1	.2
shredded, ½ cup	4	.5	.7	.1	0	2	.7
shredded (*Dole*),							
1½ cups	18	1.0	2.0	1.0	0	40	1.0
iceberg:							
1 head, 6″ diam.	70	5.4	11.3	1.0	0	48	7.5
1 leaf, .7 oz.	3	.2	.4	<.1	0	2	.3
precut (*Dole*), 3 oz.	15	1.0	3.0	0	0	15	1.0
leaf, shredded (*Dole*),							
1½ cups	12	1.0	1.0	0	0	40	1.0
looseleaf, shredded,							
½ cup	5	.4	1.0	.1	0	3	.5
Lima beans, ½ cup, except as noted:							
fresh:							
raw, trimmed . . .	88	5.3	15.7	.7	0	6	3.8
boiled, drained . . .	104	5.8	20.1	.3	0	14	4.5
mature:							
baby, boiled	115	7.3	21.2	.3	0	2	7.0
large, boiled	108	7.3	19.6	.4	0	2	6.6
canned:							
(*Goya*)	76	5.0	18.0	0	0	355	5.4
(*Green Giant/Joan of Arc* Butterbeans)	90	6.0	16.0	0	0	450	5.0
(*S&W* Butterbeans)	70	6.0	18.0	0	0	440	5.0
(*Stokely*)	100	5.0	15.0	1.0	0	380	4.0
(*Stokely* No Salt)	100	5.0	15.0	1.0	0	10	4.0
(*Van Camp's* Butterbeans)	110	8.0	22.0	.5	0	430	7.0
baby (*Allens* Butterbeans)	120	7.0	22.0	.5	0	460	6.0

Food and Measure	cal.	prot. (gms)	carbo. (gms)	fat (gms)	chol. (mgs)	sod. (mgs)	fiber (gms)
Lima beans, canned *(cont.)*							
green (*Allens/East Texas Fair/Sunshine* Limas/Butterbeans)	120	7.0	23.0	.5	0	370	8.0
green (*Del Monte*)	80	4.0	15.0	0	0	360	4.0
green (*Goya*)	90	5.0	15.0	.5	0	330	4.0
green and white (*Allens*)	110	6.0	20.0	1.0	0	280	9.0
large (*Allens* Butterbeans)	120	7.0	20.0	1.0	0	290	7.0
mature, baby, green or butterbeans (*Stokely*)	110	6.0	19.0	.5	0	350	3.0
w/bacon, baby green (*Trappey's* Limas)	120	6.0	22.0	1.0	0	330	6.0
w/bacon, baby white (*Trappey's* Limas)	130	8.0	21.0	1.5	0	350	6.0
w/ham and sauce (*Nalley*), 1 cup	240	17.0	34.0	5.0	15	1070	15.0
w/sausage, large white (*Trappey's* Butterbeans) . . .	110	6.0	21.0	1.0	0	300	6.0
frozen:							
baby (*Green Giant Harvest Fresh*) . .	80	4.0	15.0	0	0	130	4.0
baby (*Seabrook*) . .	110	6.0	22.0	0	0	140	5.0
baby (*Stilwell*) . . .	110	6.0	22.0	0	0	140	5.0
baby, butter sauce (*Green Giant*), ⅔ cup	120	6.0	18.0	4.0	<5	330	6.0
Fordhook (*Stilwell*)	90	6.0	17.0	0	0	110	5.0
plain or speckled (*Stilwell* Butterbeans)	100	6.0	20.0	0	0	130	4.0
Lime:							
2"-diam. lime	20	.5	7.1	.1	0	1	1.9
peeled, seeded, 1 oz.	9	.2	3.0	.1	0	1	.8

Food and Measure	cal.	prot. (gms)	carbo. (gms)	fat (gms)	chol. (mgs)	sod. (mgs)	fiber (gms)
Lime juice:							
fresh, 1 tbsp.	4	.1	1.4	<.1	0	tr.	.1
bottled or chilled							
(*ReaLime*), 1 tsp.	0	0	0	0	0	0	0
sweetened (*Rose's*),							
1 tsp.	10	0	2.0	0	0	0	0
Lime drink, 8 fl. oz.:							
(*After the Fall* Key							
West)	100	1.0	25.0	0	0	10	0
(*R.W. Knudsen* Cactus							
Cooler)	120	0	29.0	0	0	35	0
frozen* (*Minute Maid*							
Limeade)	100	0	26.0	0	0	0	0
Ling, meat only:							
raw, 4 oz.	99	21.5	0	.7	n.a.	153	0
baked, broiled, or mi-							
crowaved, 4 oz. . .	126	27.6	0	.9	n.a.	196	0
Ling cod, meat only:							
raw, 4 oz.	96	20.0	0	1.2	59	67	0
baked, broiled, or mi-							
crowaved, 4 oz. . .	124	25.7	0	1.5	76	86	0
Linguine, plain:							
dry, see "Pasta"							
refrigerated, 1¼ cup:							
(*Contadina*)	260	10.0	47.0	4.0	95	30	2.0
tomato herb (*Con-*							
tadina)	250	10.0	45.0	3.5	85	30	2.0
Linguine entree, fro-							
zen, 1 pkg.:							
w/shrimp and clams:							
(*The Budget Gour-*							
met Light &							
Healthy)	280	14.0	38.0	8.0	70	800	3.0
marinara (*The Bud-*							
get Gourmet) . .	300	13.0	37.0	11.0	55	760	4.0
w/tomato sauce and							
sausage (*The Bud-*							
get Gourmet) . . .	360	15.0	43.0	14.0	25	610	5.0

Food and Measure	cal.	prot. (gms)	carbo. (gms)	fat (gms)	chol. (mgs)	sod. (mgs)	fiber (gms)
Linguine entree, mix,							
w/chicken, broccoli							
(*Noodle-Roni*),							
1 cup*	370	11.0	49.0	16.0	5	1000	2.0
Liquor[1], 1 fl. oz.:							
80 proof	65	0	tr.	0	0	tr.	0
90 proof	74	0	tr.	0	0	tr.	0
100 proof	83	0	tr.	0	0	tr.	0
Little Caesars:							
Baby Pan!Pan!, 2 sqs.	616	32.7	67.3	24.2	47	1466	3.7
Crazy Bread, 1 pc. . .	106	3.3	15.9	3.4	0	114	.6
Crazy Sauce, 6 oz. . .	74	4.5	13.7	.4	0	381	5.3
Pan!Pan!, 1 medium							
slice:							
cheese only	181	9.4	22.1	6.1	15	379	1.2
pepperoni	199	10.6	22.2	7.7	15	452	1.2
Pizza!Pizza!, 1 me-							
dium slice:							
cheese only	201	11.2	23.8	7.0	17	281	1.3
pepperoni	220	12.0	23.9	8.7	17	358	1.3
salads, individual:							
antipasto	176	11.5	7.4	11.8	19	542	2.4
Caesar	140	9.4	13.6	5.4	11	372	1.9
Greek	168	9.1	12.3	9.6	37	653	3.2
tossed	116	4.8	19.3	3.0	0	170	3.0
dressings, 1.5 oz.:							
blue cheese	160	0	7.9	13.8	17	600	0
Caesar	255	0	2.6	26.5	13	404	0
French	166	0	6.0	15.7	0	553	0
Greek	268	0	.4	29.9	9	202	0
Itialian	200	0	3.0	20.8	12	468	0
Italian, fat free . . .	15	0	3.0	0	0	420	0
ranch	221	0	4.7	20.8	12	468	0
Thousand Island . .	183	0	6.4	17.0	30	542	0
sandwich, cold:							
ham and cheese . .	728	30.4	71.0	35.3	54	1602	3.2

[1] *Includes all pure distilled liquors: bourbon, brandy, gin, rum, Scotch, vodka, etc.*

Food and Measure	cal.	prot. (gms)	carbo. (gms)	fat (gms)	chol. (mgs)	sod. (mgs)	fiber (gms)
Italian	740	28.6	71.3	37.2	62	1831	3.2
veggie	647	21.7	74.2	29.0	29	1195	4.2
sandwich, hot:							
Cheeser	822	39.8	75.2	39.4	58	2244	4.9
Meatsa	1036	55.4	75.3	55.5	130	3302	5.4
pepperoni	899	42.8	73.6	47.2	58	2428	3.9
supreme	894	40.8	77.1	45.8	70	2367	3.9
veggie	669	33.4	78.7	23.9	58	1534	5.8
Liver:							
beef, pan-fried, 4 oz.	246	30.3	8.9	9.1	547	120	0
chicken:							
raw (*Tyson*), 4 oz.	140	18.0	2.0	7.0	405	65	0
simmered, 4 oz. . .	178	27.6	1.0	6.2	716	58	0
simmered, chopped,							
1 cup	219	34.1	1.2	7.6	883	71	0
duck, raw, 1 oz. . . .	39	5.3	1.0	1.3	146	n.a.	0
goose, raw, 1 oz. . .	38	4.6	1.8	1.2	n.a.	40	0
lamb, pan-fried, 4 oz.	270	29.0	4.3	14.3	559	141	0
pork, braised, 4 oz.	187	29.5	4.3	5.0	403	56	0
turkey, simmered:							
4 oz.	192	27.2	3.9	6.7	710	73	0
chopped, 1 cup . .	237	33.6	4.8	8.3	876	89	0
veal (calves), braised,							
4 oz.	187	24.5	3.1	7.8	636	60	0
Liver cheese (*Oscar Mayer*), 1.3-oz. slice	120	6.0	1.0	10.0	80	420	0
Liver pâté, see "Liverwurst" and "Pâté"							
Liverwurst (see also "Braunschweiger"), 2 oz. or ¼ cup:							
(*Boar's Head* Strassburger/Smoked) . .	170	8.0	0	15.0	85	560	0
(*Underwood*)	160	7.0	3.0	14.0	65	380	1.0
pâté (*Boar's Head*)	150	9.0	0	12.0	55	470	0
spread (*Hormel*) . . .	130	8.0	2.0	10.0	70	650	0
Lobster, northern, meat only:							
raw, 4 oz.	102	21.3	.6	1.0	108	n.a.	0

Food and Measure	cal.	prot. (gms)	carbo. (gms)	fat (gms)	chol. (mgs)	sod. (mgs)	fiber (gms)
Lobster *(cont.)*							
boiled or steamed:							
4 oz.	111	23.2	1.5	.7	82	431	0
1 cup, 5.1 oz. . . .	142	29.7	1.9	.9	104	551	0
"Lobster," imitation, frozen or refrigerated:							
chunks, ½ cup, 3 oz.:							
(*Captain Jac Lobster Tasties*)	90	9.0	12.0	.5	10	510	0
(*Louis Kemp Lobster Delights*) . .	80	8.0	11.0	0	5	610	0
salad style (*Louis Kemp Lobster Delights*), ½ cup, 3 oz.	80	8.0	11.0	0	5	600	0
tail style (*Captain Jac Lobster Tasties*), 4-oz. tail	100	8.0	16.0	0	5	300	3.0
Lobster, spiny, see "Spiny lobster"							
Lobster sauce, rock, (*Progresso*), ½ cup	100	3.0	6.0	7.0	5	430	2.0
Loganberry:							
fresh, 1 cup	89	1.4	21.5	.9	0	1	n.a.
frozen, ½ cup	40	1.1	9.6	.2	0	1	3.6
Long John Silver's:							
clams, 3 oz.	300	11.0	31.0	17	40	670	5.0
chicken:							
batter-dipped, 1 pc.	120	8.0	11.0	6.0	15	400	3.0
Flavorbaked, 1 pc.	110	19.0	<1.0	3.0	55	600	<1.0
popcorn, 3.3 oz.	250	15.0	17.0	14.0	35	590	1.0
fish:							
batter-dipped, 1 pc.	170	11.0	12.0	11.0	30	470	5.0
Flavorbaked, 1 pc.	90	14.0	1.0	2.5	35	320	0
popcorn, 3.6 oz.	290	13.0	27.0	14.0	20	1090	1.0

Food and Measure	cal.	prot. (gms)	carbo. (gms)	fat (gms)	chol. (mgs)	sod. (mgs)	fiber (gms)
shrimp:							
batter-dipped,							
1 pc.	35	1.0	2.0	2.5	10	95	0
popcorn, 3.3 oz.	280	11.0	27.0	15.0	85	920	1.0
sandwiches, 1 pc.:							
chicken, *Flavorbaked*	290	24.0	27.0	10.0	60	970	2.0
fish, batter-dipped,							
w/out sauce . . .	320	17.0	40.0	13.0	30	800	6.0
fish, *Flavorbaked*	320	23.0	28.0	14.0	55	930	2.0
Ultimate Fish	430	18.0	44.0	21.0	35	1340	3.0
sides, 1 serving:							
cheese sticks,							
1.6 oz.	160	6.0	12.0	9.0	10	360	<1.0
coleslaw	140	1.0	20.0	6.0	0	260	3.0
corn cobbette,							
1 pc.:							
w/butter	140	3.0	19.0	8.0	0	0	0
plain	80	3.0	19.0	.5	0	0	0
fries, 3 oz.	250	3.0	28.0	15.0	0	500	3.0
green beans	30	2.0	5.0	.5	<5	310	2.0
hushpuppy, 1 pc.	60	1.0	9.0	2.5	0	25	0
potato, baked . . .	210	4.0	49.0	0	0	10	3.0
rice pilaf	140	3.0	26.0	3.0	0	210	<1.0
side salad	25	1.0	4.0	0	0	15	<1.0
dressings:							
French, fat free,							
1½ oz.	50	0	14.0	0	0	360	0
Italian, 1 oz.	130	0	2.0	14.0	0	280	0
ranch, 1 oz.	170	0	1.0	18.0	5	260	0
ranch, fat free,							
1½ oz.	50	2.0	13.0	0	0	380	0
Thousand Island,							
1 oz.	110	0	5.0	10.0	15	280	0
sauces/condiments:							
honey mustard,							
.4 oz.	20	0	5.0	0	0	60	0
malt vinegar, .3 oz.	0	0	0	0	0	15	0
margarine, .2 oz.	35	0	0	4.0	0	35	0
shrimp sauce, .4 oz.	15	0	3.0	0	0	180	0

Food and Measure	cal.	prot. (gms)	carbo. (gms)	fat (gms)	chol. (mgs)	sod. (mgs)	fiber (gms)
Long John Silver's, sauces/condiments *(cont.)*							
sour cream, 1 oz.	60	<1.0	1.0	6.0	15	15	0
sweet 'n' sour,							
.4 oz.	20	0	5.0	0	0	45	0
tartar sauce, .4 oz.	35	0	5.0	1.5	0	35	0
Longan, shelled:							
fresh, seeded, 1 oz.	17	.4	4.3	<.1	0	<1	.3
dried, 1 oz.	81	1.4	21.0	.1	0	14	<1.0
Loquat:							
1 medium, .6 oz. . . .	5	<.1	1.2	<.1	0	<1	.2
peeled, seeded, 1 oz.	13	.1	3.4	.1	0	<1	.5
(*Frieda's*), 3.5 oz. . . .	48	.4	12.4	.2	0	0	n.a.
Lotus root:							
raw, trimmed, 1 oz.	16	.7	4.9	<.1	0	11	1.4
boiled, drained, 4 oz.	75	1.8	18.2	.1	0	51	3.5
Lotus seed:							
raw, 1 oz.	25	1.2	4.9	.2	0	<1	n.a.
dried, 1 oz.	94	4.4	18.3	.6	0	1	n.a.
fried, 1 cup	106	4.9	20.6	.6	0	1	n.a.
Lox, see "Salmon, smoked"							
Lunch combinations (*Lunchables*), 1 pkg.:							
bologna/American . .	470	17.0	22.0	35.0	85	1580	<1.0
bologna/wild cherry	530	13.0	60.0	28.0	60	1120	<1.0
chicken/turkey deluxe	390	21.0	24.0	23.0	70	1820	<1.0
ham/cheddar	360	20.0	21.0	21.0	75	1760	<1.0
ham/Swiss	340	21.0	20.0	20.0	70	1790	<1.0
ham/fruit punch . . .	440	15.0	54.0	20.0	50	1270	<1.0
ham/fruit punch, low fat	360	17.0	52.0	10.0	35	1150	0
ham/*Surfer Cooler* . .	380	18.0	57.0	10.0	35	1380	<1.0
pizza, mozzarella:							
cheddar	330	18.0	33.0	14.0	35	870	2.0
fruit punch	480	18.0	65.0	17.0	35	900	2.0
pizza/pepperoni:							
mozzarella	330	17.0	32.0	15.0	35	850	2.0
orange	480	18.0	65.0	17.0	35	900	2.0

Food and Measure	cal.	prot. (gms)	carbo. (gms)	fat (gms)	chol. (mgs)	sod. (mgs)	fiber (gms)
salami/American . . .	420	19.0	21.0	29.0	80	1690	<1.0
turkey/cheddar	350	20.0	22.0	20.0	70	1750	1.0
turkey/ham	370	21.0	25.0	21.0	65	1930	<1.0
turkey/Monterey Jack	350	21.0	19.0	21.0	75	1700	1.0
turkey/*Pacific Cooler*	450	16.0	53.0	20.0	50	1330	1.0
turkey/*Pacific Cooler,* low fat	360	17.0	55.0	9.0	30	1280	<1.0
turkey/*Surfer Cooler*	430	14.0	61.0	15.0	45	1240	0
Lunch meat (see also specific listings), spiced loaf (*Oscar Mayer*), 1-oz. slice	70	4.0	2.0	5.0	20	340	0
Lunch meat, canned: (*Spam*), 2 oz.	170	7.0	0	16.0	40	750	0
(*Spam* Less Salt), 2 oz.	170	7.0	0	16.0	40	560	0
(*Spam* Lite), 2 oz. . . .	110	9.0	0	8.0	45	560	0
spread (*Spam*), 2 oz.	100	8.0	1.0	11.0	40	580	0
Lunch "meat," vegetarian, canned (*Loma Linda Nuteena*), ³⁄₈″ slice	160	6.0	6.0	13.0	0	120	2.0
Lupin, boiled, ½ cup	98	12.9	8.2	2.4	0	3	2.3
Lupinin beans, in jars (*Canto*), ¼ cup . .	30	3.0	3.0	0	0	1420	3.0
Lychee, shelled, 1 oz.:							
raw, seeded	19	.2	4.7	.1	0	<1	.4
raw, peeled (*Frieda's*)	18	.3	4.6	.1	0	1	n.a.
dried	79	1.1	20.0	.3	0	1	1.3

M

Food and Measure	cal.	prot. (gms)	carbo. (gms)	fat (gms)	chol. (mgs)	sod. (mgs)	fiber (gms)
Macadamia nut:							
raw (*Frieda's*), 1 oz.	196	2.2	4.5	20.3	0	n.a.	n.a.
dried, shelled:							
1 oz.	199	2.4	3.9	20.9	0	1	2.6
1 cup	940	11.1	18.4	98.8	0	6	12.5
oil-roasted, 1 oz. . . .	204	2.1	3.7	21.7	0	2	n.a.
Macaroni (see also "Pasta"):							
uncooked:							
2 oz.	211	7.3	42.6	.9	0	4	1.4
(*Creamette*), 2 oz.	210	7.0	42.0	1.0	0	0	2.0
elbow, 1 cup	389	13.4	78.4	1.7	0	8	2.5
elbow, regular or whole wheat (*Eden*), 2 oz. . .	210	10.0	39.0	1.5	0	0	6.0
elbow (*Goya* Coditos), 2 oz.	210	6.0	45.0	1.0	0	0	0
cooked:							
4 oz.	160	5.4	32.1	.8	0	1	1.8
elbow, 1 cup	197	6.7	39.7	.9	0	1	2.2
small shells, 1 cup	162	5.5	32.6	.8	0	1	1.8
spirals, 1 cup . . .	189	6.4	38.0	.9	0	1	2.1
vegetable (tricolor), 4 oz.	145	5.1	30.2	.1	0	7	4.9
whole-wheat, 4 oz.	141	6.0	30.1	.6	0	3	5.0
Macaroni dinner, and cheese, frozen (*Swanson* Budget), 1 pkg.	320	17.0	43.0	11.0	20	960	6.0

Food and Measure	cal.	prot. (gms)	carbo. (gms)	fat (gms)	chol. (mgs)	sod. (mgs)	fiber (gms)
Macaroni entree, canned, 7½ oz., except as noted:							
and beef:							
(*Kid's Kitchen* Beefy)	190	11.0	23.0	6.0	30	790	2.0
(*Kid's Kitchen* Cheezy Mac & Beef)	260	15.0	34.0	7.0	30	800	1.0
(*Libby's Diner*), 7¾ oz.	220	9.0	31.0	9.0	20	760	5.0
and cheese:							
(*Chef Boyardee* Bowl)	160	7.0	31.0	1.0	15	920	2.0
(*Franco-American*), 1 cup	200	11.0	29.0	7.0	10	1060	4.0
(*Hormel* Micro Cup)	260	11.0	30.0	11.0	35	690	1.0
(*Libby's Diner*), 7¾ oz.	320	12.0	25.0	20.0	30	1400	2.0
(*Kid's Kitchen*) . . .	260	11.0	30.0	11.0	35	690	1.0
chili, see "Chili"							
Macaroni entree, frozen, 1 pkg., except as noted:							
and beef:							
(*Banquet* Bake at Home), 8-oz. cup	230	13.0	31.0	7.0	25	810	3.0
(*Kid Cuisine* Rip-Roaring)	370	12.0	58.0	15.0	20	770	5.0
(*Lean Cuisine*) . . .	280	13.0	40.0	8.0	25	550	3.0
(*Marie Callender's*)	310	12.0	40.0	11.0	15	680	5.0
(*Nalley*)	250	10.0	22.0	14.0	50	920	4.0
(*Stouffer's*)	420	20.0	40	20.0	50	1530	5.0
(*Weight Watchers*)	220	13.0	32.0	4.5	15	560	4.0
casserole (*Healthy Choice*)	200	14.0	34.0	10.0	15	450	5.0
casserole (*Swanson*)	270	8.0	39.0	5.0	35	1060	2.0
broccoli (*Swanson Mac & More*) . . .	220	12.0	28.0	8.0	20	760	2.0

Food and Measure	cal.	prot. (gms)	carbo. (gms)	fat (gms)	chol. (mgs)	sod. (mgs)	fiber (gms)
Macaroni entree, frozen *(cont.)*							
and cheese:							
(*Amy's*)	450	22.0	58.0	9.0	n.a.	430	n.a.
(*Banquet*)	350	13.0	47.0	12.0	20	960	5.0
(*Banquet* Bake at							
Home), 8 oz. . .	300	14.0	39.0	10.0	25	1190	2.0
(*Banquet* Family),							
1 cup	210	8.0	33.0	5.0	10	1290	4.0
(*The Budget Gour-*							
met Homestyle)	400	17.0	38.0	20.0	45	1320	4.0
(*The Budget Gour-*							
met Side Dish),							
6 oz.	270	11.0	27.0	13.0	40	600	1.0
(*Healthy Choice*) . .	290	15.0	45.0	4.0	20	470	6.0
(*Kid Cuisine* Magi-							
cal)	420	10.0	68.0	12.0	25	920	3.0
(*Lean Cuisine*) . . .	270	13.0	39.0	7.0	20	550	2.0
(*Marie Callender's*)	420	20.0	47.0	17.0	40	1410	3.0
(*Morton*)	200	7.0	35.0	3.0	10	600	2.0
(*Morton* 16/28 oz.),							
1 cup	230	9.0	40.0	4.0	5	1000	3.0
(*Stouffer's*), ½ of							
12-oz. pkg. . . .	330	14.0	31.0	17.0	30	940	2.0
(*Stouffer's*), ⅕ of							
40-oz. pkg. . . .	310	13.0	29.0	16.0	30	970	2.0
(*Swanson* Entree)	280	15.0	36.0	10.0	20	1050	2.0
(*Swanson* Entree),							
1 cup	260	14.0	34.0	9.0	20	990	2.0
(*Swanson Mac &*							
More Classic) . .	240	14.0	30.0	9.0	20	800	2.0
(*Tabatchnik* Side							
Dish)	280	14.0	30.0	12.0	26	840	2.0
(*Weight Watchers*)	280	13.0	42.0	7.0	25	590	4.0
bake casserole,							
3-cheese (*Swan-*							
son)	400	22.0	53.0	14.0	20	1580	3.0
and broccoli (*Lean*							
Cuisine Lunch Ex-							
press)	240	12.0	35.0	6.0	15	460	5.0

Food and Measure	cal.	prot. (gms)	carbo. (gms)	fat (gms)	chol. (mgs)	sod. (mgs)	fiber (gms)
w/cheddar and Parmesan (*The Budget Gourmet* Light & Healthy)	340	8.0	48.0	8.0	25	760	2.0
cheddar, white (*Swanson Mac & More*)	200	11.0	27.0	7.0	10	790	2.0
pie (*Banquet*) . . .	200	7.0	35.0	3.0	10	600	2.0
salsa (*Swanson Mac & More*)	210	12.0	27.0	8.0	15	870	2.0
Italiano (*Swanson Mac & More*) . . .	180	8.0	25.0	5.0	15	480	2.0
soy cheeze (*Amy's*)	360	16.0	42.0	14.0	0	500	4.0
Macaroni entree mix, dry, except as noted:							
and cheese:							
(*Creamette*), ⅓ pkg.	250	9.0	48.0	2.0	<5	640	2.0
(*Kraft* Original Dinner), 2½ oz. . . .	260	11.0	47.0	2.5	10	560	1.0
(*Kraft* Original Deluxe Dinner), 3½ oz.	320	14.0	44.0	10.0	25	730	1.0
(*Kraft Thick'n Creamy*), 2½ oz.	260	11.0	48.0	2.5	10	560	2.0
Alfredo (*Annie's*), ½ cup	200	8.0	33.0	3.5	10	270	1.0
all varieties, except original and white cheddar (*Kraft* Dinner), 2½ oz.	260	12.0	47.0	3.0	10	600	1.0
cheddar (*Golden Grain*), 1 cup* . .	340	8.0	40.0	17.0	5	680	2.0
cheddar, white, mild (*Kraft* Dinner), 2½ oz.	260	11.0	47.0	3.0	10	560	1.0
cheddar or Parmesan (*Fantastic*), ⅜ cup	200	8.0	40.0	1.5	0	550	5.0

Food and Measure	cal.	prot. (gms)	carbo. (gms)	fat (gms)	chol. (mgs)	sod. (mgs)	fiber (gms)
Macaroni entree mix, and cheese *(cont.)*							
rotini, w/broccoli							
(*Velveeta*), 4½ oz.	400	18.0	46.0	16.0	45	1240	2.0
shells (*Velveeta*							
Original), 4 oz.	360	16.0	44.0	13.0	40	1030	1.0
shells, w/bacon							
(*Velveeta*), 4 oz.	360	17.0	43.0	14.0	40	1140	1.0
shells, w/salsa							
(*Velveeta* Origi-							
nal), 4 oz.	380	17.0	47.0	14.0	40	1180	2.0
three cheese (*Knorr*							
Cup), 1 pkg. . . .	240	8.0	40.0	5.0	15	810	2.0
Macaroni and							
cheese, see "Maca-							
roni dinner" and							
"Macaroni entree"							
Mace, ground:							
1 tsp.	8	.1	.9	.6	0	1	.1
(*McCormick*), ¼ tsp.	2	0	.2	.1	0	<1	.1
Mackerel, meat only:							
Atlantic:							
raw, 4 oz.	232	21.1	0	15.8	80	102	0
baked, broiled, or							
microwaved, 4 oz.	297	27.0	0	20.2	85	94	0
king:							
raw, 4 oz.	119	23.0	0	2.3	61	179	0
baked, broiled, or							
microwaved, 4 oz.	152	29.5	0	2.9	77	230	0
Pacific and jack:							
raw, 4 oz.	179	22.8	0	9.0	53	98	0
baked, broiled, or							
microwaved, 4 oz.	228	29.2	0	11.5	68	125	0
Spanish:							
raw, 4 oz.	158	21.9	0	7.2	86	67	0
baked, broiled, or							
microwaved, 4 oz.	179	26.8	0	7.2	83	75	0
smoked (*Spence &*							
Co.), 2 oz.	180	13.0	0	15.0	30	840	0

Food and Measure	cal.	prot. (gms)	carbo. (gms)	fat (gms)	chol. (mgs)	sod. (mgs)	fiber (gms)
Mackerel, canned, boneless, drained:							
jack, 4 oz.	177	26.3	0	7.1	90	430	0
skinless (*Reese*), 4.375-oz. can . . .	240	20.0	0	18.0	40	470	0
Madras sauce, see "Curry sauce"							
Mahi mahi:							
fresh, see "Dolphinfish"							
frozen, fillet (*Peter Pan*), 4 oz.	100	24.0	0	.5	50	280	0
Mai tai drink mixer, bottled (*Mr. & Mrs. "T"*), 4.5 fl. oz. . .	140	0	33.0	0	0	65	0
Malt beverage (*Goya*), 12 fl. oz.	280	1.0	39.0	0	0	80	0
Malt cooler (*Bartles & Jaymes*), 12-oz. bottle:							
berry	210	0	33.0	0	0	5	0
black cherry	200	0	32.0	0	0	5	0
Fuzzy Navel	230	0	39.0	0	0	5	0
iced tea, Long Island	250	0	43.0	0	0	20	0
Mai Tai	240	0	40.0	0	0	5	0
margarita	260	0	46.0	0	0	40	0
original	190	0	29.0	0	0	0	0
peach	210	0	33.0	0	0	5	0
piña colada	270	0	48.0	0	0	5	0
sangria, red	200	0	31.0	0	0	5	0
strawberry	210	0	33.0	0	0	5	0
strawberry daiquiri	220	0	36.0	0	0	5	0
tropical	230	0	37.0	0	0	5	0
Malted milk powder, 3 tbsp.:							
natural:							
(*Kraft*)	80	1.0	17.0	1.0	0	40	<1.0
(*Nestlé* Original) . .	90	3.0	15.0	2.0	5	85	<1.0

Food and Measure	cal.	prot. (gms)	carbo. (gms)	fat (gms)	chol. (mgs)	sod. (mgs)	fiber (gms)
Malted milk powder *(cont.)*							
chocolate:							
(*Kraft*)	90	3.0	15.0	2.0	5	85	0
(*Nestlé*)	90	1.0	18.0	1.0	0	40	<1.0
Mammy apple:							
fresh, peeled, seeded,							
1 oz.	14	.1	3.5	.1	0	4	.9
frozen, chunks							
(*Goya*), ⅓ pkg. . .	140	2.0	32.0	0	0	10	10.0
Mandioca, see							
"Yuca"							
Mango:							
fresh:							
10.6-oz. fruit	135	1.1	35.2	.6	0	4	3.7
peeled (*Frieda's*),							
1 oz.	19	.2	4.8	.1	0	2	n.a.
peeled, sliced,							
½ cup	54	.4	14.0	.2	0	2	1.5
dried (*Sonoma*), 2 oz.	180	0	44.0	1.0	0	50	0
frozen, chunks							
(*Goya*), ⅓ pkg. . .	100	1.0	24.0	0	0	10	2.0
Mango drink,							
8 fl. oz.:							
(*Snapple* Madness)	110	0	29.0	0	0	10	0
(*Snapple* Madness							
Diet)	20	0	5.0	0	0	10	0
(*Tree Top* More							
Mango)	120	0	29.0	0	0	25	0
tangerine (*Veryfine*)	110	0	27.0	0	0	5	0
Mango juice,							
8 fl. oz.:							
(*After the Fall* Mon-							
tage)	110	1.0	27.0	0	0	10	0
peach (*R.W. Knudsen*)	120	0	30.0	0	0	50	0
Mango nectar:							
(*Goya*), 12 fl. oz. . .	230	0	56.0	0	0	15	2.0
(*Libby's/Kern's*),							
8 fl. oz.	150	0	36.0	0	0	5	0

Food and Measure	cal.	prot. (gms)	carbo. (gms)	fat (gms)	chol. (mgs)	sod. (mgs)	fiber (gms)
orange (*Kern's*),							
8 fl. oz.	140	0	35.0	0	0	10	0
Manhattan mixer,							
bottled (*Holland*							
House/Mr. & Mrs.							
"T"), 2 fl. oz. . . .	60	0	15.0	0	0	10	0
Manicotti, frozen,							
2 pcs.:							
(*Celentano*), 7 oz. . .	410	20.0	40.0	19.0	100	630	7.0
mini (*Celentano*),							
4.8 oz.	110	17.0	32.0	12.0	66	500	n.a.
Manicotti entree, fro-							
zen, 1 pkg., except							
as noted:							
cheese:							
(*Celentano*)	450	24.0	41.0	21.0	85	910	9.0
(*Celentano*), ½ of							
14-oz. pkg. . . .	310	17.0	27.0	15.0	75	670	6.0
(*Celentano* Great							
Choice)	250	16.0	41.0	2.5	20	650	3.0
(*Celentano* Value							
Pack), 2 pcs.,							
8 oz.	320	17.0	28.0	15.0	75	690	6.0
(*Stouffer's*)	340	18.0	32.0	16.0	50	810	7.0
(*Weight Watchers*)	260	17.0	31.0	7.0	30	570	5.0
w/meat sauce (*The*							
Budget Gourmet)	420	18.0	38.0	22.0	85	810	4.0
three cheese							
(*Healthy Choice*)	310	16.0	41.0	9.0	20	450	7.0
Florentine:							
(*Celentano*)	220	13.0	28.0	6.0	0	660	4.0
(*Celentano* Great							
Choice)	230	15.0	29.0	6.0	35	600	5.0
Manioc, see "Yuca"							

Food and Measure	cal.	prot. (gms)	carbo. (gms)	fat (gms)	chol. (mgs)	sod. (mgs)	fiber (gms)
Maple syrup (see also "Pancake syrup") (*Cary's/Maple Orchard's/Mac-Donald's* Pure), ¼ cup	210	0	52.0	0	0	15	0
Margarine, 1 tbsp.:							
(*Mazola*)	100	0	0	11.0	0	100	0
(*Mazola* Light)	50	0	0	6.0	0	130	0
(*Mazola* Unsalted) . .	100	0	0	11.0	0	0	0
(*Nucoa*)	100	0	0	11.0	0	160	0
(*Smart Beat* Nonfat)	10	0	1.0	0	0	90	0
(*Smart Beat* Super Light/Trans Fat Free)	20	0	0	2.0	0	105	0
(*Smart Beat* Unsalted)	25	0	0	2.5	0	0	0
blend, see "spread," below							
soft:							
(*Chiffon* Tub) . . .	100	0	0	11.0	0	105	0
(*Parkay* Tub)	100	0	0	11.0	0	105	0
(*Parkay* Diet Tub)	50	0	0	6.0	0	110	0
spread:							
(*Kraft* Touch of Butter Stick)	90	0	0	10.0	0	110	0
(*Kraft* Touch of Butter Tub)	60	0	0	7.0	0	110	0
(*Mazola* Light) . . .	50	0	0	6.0	0	100	0
(*Parkay* Stick 53%)	70	0	0	7.0	0	120	0
(*Parkay* Stick 70%)	90	0	0	10.0	0	110	0
(*Parkay* Tub 50%)	60	0	0	7.0	0	110	0
(*Parkay Light* Tub 40%)	50	0	0	6.0	0	120	0
squeeze:							
(*Kraft Touch O Butter*)	80	0	0	9.0	0	115	0
(*Parkay*)	80	0	0	9.0	0	120	0
(*Smart Beat Smart Squeeze*)	5	0	1.0	0	0	100	0

Food and Measure	cal.	prot. (gms)	carbo. (gms)	fat (gms)	chol. (mgs)	sod. (mgs)	fiber (gms)
whipped:							
(*Chiffon* Tub) . . .	70	0	0	7.0	0	70	0
(*Parkay* Tub)	70	0	0	7.0	0	70	0
Margarita mixer:							
bottled:							
(*Holland House/Mr. & Mrs. "T"*),							
4 fl. oz.	130	0	29.0	0	0	40	0
strawberry (*Holland House/Mr. & Mrs. "T"*), 3.5 fl. oz.	150	0	34.0	0	0	20	0
frozen* (*Bacardi*),							
8 fl. oz.	90	0	25.0	0	0	0	0
mix (*Bar-Tenders*),							
2 pkts., .9 oz. . . .	90	0	21.0	0	0	70	0
Marinade (see also "Stir-fry sauce" and specific listings), 1 tbsp., except as noted:							
(*House of Tsang* Classic), ½ tbsp.	15	0	4.0	0	0	350	0
(*House of Tsang* Mandarin)	25	0	6.0	0	0	680	0
Hawaiian (*Lawry's*)	20	0	4.0	0	0	250	0
lemon butter dill, seafood (*Ken's Steak House*)	50	0	3.0	4.5	0	95	0
lemon pepper (*Lawry's*)	10	0	1.0	.5	0	380	0
red wine (*Lawry's*)	5	0	1.0	0	0	270	0
and stir-fry sauce (*Mary Rose* Sari)	5	0	1.0	0	0	440	0
Marinade seasoning mix, meat (*Lawry's* Carne Asada), 1 tsp.	5	0	1.0	0	0	590	0
Marjoram, dried:							
1 tsp.	2	.1	.4	<.1	0	<1	.1
(*McCormick*), ¼ tsp.	1	0	.2	0	0	<1	.1

Food and Measure	cal.	prot. (gms)	carbo. (gms)	fat (gms)	chol. (mgs)	sod. (mgs)	fiber (gms)
Marmalade, see "Jam and pre- serves"							
Marrow squash, raw, trimmed, 1 oz. . . .	4	.2	1.0	<.1	0	n.a.	<1.0
Marshmallow top- ping, 2 tbsp.:							
(*Smucker's*)	120	0	29.0	0	0	0	0
creme (*Kraft*)	40	0	10.0	0	0	10	0
all varieties (*Marsh- mallow Fluff*)	60	0	5.0	0	0	20	0
Masa, see "Corn- meal"							
Matzo, see "Crack- ers"							
Mayonnaise, 1 tbsp.:							
(*Best Foods* Real) . .	100	0	0	11.0	5	90	0
(*Blue Plate*)	100	0	0	11.0	10	80	0
(*Hellmann's* Real) . .	100	0	0	11.0	5	80	0
(*Hellmann's/Best Foods* Light)	50	0	1.0	5.0	5	115	0
(*Hellmann's/Best Foods* Low Fat) . .	25	0	4.0	1.0	0	140	0
(*Kraft* Real)	100	0	0	11.0	10	75	0
(*Master Choice*) . . .	100	0	0	2.0	5	80	0
(*Nalley* Real)	100	0	0	11.0	5	85	0
(*Nalley* Light)	50	0	5.0	10.0	10	100	0
(*Smart Beat Super Light* Reduced Fat)	35	0	2.0	3.0	0	110	0
(*Weight Watchers* Light)	25	0	1.0	2.0	5	130	0
(*Weight Watchers* Light Low Sodium)	25	0	1.0	2.0	5	40	0
canola (*Smart Beat* Reduced Fat) . . .	35	0	2.0	3.0	0	110	0
dressing:							
(*Kraft Free*)	10	0	2.0	0	0	105	0
(*Kraft Light*)	50	0	1.0	5.0	0	110	0

Food and Measure	cal.	prot. (gms)	carbo. (gms)	fat (gms)	chol. (mgs)	sod. (mgs)	fiber (gms)
(*Miracle Whip* Salad)	70	0	2.0	7.0	5	85	0
(*Miracle Whip Free*)	15	0	3.0	0	0	120	0
(*Miracle Whip* Light)	40	0	3.0	3.0	0	120	0
(*Smart Beat* Nonfat)	10	0	3.0	0	0	135	0
(*Spin Blend*)	60	0	3.0	5.0	5	110	0
(*Spin Blend* Nonfat)	15	0	3.0	0	0	110	0
(*Weight Watchers* Nonfat)	10	0	3.0	0	0	105	0
whipped (*Weight Watchers* Nonfat)	15	0	3.0	0	0	95	0
tofu (*Nayonaise*) . . .	35	0	1.0	3.0	0	105	0
McDonald's, 1 serving:							
breakfast biscuit:							
plain	260	4.0	32.0	13.0	0	840	1.0
bacon, egg, and cheese	440	17.0	33.0	26.0	235	1310	1.0
sausage	430	10.0	32.0	29.0	35	1130	1.0
sausage and egg	520	16.0	33.0	35.0	245	1220	1.0
breakfast burrito . . .	320	13.0	23.0	20.0	195	600	1.0
breakfast dishes:							
eggs, scrambled, 2	170	13.0	1.0	12.0	425	190	0
hash browns	130	1.0	14.0	8.0	0	330	1.0
hotcakes:							
plain	310	9.0	53.0	7.0	15	610	2.0
w/syrup, margarine	580	9.0	100.0	16.0	15	760	2.0
sausage	170	6.0	0	16.0	35	290	0
breakfast muffin:							
English	140	4.0	25.0	2.0	0	220	1.0
Egg McMuffin . . .	290	17.0	27.0	13.0	235	730	1.0
Sausage McMuffin	360	13.0	26.0	23.0	45	750	1.0
Sausage McMuffin, w/egg	440	19.0	27.0	29.0	255	820	1.0
danish and muffin:							
apple bran muffin	170	4.0	38.0	0	0	200	1.0
apple danish	360	5.0	51.0	16.0	40	290	1.0

Food and Measure	cal.	prot. (gms)	carbo. (gms)	fat (gms)	chol. (mgs)	sod. (mgs)	fiber (gms)
McDonald's, danish and muffin (cont.)							
cheese danish . . .	410	7.0	47.0	22.0	70	340	0
cinnamon raisin danish	430	5.0	56.0	22.0	50	280	1.0
cinnamon roll . . .	400	7.0	47.0	20.0	75	340	2.0
raspberry danish	400	5.0	58.0	16.0	45	300	1.0
sandwiches:							
Arch Deluxe	570	29.0	43.0	31.0	90	1110	4.0
Arch Deluxe, w/bacon	610	33.0	43.0	34.0	100	1250	4.0
Big Mac	530	25.0	47.0	28.0	80	880	3.0
cheeseburger . . .	320	15.0	35.0	14.0	45	770	2.0
Filet-O-Fish	360	14.0	40.0	16.0	35	690	2.0
hamburger	270	12.0	34.0	10.0	30	530	2.0
McChicken	510	17.0	44.0	30.0	50	820	2.0
McGrilled Chicken Classic	260	24.0	33.0	4.0	45	500	2.0
Quarter Pounder . .	430	23.0	37.0	21.0	70	730	2.0
Quarter Pounder, w/cheese	530	28.0	38.0	30.0	95	1160	2.0
Chicken McNuggets:							
4 pcs.	190	12.0	10.0	11.0	40	340	0
6 pcs.	290	18.0	15.0	17.0	60	510	0
9 pcs.	430	27.0	23.0	26.0	90	770	0
McNuggets sauce pkt.:							
barbecue	45	0	10.0	0	0	250	0
honey	45	0	12.0	0	0	0	0
honey mustard . .	50	0	3.0	4.5	10	85	0
hot mustard	60	1.0	7.0	3.5	5	240	<1.0
sweet and sour . .	50	0	11.0	0	0	140	0
french fries:							
small	210	3.0	26.0	10.0	0	135	2.0
large	450	6.0	57.0	22.0	0	290	5.0
Super Size	540	8.0	68.0	26.0	0	350	6.0
salads:							
chicken, fajita . . .	160	20.0	9.0	6.0	65	400	3.0
garden	80	6.0	7.0	4.0	140	60	2.0

Food and Measure	cal.	prot. (gms)	carbo. (gms)	fat (gms)	chol. (mgs)	sod. (mgs)	fiber (gms)
salad bacon bits,							
1 pkg.	15	1.0	0	1.0	5	90	0
salad croutons, 1 pkg.	50	1.0	7.0	1.5	0	125	0
salad dressing,							
1 pkg.:							
blue cheese	190	2.0	8.0	17.0	30	650	0
ranch	230	1.0	10.0	21.0	20	550	0
red French, reduced							
calorie	160	0	23.0	8.0	0	490	0
Thousand Island . .	190	1.0	16.0	13.0	25	510	1.0
vinaigrette, lite . . .	50	0	9.0	2.0	0	240	0
desserts and shakes:							
baked apple pie . .	260	3.0	34.0	13.0	0	200	<1.0
McDonaldland Cook-							
ies, 1 pkg.	260	4.0	41.0	9.0	0	270	1.0
shake, small:							
chocolate	340	12.0	64.0	5.0	25	300	1.0
strawberry . . .	340	12.0	63.0	5.0	25	220	0
vanilla	340	11.0	62.0	5.0	25	220	0
sundae, hot fudge	290	8.0	53.0	5.0	5	240	2.0
sundae nuts, 1/4 oz.	40	2.0	2.0	3.5	0	0	0
yogurt, frozen,							
lowfat:							
cone, vanilla . .	120	4.0	24.0	.5	5	115	0
hot caramel sun-							
dae	310	7.0	62.0	3.0	5	250	<1.0
strawberry sun-							
dae	240	6.0	51.0	1.0	5	170	<1.0
Meat, see specific							
listings							
Meat, canned (see							
also "Meat							
spread"):							
potted (*Goya*), 1/4 cup	60	8.0	0	6.0	60	600	0
potted (*Hormel*), 2 oz.	100	7.0	1.0	7.0	50	580	0
potted or deviled							
(*Libby's*), 3 oz. . .	160	11.0	0	13.0	90	620	0

Food and Measure	cal.	prot. (gms)	carbo. (gms)	fat (gms)	chol. (mgs)	sod. (mgs)	fiber (gms)
"Meat," ground, frozen (*Morningstar Farms* Ground Meatless), ½ cup	60	10.0	4.0	0	0	260	2.0
Meat, lunch, see "Lunch meat" and specific listings							
Meat, potted, see "Meat, canned"							
Meat loaf dinner, frozen, 1 pkg.:							
(*Banquet*)	650	29.0	49.0	38.0	85	2140	10.0
(*Healthy Choice*) . . .	320	16.0	46.0	8.0	35	460	7.0
(*Marie Callender's*)	540	23.0	44.0	30.0	80	1230	7.0
(*Swanson*)	380	25.0	44.0	16.0	35	1160	5.0
(*Swanson* Budget) . .	330	29.0	29.0	19.0	25	970	4.0
(*Swanson Hungry Man*)	610	43.0	65.0	28.0	45	1950	6.0
Meat loaf entree, frozen, 1 pkg.:							
(*Banquet* Homestyle)	280	12.0	23.0	17.0	40	1100	4.0
w/whipped potato: (*Lean Cuisine*) . . .	250	22.0	25.0	7.0	45	570	5.0
(*Stouffer's* Homestyle)	390	20.0	24.0	24.0	80	910	3.0
tomato sauce w/ (*Morton*)	250	9.0	24.0	13.0	20	1110	5.0
w/sauce and vegetables (*Swanson*) . .	260	18.0	20.0	12.0	50	860	7.0
"Meat" loaf mix, vegetarian (*Natural Touch*), ¼ cup	100	14.0	10.0	.5	0	700	7.0
Meat loaf seasoning mix:							
(*Durkee* Pouch), ⅑ pkt.	20	.5	3.0	0	0	360	0
(*Durkee/French's* Roasting Bag), ⅛ pkg.	15	2.0	2.0	0	0	500	0

Food and Measure	cal.	prot. (gms)	carbo. (gms)	fat (gms)	chol. (mgs)	sod. (mgs)	fiber (gms)
(*Lawry's*), 1 tbsp. . .	35	<1.0	7.0	0	0	430	0
Meat seasoning (*Aromat*), ¼ tsp.	0	0	0	0	0	230	0
Meat spread (see also specific listings), (*Oscar Mayer* Sandwich Spread), 2 oz.	130	4.0	8.0	10.0	25	460	0
Meat tenderizer, unseasoned (*Tone's*), 1 tsp.	7	0	1.2	.2	0	1760	tr.
Meat turnover, see "Empanadilla"							
"Meatball," vegetarian, w/gravy, canned (*Loma Linda Tender Rounds*), 6 pcs.	120	14.0	5.0	5.0	0	330	3.0
Meatball entree, frozen, 1 pkg.:							
kofta curry (*Deep*) . .	245	6.0	20.0	16.0	17	600	3.0
and spaghetti, see "Spaghetti entree"							
Swedish:							
(*The Budget Gourmet*)	550	22.0	40.0	34.0	150	1050	3.0
(*Healthy Choice*) . .	320	22.0	37.0	9.0	65	600	5.0
(*Stouffer's*)	440	23.0	36.0	23.0	85	840	3.0
(*Weight Watchers*)	280	18.0	34.0	8.0	30	510	3.0
w/broccoli (*Stouffer's Lunch Express*)	360	15.0	32.0	19.0	30	900	3.0
w/pasta (*Lean Cuisine*)	290	22.0	32.0	8.0	55	590	3.0
w/pasta (*Stouffer's Lunch Express*)	530	19.0	41.0	32.0	65	1010	3.0
Meatball seasoning mix, Italian (*Durkee* Pouch), ⅕ pkt. . .	20	1.0	3.0	0	0	360	0

Food and Measure	cal.	prot. (gms)	carbo. (gms)	fat (gms)	chol. (mgs)	sod. (mgs)	fiber (gms)
Meatball stew, canned:							
(*Dinty Moore*), 1 cup	270	13.0	18.0	16.0	35	1110	3.0
(*Dinty Moore* Cup), 7.5 oz.	250	12.0	16.0	15.0	30	990	2.0
Melon balls, frozen:							
(*Stilwell*), 1 cup . . .	50	1.0	14.0	0	0	15	.5
cantaloupe/honeydew, ½ cup	28	.7	6.9	.2	0	27	.6
Melon drink blend (*Tree Top* Wonder Melon), 8 fl. oz. . . .	120	0	30.0	0	0	25	0
Melonberry juice cocktail (*Snapple*), 8 fl. oz.	120	0	29.0	0	0	10	0
Menudo, canned (*Goya*), 1 cup . . .	200	14.0	12.0	9.0	0	1250	2.0
Menudo seasoning mix (*Gebhardt*), ¼ tsp.	0	0	0	0	0	45	0
Mesquite sauce (*S&W*), 1 tbsp. . . .	10	0	3.0	0	0	400	0
Mesquite seasoning butter (*Tone's*), ¼ tsp.	0	0	0	0	0	125	0
Mexican beans (see also "Chili beans"), canned, ½ cup:							
(*Allens/Brown Beauty*)	120	7.0	21.0	1.0	0	300	8.0
(*Chi-Chi's* Ranchero)	100	6.0	18.0	.5	0	540	3.0
(*Green Giant/Joan of Arc*)	120	6.0	21.0	1.5	0	530	5.0
(*Old El Paso* Mexe Beans)	110	7.0	19.0	.5	0	630	7.0
(*Stokely* Red)	110	7.0	21.0	.5	0	600	6.0
w/jalapeños:							
(*Brown Beauty*) . .	120	7.0	21.0	1.0	0	370	7.0
(*Trappey's* Mexi-Beans)	130	7.0	22.0	1.5	0	460	8.0

Food and Measure	cal.	prot. (gms)	carbo. (gms)	fat (gms)	chol. (mgs)	sod. (mgs)	fiber (gms)
Mexican dinner (see also specific listings), frozen, 1 pkg.:							
(*Patio*)	430	15.0	59.0	15.0	20	1840	13.0
(*Patio* Fiesta)	340	13.0	51.0	9.0	15	1760	11.0
(*Patio* Ranchera) . . .	410	13.0	55.0	15.0	25	2400	14.0
style:							
(*Banquet*)	820	28.0	100.0	34.0	50	2060	20.0
(*Swanson* Budget)	400	25.0	52.0	16.0	20	1350	7.0
(*Swanson* Hungry Man)	780	55.0	86.0	36.0	60	2120	12.0
combination (*Swanson*)	470	28.0	57.0	18.0	20	1620	8.0
Mexican entree (see also specific listings), frozen, 1 pkg.:							
(*Banquet*)	400	14.0	56.0	13.0	15	1520	10.0
combination (*Banquet*)	380	15.0	55.0	11.0	15	1370	9.0
Mexican seasoning:							
(*Chi-Chi's* Mix), 1 tsp.	10	0	1.0	0	0	290	0
(*Tone's*), 1 tsp. . . .	6	.3	1.3	.1	tr.	4185	.4
w/coriander (*Goya* Sazon), ¼ tsp. . . .	0	0	0	0	0	170	0
w/saffron (*Goya* Sazon), ¼ tsp. . . .	0	0	0	0	0	150	0
Milk, 8 fl. oz.:							
buttermilk, cultured	99	8.1	11.7	2.2	9	257	0
whole, 3.3% fat . . .	150	8.0	11.4	8.2	33	120	0
lowfat:							
2% fat	121	8.1	11.7	4.7	18	122	0
2%, protein fortified	137	9.7	13.5	4.9	19	145	0
1% fat	102	8.0	11.7	2.6	10	123	0
1%, protein fortified	119	9.7	13.6	2.9	10	143	0
skim	86	8.4	11.9	.4	4	126	0

Food and Measure	cal.	prot. (gms)	carbo. (gms)	fat (gms)	chol. (mgs)	sod. (mgs)	fiber (gms)
Milk, canned,							
2 tbsp.:							
condensed, sweet-							
ened:							
(*Borden*)	130	3.0	23.0	3.0	10	40	0
(*Carnation*)	130	3.0	22.0	3.0	10	45	0
(*Eagle/Magnolia*							
Brand/Meadow							
Gold/Star)	130	3.0	23.0	3.0	10	40	0
(*Goya*)	130	3.0	22.0	3.0	5	45	0
lowfat (*Borden*) . .	120	3.0	23.0	1.5	5	40	0
lowfat (*Eagle*) . . .	120	3.0	23.0	1.5	5	40	0
skim (*Borden* Fat							
Free)	110	3.0	24.0	0	0	40	0
skim (*Eagle* Fat							
Free)	110	3.0	24.0	0	<5	40	0
evaporated:							
(*Carnation*)	40	2.0	3.0	2.5	10	35	0
(*Pet*)	40	2.0	3.0	2.0	5	30	0
lowfat (*Carnation*)	25	2.0	3.0	.5	5	35	0
skim (*Carnation*) . .	25	2.0	4.0	0	0	40	0
skim (*Pet*)	25	2.0	3.0	0	<5	35	0
Milk, chocolate, see							
"Chocolate milk"							
Milk, dry:							
buttermilk:							
sweet cream, 1 cup	464	41.2	58.8	6.9	83	621	0
sweet cream,							
1 tbsp.	25	2.2	3.2	.4	5	34	0
whole, 1 oz.	141	7.5	10.9	7.6	27	105	0
whole, 1 cup	635	33.7	49.2	34.2	124	475	0
nonfat:							
regular, 1 cup . . .	435	43.4	62.4	.9	24	642	0
instant, 3.2-oz. pkt.	244	23.9	35.5	.5	12	373	0
(*Carnation*), ⅓ cup	80	8.0	12.0	0	<5	125	0
Milk, goat's, 1 cup	168	8.7	10.9	10.1	28	122	0

Food and Measure	cal.	prot. (gms)	carbo. (gms)	fat (gms)	chol. (mgs)	sod. (mgs)	fiber (gms)
"Milk," nondairy (see also "Soy beverage"), 8 fl. oz.:							
(*EdenBlend*)	120	7.0	16.0	3.0	0	85	0
(*EdenRice*)	110	1.0	21.0	3.0	0	85	0
(*Rice Dream* Original)	120	1.0	25.0	2.0	0	90	0
chocolate (*Rice Dream*)	160	1.0	35.0	2.5	0	100	0
vanilla (*Rice Dream*)	130	1.0	28.0	2.0	0	90	0
Milk, sheep's, 1 cup	264	14.7	13.1	17.2	n.a.	108	0
Milk beverage, flavored (see also specific flavors):							
Butterfinger (*Nestlé Quik*), 8 fl. oz. . . .	200	8.0	30.0	5.0	20	120	1.0
shake, root beer (*Nestlé Killer*), 14 oz. . .	460	13.0	67.0	15.0	70	220	4.0
Milkfish, meat only:							
raw, 4 oz.	168	23.3	0	7.6	59	n.a.	0
baked, broiled, or microwaved, 4 oz. . .	215	29.8	0	9.8	76	n.a.	0
Milkshake, see "Milk beverage, flavored" and specific flavors							
Millet:							
raw, 1 oz.	107	3.1	20.7	1.2	0	1	2.4
cooked, 4 oz.	135	4.0	26.8	1.1	0	2	1.5
hulled (*Arrowhead Mills*), ¼ cup . . .	150	5.0	34.0	1.5	0	0	3.0
Millet flour (*Arrowhead Mills*), ¼ cup	110	4.0	26.0	1.0	0	0	2.0
Mincemeat, see "Pie filling"							
Mint sauce (*Crosse & Blackwell*), 1 tsp.	5	0	1.0	0	0	0	0
Miso, soy:							
1 oz.	58	3.3	7.9	1.7	0	1034	1.5
½ cup	284	16.3	38.6	8.4	0	5032	7.6
(*Eden* Hacho), 1 tbsp.	35	3.0	2.0	1.5	0	600	1.0

Food and Measure	cal.	prot. (gms)	carbo. (gms)	fat (gms)	chol. (mgs)	sod. (mgs)	fiber (gms)
Miso *(cont.)*							
w/barley (*Eden* Organic Mugi), 1 tbsp.	25	2.0	3.0	1.0	0	760	1.0
w/rice, 1 tbsp.:							
(*Eden* Kome)	25	2.0	3.0	1.0	0	850	<1.0
brown (*Eden* Genmai)	25	2.0	3.0	1.0	0	810	<1.0
white (*Eden* Shiro)	35	2.0	5.0	1.0	0	410	1.0
Mocha drink:							
chilled (*Nestlé Mocha Cooler*), 1 cup . . .	170	7.0	25.0	4.0	15	150	0
canned, cafe (*Carnation Instant Breakfast*), 10 fl. oz. . .	220	12.0	35.0	2.5	5	230	1.0
mix, see "Coffee, flavored, mix"							
Molasses, 1 tbsp.:							
(*Grandma's* 4-Star)	50	0	14.0	0	0	0	0
bead (*La Choy*) . . .	50	0	12.0	0	0	50	0
blackstrap (*New Morning*)	60	<1.0	13.0	0	0	20	0
dark or light (*Br'er Rabbit*)	60	0	14.0	0	0	15	0
gold (*Grandma's*) . .	50	0	14.0	0	0	0	0
green (*Grandma's*)	50	0	12.0	0	0	10	0
Monkfish, meat only:							
raw, 4 oz.	86	16.4	0	1.7	29	21	0
baked, broiled, or microwaved, 4 oz. . .	110	21.0	0	2.2	36	26	0
Monosodium glutamate (*Tone's*), 1 tsp.	0	0	0	0	0	638	0
Mortadella, 2 oz.:							
(*Boar's Head Cinghiale*)	160	9.0	0	14.0	30	560	0
w/pistachios (*Boar's Head Cinghiale*) . .	170	9.0	3.0	14.0	30	560	0
Mothbean, boiled, 4 oz.	133	8.9	23.8	.6	0	11	n.a.

Food and Measure	cal.	prot. (gms)	carbo. (gms)	fat (gms)	chol. (mgs)	sod. (mgs)	fiber (gms)
Mother's loaf, pork,							
1 oz.	80	3.4	2.1	6.3	13	320	0
Mousse, see "Pudding mix"							
Muffin, 1 pc., except as noted:							
(*Arnold Bran'nola*) . .	130	6.0	29.0	1.5	0	160	3.0
(*Arnold* Extra Crisp)	120	4.0	25.0	1.0	0	190	1.0
almond poppyseed (*Aunt Fanny's*),							
2 pcs.	310	3.0	45.0	13.0	15	250	1.0
apple:							
(*Awrey's*), 1½ oz.	130	2.0	18.0	6.0	20	220	0
(*Awrey's*), 2½ oz.	250	2.0	28.0	14.0	55	100	0
bran (*Aunt Fanny's*),							
2 pcs.	290	4.0	45.0	11.0	15	220	2.0
banana nut:							
(*Aunt Fanny's*),							
2 pcs.	320	4.0	44.0	14.0	15	240	1.0
(*Awrey's* Grande)	400	7.0	46.0	22.0	90	440	2.0
(*Tastykake*), ½ pc.,							
2 oz.	120	4.0	26.0	13.0	35	220	1.0
(*Tastykake* Family)	220	3.0	33.0	6.0	5	210	1.0
mini (*Hostess*),							
5 pcs.	260	3.0	28.0	16.0	40	160	<1.0
blueberry:							
(*Aunt Fanny's*),							
2 pcs.	290	3.0	45.0	11.0	15	230	1.0
(*Awrey's*), 1½ oz.	130	2.0	19.0	5.0	10	180	<1.0
(*Awrey's*), 2½ oz.	210	3.0	30.0	7.0	20	280	1.0
(*Awrey's* Grande)	340	5.0	43.0	16.0	90	310	1.0
(*Entenmann's*) . . .	160	2.0	24.0	7.0	40	210	<1.0
(*Entenmann's* Fat Free)	120	2.0	26.0	0	0	220	<1.0
(*Tastykake*), ½ pc.,							
2 oz.	230	3.0	30.0	11.0	30	160	1.0
(*Tastykake* Family)	170	3.0	27.0	6.0	35	300	1.0
(*Tastykake* Low Fat),							
½ pc., 2 oz. . . .	150	2.0	32.0	2.0	0	230	1.0

Food and Measure	cal.	prot. (gms)	carbo. (gms)	fat (gms)	chol. (mgs)	sod. (mgs)	fiber (gms)
Muffin, blueberry *(cont.)*							
loaf *(Hostess)*, 3.8 oz.	440	5.0	62.0	19.0	80	460	2.0
mini *(Hostess)*, 5 pcs.	240	3.0	30.0	13.0	40	180	<1.0
top *(Awrey's)*, 2½ oz.	210	3.0	31.0	8.0	20	290	1.0
carrot raisin *(Awrey's Grande)*	360	6.0	59.0	11.0	60	370	2.0
cheese streusel *(Awrey's Grande)* . . .	380	8.0	48.0	17.0	95	380	1.0
chocolate chip:							
chocolate *(Awrey's Grande)*	460	6.0	51.0	26.0	100	450	1.0
mini *(Hostess)*, 5 pcs.	260	3.0	29.0	15.0	35	170	1.0
cinnamon apple, mini *(Hostess)*, 5 pcs.	260	3.0	28.0	16.0	45	180	<1.0
corn:							
(Awrey's), 1½ oz.	130	2.0	20.0	4.0	10	210	<1.0
(Awrey's), 2½ oz.	220	4.0	33.0	8.0	25	430	<1.0
(Tastykake), ½ pc., 2 oz.	220	4.0	30.0	11.0	30	160	1.0
(Tastykake Golden Family)	190	4.0	31.0	6.0	40	280	1.0
cranberry orange *(Tastykake Low Fat)*, ½ pc., 2 oz.	160	2.0	33.0	2.0	0	240	1.0
cranberry nut *(Awrey's)*	120	2.0	20.0	4.0	10	210	0
English:							
(Awrey's)	140	5.0	28.0	1.0	0	230	2.0
(Pepperidge Farm)	130	5.0	26.0	1.0	0	250	2.0
(Roman Meal) . . .	135	6.0	27.0	2.0	0	290	2.0
(Tastykake)	130	5.0	26.0	.5	0	250	2.0
(Thomas')	120	4.0	25.0	1.0	0	200	1.0
blueberry *(Thomas')*	140	4.0	31.0	1.0	0	200	2.0
cinnamon raisin *(Pepperidge Farm)*	140	5.0	28.0	1.0	0	230	2.0

Food and Measure	cal.	prot. (gms)	carbo. (gms)	fat (gms)	chol. (mgs)	sod. (mgs)	fiber (gms)
cinnamon raisin							
(*Tastykake*) . . .	110	3.0	20.0	1.0	0	170	3.0
cranberry (*Thomas'*)	140	4.0	31.0	1.0	0	210	2.0
honey wheat							
(*Thomas'*)	110	5.0	24.0	1.0	0	190	3.0
oat bran (*Thomas'*)	120	4.0	26.0	1.0	0	210	2.0
raisin (*Thomas'*) . .	140	4.0	31.0	1.0	0	170	1.0
sandwich size							
(*Thomas'* 4 Pack)	190	7.0	38.0	2.0	0	280	2.0
sandwich size							
(*Thomas'* Twin)	190	7.0	41.0	1.5	0	300	2.0
seven grain (*Pep-*							
peridge Farm) . .	130	5.0	26.0	1.0	0	230	2.0
sourdough (*Pepper-*							
idge Farm)	130	5.0	26.0	1.0	0	250	2.0
sourdough (*Tas-*							
tykake)	130	5.0	25.0	1.0	0	210	2.0
sourdough							
(*Thomas'*)	120	4.0	25.0	1.0	0	190	1.0
sourdough, sand-							
wich size							
(*Thomas' Em's*)	200	7.0	41.0	2.0	0	310	2.0
wheat, sandwich							
size (*Thomas'*							
Em's)	180	8.0	39.0	1.5	0	300	4.0
lemon poppyseed:							
(*Awrey's*)	170	2.0	19.0	10.0	35	65	0
(*Awrey's* Grande)	390	5.0	41.0	23.0	85	280	<1.0
oat bran:							
(*Hostess*)	160	2.0	22.0	8.0	0	150	<1.0
banana nut (*Host-*							
ess)	150	2.0	22.0	6.0	0	160	1.0
onion, sandwich size							
(*Thomas' Em's*) . .	180	6.0	40.0	1.5	0	270	2.0
raisin (*Arnold*)	150	5.0	32.0	1.0	0	160	1.0
raisin bran:							
(*Awrey's*), 1½ oz.	110	2.0	18.0	4.0	15	270	1.0
(*Awrey's*), 2½ oz.	190	3.0	30.0	7.0	20	280	2.0
(*Awrey's* Grande)	350	5.0	47.0	16.0	90	310	4.0

Food and Measure	cal.	prot. (gms)	carbo. (gms)	fat (gms)	chol. (mgs)	sod. (mgs)	fiber (gms)
Muffin, raisin bran *(cont.)*							
(*Tastykake* Low Fat),							
½ pc., 2 oz.	170	3.0	38.0	2.0	0	230	3.0
top (*Awrey's*) . . .	190	3.0	30.0	7.0	20	280	1.0
sourdough *Arnold*)	120	4.0	25.0	1.0	0	200	1.0
Muffin, frozen or re-							
frigerated, 1 pc.:							
apple oatmeal (*Pep-*							
peridge Farm							
Wholesome Choice)	160	4.0	28.0	3.5	0	190	3.0
banana nut (*Weight*							
Watchers)	180	3.0	34.0	4.0	15	260	5.0
blueberry:							
(*Pepperidge Farm*							
Wholesome							
Choice)	140	3.0	27.0	2.5	0	190	2.0
(*Weight Watchers*)	180	3.0	33.0	4.0	15	270	2.0
bran:							
harvest honey							
(*Weight Watchers*)	220	3.0	42.0	4.5	5	180	5.0
w/raisins (*Pepper-*							
idge Farm Whole-							
some Choice) . .	150	4.0	30.0	2.5	0	260	4.0
chocolate chocolate							
chip (*Weight Watch-*							
ers)	200	4.0	39.0	4.0	5	250	1.0
corn (*Pepperidge*							
Farm Wholesome							
Choice)	150	4.0	27.0	3.0	0	190	1.0
English:							
(*Thomas'*)	120	4.0	25.0	1.0	0	200	1.0
honey wheat							
(*Thomas'*)	110	5.0	24.0	1.0	0	190	3.0
Muffin mix, dry:							
blueberry:							
wild (*Betty Crocker*							
Fat Free), 3 tbsp.	120	1.0	27.0	0	0	190	0
wild (*Betty Crocker*),							
¼ cup	140	2.0	29.0	1.5	0	210	0

Food and Measure	cal.	prot. (gms)	carbo. (gms)	fat (gms)	chol. (mgs)	sod. (mgs)	fiber (gms)
bran:							
multi (*Buckeye*),							
¹/₁₂ pkg.	110	2.0	25.0	1.0	0	280	2.0
wheat (*Arrowhead*							
Mills), ¹/₃ cup dry	150	7.0	26.0	2.0	0	160	7.0
oat (*Arrowhead*							
Mills), ¹/₃ cup dry	160	7.0	23.0	4.0	0	310	7.0
corn (*Flako*), ¹/₃ cup	160	2.0	29.0	4.0	0	380	1.0
lemon poppy seed							
(*Betty Crocker*),							
¹/₄ cup	150	2.0	30.0	2.0	0	220	0
Muffin sandwich, see							
"Egg breakfast							
sandwich"							
Mulberry:							
10 berries, ¹/₂ oz. . .	7	.2	1.5	.1	0	2	.3
¹/₂ cup	31	1.0	6.9	.3	0	7	1.2
Mullet, striped, meat							
only:							
raw, 4 oz.	133	22.0	0	4.3	56	74	0
baked, broiled, or mi-							
crowaved, 4 oz. . .	170	28.1	0	5.5	71	81	0
Mung beans:							
dry (*Arrowhead Mills*),							
¹/₄ cup	160	11.0	28.0	.5	0	0	9.0
boiled, ¹/₂ cup	107	7.1	19.3	.4	0	2	7.7
Mung beans,							
sprouted:							
raw, 1 oz.	9	.9	1.7	.1	0	2	.5
raw (*Jonathan's*),							
1 cup	30	3.0	4.0	.5	0	5	.5
boiled, drained, ¹/₂ cup	13	1.3	2.6	.1	0	6	.9
Mungo beans, boiled,							
¹/₂ cup	95	6.8	16.5	.5	0	7	5.8
Mushroom:							
fresh:							
raw, pcs., ¹/₂ cup	9	.7	1.6	.2	0	1	.4

Food and Measure	cal.	prot. (gms)	carbo. (gms)	fat (gms)	chol. (mgs)	sod. (mgs)	fiber (gms)
Mushroom, fresh *(cont.)*							
boiled,							
drained, pcs.,							
½ cup	21	1.7	4.0	.4	0	2	1.7
canned:							
all varieties, except							
w/garlic (*BinB*),							
4¼-oz. can . . .	30	3.0	4.0	0	0	460	2.0
all varieties (*Green*							
Giant), ½ cup . .	30	3.0	4.0	0	0	440	2.0
w/garlic, sliced							
(*BinB*),							
4¼-oz. can . . .	35	3.0	4.0	.5	0	410	1.0
freeze-dried (*Tone's*),							
⅓ cup	15	1.0	2.0	0	0	0	1.0
Mushroom, breaded,							
frozen (*Empire* Ko-							
sher), 7 pcs.,							
2.9 oz.	90	4.0	16.0	1.0	0	390	1.0
Mushroom, enoki:							
trimmed, 1 oz.	10	.4	2.2	.1	0	1	<1.0
1 large, 4⅛" long . .	2	.1	.4	<.1	0	<1	<1.0
Mushroom, Japanese							
honey, trimmed							
(*Frieda's*), 1 oz. . .	9	.6	1.2	<.1	0	n.a.	n.a.
Mushroom, oyster,							
fresh or dried							
(*Frieda's*), 1 oz. . .	7	.6	1.3	.1	0	1	.2
Mushroom, porto-							
bello:							
fresh (*Frieda's*), 1 oz.	8	.8	1.2	.1	0	4	<1.0
dried (*Frieda's*), ½ oz.	13	2.5	4.0	0	0	5	n.a.
Mushroom, shiitake:							
fresh:							
raw (*Frieda's*), 1 oz.	48	2.1	3.2	.3	0	<5	.7
cooked, 4 medium							
or ½ cup pcs. . .	40	1.1	10.4	.2	0	3	1.5
dried, 4 medium,							
½ oz.	44	1.4	11.3	.2	0	2	1.7

Food and Measure	cal.	prot. (gms)	carbo. (gms)	fat (gms)	chol. (mgs)	sod. (mgs)	fiber (gms)
Mushroom, Yamabiko honshimeji							
(*Frieda's*), 1 oz. . .	3	.6	1.2	.1	0	n.a.	n.a.
Mushroom pilaf, freeze-dried, w/vegetables (*Al-pineAire*), 1½ cups	373	41.0	77.0	2.0	0	2196	n.a.
Mushroom gravy, ¼ cup:							
(*Franco-American*) . .	20	2.0	3.0	1.0	5	300	0
country or w/wine (*Pepperidge Farm*)	30	1.0	4.0	.5	<5	300	0
creamy (*Franco-American*)	20	2.0	4.0	1.0	<5	310	0
Mushroom gravy mix:							
(*Durkee*), ¼ cup* . .	15	.5	3.0	0	0	230	0
(*French's*), ¼ cup*	10	0	3.0	.5	0	250	0
(*Loma Linda Gravy Quik*), 1 tbsp. . . .	15	<1.0	3.0	0	0	300	0
brown (*Durkee*), ¼ cup*	15	1.0	3.0	0	0	300	0
hunter (*Knorr*), 1 tbsp.	25	1.0	4.0	1.0	0	270	0
Mushroom sauce (*House of Tsang*), 1 tbsp.	10.0	0	2.0	.5	0	210	0
Mushroom sauce mix (*Knorr*), ⅕ pkg. . .	20	<1.0	2.0	1.0	0	200	0
Mussel, blue, meat only:							
raw, 4 oz.	98	13.5	4.2	2.5	32	324	0
raw, 1 cup	129	17.9	5.5	3.4	42	429	0
boiled or steamed, 4 oz.	195	27.0	8.4	5.1	64	418	0
Mustard, in jars, 1 tsp., except as noted:							
all varieties (*Hebrew National* Deli) . . .	0	0	0	0	0	65	0

Food and Measure	cal.	prot. (gms)	carbo. (gms)	fat (gms)	chol. (mgs)	sod. (mgs)	fiber (gms)
Mustard *(cont.)*							
(*Boar's Head* Deli) . .	0	0	0	0	0	40	0
(*French's* Yellow) . .	0	0	0	0	0	55	0
(*Grey Poupon* Deli)	5	0	0	0	0	50	0
(*Grey Poupon* Spicy)	5	<1.0	<1.0	0	0	60	0
(*Gulden's* Spicy) . . .	0	0	0	0	0	50	0
(*Kraft* Pure)	0	0	0	0	0	60	0
Chinese (*House of*							
Tsang), 1 pkt. . . .	15	0	<1.0	1.0	0	110	0
Dijon:							
(*Grey Poupon*) . . .	5	<1.0	<1.0	0	0	120	0
(*Roland* Extra							
Strong)	10	0	0	.5	0	130	0
horseradish (*Kraft*)	0	0	0	0	0	55	0
hot (*Eden*)	0	0	<1.0	0	0	65	0
hot (*Nance's*)	15	0	2.0	1.0	0	90	0
sharp (*Nance's*) . . .	15	0	2.0	1.0	0	95	0
Mustard blend (*Best*							
Foods/Hellmann's							
Dijonnaise), 1 tsp.	5	0	1.0	0	0	70	0
Mustard greens,							
½ cup, except as							
noted:							
fresh, chopped:							
raw, 1 oz. or ½ cup	7	.8	1.4	.1	0	7	.6
boiled, drained . . .	11	1.6	1.5	.2	0	11	1.4
canned (*Allens/Sun-*							
shine)	30	1.0	5.0	.5	0	10	3.0
frozen, chopped:							
(*Seabrook*), 3 oz.	30	2.0	2.0	0	0	20	2.0
Mustard powder,							
1 tsp.	9	.5	.3	.6	0	<1	<1.0
Mustard sauce mix,							
herb (*Knorr*),							
1 tbsp.	4	2.0	5.0	1.5	0	380	0
Mustard seeds:							
1 tsp.	15	.8	1.2	1.0	0	<1	<1.0
(*McCormick*), ¼ tsp.	2	.2	.2	.2	0	0	.1

Food and Measure	cal.	prot. (gms)	carbo. (gms)	fat (gms)	chol. (mgs)	sod. (mgs)	fiber (gms)
Mustard spinach:							
raw, chopped, ½ cup	17	1.7	2.9	.2	0	n.a.	n.a.
boiled, drained,							
chopped, ½ cup . .	14	1.5	2.5	.2	0	n.a.	n.a.
Mustard tallow,							
1 tbsp.	115	0	0	12.8	13	0	0

N

Food and Measure	cal.	prot. (gms)	carbo. (gms)	fat (gms)	chol. (mgs)	sod. (mgs)	fiber (gms)
Nacho dip (see also "Cheese dip"), mild (*Guiltless Gourmet*), 2 tbsp.	25	1.0	5.0	0	0	150	0
Nacho dip mix, (*Knorr*), ½ tsp. . . .	10	0	1.0	0	0	140	0
Nacho pepper, see "Pepper, jalapeño" and "Pepper, nacho"							
Natto, ½ cup	187	15.6	12.6	9.7	0	6	4.8
Navy beans, ½ cup:							
boiled	129	7.9	24.0	.5	0	1	3.3
canned:							
w/liquid	148	9.9	26.8	.6	0	587	6.7
(*Allens*)	110	6.0	19.0	1.0	0	380	6.0
(*Eden* Organic) . .	100	6.0	18.0	.5	0	15	7.0
(*Stokely*)	110	6.0	19.0	.5	0	350	3.0
bacon or bacon/ jalapeño (*Trappey's*)	110	6.0	17.0	1.5	0	420	7.0
Navy beans, sprouted, raw, ½ cup	35	3.2	6.8	.4	0	n.a.	n.a.
Nectarine:							
1 medium, 2½" diam.	67	1.3	16.0	.6	0	<1	2.2
sliced, ½ cup	34	.7	8.1	.3	0	<1	1.1
New England brand sausage (*Oscar Mayer*), 1.6 oz. . .	60	8.0	1.0	2.5	25	570	0

Food and Measure	cal.	prot. (gms)	carbo. (gms)	fat (gms)	chol. (mgs)	sod. (mgs)	fiber (gms)
Newburg sauce mix							
(*Knorr*), ⅓ pkg. . . .	30	1.0	5.0	1.0	0	350	0
Noodle, Chinese:							
(*Nasoya*), 1 cup,							
2¾ oz.	210	8.0	43.0	1.0	10	440	2.0
cellophane or long							
rice, dry, 2 oz. . . .	199	.1	48.8	<.1	0	6	<1.0
chow mein:							
½ cup	119	1.9	13.0	6.9	0	99	.9
(*Mee Tu*), ⅔ cup	120	3.0	17.0	4.5	0	220	0
(*La Choy*), ½ cup	140	3.0	19.0	6.0	0	220	1.0
crispy, wide (*La*							
Choy), ½ cup . . .	150	2.0	17.0	8.0	0	260	1.0
egg, dried (*House of*							
Tsang), 2 oz.	200	7.0	43.0	0	0	120	1.0
rice (*La Choy*), ½ cup	120	2.0	21.0	3.0	0	380	0
Noodle, egg:							
uncooked, 2 oz.:							
(*Creamette/Penn*							
Dutch)	210	8.0	39.0	2.5	55	20	1.0
(*Kluski*)	220	8.0	40.0	3.0	55	n.a.	1.0
(*Manischewitz*) . . .	210	6.0	42.0	1.5	45	25	1.0
all varieties (*Crea-*							
mette/Goodman's)	220	8.0	40.0	3.0	55	15	1.0
all varieties (*Eden*							
Organic)	220	10.0	42.0	2.0	60	5	2.0
bow-ties (*Mueller's*)	220	8.0	38.0	3.0	60	10	1.0
and spinach (*Prince*							
Paglia E Fieno)	220	8.0	41.0	3.0	55	15	2.0
yolk-free (*Borden*)	210	8.0	41.0	1.0	0	25	1.0
cooked:							
1 cup	212	7.6	39.7	2.4	53	11	1.8
spinach, 1 cup . . .	211	8.1	38.8	2.5	52	20	3.7
Noodle, egg-free,							
frozen (*Morningstar*							
Farms Homestyle),							
½ cup	160	5.0	33.0	0	0	10	1.0

Food and Measure	cal.	prot. (gms)	carbo. (gms)	fat (gms)	chol. (mgs)	sod. (mgs)	fiber (gms)
Noodle, Japanese,							
dry, except as							
noted:							
(*Nasoya*), 1 cup,							
2¾ oz.	210	8.0	43.0	.5	0	440	2.0
soba, 2 oz.:							
buckwheat (*Eden*							
100%)	200	5.0	41.0	1.5	0	30	3.0
buckwheat (*Eden*							
40%)	190	8.0	37.0	1.0	0	490	3.0
lotus root (*Eden*)	190	9.0	37.0	1.0	0	470	4.0
mugwort (*Eden*) . .	190	8.0	37.0	.5	0	550	2.0
wild yam (*Eden*) . .	190	9.0	37.0	.5	0	510	2.0
soba, cooked, 1 cup	113	5.8	24.4	.1	0	40	n.a.
somen:							
2 oz.	203	6.5	42.2	.5	0	1049	2.4
cooked, 1 cup . . .	230	7.0	48.5	.3	0	284	n.a.
spinach (*Nasoya*),							
1 cup, 2¾ oz. . . .	210	8.0	42.0	.5	0	440	3.0
udon:							
(*Eden*), 2 oz.	190	8.0	37.0	1.5	0	660	3.0
cooked, 4 oz. . . .	115	2.8	23.0	.6	0	51	n.a.
udon, brown rice,							
(*Eden*), 2 oz.	190	8.0	38.0	1.0	0	510	2.0
Noodle dishes,							
canned or frozen,							
see "Noodle entree"							
Noodle dishes, mix,							
½ pkg. dry, except							
as noted:							
Alfredo:							
(*Lipton* Noodles &							
Sauce)	250	10.0	38.0	7.0	75	940	1.0
carbonara (*Lipton*							
Noodles & Sauce)	260	10.0	38.0	7.0	85	890	2.0
broccoli (*Lipton*							
Noodles & Sauce)	260	10.0	39.0	7.0	75	940	2.0
beef (*Lipton* Noodles							
& Sauce)	220	8.0	42.0	3.5	60	930	2.0

Food and Measure	cal.	prot. (gms)	carbo. (gms)	fat (gms)	chol. (mgs)	sod. (mgs)	fiber (gms)
broccoli, 1 cup*:							
au gratin (*Noodle Roni*)	290	11.0	39.0	10.0	10	850	2.0
and mushroom (*Noodle Roni*) . .	460	13.0	49.0	24.0	5	1250	3.0
butter:							
(*Lipton* Noodles & Sauce)	260	8.0	40.0	8.0	65	910	2.0
and herb (*Lipton* Noodles & Sauce)	250	9.0	41.0	7.0	65	860	2.0
cheddar:							
(*Kraft* Dinner), 2.5 oz.	270	12.0	45.0	4.5	70	590	1.0
(*Master-A-Meal*), 1/5 pkg.	180	6.0	30.0	4.0	35	680	0
(*Nissin* Noodles and Sauce), 2.5 oz.	330	6.0	43.0	15.0	<5	940	2.0
bacon (*Lipton* Noodles & Sauce) . .	230	9.0	38.0	4.5	65	930	2.0
mild (*Noodle Roni*), 1 cup*	300	11.0	40.0	11.0	10	880	2.0
cheese (*Lipton* Noodles & Sauce) . . .	250	10.0	44.0	4.5	65	850	1.0
chicken/chicken flavor:							
(*Kraft* Dinner), 2.5 oz.	270	10.0	45.0	5.0	60	1350	1.0
(*Lipton* Noodles & Sauce)	230	8.0	41.0	4.5	60	760	2.0
(*Nissin* Noodles and Sauce), 2.4 oz.	330	7.0	41.0	15.0	10	940	4.0
(*Noodle Roni*), 1 cup*	320	10.0	40.0	13.0	5	1020	2.0
broccoli (*Lipton* Noodles & Sauce)	220	9.0	40.0	4.0	60	750	2.0
creamy (*Lipton* Noodles & Sauce) . .	230	9.0	39.0	6.0	65	710	2.0
tetrazzini (*Lipton* Noodles & Sauce)	220	8.0	37.0	5.0	65	850	2.0

Food and Measure	cal.	prot. (gms)	carbo. (gms)	fat (gms)	chol. (mgs)	sod. (mgs)	fiber (gms)
Noodle dishes, mix *(cont.)*							
garlic, creamy (*Noodle*							
Roni), 1 cup* . . .	500	12.0	49.0	29.0	10	1170	2.0
herb and butter (*Noo-*							
dle Roni), 1 cup*	500	12.0	51.0	28.0	5	1150	2.0
Oriental:							
(*Knorr* Cup), 1 pkg.	210	7.0	39.0	3.0	20	830	2.0
(*Noodle Roni*),							
1 cup*	290	7.0	38.0	12.0	0	900	2.0
Parmesan:							
(*Lipton* Noodles &							
Sauce)	250	10.0	37.0	8.0	70	750	2.0
(*Noodle Roni*							
Parmesano),							
1 cup*	400	14.0	49.0	17.0	10	950	2.0
Romanoff:							
(*Lipton* Noodles &							
Sauce)	260	9.0	41.0	7.0	70	920	2.0
(*Noodle Roni*),							
1 cup*	410	13.0	47.0	19.0	10	1240	2.0
sour cream and chive							
(*Lipton* Noodles &							
Sauce)	260	8.0	41.0	8.0	70	800	2.0
Stroganoff:							
(*Lipton* Noodles &							
Sauce)	210	9.0	37.0	4.0	65	850	2.0
(*Noodle Roni*),							
1 cup*	370	14.0	48.0	14.0	10	1250	2.0
tomato, Italian (*Nissin*							
Noodles & Sauce),							
2.4 oz.	320	7.0	42.0	14.0	<5	940	3.0
Noodle entree,							
canned, 1 cup, ex-							
cept as noted:							
w/beef:							
(*Hunt's* Homestyle)	150	10.0	22.0	4.0	15	1240	5.0
(*La Choy* Bi-Pack)	150	12.0	24.0	1.0	15	1100	3.0

Food and Measure	cal.	prot. (gms)	carbo. (gms)	fat (gms)	chol. (mgs)	sod. (mgs)	fiber (gms)
w/chicken:							
(*Dinty Moore*),							
7½ oz.	200	8.0	21.0	9.0	40	1140	1.0
(*Hormel* Micro Cup),							
7½ oz.	200	8.0	21.0	9.0	40	1140	1.0
(*Hormel* Micro Cup),							
10½ oz.	270	12.0	31.0	11.0	40	1630	3.0
(*La Choy* Bi-Pack)	160	10.5	23.0	4.0	15	1165	4.0
(*Nalley* Dinner) . .	160	9.0	19.0	6.0	15	1240	2.0
(*Nalley* Dinner),							
7½ oz.	140	9.0	19.0	3.0	20	930	2.0
cacciatore or regular							
(*Hunt's* Home-							
style)	175	12.0	21.0	6.0	37	1280	2.0
w/mushrooms							
(*Hunt's* Home-							
style)	200	10.0	32.0	4.5	25	910	3.5
w/franks (*Van Camp's*							
Noodle Weenee),							
1 can	230	7.0	34.0	8.0	20	680	1.0
rings (*Kid's Kitchen*),							
7.5 oz.	150	11.0	16.0	5.0	20	860	1.0
sweet and sour,							
w/chicken (*La Choy*							
Entree)	260	7.0	49.0	3.0	10	700	9.0
w/vegetables:							
(*La Choy* Entree)	130	5.0	27.0	1.0	0	1310	3.0
and beef (*La Choy*							
Entree)	160	7.0	27.0	3.0	5	1330	3.0
and chicken (*La*							
Choy Entree) . .	160	10.0	24.0	3.0	20	860	1.0
Noodle entree, fro-							
zen, 1 pkg., except							
as noted:							
and beef (*Banquet*							
Family), 1 cup . . .	140	11.0	16.0	4.0	35	1120	2.0
and chicken:							
(*Banquet* Bake at							
Home), 8-oz. cup	210	10.0	24.0	9.0	25	810	2.0

Food and Measure	cal.	prot. (gms)	carbo. (gms)	fat (gms)	chol. (mgs)	sod. (mgs)	fiber (gms)
Noodle entree, frozen, and chicken *(cont.)*							
escalloped (*Marie Callender's*), 6½ oz.	270	10.0	22.0	16.0	20	670	1.0
escalloped, and turkey (*The Budget Gourmet*)	440	19.0	44.0	20.0	115	840	2.0
kung pao, and vegetables (*Weight Watchers*)	260	8.0	35.0	10.0	5	690	5.0
Romanoff (*Stouffer's*)	490	18.0	48.0	25.0	60	1400	4.0
Nopales, see "Cactus leaves"							
Nori, see "Seaweed"							
Nut topping (see also specific listings) (*Planters*), 2 tbsp.	100	3.0	3.0	9.0	0	0	1.0
Nutmeg, ground:							
1 tsp.	12	.1	1.1	.8	0	tr.	.1
(*McCormick*), ¼ tsp.	3	0	.3	.2	0	<1	.1
Nuts, see specific listings							
Nuts, mixed, 1 oz., except as noted:							
dry-roasted:							
w/peanuts	169	4.9	7.2	14.6	0	3	2.6
w/peanuts, salted	169	4.9	7.2	14.6	0	190	2.6
(*Planters*)	170	6.0	7.0	14.0	0	250	2.0
honey-roasted (*Planters*)	140	5.0	9.0	13.0	0	85	2.0
oil-roasted:							
w/peanuts	175	4.8	6.1	16.0	0	3	2.8
w/peanuts, salted	175	4.8	6.1	16.0	0	185	2.8
(*Paradise/White Swan*), ¼ cup, 1.2 oz.	210	7.0	6.0	18.0	0	40	4.0
(*Planters*)	170	6.0	5.0	15.0	0	115	2.0
(*Planters* Deluxe)	170	5.0	6.0	16.0	0	110	2.0

Food and Measure	cal.	prot. (gms)	carbo. (gms)	fat (gms)	chol. (mgs)	sod. (mgs)	fiber (gms)
(*Planters* Lightly Salted)	170	6.0	6.0	15.0	0	55	2.0
(*Planters* Unsalted)	170	6.0	6.0	15.0	0	0	3.0
no Brazils (*Planters* 3½ oz.)	170	5.0	6.0	15.0	0	110	2.0
no Brazils (*Planters* Lightly Salted) . .	170	6.0	6.0	15.0	0	55	2.0
no peanuts (*Paradise/White Swan Deluxe*), ¼ cup, 1.2 oz.	220	6.0	7.0	18.0	0	60	4.0
cashews, w/almonds: macadamias (*Planters* Select)	170	4.0	6.0	16.0	0	90	2.0
pecans (*Planters* Select)	170	4.0	7.0	15.0	0	95	2.0
sesame, oil-roasted (*Planters*)	150	5.0	9.0	12.0	0	240	2.0
tamari-roasted (*Eden*)	170	8.0	9.0	11.0	0	55	3.0

O

Food and Measure	cal.	prot. (gms)	carbo. (gms)	fat (gms)	chol. (mgs)	sod. (mgs)	fiber (gms)
Oat (see also "Cereal"):							
whole grain, 1 oz. . . .	110	4.8	18.8	2.0	0	1	n.a.
flakes, rolled (*Arrowhead Mills*), ⅓ cup	130	5.0	23.0	2.5	0	0	4.0
rolled or oatmeal:							
dry, 1 oz.	109	4.5	19.0	1.8	0	1	2.9
cooked, 1 cup . . .	145	6.0	25.2	2.4	0	1	n.a.
steel cut (*Arrowhead Mills*), ¼ cup . . .	170	6.0	29.0	3.0	0	0	5.0
Oat bran, dry:							
1 oz.	70	4.9	18.8	2.0	0	1	4.5
(*Arrowhead Mills*), ⅓ cup	150	8.0	23.0	2.5	0	0	7.0
Oat flour (*Arrowhead Mills*), ⅓ cup . . .	120	5.0	20.0	2.0	0	0	4.0
Oat groats (*Arrowhead Mills*), ¼ cup	160	6.0	29.0	.5	0	0	4.0
Ocean perch, Atlantic, meat only:							
raw, 4 oz.	107	21.1	0	1.9	48	85	0
baked, broiled, or microwaved, 4 oz. . .	137	27.1	0	2.4	61	109	0
Octopus, meat only:							
raw, 4 oz.	93	16.9	2.5	1.2	55	n.a.	0
boiled or steamed, 4 oz.	186	33.8	5.0	2.4	109	n.a.	0
Octopus, canned:							
(*Goya*), ¼ cup	140	11.0	3.0	9.0	25	410	0
in garlic sauce (*Goya*), ¼ cup . . .	150	13.0	3.0	9.0	25	410	0

Food and Measure	cal.	prot. (gms)	carbo. (gms)	fat (gms)	chol. (mgs)	sod. (mgs)	fiber (gms)
a la marinara (*Goya*), ¼ cup	180	9.0	4.0	14.0	25	410	0
in olive oil (*Goya*), ¼ cup	150	11.0	3.0	9.0	25	410	0
spiced, in red sauce (*Reese*), 2 oz. . . .	120	7.0	4.0	8.0	0	430	0
Oheloberry, ½ cup	20	.3	4.8	.2	0	1	n.a.
Oil, 1 tbsp., except as noted:							
all varieties and blends (*Wesson*)	122	0	0	13.6	0	0	0
almond, canola, cocoa butter, corn, cotton- seed, hazelnut, nut- meg butter, oat, palm, or poppyseed	120	0	0	13.6	0	0	0
avocado or mustard	124	0	0	14.0	0	0	0
butter oil	112	<.1	0	12.7	33	n.a.	0
coconut	117	0	0	13.6	0	0	0
cod liver	123	0	0	13.6	78	n.a.	0
corn, all varieties (*Goya*)	120	0	0	14.0	0	0	0
corn or canola/corn (*Mazola*)	120	0	0	14.0	0	0	0
herring	123	0	0	13.6	104	n.a.	0
olive, peanut, saf- flower, sesame, soy- bean, sunflower, vegetable, or walnut	120	0	0	14.0	0	0	0
Oriental cooking (*House of Tsang Mongolian Fire/Sai- gon Sizzle*), 1 tsp.	45	0	0	5.0	0	0	0
peanut or popcorn (*Planters*)	120	0	0	14.0	0	0	0
popcorn, popping and topping (*Orville Redenbacher*) . . .	120	0	0	13.5	0	0	0
salmon	123	0	0	13.6	66	n.a.	0

Food and Measure	cal.	prot. (gms)	carbo. (gms)	fat (gms)	chol. (mgs)	sod. (mgs)	fiber (gms)
Oil *(cont.)*							
sardine	123	0	0	13.6	97	n.a.	0
sesame, regular or							
hot pepper (*Eden*)	130	0	0	14.0	0	0	0
sesame, regular or							
hot chili (*House of*							
Tsang), 1 tsp. . . .	45	0	0	5.0	0	0	0
wok (*House of Tsang*)	130	0	0	14.0	0	0	0
Oil substitute (*Baking*							
Healthy), 1 tbsp. . .	30	0	7.0	0	0	7	0
Okra:							
fresh:							
raw, sliced, ½ cup	19	1.0	3.8	.1	0	4	1.3
boiled, drained,							
8 pods, 3″ × ⅝″	27	1.6	6.1	.1	0	5	2.1
boiled drained,							
sliced, ½ cup . .	25	1.5	5.8	.1	0	4	2.0
canned, ½ cup:							
cut (*Allens/Trap-*							
pey's)	25	1.0	6.0	0	0	400	3.0
w/tomatoes (*Allens/*							
Trappey's)	25	1.0	5.0	0	0	380	3.0
w/tomatoes and							
corn (*Allens/Trap-*							
pey's)	30	<1.0	6.0	0	0	280	4.0
creole gumbo (*Trap-*							
pey's)	35	2.0	6.0	0	0	290	3.0
frozen:							
boiled, drained,							
sliced, ½ cup . .	34	1.9	7.5	.3	0	3	2.6
whole (*Seabrook*),							
9 pods, 3 oz. . .	25	1.0	5.0	0	0	35	3.0
whole (*Stilwell*),							
9 pods, 3 oz. . .	35	1.0	6.0	.5	0	15	4.0
cut (*Stilwell*),							
¾ cup	25	2.0	4.0	0	0	15	3.0
and tomatoes							
(*Stilwell*), ⅔ cup	25	1.0	5.0	0	0	20	3.0

Food and Measure	cal.	prot. (gms)	carbo. (gms)	fat (gms)	chol. (mgs)	sod. (mgs)	fiber (gms)
Old-fashioned drink mixer, bottled (*Holland House*), 2 fl. oz.	80	0	20.0	0	0	15	0
Old-fashioned loaf (*Oscar Mayer*), 1 oz.	60	4.0	2.0	5.0	15	340	0
Olive, pickled, ½ oz., except as noted:							
black, see "ripe," below							
Calamata:							
(*Krinos*), 3 pcs. . .	45	0	2.0	4.0	0	270	0
(*Zorba*), 5 pcs. . .	90	1.0	2.0	9.0	0	260	0
green, w/pits:							
10 small	33	.4	.4	3.6	0	686	.7
10 large	45	.5	.5	4.9	0	926	1.0
10 giant	76	.9	.9	8.3	0	1572	1.7
green, pitted, 1 oz.	33	.4	.4	3.6	0	680	.7
green, cracked (*Krinos*)	20	0	2.0	1.0	0	410	0
green, queen/Spanish:							
(*S&W*), 2 pcs. . . .	20	0	1.0	2.0	0	220	0
(*Zorba*), 2 pcs. . .	25	<1.0	1.0	2.0	0	230	0
ripe, pitted:							
California (*Vlasic*), 1 tsp. chopped or 4–6 pcs.	25	0	1.0	2.5	0	115	0
(*Lindsay*), 6 small, 5 medium, 4 large, or 1⅓ tbsp. chopped	25	0	1.0	2.5	0	115	0
(*S&W*), 3 extra large	25	0	1.0	2.5	0	110	0
(*S&W*), 3 jumbo	25	0	1.0	2.0	0	135	0
(*Vlasic*), 4 large . .	25	0	1.0	2.5	0	55	0
(*Vlasic*), 6 small . .	25	0	1.0	2.5	0	115	0
Spanish (*Vlasic*), 8 small	20	0	1.0	2.0	0	280	0

Food and Measure	cal.	prot. (gms)	carbo. (gms)	fat (gms)	chol. (mgs)	sod. (mgs)	fiber (gms)
Olive *(cont.)*							
ripe, w/pits:							
(*Lindsay*), 5 medium or 4 large	25	0	0	2.5	0	125	0
(*S&W*), 1 super colossal	15	0	1.0	1.5	0	80	0
ripe, oil-cured:							
(*Krinos*)	70	0	3.0	6.0	0	390	0
(*Progresso*), 6 pcs.	80	0	3.0	6.0	0	330	1.0
ripe, Greek:							
10 medium	65	.4	1.7	6.9	0	631	0
10 extra large . . .	89	.6	2.3	9.5	0	868	0
pitted, 1 oz.	96	.6	2.5	10.2	0	932	0
(*Krinos*)	35	0	2.0	3.0	0	320	0
(*Krinos* Alfonso) . .	30	0	1.0	3.0	0	360	0
(*Krinos* Nafplion)	20	0	2.0	1.0	0	300	0
(*Zorba*), 1.7-oz. pc.	60	0	6.0	4.0	0	540	0
royal (*Krinos*)	30	0	1.0	2.5	0	290	0
salad (*Goya*), ¼ cup	25	0	0	2.5	0	330	0
stuffed, Manzanilla:							
(*Goya*), 4 pcs. . . .	25	0	0	2.0	0	230	0
(*Lindsay*), 5 pcs.	25	0	1.0	2.5	0	330	0
(*S&W*), 3 pcs. . . .	25	0	1.0	2.0	0	240	0
stuffed, queen:							
(*Goya*), 2 pcs. . . .	20	0	0	1.5	0	260	0
(*Lindsay*), 2 pcs.	15	0	1.0	1.5	0	310	0
(*S&W*, 4¾ oz.), 2 pcs.	15	0	1.0	1.5	0	250	0
(*S&W*, 7 oz.), 2 pcs.	20	0	1.0	1.5	0	290	0
(*S&W*, 10 oz.), 1 pc.	10	0	1.0	1.0	0	180	0
queen (*Vlasic*) . . .	20	0	1.0	1.5	0	340	0
stuffed, w/tuna (*Goya*), 4 pcs. . .	25	0	1.0	2.5	0	240	0
Olive loaf (*Boar's Head*), 2 oz.	130	6.0	<1.0	12.0	20	630	0
Olive oil, see "Oil"							

Food and Measure	cal.	prot. (gms)	carbo. (gms)	fat (gms)	chol. (mgs)	sod. (mgs)	fiber (gms)
Olive salad, drained							
(*Progresso*), 2 tbsp.	25	0	1.0	2.5	0	360	1.0
Omelet, see "Egg							
breakfast"							
Onion, mature:							
fresh or stored:							
raw, 1 oz.	11	.3	2.4	<.1	0	1	.5
raw, chopped,							
½ cup	30	.9	6.9	0.1	0	2	1.4
raw, chopped,							
1 tbsp.	4	.1	.9	<.1	0	tr.	.2
boiled, drained,							
chopped, ½ cup	47	1.4	10.7	.2	0	3	1.5
canned or in jars:							
whole (*Green Gi-*							
ant), ½ cup . . .	35	<1.0	3.0	0	0	410	1.0
whole (*S&W*),							
½ cup	40	0	8.0	0	0	410	1.0
cocktail (*Crosse &*							
Blackwell),							
1 tbsp.	5	0	1.0	0	0	250	0
cocktail (*S&W*							
4 oz.), 12 pcs.,							
1.1 oz.	5	0	1.0	0	0	300	0
cocktail (*S&W*							
16 oz.), 8 pcs.,							
1.1 oz.	5	0	1.0	0	0	300	0
sweet, in sauce							
(*Boar's Head* Vid-							
alia), 1 tbsp. . . .	10	0	2.0	0	0	15	0
wild, marinated,							
(*Krinos* Volvi),							
1 oz.	15	0	2.0	.5	0	230	1.0
frozen, chopped:							
(*Ore-Ida*), ¾ cup	25	<1.0	6.0	0	0	15	1.0
boiled, drained,							
1 tbsp.	4	.1	1.0	<.1	0	2	.2
frozen rings, see "On-							
ion rings"							

Food and Measure	cal.	prot. (gms)	carbo. (gms)	fat (gms)	chol. (mgs)	sod. (mgs)	fiber (gms)
Onion, cocktail, see "Onion"							
Onion, dried:							
flakes, 1 tbsp.	16	.5	4.2	<.1	0	1	.5
minced, 1 tsp.	7	.2	1.9	0	0	<1	.2
Onion, green (scal-lion), raw, trimmed, w/top:							
chopped, ½ cup . . .	16	.9	3.7	.1	0	8	1.3
chopped, 1 tbsp. . .	2	.1	.4	<.1	0	1	.2
freeze-dried (*McCor-mick*), ¼ tsp.	1	0	.2	0	0	<1	.1
Onion, Welsh, 1 oz.	10	.5	1.8	.1	0	n.a.	<1.0
Onion dip, 2 tbsp.:							
creamy (*Kraft* Pre-mium)	45	<1.0	2.0	4.0	10	160	0
French:							
(*Breakstone's*) . . .	50	1.0	2.0	4.0	20	160	0
(*Frito-Lay*)	60	1.0	4.0	5.0	15	230	0
(*Heluva* Good) . . .	50	1.0	2.0	5.0	20	160	0
(*Heluva* Good Light)	35	1.0	3.0	2.0	10	180	0
(*Heluva* Good Free)	25	1.0	3.0	0	0	200	0
(*Knudsen* Premium)	50	1.0	2.0	4.0	20	160	0
(*Kraft*)	60	1.0	4.0	4.0	0	230	0
(*Kraft* Premium) . .	50	<1.0	2.0	4.0	10	160	0
(*Nalley*)	100	1.0	3.0	10.0	15	250	0
(*Old Dutch*)	50	1.0	3.0	4.0	10	150	0
(*Ruffles*)	70	1.0	4.0	5.0	0	240	1.0
(*Ruffles* Low Fat)	40	2.0	6.0	1.0	0	230	<1.0
(*Sealtest*)	50	1.0	2.0	4.0	20	160	0
green (*Kraft*)	60	1.0	4.0	4.0	0	190	0
sour cream and (*Lay's*)	40	1.0	6.0	1.0	<5	230	<1.0
toasted (*Breakstone's*)	50	1.0	2.0	4.0	20	180	0
Onion dip mix, and chive (*Knorr*), ½ tsp.	5	0	1.0	0	0	110	0

Food and Measure	cal.	prot. (gms)	carbo. (gms)	fat (gms)	chol. (mgs)	sod. (mgs)	fiber (gms)
Onion gravy, ¼ cup:							
roasted, and garlic							
(*Pepperidge Farm*)	25	2.0	4.0	1.0	<5	350	0
zesty (*Heinz* Home							
Style)	20	1.0	.5	0	0	330	0
mix*:							
(*Durkee*)	10	.5	3.0	0	0	310	0
(*French's*)	15	0	4.0	1.0	0	260	0
(*Loma Linda* Gravy							
Quik)	20	<1.0	3.0	0	0	230	0
brown (*Durkee*) . .	15	1.0	4.0	0	0	290	0
brown, Lyonnaise							
(*Knorr*)	20	1.0	4.0	.5	0	320	0
Onion powder:							
1 tsp.	10	.3	2.4	0	0	2	.2
(*McCormick*), ¼ tsp.	3	.1	.6	0	0	<1	.1
(*Tone's*), ¼ tsp. . . .	5	0	1.0	0	0	0	0
Onion rings, frozen:							
(*Mrs. Paul's* Old Fash-							
ioned), 7 rings . . .	230	18.0	29.0	12.0	0	450	1.0
(*Ore-Ida* Classic),							
4 rings	220	4.0	26.0	12.0	0	510	2.0
(*Ore-Ida* Gourmet),							
4 rings	220	3.0	26.0	11.0	0	510	2.0
(*Ore-Ida Onion Ring-*							
ers), 6 rings	230	3.0	26.0	13.0	0	300	2.0
Onion salt:							
(*Durkee* California),							
½ tsp.	0	0	0	0	0	290	0
(*Tone's*), 1 tsp. . . .	1	.1	.4	tr.	0	1599	<.1
Onion sprouts:							
(*Jonathan's*), 1 cup	30	1.0	5.0	0	0	5	2.0
(*Shaw's* Premium							
Salad), 2 oz.	11	1.0	0	<1.0	0	85	3.0
Opossum, meat only,							
roasted, 4 oz. . . .	251	34.2	0	11.6	n.a.	n.a.	0
Orange:							
California navel:							
2⅞″ orange	65	1.4	16.3	.1	0	1	3.4

Food and Measure	cal.	prot. (gms)	carbo. (gms)	fat (gms)	chol. (mgs)	sod. (mgs)	fiber (gms)
Orange, California navel *(cont.)*							
sections w/out							
membrane, ½ cup	38	.9	9.6	.1	0	1	2.0
California Valencia:							
2⅝″ orange	59	1.3	14.4	.4	0	0	2.9
sections w/out							
membrane, ½ cup	44	.9	10.7	.3	0	0	2.2
Florida:							
2 ¹¹⁄₁₆″ orange . . .	69	1.1	17.4	.3	0	1	3.6
sections w/out							
membrane, ½ cup	42	.7	10.7	.2	0	1	2.2
Orange, Mandarin,							
see "Tangerine"							
Orange drink,							
8 fl. oz., except as							
noted:							
(*Bright & Early*) . . .	120	0	30.0	0	0	30	0
(*Capri Sun*),							
6.75 fl. oz.	100	0	26.0	0	0	20	0
(*Hi-C*)	120	0	32.0	0	0	25	0
(*Lincoln*)	130	0	33.0	0	0	80	0
orangeade (*Snapple*)	120	0	29.0	0	0	10	0
punch (*Kool-Aid*							
Bursts), 6.75 fl. oz.	100	0	24.0	0	0	30	0
tropical (*Farmers Mar-*							
ket)	120	0	29.0	0	0	0	0
Orange drink blends,							
8 fl. oz.:							
cranberry:							
(*Tropicana Twister*)	130	0	32.0	0	0	15	0
(*Tropicana Twister*							
Light)	30	0	7.0	0	0	20	0
guava nectar (*Kern's*)	150	0	36.0	0	0	10	0
peach (*Tropicana*							
Twister)	120	0	31.0	0	0	20	0
pineapple (*Lincoln*)	130	0	32.0	0	0	70	0
punch (*Minute Maid*)	120	0	33.0	0	0	30	0
raspberry:							
(*Tropicana Twister*)	120	0	31.0	0	0	20	0

Food and Measure	cal.	prot. (gms)	carbo. (gms)	fat (gms)	chol. (mgs)	sod. (mgs)	fiber (gms)
(*Tropicana Twister* Light)	35	0	9.0	0	0	20	0
strawberry-banana:							
(*Tropicana Twister*)	120	0	29.0	0	0	20	0
(*Tropicana Twister* Light)	35	<1.0	9.0	0	0	20	0
strawberry-guava							
(*Tropicana Twister*)	120	0	29.0	0	0	20	0
Orange drink mix*, 8 fl. oz.:							
(*Kool-Aid* w/sugar)	60	0	16.0	0	0	5	0
(*Tang*)	100	0	24.0	0	0	0	0
(*Tang* Sugar Free) . .	5	0	1.0	0	0	0	0
Orange juice, 8 fl. oz., except as noted:							
fresh, 6 fl. oz.	83	1.3	19.3	.4	0	2	.4
(*Apple & Eve*), 10 fl. oz.	130	3.0	32.0	0	0	5	0
(*Dole*), 10 fl. oz. . . .	140	2.0	33.0	0	0	25	0
(*Minute Maid* Box)	120	0	28.0	0	0	25	0
(*R.W. Knudsen*) . . .	100	2.0	23.0	0	0	35	0
(*S&W*), 6-fl.-oz. can	90	1.0	22.0	0	0	0	0
(*Tree Top*)	120	0	28.0	0	0	25	0
(*Tree Top*), 11.5 fl. oz.	170	0	40.0	0	0	35	0
(*Tropicana* Pure Premium)	110	<1.0	27.0	0	0	0	0
(*Tropicana* Pure Premium + Fiber) . . .	120	<1.0	30.0	0	0	0	2.5
(*Tropicana* Ruby Red Pure Premium) . .	120	<1.0	28.0	0	0	0	0
(*Veryfine*)	120	1.0	24.0	0	0	35	0
(*Veryfine*), 11.5 fl. oz.	170	3.0	34.0	0	0	50	0
chilled:							
all varieties, except calcium rich and not concentrate (*Minute Maid* Premium)	110	0	27.0	0	0	25	0

Food and Measure	cal.	prot. (gms)	carbo. (gms)	fat (gms)	chol. (mgs)	sod. (mgs)	fiber (gms)
Orange juice, chilled *(cont.)*							
calcium rich (*Minute Maid* Premium)	120	0	27.0	0	0	25	0
not concentrate (*Minute Maid* Premium)	110	0	27.0	0	0	0	0
frozen*:							
all varieties, except calcium rich (*Minute Maid* Premium)	110	0	27.0	0	0	0	0
calcium rich (*Minute Maid* Premium)	120	0	27.0	0	0	0	0
Orange juice blends, 8 fl. oz.:							
kiwi-passion fruit (*Tropicana* Tropics)	100	<1.0	26.0	0	0	15	0
mango (*R.W. Knudsen*)	120	0	30.0	0	0	50	0
peach-mango (*Tropicana* Tropics) . . .	110	<1.0	28.0	0	0	15	0
pineapple (*Tropicana* Tropics)	100	<1.0	27.0	0	0	15	0
punch:							
(*Juicy Juice*)	120	0	30.0	0	0	10	0
(*Veryfine* Juice-Ups)	140	0	35.0	0	0	15	0
Orange juice float (*R.W. Knudsen*), 8 fl. oz.	140	1.0	33.0	0	0	60	0
Orange peel:							
peel, 1 tbsp.	—[1]	.1	1.5	<.1	0	0	.2
candied, 1.1 oz.:							
(*S&W*), 58 pcs. . .	80	0	23.0	0	0	35	2.0
diced (*Paradise/ White Swan*), 2 tbsp.	90	0	23.0	0	0	15	2.0

[1] *Cannot be calculated; no digestibility value for peel.*

Food and Measure	cal.	prot. (gms)	carbo. (gms)	fat (gms)	chol. (mgs)	sod. (mgs)	fiber (gms)
Orange sauce, mandarin (*Ka-Me*), 2 tbsp.	80	0	21.0	0	0	430	0
Oregano, dried:							
1 tsp.	3	.1	.5	0	0	0	.1
(*McCormick*), ¼ tsp.	2	0	.3	0	0	<1	.2
Mexican (*McCormick*), ¼ tsp.	1	0	.2	0	0	0	.1
Oriental sauce (see also "Stir-fry sauce" and specific listings, 1 tsp., except as noted:							
(*House of Tsang* Chow Chow)	5	0	0	0	0	150	0
(*House of Tsang* Imperial), 1 tbsp. . . .	25	0	5.0	0	0	410	0
(*House of Tsang* Namasu)	10	0	2.0	0	0	170	0
brown, spicy (*House of Tsang*)	15	0	3.0	0	0	125	0
hot and spicy (*House of Tsang* Hunan) . .	5	0	0	0	0	35	0
Oriental 5-spice (*Tone's*), 1 tsp. . .	9	.3	1.9	.3	0	2	.5
Oriental sauce, see specific listings							
Oyster, meat only, 4 oz., except as noted:							
Eastern, wild:							
raw, 1 lb.	310	32.0	17.7	11.1	238	957	0
raw, 6 medium, 3 oz.	57	5.9	3.3	2.1	44	177	0
baked, broiled, or microwaved . . .	82	9.4	5.4	2.2	56	277	0
steamed or poached	155	16.0	8.9	5.6	119	478	0
Eastern, farmed:							
raw	67	5.9	6.3	1.8	29	202	0

Food and Measure	cal.	prot. (gms)	carbo. (gms)	fat (gms)	chol. (mgs)	sod. (mgs)	fiber (gms)
Oyster, Eastern, farmed *(cont.)*							
baked, broiled, or							
microwaved . . .	90	7.9	8.3	2.4	43	185	0
Pacific:							
raw	93	10.7	5.6	2.6	n.a.	120	0
raw, boiled, or							
steamed, 1 me-							
dium	41	4.7	2.5	1.2	n.a.	53	0
boiled or steamed	185	21.4	11.2	5.2	n.a.	240	0
Oyster, canned:							
Eastern, wild:							
w/liquid, 4 oz. . . .	78	8.0	4.4	2.8	62	127	0
w/liquid, 1 cup . .	170	17.5	9.7	6.1	136	277	0
whole (*S&W*), 2 oz.	70	8.0	2.0	3.0	20	160	2.0
smoked:							
(*Reese* Petite), 2 oz.	110	8.0	6.0	6.0	50	220	0
(*S&W*), 2 oz. . . .	100	10.0	6.0	6.0	40	210	4.0
Oyster plant, see							
"Salsify"							
Oyster and shrimp							
sauce (*TryMe* Carib-							
bean Clipper), 1 tsp.	10	0	2.0	0	0	140	0
Oyster stew, see							
"Soup"							

P

Food and Measure	cal.	prot. (gms)	carbo. (gms)	fat (gms)	chol. (mgs)	sod. (mgs)	fiber (gms)
Palm, hearts of, canned:							
(*Haddon House*), 4.5 oz.	20	2.0	3.0	0	0	450	2.0
(*Goya*), ½ cup	25	2.0	4.0	.5	0	450	2.0
Pancake, frozen, 3 pcs., except as noted:							
(*Aunt Jemima* Lowfat)	130	4.0	33.0	1.5	0	580	8.0
(*Aunt Jemima* Original)	200	6.0	40.0	3.0	15	700	2.0
(*Downyflake*)	270	5.0	47.0	7.0	5	700	2.0
(*Hungry Jack* Microwave Original) . . .	240	5.0	47.0	4.0	10	550	1.0
blueberry:							
(*Aunt Jemima*) . . .	210	6.0	40.0	3.5	15	670	2.0
(*Hungry Jack* Microwave)	230	5.0	45.0	3.5	10	550	1.0
buttermilk:							
(*Aunt Jemima*) . . .	180	5.0	34.0	3.0	15	590	2.0
(*Hungry Jack* Microwave)	240	5.0	46.0	4.0	10	580	1.0
mini (*Hungry Jack* Microwave), 11 pcs.	230	5.0	44.0	4.0	10	550	1.0
Pancake breakfast, frozen, 1 pkg.:							
(*Swanson Kids Breakfast Blast* Mini) . .	320	12.0	54.0	8.0	45	640	2.0
w/bacon (*Swanson Great Starts*)	400	31.0	42.0	20.0	100	1030	1.0

Food and Measure	cal.	prot. (gms)	carbo. (gms)	fat (gms)	chol. (mgs)	sod. (mgs)	fiber (gms)
Pancake breakfast *(cont.)*							
w/sausage (*Swanson Great Starts*)	490	38.0	52.0	25.0	90	950	3.0
silver dollar:							
eggs and (*Swanson Great Starts*) . . .	250	22.0	22.0	14.0	290	540	1.0
and sausage (*Swanson Great Starts*)	340	28.0	36.0	18.0	70	670	1.0
Pancake mix, ⅓ cup dry, except as noted:							
(*Aunt Jemima* Original)	150	4.0	34.0	.5	0	620	1.0
(*Aunt Jemima* Complete)	190	6.0	39.0	2.0	0	470	1.0
(*Hungry Jack* Original)	150	3.0	32.0	1.5	0	640	<1.0
(*Hungry Jack* Premeasured), ½ pkt.	200	5.0	38.0	3.5	0	780	1.0
(*Hungry Jack Extra Lights*)	160	3.0	33.0	1.5	0	590	<1.0
(*Hungry Jack Hungry Lights* Complete)	150	4.0	30.0	2.0	0	600	<1.0
buckwheat:							
(*Arrowhead Mills*)	140	8.0	25.0	1.5	0	220	5.0
(*Aunt Jemima*), ¼ cup	120	5.0	28.0	1.0	0	560	4.0
buttermilk:							
(*Arrowhead Mills*), ¼ cup	120	5.0	25.0	.5	<5	350	2.0
(*Aunt Jemima* Complete)	190	6.0	38.0	2.0	10	480	2.0
(*Aunt Jemima* Complete Reduced Calorie)	140	8.0	30.0	1.5	15	510	5.0
(*Hungry Jack*) . . .	160	4.0	33.0	1.5	0	650	<1.0
(*Hungry Jack* Complete)	160	4.0	32.0	1.5	<5	560	<1.0

Food and Measure	cal.	prot. (gms)	carbo. (gms)	fat (gms)	chol. (mgs)	sod. (mgs)	fiber (gms)
corn, blue (*Arrowhead Mills*)	150	4.0	28.0	2.0	0	130	3.0
gluten-free (*Arrowhead Mills*), ¼ cup	130	4.0	24.0	2.0	0	180	5.0
kamut (*Arrowhead Mills*), ¼ cup . . .	130	7.0	26.0	1.0	0	330	4.0
multigrain (*Arrowhead Mills*), ¼ cup . . .	120	5.0	24.0	.5	0	260	3.0
oat bran (*Arrowhead Mills*)	140	4.0	25.0	1.5	0	160	6.0
wild rice (*Arrowhead Mills*)	140	3.0	30.0	1.0	0	65	0
whole grain (*Arrowhead Mills*), ¼ cup	120	5.0	24.0	.5	0	260	4.0
whole wheat (*Aunt Jemima*), ¼ cup . . .	130	6.0	28.0	.5	0	560	3.0
Pancake syrup (see also "Maple syrup"), ¼ cup, except as noted:							
table blends:							
1 tbsp.	57	0	15.0	0	0	17	0
w/butter, 1 tbsp. . . .	59	0	14.8	.3	1	20	0
w/2% maple, 1 tbsp.	53	0	13.9	0	0	12	0
(*Aunt Jemima*)	210	0	53.0	0	0	120	0
(*Aunt Jemima* Lite)	100	0	27.0	0	0	160	0
(*Country Kitchen*) . .	200	0	53.0	0	0	110	0
(*Country Kitchen Lite*)	100	0	26.0	0	0	160	0
(*Golden Griddle*) . . .	220	0	57.0	0	0	55	0
(*Hungry Jack*)	210	0	17.0	0	0	90	0
(*Hungry Jack* Lite) . .	100	0	8.0	0	0	180	<1.0
(*Karo*)	240	0	60.0	0	0	85	0
(*Log Cabin*)	200	0	52.0	0	0	60	0
(*Log Cabin Lite*) . . .	100	0	26.0	0	0	180	0
(*Mrs. Richardson's*)	210	0	52.0	0	0	115	0
(*Mrs. Richardson's* Lite)	100	0	26.0	0	0	160	0

Food and Measure	cal.	prot. (gms)	carbo. (gms)	fat (gms)	chol. (mgs)	sod. (mgs)	fiber (gms)
Pancake syrup *(cont.)*							
(*Smucker's* Diet							
Breakfast Syrup),							
1 oz.	20	0	4.0	0	0	35	0
butter flavor:							
(*Aunt Jemima* Rich)	210	0	52.0	0	0	170	0
(*Aunt Jemima* But-							
terlite)	100	0	26.0	0	0	150	0
(*Country Kitchen*)	200	0	53.0	0	0	200	0
maple (*Hungry*							
Jack)	210	0	17.0	0	0	90	0
maple (*Hungry Jack*							
Lite)	100	0	8.0	0	0	180	<1.0
or maple (*S&W* Re-							
duced Calorie) . .	60	0	15.0	0	0	105	0
Pancreas, braised:							
beef, 4 oz.	307	30.7	0	19.5	n.a.	68	0
lamb, 4 oz.	265	25.9	0	17.1	454	59	0
pork, 4 oz.	248	32.3	0	12.2	357	48	0
veal (calf), 4 oz. . . .	290	33.0	0	16.6	n.a.	n.a.	0
Papaya:							
fresh:							
1-lb. fruit,							
3½" × 5⅛" . . .	117	1.9	29.8	.4	0	8	5.5
peeled, cubed,							
½ cup	27	.4	6.9	.1	0	2	1.3
peeled (*Frieda's*),							
1 oz.	11	.2	2.8	<.1	0	1	n.a.
dried (*Sonoma*),							
2 pcs., 2 oz.	200	0	41.0	4.0	0	60	6.0
frozen, slices (*Goya*),							
⅓ pkg.	50	1.0	11.0	0	0	12	2.0
Papaya, creamed							
(*R.W. Knudsen*),							
2 fl. oz.	40	0	10.0	0	0	10	0
Papaya drink,							
8 fl. oz., except as							
noted:							
(*Farmer's Market*) . .	130	1.0	32.0	0	0	0	0

Food and Measure	cal.	prot. (gms)	carbo. (gms)	fat (gms)	chol. (mgs)	sod. (mgs)	fiber (gms)
colada (*Snapple*) . . .	120	0	29.0	0	0	10	0
juice (*After the Fall*							
Pele's)	100	1.0	25.0	0	0	15	0
nectar:							
(*Goya*), 12 fl. oz.	220	0	56.0	0	0	25	1.0
(*Libby's/Kern's*),							
11.5 fl. oz.	210	<1.0	51.0	0	0	10	0
(*R.W. Knudsen*) . .	130	0	34.0	0	0	35	0
(*Santa Cruz*)	110	0	28.0	0	0	35	0
punch (*Lincoln*) . . .	130	0	32.0	0	0	75	0
Pappadum, 1 oz.:							
(*Patak's*), 3 pcs. . . .	80	6.0	13.0	.5	0	819	3.0
snack crisps (*Tama-*							
rind Tree), 30 pcs.	140	4.0	16.0	6.0	0	570	1.0
Paprika:							
1 tsp.	6	.3	1.2	.3	0	1	.6
(*McCormick*), ¼ tsp.	2	.1	.3	.1	0	<1	.2
Parsley:							
fresh:							
10 sprigs	4	.3	.6	.1	0	6	.3
chopped, ½ cup . .	11	.9	1.9	.2	0	17	1.0
dried:							
1 tsp.	1	.1	.2	.1	0	1	.2
(*McCormick*),							
¼ tsp.	<1	0	0	0	0	<1	0
freeze-dried, 1 tbsp.	1	.1	.2	<.1	0	2	.2
Parsley root, 1 oz.	3	.8	.7	.2	0	28	.4
Parsnip:							
raw, sliced, ½ cup	50	.8	12.1	.2	0	7	3.3
boiled, drained:							
1 medium, 9″ . . .	130	2.1	31.3	.5	0	17	6.4
sliced, ½ cup . . .	63	1.0	15.2	.2	0	8	3.1
Passion fruit:							
fresh, purple:							
1 medium	18	.4	4.2	.1	0	n.a.	1.9
trimmed, 1 oz. . . .	27	.6	6.6	.2	0	n.a.	2.9
(*Frieda's*), 3.5 oz.	90	2.2	21.2	.7	0	28	n.a.
frozen, chunks							
(*Goya*), ⅓ pkg. . .	70	2.0	15.0	0	0	35	2.0

Food and Measure	cal.	prot. (gms)	carbo. (gms)	fat (gms)	chol. (mgs)	sod. (mgs)	fiber (gms)
Passion fruit juice:							
fresh:							
purple, 6 fl. oz. . .	95	.7	25.2	.1	0	n.a.	.4
yellow, 6 fl. oz. . .	111	1.2	26.8	.3	0	11	.4
(*Snapple*), 10 fl. oz.	160	0	39.0	0	0	20	0
Passion fruit-mango							
drink (*Heinke's*),							
8 fl. oz.	130	0	33.0	0	0	25	0
Pasta, dry (see also							
"Macaroni" and							
specific listings),							
uncooked, 2 oz.:							
plain	211	7.3	42.6	.9	0	4	1.4
all varieties:							
(*Creamette/Prince*)	210	7.0	42.0	1.0	0	0	2.0
(*Delverde*)	200	7.0	41.0	.5	0	0	1.0
(*Goya* Estrellas) . .	210	6.0	45.0	1.0	0	0	0
(*Mueller's*)	210	7.0	42.0	1.0	0	0	1.0
w/egg (*Herb's*) . . .	220	10.0	42.0	2.0	60	5	2.0
kamut (*Eden*) . . .	210	10.0	38.0	1.5	0	0	6.0
fettuccine (*Prince*) . .	220	8.0	40.0	3.0	55	15	1.0
kudzu and sweet po-							
tato (*Eden*)	190	0	47.0	0	0	0	0
linguine, tomato-basil							
(*Prince*)	200	7.0	41.0	1.0	0	15	2.0
mung bean (*Eden*) . .	190	0	47.0	0	0	5	0
noodle-style, yolk free							
(*Mueller's*)	210	8.0	42.0	1.0	0	10	1.0
penne, tomato-pep-							
per-basil (*Prince*)	210	8.0	41.0	1.0	0	15	2.0
ribbons:							
durum wheat, all va-							
rieties (*Eden*) . .	220	8.0	44.0	1.0	0	0	3.0
regular or spinach,							
whole wheat							
(*Eden*)	200	8.0	40.0	1.5	0	10	7.0
rice (*Eden*)	200	5.0	44.0	.5	0	5	0
sesame rice spirals							
(*Eden*)	200	10.0	37.0	2.0	0	0	6.0

Food and Measure	cal.	prot. (gms)	carbo. (gms)	fat (gms)	chol. (mgs)	sod. (mgs)	fiber (gms)
shells (*Goya* Conchas)	210	6.0	45.0	1.0	0	0	0
spaghetti:							
(*Eden*)	210	7.0	42.0	1.0	0	10	2.0
(*Prince* Square/Thin)	200	8.0	40.0	1.0	0	20	2.0
parsley-garlic (*Eden*)	210	7.0	42.0	1.0	0	10	2.0
whole wheat (*Eden*)	210	10.0	39.0	1.5	0	0	6.0
tri-color (*Mueller's*)	210	7.0	42.0	1.0	0	10	1.0
vegetable rotini, spirals, shells (*Eden/ Herb's*)	210	7.0	42.0	1.0	0	10	2.0
vegetable spirals, whole wheat (*Eden*)	210	10.0	39.0	1.5	0	0	6.0
Pasta, cooked, 1 cup:							
plain	197	6.7	39.7	.9	0	1	2.4
corn	176	3.7	39.1	1.0	0	1	3.4
spinach	183	6.4	36.6	.9	0	20	n.a.
whole wheat	174	7.5	37.2	.6	0	4	6.3
Pasta, refrigerated, (see also specific pasta listings) plain:							
uncooked:							
w/egg, 2 oz.	163	6.4	31.0	1.3	41	15	2.0
spinach, w/egg, 2 oz.	164	6.4	31.6	1.2	41	15	n.a.
cooked:							
w/egg, 4 oz.	149	5.8	28.3	1.2	37	7	n.a.
spinach, w/egg, 4 oz.	147	5.7	28.4	1.1	37	7	n.a.
Pasta dinner, see specific listings							
Pasta dishes, frozen (see also "Pasta entree, frozen"):							
Alfredo:							
(*Green Giant Pasta Accents*), 2 cups	210	9.0	25.0	8.0	15	480	4.0

Food and Measure	cal.	prot. (gms)	carbo. (gms)	fat (gms)	chol. (mgs)	sod. (mgs)	fiber (gms)
Pasta dishes, frozen, Alfredo *(cont.)*							
w/broccoli (*The Budget Gourmet Side Dish*), 5.8 oz.	230	9.0	23.0	11.0	30	670	1.0
cheddar:							
creamy (*Green Giant Pasta Accents*), 2⅓ cups	250	9.0	44.0	8.0	15	700	5.0
white (*Green Giant Pasta Accents*), 1¾ cups	300	10.0	38.0	12.0	20	570	4.0
garden herb (*Green Giant Pasta Accents*), 2 cups . . .	230	9.0	32.0	7.0	15	750	7.0
garlic (*Green Giant Pasta Accents*), 2 cups	260	7.0	36.0	10.0	15	640	5.0
Florentine (*Green Giant Pasta Accents*), 2 cups	310	13.0	44.0	9.0	20	910	5.0
primavera (*Green Giant Pasta Accents*), 2¼ cups	320	13.0	40.0	12.0	20	500	7.0
Pasta dishes, mix (see also specific pasta listings), dry, ½ pkg., except as noted:							
cheese:							
cheddar broccoli (*Lipton* Pasta & Sauce)	260	9.0	46.0	3.5	10	870	1.0
four, corkscrews (*Noodle-Roni*), 1 cup*	410	13.0	49.0	19.0	10	1040	2.0
three (*Lipton* Pasta & Sauce)	240	9.0	41.0	5.0	10	870	1.0

Food and Measure	cal.	prot. (gms)	carbo. (gms)	fat (gms)	chol. (mgs)	sod. (mgs)	fiber (gms)
chicken:							
herb Parmesan							
(*Golden Saute*)	230	8.0	45.0	3.0	<5	830	3.0
primavera (*Lipton*							
Pasta & Sauce)	220	7.0	40.0	3.0	5	730	1.0
stir-fry (*Golden*							
Saute)	220	7.0	45.0	2.0	0	850	2.0
garlic:							
butter (*Golden*							
Saute)	210	6.0	41.0	3.0	5	790	2.0
creamy (*Lipton*							
Pasta & Sauce)	260	8.0	45.0	6.0	10	840	1.0
creamy, corkscrews							
(*Noodle-Roni*),							
1 cup*	420	9.0	40.0	25.0	5	1020	2.0
and herb (*Spice Is-*							
lands Quick Meal),							
1 pkg.	160	6.0	32.0	1.5	25	420	<1.0
herb, tomato (*Lipton*							
Pasta & Sauce) . .	240	9.0	48.0	2.0	0	690	3.0
mixed (*Buckeye*							
Oceans of), 2 oz.	210	7.0	42.0	1.0	0	0	2.0
primavera:							
(*Knorr* Cup), 1 pkg.	210	6.0	36.0	4.5	10	840	2.0
(*Lipton* Pasta &							
Sauce)	240	8.0	42.0	5.0	10	880	2.0
(*Spice Islands* Quick							
Meal), 1 pkg. . .	170	8.0	32.0	1.5	25	490	1.0
salad:							
(*Buckeye* Sunny							
Day), 1/10 pkg. . .	130	4.0	23.0	2.0	0	75	1.0
Caesar (*Kraft*),							
2.5 oz.	350	7.0	30.0	22.0	15	650	2.0
garden primavera							
(*Kraft*), 2.5 oz.	280	8.0	34.0	12.0	<5	730	2.0
hearty (*Buckeye*),							
1/8 pkg.	140	5.0	27.0	1.0	0	120	1.0
Italian, light (*Kraft*),							
2.5 oz.	190	8.0	34.0	2.0	<5	660	2.0

Food and Measure	cal.	prot. (gms)	carbo. (gms)	fat (gms)	chol. (mgs)	sod. (mgs)	fiber (gms)
Pasta dishes, mix, salad *(cont.)*							
Italian herb (*Fantastic*), ⅔ cup . . .	170	7.0	34.0	1.5	0	380	2.0
Parmesan peppercorn (*Kraft*), 2.5 oz.	360	8.0	28.0	25.0	20	610	2.0
ranch, classic, w/bacon (*Kraft*), 2.5 oz.	360	7.0	30.0	23.0	15	500	2.0
seasoned (*Buckeye Sunny*), ⅑ pkg.	140	5.0	26.0	2.0	0	50	1.0
spicy Oriental (*Fantastic*), ⅔ cup . .	200	7.0	37.0	3.0	0	420	3.0
spinach and mushroom (*Spice Islands Quick Meal*), 1 pkg.	160	6.0	29.0	2.0	5	490	<1.0
tomato, creamy, 1 pkg.:							
basil (*Spice Islands Quick Meal*) . . .	190	6.0	40.0	1.0	0	520	1.0
twists (*Knorr* Cup)	230	8.0	41.0	4.0	10	800	2.0
Pasta entree, canned (see also specific listings):							
spirals, and chicken *Libby's Diner*), 7¾ oz.	130	8.0	16.0	4.0	15	980	4.0
twists (*Franco-American*), 1 cup	250	8.0	41.0	5.0	10	1160	2.0
Pasta entree, freeze-dried:							
primavera (*Mountain House*), 1 cup . . .	220	10.0	32.0	6.0	20	690	4.0
Roma (*AlpineAire*), 1⅓ cups	328	18.0	47.0	1.0	n.a.	686	n.a.

Food and Measure	cal.	prot. (gms)	carbo. (gms)	fat (gms)	chol. (mgs)	sod. (mgs)	fiber (gms)
Pasta entree, frozen, (see also "Pasta dishes, frozen" and specific pasta listings), 1 pkg., except as noted:							
cheddar bake w/ (*Lean Cuisine*) . . .	220	12.0	29.0	6.0	20	560	3.0
cheddar and broccoli (*Banquet*)	350	12.0	48.0	12.0	15	900	6.0
and chicken marinara (*Lean Cuisine Lunch Express*)	270	15.0	38.0	6.0	20	540	4.0
marinara twist (*Lean Cuisine*)	240	10.0	42.0	3.0	5	440	4.0
primavera, w/chicken (*Marie Callender's*), 1 cup	310	12.0	22.0	19.0	25	450	3.0
rings (*Swanson Fun Feast* Razzlin') . . .	380	18.0	57.0	12.0	25	780	4.0
sausage and peppers (*Banquet*)	340	11.0	43.0	13.0	10	840	7.0
and spinach Romano (*Weight Watchers*)	240	11.0	32.0	8.0	5	510	4.0
w/tomato basil sauce (*Weight Watchers*)	260	12.0	33.0	9.0	10	360	5.0
and tuna casserole (*Lean Cuisine Lunch Express*)	280	18.0	39.0	6.0	20	590	4.0
and turkey Dijon (*Lean Cuisine Lunch Express*)	270	16.0	37.0	6.0	30	570	6.0
vegetable Italiano (*Healthy Choice*) . .	240	9.0	48.0	1.0	0	480	6.0
wheels and cheese (*Swanson Fun Feast*)	390	17.0	60.0	11.0	15	1110	8.0

Food and Measure	cal.	prot. (gms)	carbo. (gms)	fat (gms)	chol. (mgs)	sod. (mgs)	fiber (gms)
Pasta entree, frozen *(cont.)*							
wide ribbon w/ricotta							
(*The Budget Gourmet*)	420	16.0	41.0	22.0	65	620	2.0
Pasta flour, see							
"Semolina flour"							
Pasta salad, see							
"Pasta dishes, mix"							
Pasta sauce, tomato							
(see also "Tomato							
sauce" and specific							
sauce listings),							
½ cup:							
(*Campbell's*)	120	2.0	25.0	1.5	<5	550	2.0
(*Campbell's* Home-							
style)	90	2.0	18.0	1.0	0	510	2.0
(*Del Monte*)	60	2.0	14.0	1.0	0	500	3.0
(*Eden* Organic) . . .	80	3.0	12.0	2.5	0	320	3.0
(*Eden* Organic No							
Salt)	80	3.0	12.0	2.5	0	10	3.0
(*Healthy Choice*) . . .	50	2.0	10.0	.5	0	390	2.5
(*Hunt's* Homestyle)	55	2.0	7.0	2.5	0	595	1.5
(*Hunt's* Old Country)	55	2.0	7.0	2.5	0	540	3.0
(*Hunt's* Original) . . .	65	2.0	11.0	2.5	0	620	4.0
(*Paesana* Casalinga)	70	0	7.0	4.0	0	440	1.0
(*Patsy's* Fileto di							
Pomodoro)	90	2.0	7.0	6.0	0	430	2.0
(*Pomodoro Fresca*							
Solo)	25	1.0	6.0	0	0	10	1.0
(*Porino's*)	130	2.0	11.0	10.0	0	560	3.0
(*Prego*)	140	1.5	23.0	4.5	5	610	2.0
(*Prego* Low Sodium)	110	1.5	11.0	6.0	0	25	3.0
(*Prego Extra Chunky*							
Supreme Tomato)	120	2.0	20.0	3.0	0	580	3.0
(*Pritikin* Original) . .	60	2.0	7.0	.5	0	30	2.0
(*Progresso*)	100	3.0	12.0	4.5	<5	620	2.0
w/basil:							
(*Barilla*)	70	2.0	10.0	2.5	0	570	3.0
(*Classico* Di Napoli)	50	2.0	8.0	1.0	0	410	2.0

Food and Measure	cal.	prot. (gms)	carbo. (gms)	fat (gms)	chol. (mgs)	sod. (mgs)	fiber (gms)
(*Del Monte*)	60	2.0	11.0	1.0	0	480	<1.0
(*Del Monte* D'Italia)	50	2.0	9.0	1.5	0	390	<1.0
(*Hunt's* Classic) . .	50	2.0	7.5	2.0	0	615	4.0
(*Porino's*)	100	1.0	14.0	6.0	0	320	1.0
(*Prego*)	110	2.0	19.0	3.0	0	420	3.0
zesty (*Prego Extra Chunky*)	110	2.0	22.0	1.5	0	510	3.0
w/beef, ground (*Campbell's*)	100	2.0	19.0	1.5	<1	600	2.0
cheese, wine and herbs (*Porino's*) . .	150	3.0	19.0	9.0	0	180	n.a.
beef or beef and pork (*Porino's*)	120	2.0	13.0	7.0	0	620	2.0
cheese, four:							
(*Classico* Di Parma)	70	2.0	7.0	4.0	<5	480	1.0
(*Del Monte* D'Italia)	60	2.0	8.0	2.0	0	370	<1.0
cheese, three (*Prego*)	100	2.0	20.0	2.0	0	480	3.0
cheese and garlic, Italian (*Hunt's*) . . .	65	3.0	9.0	2.5	<5	690	2.0
fra diavolo (*Patsy's*)	120	3.0	11.0	1.0	0	440	3.0
garden:							
(*Porino's* Chunky)	150	2.0	17.0	9.0	0	390	2.0
(*Porino's* Gardina Fresca)	110	2.0	11.0	7.0	0	540	2.0
(*Pritikin* Chunky) . .	50	2.0	6.0	.5	0	30	2.0
combination (*Prego Extra Chunky*) . .	90	2.0	16.0	1.0	0	480	3.0
style (*Del Monte*)	60	2.0	11.0	1.0	0	510	<1.0
garlic (*Prego Extra Chunky* Supreme)	130	2.0	23.0	3.0	0	570	3.0
garlic and cheese (*Prego Extra Chunky*)	130	2.0	22.0	3.5	0	610	3.0
garlic and herb:							
(*Del Monte*)	60	2.0	11.0	1.5	0	490	<1.0
(*Healthy Choice*) . .	50	2.0	10.0	.5	0	390	2.5
(*Hunt's* Old Country)	65	2.5	9.0	3.0	0	520	3.5

Food and Measure	cal.	prot. (gms)	carbo. (gms)	fat (gms)	chol. (mgs)	sod. (mgs)	fiber (gms)
Pasta sauce *(cont.)*							
garlic and onion:							
(*Del Monte*)	60	2.0	13.0	1.0	0	460	2.0
(*Healthy Choice* Extra Chunky) . . .	40	2.0	8.0	0	0	370	1.0
(*Hunt's* Chunky) . .	60	1.5	12.5	1.0	0	525	1.5
(*Hunt's* Classic) . .	60	2.0	10.0	2.0	0	600	2.0
extra (*Campbell's*)	60	2.0	12.0	1.0	0	370	2.0
green pepper and mushroom (*Del Monte*)	60	2.0	12.0	1.0	0	390	3.0
hot (*Pomodoro Fresca* Cayenne)	40	1.0	6.0	1.5	0	230	1.0
Italian:							
herb (*Del Monte*)	60	2.0	12.0	1.0	0	520	<1.0
spice (*Aunt Millie's* Family Style) . .	90	3.0	16.0	1.5	0	650	2.0
style (*Campbell's*)	120	2.0	25.0	1.5	<5	550	2.0
marinara:							
(*Aunt Millie's*) . . .	70	2.0	9.0	3.0	0	320	2.0
(*Barilla*)	80	2.0	10.0	4.0	0	450	3.0
(*Campbell's*)	90	2.0	18.0	1.0	0	510	2.0
(*Colavita*)	65	3.0	11.0	0	0	480	3.0
(*Del Monte* D'Italia Classic)	50	2.0	9.0	1.5	0	510	<1.0
(*Hunt's* Chunky) . .	60	1.5	12.0	1.5	0	525	1.5
(*Paesana*)	115	2.0	9.0	8.0	0	480	2.0
(*Patsy's*)	120	3.0	11.0	6.0	0	440	3.0
(*Prego*)	110	2.0	12.0	6.0	0	670	3.0
(*Prince* Chunky) . .	70	2.0	13.0	1.5	0	610	2.0
(*Prince* Traditional)	50	3.0	9.0	.5	0	580	2.0
(*Pritikin*)	60	3.0	4.0	0	0	260	2.0
(*Progresso*)	90	2.0	8.0	4.5	<5	480	2.0
(*Progresso* Authentic)	100	3.0	9.0	5.0	<5	440	5.0
(*Rao's Homemade*)	60	5.0	4.0	4.0	0	375	2.0
w/pizza paste (*Aunt Millie's*)	70	2.0	9.0	2.5	0	330	3.0

Food and Measure	cal.	prot. (gms)	carbo. (gms)	fat (gms)	chol. (mgs)	sod. (mgs)	fiber (gms)
meat/meat flavor:							
(*Aunt Millie's*) . . .	80	3.0	9.0	3.0	<5	330	2.0
(*Aunt Millie's* Family Style)	100	3.0	16.0	2.5	<5	670	2.0
(*Del Monte*)	70	3.0	13.0	2.0	<5	510	3.0
(*Healthy Choice*) . .	50	2.5	8.0	1.0	<5	385	2.0
(*Hunt's* Homestyle)	55	2.0	7.0	2.5	<5	595	1.5
(*Hunt's* Old Country)	55	2.5	7.0	2.5	<5	475	2.5
(*Hunt's* Original) . .	65	2.0	11.0	2.5	<5	605	2.0
(*Prego*)	140	2.0	21.0	6.0	5	500	3.0
(*Prince* Chunky) . .	90	2.0	13.0	3.0	<5	620	2.0
(*Progresso*)	100	4.0	12.0	4.5	5	610	3.0
mushroom:							
(*Aunt Millie's*) . . .	70	2.0	10.0	2.0	0	280	2.0
(*Aunt Millie's* Family Style)	80	3.0	16.0	1.0	0	530	3.0
(*Campbell's*)	100	2.0	22.0	1.0	0	530	2.0
(*Del Monte*)	70	2.0	15.0	1.0	0	520	2.0
(*Healthy Choice*) . .	50	2.0	10.0	.5	0	390	2.5
(*Healthy Choice* Extra Chunky) . . .	40	2.0	8.0	0	0	350	1.0
(*Hunt's* Homestyle)	55	2.0	7.0	2.5	0	585	1.5
(*Hunt's* Original) . .	65	2.0	11.0	2.5	0	605	2.0
(*Hunt's* Old Country)	55	2.0	7.0	2.5	0	540	3.0
(*Prego*)	150	2.0	23.0	5.0	0	670	3.0
(*Prego Extra Chunky* Supreme)	130	2.0	21.0	4.5	5	490	3.0
(*Prince* Chunky) . .	70	2.0	13.0	1.5	0	670	2.0
(*Progresso*)	100	3.0	12.0	4.5	<5	580	4.0
(*Weight Watchers*)	60	2.0	11.0	0	0	420	4.0
and garlic (*Barilla*)	80	1.0	9.0	3.5	0	500	3.0
and garlic (*Campbell's*)	90	2.0	19.0	1.0	0	540	2.0
and garlic (*Healthy Choice* Super Chunky)	45	3.0	9.0	0	0	410	3.0

Food and Measure	cal.	prot. (gms)	carbo. (gms)	fat (gms)	chol. (mgs)	sod. (mgs)	fiber (gms)
Pasta sauce, mushroom *(cont.)*							
and green pepper *(Prego Extra Chunky)*	120	2.0	18.0	4.5	5	430	6.0
and onion *(Prego Extra Chunky)* . .	110	5.0	18.0	3.0	5	500	3.0
Parmesan *(Prego)*	120	2.0	19.0	3.5	10	570	3.0
and ripe olive *(Classico Di Sicilia)* . .	50	2.0	8.0	1.0	0	490	2.0
and tomato *(Prego Extra Chunky)* . .	110	2.0	19.0	3.0	0	510	3.0
w/spice, extra *(Prego Extra Chunky)*	120	2.0	19.0	4.0	0	510	3.0
and sweet peppers *(Healthy Choice Super Chunky)*	45	2.0	9.0	0	0	365	1.0
olive, black, and mushrooms *(Porino's)*	100	1.0	14.0	6.0	0	340	1.0
olive, green and black *(Barilla)*	100	2.0	9.0	6.0	0	710	3.0
w/olives and mushrooms *(Classico Di Sicilia)*	50	2.0	8.0	1.0	0	490	2.0
onion and garlic:							
(Classico Di Sorrento)	80	2.0	9.0	4.0	0	410	2.0
(Porino's)	100	1.0	14.0	5.0	0	320	1.0
(Prego)	110	2.0	19.0	3.0	0	420	3.0
(Prego Extra Chunky)	110	2.0	19.0	3.5	5	480	3.0
oregano, zesty *(Prego Extra Chunky)* . . .	140	5.0	25.0	3.0	0	580	3.0
w/Parmesan:							
(Hunt's Classic) . .	50	2.0	8.0	2.0	0	635	2.0
(Prego)	120	2.0	19.0	3.0	5	570	3.0
pepper, sweet or red:							
and garlic *(Barilla)*	70	2.0	8.0	3.5	0	580	3.0

Food and Measure	cal.	prot. (gms)	carbo. (gms)	fat (gms)	chol. (mgs)	sod. (mgs)	fiber (gms)
and onion (*Classico Di Salerno*) . . .	70	1.0	8.0	4.0	0	380	3.0
and onion (*Porino's*)	100	1.0	14.0	5.0	0	310	1.0
red (*Del Monte D'Italia*)	50	2.0	9.0	1.5	0	510	<1.0
and Italian sausage (*Aunt Millie's*) . .	60	3.0	8.0	2.0	5	350	2.0
spicy (*Barilla*) . . .	80	2.0	9.0	3.5	0	570	3.0
spicy (*Classico* Di Roma Arrabbiata)	60	2.0	6.0	2.5	0	270	2.0
w/pesto (*Classico* Di Genoa)	110	4.0	10.0	6.0	<5	450	2.0
sausage, Italian:							
(*Hunt's*)	75	2.5	12.0	3.0	<5	595	2.0
and fennel (*Classico D'Abruzzi*)	90	4.0	7.0	5.0	10	430	2.0
sausage and pepper:							
(*Prego Extra Chunky*)	180	2.0	22.0	9.0	10	570	3.0
and mushroom (*Porino's*)	150	3.0	20.0	8.0	0	340	n.a.
spinach and cheese (*Classico* Di Firenze)	80	3.0	8.0	4.5	<5	490	2.0
sun-dried tomato (*Classico* Di Capri)	80	2.0	8.0	4.5	0	430	2.0
w/vegetables:							
(*Hunt's* Chunky) . .	65	1.5	13.0	1.0	0	530	2.0
(*Prego Extra Chunky* Supreme)	90	2.0	15.0	3.0	5	490	3.0
Italian (*Healthy Choice* Extra Chunky)	40	2.0	8.0	0	0	380	1.0
Italian (*Hunt's* Old Country)	65	2.5	9.0	2.5	0	615	3.0
primavera (*Healthy Choice* Super Chunky)	45	2.0	9.0	0	0	360	1.0

Food and Measure	cal.	prot. (gms)	carbo. (gms)	fat (gms)	chol. (mgs)	sod. (mgs)	fiber (gms)
Pasta sauce *(cont.)*							
zucchini and Parme-							
san (*Classico* Di Mi-							
lano)	70	3.0	9.0	2.5	0	470	2.0
Pasta sauce, refriger-							
ated, tomato,							
½ cup:							
chunky tomato (*Con-*							
tadina Fat Free) . .	45	2.0	9.0	0	0	690	2.0
marinara (*Contadina*)	80	2.0	10.0	4.0	0	560	3.0
roasted garlic and ar-							
tichoke (*Monterey*							
Pasta Company) . .	70	2.0	8.0	3.0	0	620	2.0
Pasta sauce mix (see							
also specific list-							
ings):							
(*Knorr* Parma Rosa),							
2 tbsp.	60	2.0	8.0	2.0	<5	530	0
(*Lawry's*), 1 tbsp. . . .	35	<1.0	6.0	1.0	0	680	0
garlic and herb:							
(*Knorr*), ⅓ pkg. . . .	70	1.0	7.0	3.5	0	840	0
(*Spice Islands*),							
¼ pkg.	15	.5	3.0	2.5	0	380	0
w/mushroom flavor							
(*McCormick*),							
1 tbsp.	25	0	5.0	0	0	490	0
primavera (*Spice Is-*							
lands Pouch),							
⅕ pkg.	30	0	3.0	1.5	5	440	0
salad (*Durkee* Pouch),							
2 tsp.	10	.5	2.0	0	0	200	0
spaghetti:							
(*Durkee*), ½ cup*	15	0	5.0	0	0	390	0
(*Durkee* Family),							
2 tsp.	20	.5	4.0	0	0	560	0
American style							
(*Durkee*), ½ cup*	15	0	6.0	0	0	170	0
w/mushrooms							
(*Durkee*), ½ cup*	15	.5	4.0	0	0	520	0

Food and Measure	cal.	prot. (gms)	carbo. (gms)	fat (gms)	chol. (mgs)	sod. (mgs)	fiber (gms)
zesty (*Durkee*),							
2 tsp.	20	.5	5.0	0	0	350	0
Pastrami, 2 oz.:							
(*Healthy Deli*)	80	11.0	2.0	3.0	30	480	0
(*Hebrew National*) . .	80	12.0	0	3.0	30	510	0
brisket or Romanian							
(*Boar's Head*) . . .	90	12.0	2.0	4.0	30	620	0
round (*Boar's Head*)	70	12.0	<1.0	2.5	30	530	0
round (*Hebrew Na-*							
tional)	70	10.0	0	3.0	25	440	0
turkey, see "Turkey							
pastrami"							
Pastry, see specific							
listings							
Pastry shell (see also							
"Pie crust"):							
dough (*Goya* Discos),							
1 pc.	120	4.0	20.0	3.0	0	90	0
patty (*Pepperidge*							
Farm), 1 shell . . .	230	3.0	23.0	14.0	0	135	2.0
sheet, puff (*Pepper-*							
idge Farm), ⅙ sheet	200	3.0	23.0	11.0	0	135	3.0
tart:							
(*Oronoque*), 3″ shell	140	2.0	11.0	9.0	0	130	0
(*Pet-Ritz*), 3″ shell	140	2.0	11.0	9.0	0	130	0
(*Pet-Ritz*),							
¼ of 6″ shell . .	110	2.0	9.0	7.0	0	105	0
Pastry filling (see							
also "Pie filling"),							
canned, 2 tbsp.:							
almond (*Solo*)	120	1.0	23.0	2.5	0	45	2.0
apple, Dutch (*Solo*)	80	0	20.0	0	0	45	1.0
apricot (*Solo*)	80	0	17.0	0	0	20	1.0
blueberry, wild (*Solo*)	80	0	17.0	0	0	25	1.0
cherry (*Solo*)	80	0	20.0	0	0	25	1.0
date (*Solo*)	100	0	22.0	0	0	40	3.0
nut, fancy (*Solo*) . .	140	1.0	25.0	5.0	0	55	5.0
pecan (*Solo*)	130	1.0	24.0	4.0	0	50	1.0
pineapple (*Solo*) . . .	80	0	19.0	0	0	20	1.0

Food and Measure	cal.	prot. (gms)	carbo. (gms)	fat (gms)	chol. (mgs)	sod. (mgs)	fiber (gms)
Pastry filling *(cont.)*							
poppy seed (*Solo*) . .	140	2.0	30.0	4.0	0	30	3.0
prune plum (*Solo*) . .	70	0	18.0	0	0	25	1.0
raspberry, red (*Solo*)	80	0	19.0	0	0	25	1.0
strawberry (*Solo*) . .	70	0	18.0	0	0	20	1.0
Pâté (see also "Liver-wurst"), canned:							
1 oz.	90	4.0	.4	7.9	n.a.	198	0
1 tbsp.	41	1.9	.2	3.6	n.a.	91	0
chicken liver:							
1 oz.	57	3.8	1.9	3.7	n.a.	n.a.	0
1 tbsp.	26	1.8	.9	1.7	n.a.	n.a.	0
goose liver:							
smoked, 1 oz. . . .	131	3.2	1.3	12.4	43	n.a.	0
smoked, 1 tbsp. . .	60	1.5	.6	5.7	20	n.a.	0
liver (*Sells*), ¼ cup	160	7.0	3.0	14.0	65	380	1.0
Pâté, vegetarian (*Bonavita* Swiss),							
1 oz.	61	2.0	3.0	4.0	0	160	0
Pea pods, Chinese, see "Peas, edible-podded"							
Peach:							
fresh:							
2½" peach, 4 per lb.	37	.6	9.7	.1	0	tr.	1.7
sliced, ½ cup. . . .	37	.6	9.4	.1	0	1	1.7
canned, see "Peach, canned"							
dried:							
(*Sonoma*), 3–5 pcs., 1.4 oz.	120	1.0	31.0	0	0	0	1.0
sulfured, halves, ½ cup	192	2.9	49.1	.6	0	6	6.6
sulfured, 10 halves, 4.6 oz.	311	4.7	79.7	1.0	0	9	10.7
sun-dried (*Del Monte*), 1.4 oz., ⅓ cup	90	1.0	26.0	0	0	0	5.0

Food and Measure	cal.	prot. (gms)	carbo. (gms)	fat (gms)	chol. (mgs)	sod. (mgs)	fiber (gms)
frozen, sliced, sweet-							
ened, ½ cup	118	.8	30.0	.2	0	8	1.8
Peach, canned,							
½ cup, halves or							
slices, except as							
noted:							
(*Hunt's*)	100	1.0	24.0	0	0	10	1.0
(*S&W* Ready-Cut Cali-							
fornia Sun)	80	<1.0	20.0	0	0	20	1.0
(*S&W* Ready-Cut							
Tropical Sun) . . .	80	<1.0	19.0	0	0	15	0
w/cinnamon (*S&W*							
Sweet Memory							
Ready-Cut Sun) . .	70	<1.0	19.0	0	0	15	<1.0
in juice, cling:							
(*Del Monte* Natural)	60	0	15.0	0	0	10	1.0
(*Libby's* Lite) . . .	60	1.0	13.0	0	0	10	1.0
(*S&W* Natural) . . .	80	1.0	19.0	0	0	20	1.0
in juice or extra light							
syrup, diced (*Del*							
Monte Naturals							
Snack Cup), 4¼ oz.	60	0	15.0	0	0	15	1.0
in extra light syrup:							
cling (*Del Monte*							
Lite)	60	0	15.0	0	0	10	1.0
freestone (*Del*							
Monte Lite) . . .	60	0	14.0	0	0	10	1.0
in light syrup, diced							
(*Del Monte* Snack							
Cup), 3½ oz. . . .	70	0	17.0	0	0	10	<1.0
in heavy syrup, cling:							
(*Del Monte/Del*							
Monte Melba) . .	100	0	24.0	0	0	10	1.0
(*S&W*)	100	1.0	24.0	0	0	10	1.0
diced (*Del Monte*							
Snack Cup),							
4¼ oz.	90	0	23.0	0	0	10	1.0

Food and Measure	cal.	prot. (gms)	carbo. (gms)	fat (gms)	chol. (mgs)	sod. (mgs)	fiber (gms)
Peach, canned *(cont.)*							
in heavy syrup, free-							
stone:							
(*Del Monte*)	100	0	24.0	0	0	10	1.0
(*S&W*)	100	1.0	23.0	0	0	50	0
raspberry flavor, cling,							
in heavy syrup (*Del*							
Monte)	80	<1.0	20.0	0	0	10	<1.0
spiced (*Del Monte*							
Natural Harvest) . .	80	<1.0	21.0	0	0	10	<1.0
spiced, in heavy							
syrup:							
(*Del Monte*)	100	0	24.0	0	0	10	<1.0
(*S&W*), 4.3-oz. pc.	100	<1.0	23.0	0	0	20	<1.0
Peach, frozen, sliced:							
(*Big Valley*), ⅔ cup	50	1.0	13.0	0	0	0	2.0
(*Stilwell*), 1 cup . . .	60	1.0	14.0	0	0	0	2.0
Peach butter							
(*Smucker's*), 1 tbsp.	45	0	11.0	0	0	10	0
Peach drink, 8 fl. oz.:							
(*After the Fall*)	100	1.0	27.0	0	0	20	0
(*Farmer's Market*) . .	120	0	31.0	0	0	0	0
(*Tree Top* Quake) . .	120	0	30.0	0	0	25	0
Peach dumpling, fro-							
zen (*Pepperidge*							
Farm), 1 pc.	300	3.0	47.0	11.0	0	150	6.0
Peach juice blend:							
(*Dole* Orchard),							
8 fl. oz.	140	1.0	34.0	0	0	30	0
(*Dole* Orchard),							
10 fl. oz.	170	1.0	42.0	0	0	45	0
Peach nectar:							
(*Goya*), 8 fl. oz. . . .	150	1.0	36.0	0	0	10	3.0
(*Goya*), 12 fl. oz. . .	220	1.0	54.0	0	0	25	2.0
(*Libby's*), 8 fl. oz. . .	150	<1.0	36.0	0	0	0	0
(*Libby's/Kern's*),							
11.5 fl. oz.	210	1.0	52.0	0	0	5	0
(*R.W. Knudsen*),							
8 fl. oz.	120	0	30.0	0	0	25	0

Food and Measure	cal.	prot. (gms)	carbo. (gms)	fat (gms)	chol. (mgs)	sod. (mgs)	fiber (gms)
Peanut, shelled, 1 oz., except as noted:							
unroasted	159	7.2	4.5	13.8	0	5	2.5
boiled, salted	90	3.8	6.0	6.2	0	213	2.5
dry-roasted:							
½ cup	428	17.3	15.7	36.3	0	4	5.8
(*Little Debbie*) . . .	160	7.0	5.0	14.0	0	130	2.0
(*Planters*)	160	7.0	6.0	13.0	0	250	3.0
(*Planters* Lightly Salted)	170	8.0	5.0	14.0	0	95	3.0
(*Planters* Lightly Salted), 1-oz. pkg.	160	7.0	5.0	14.0	0	110	3.0
(*Planters* Lightly Salted), 1¾-oz. pkg. . . .	290	13.0	9.0	25.0	0	190	4.0
(*Planters* Unsalted)	160	8.0	6.0	14.0	0	0	3.0
honey-roasted:							
(*Frito-Lay*), ¼ cup	270	10.0	10.0	21.0	0	80	2.0
(*Planters*)	160	6.0	8.0	13.0	0	90	2.0
(*Smart Snackers*), .7 oz.	100	7.0	7.0	5.0	0	100	2.0
dry-roasted (*Planters*), 1.7-oz. pkg.	260	10.0	17.0	19.0	0	360	3.0
oil-roasted (*Planters* Reduced Fat) . .	130	8.0	12.0	7.0	0	150	2.0
hot (*Frito-Lay*), ¼ cup	280	12.0	6.0	21.0	0	340	4.0
hot and spicy:							
(*Planters Heat*) . .	160	7.0	5.0	14.0	0	190	2.0
(*Planters Heat*), 1.7-oz. pkg. . . .	290	12.0	9.0	25.0	0	370	4.0
(*Planters Heat*), 2-oz. pkg.	330	14.0	10.0	29.0	0	390	3.0
(*Planters Heat* Munch 'N Go Singles*), 2.5-oz. pkg.	410	18.0	13.0	36.0	0	480	6.0
oil-roasted:							
½ cup	419	19.0	13.6	35.5	0	4	6.6
(*Pennant*)	170	7.0	6.0	14.0	0	115	3.0

Food and Measure	cal.	prot. (gms)	carbo. (gms)	fat (gms)	chol. (mgs)	sod. (mgs)	fiber (gms)
Peanut, oil-roasted *(cont.)*							
(*Planters*), 2-oz. bag	340	14.0	11.0	29.0	0	290	5.0
(*Planters* Fun Size)							
2 bags, 1 oz. . . .	170	7.0	6.0	14.0	0	140	2.0
(*Planters* Lightly							
Salted),							
1¾-oz. pkg.	300	13.0	8.0	27.0	0	95	4.0
(*Planters Munch 'N*							
Go)	170	7.0	6.0	15.0	0	150	2.0
cocktail (*Planters*)	170	7.0	6.0	14.0	0	115	2.0
cocktail (*Planters*							
Lightly Salted) . .	170	7.0	5.0	15.0	0	55	2.0
cocktail (*Planters*							
Unsalted)	170	7.0	6.0	14.0	0	0	2.0
fancy (*Paradise/*							
White Swan),							
¼ cup, 1½ oz.	270	11.0	7.0	22.0	0	135	5.0
salted (*Planters*) . .	170	7.0	5.0	15.0	0	115	2.0
salted (*Planters*),							
1-oz. pkg.	170	7.0	5.0	14.5	0	110	2.0
salted (*Planters*),							
1.7-oz. pkg. . . .	290	12.0	10.0	25.0	0	250	4.0
Spanish:							
(*Planters*)	170	7.0	5.0	14.0	0	105	2.0
raw (*Planters*) . . .	150	7.0	6.0	13.0	0	180	3.0
sweet (*Planters Sweet*							
N Crunchy)	140	4.0	16.0	7.0	0	115	2.0
Peanut butter,							
2 tbsp.:							
chunky or crunchy:							
(*Adams* Natural) . .	200	10.0	5.0	16.0	0	90	1.0
(*Adams* Unsalted)	200	10.0	5.0	16.0	0	5	2.0
(*Adams No-Stir*) . .	200	10.0	4.0	16.0	0	120	2.0
(*Peter Pan*)	190	8.0	6.0	16.0	0	120	2.0
(*Peter Pan Real*)	190	9.0	5.0	16.0	0	90	4.0
(*Peter Pan*							
Whipped)	150	6.0	5.0	12.5	0	95	2.0

Food and Measure	cal.	prot. (gms)	carbo. (gms)	fat (gms)	chol. (mgs)	sod. (mgs)	fiber (gms)
(*Roasted Honey Nut* Skippy Super Chunk)	190	7.0	7.0	17.0	0	120	2.0
(*Skippy Super* Chunk)	190	8.0	6.0	17.0	0	140	2.0
(*Skippy Super* Chunk Reduced Fat)	190	8.0	13.0	12.0	0	170	1.0
(*Teddie* Super) . . .	190	8.0	7.0	16.0	0	100	3.0
spread (*Peter Pan* Smart Choice) . .	195	7.8	14.5	11.7	0	153	1.7
chunky or creamy:							
(*Arrowhead Mills*)	190	9.0	6.0	16.0	0	tr.	4.5
(*Peter Pan* Very Low Sodium) . .	195	8.0	6.0	17.5	0	<1.0	2.0
(*Roaster Fresh*) . .	166	8.0	5.0	14.0	0	97	0
(*Roaster Fresh* Un-salted)	166	8.0	5.0	14.0	0	2	0
(*Smuckers*)	190	7.0	6.0	15.0	0	160	2.0
(*Smucker's* Natural)	200	7.0	7.0	16.0	0	120	2.0
(*Smucker's* Natural No Salt)	200	7.0	7.0	16.0	0	0	2.0
creamy or smooth:							
(*Adams* Natural) . .	200	10.0	4.0	16.0	0	115	1.0
(*Adams* Unsalted)	200	10.0	5.0	15.0	0	0	2.0
(*Adams* No-Stir) . .	210	10.0	4.0	17.0	0	160	2.0
(*Peter Pan*)	190	8.0	7.0	16.0	0	150	2.0
(*Peter Pan* Real)	190	9.5	5.0	16.0	0	95	3.0
(*Peter Pan* Whipped)	150	6.0	5.0	12.5	0	120	2.0
(*Roasted Honey Nut* Skippy)	190	7.0	6.0	17.0	0	125	2.0
(*Skippy*)	190	8.0	6.0	17.0	0	150	2.0
(*Skippy* Reduced Fat)	190	8.0	14.0	12.0	0	200	1.0
(*Teddie*)	190	8.0	7.0	16.0	0	125	3.0
spread (*Peter Pan* Smart Choice) . .	180	8.0	14.5	11.0	0	190	2.0
unsalted (*Teddie*) . .	190	8.0	7.0	16.0	0	0	3.0

Food and Measure	cal.	prot. (gms)	carbo. (gms)	fat (gms)	chol. (mgs)	sod. (mgs)	fiber (gms)
Peanut butter cara-mel topping (*Smucker's*), 2 tbsp.	150	3.0	24.0	4.5	0	125	<1.0
Peanut butter and jelly (*Smucker's Goober*), 3 tbsp. . . .	230	7.0	24.0	13.0	0	160	2.0
Peanut butter snack (see also "Cracker"), graham:							
(*Mr. Peanut P.B. Crisps*), 1 oz.	140	4.0	16.0	7.0	0	90	1.0
(*Mr. Peanut P.B. Crisps*), 1.5-oz. pkg.	210	5.0	24.0	10.0	0	135	2.0
Peanut flour, 1 cup:							
defatted	196	31.3	20.8	.3	0	9	n.a.
defatted, salted . . .	196	31.3	20.8	.3	0	108	n.a.
lowfat	257	20.3	18.8	13.1	0	0	n.a.
Peanut sauce, Orien-tal:							
(*House of Tsang Bangkok Padang*), 1 tbsp.	45	1.0	4.0	2.5	0	240	0
cooking (*Kylin Singa-pore Satay*), 1/4 cup	60	2.0	7.0	3.0	0	650	<1.0
Pear:							
fresh, w/peel:							
Bartlett, 1 medium, 2 1/2 per lb.	98	.7	25.1	.7	0	1	4.0
sliced, 1/2 cup . . .	49	.3	12.5	.3	0	1	2.0
canned, see "Pear, canned"							
dried:							
2 oz.	149	1.1	39.5	.4	0	4	4.3
halves, 1/2 cup . . .	236	1.7	62.7	.6	0	5	6.8
(*Sonoma*), 3–4 pcs., 1.4 oz.	120	1.0	33.0	0	0	0	3.0
Pear, Asian, whole, 1 medium, 2 1/4" × 2 1/2" diam.	51	.6	13.0	.3	0	(0)	4.4

Food and Measure	cal.	prot. (gms)	carbo. (gms)	fat (gms)	chol. (mgs)	sod. (mgs)	fiber (gms)
Pear, canned, ½ cup halves or slices, except as noted:							
(*S&W* Ready-Cut California Sun)	80	<1.0	19.0	0	0	10	<1.0
in juice (*Libby's* Lite)	60	0	13.0	0	0	10	1.0
in juice or extra light syrup (*Del Monte* Natural/Lite)	60	0	15.0	0	0	10	1.0
in extra light syrup (*Del Monte* Snack Cup), 4¼ oz. . . .	60	0	15.0	0	0	10	1.0
in light syrup, diced (*Del Monte* Snack Cup), 3½-oz. cup	70	0	17.0	0	0	10	<1.0
in heavy syrup:							
(*Del Monte*)	100	0	24.0	0	0	10	1.0
diced (*Del Monte* Snack Cup), 4¼ oz.	90	0	23.0	0	0	10	1.0
Bartlett:							
in juice (*S&W* Natural)	80	0	21.0	0	0	10	2.0
in heavy syrup (*S&W*)	90	0	22.0	0	0	10	2.0
ginger flavor (*Del Monte* Natural) . .	90	0	22.0	0	0	10	1.0
Pear juice, 8 fl. oz.:							
(*After the Fall* Harvest)	90	0	22.0	0	0	10	0
(*After the Fall* Rouge River)	100	0	24.0	0	0	20	0
(*Heinke's*)	120	0	30.0	0	0	25	0
(*R.W. Knudsen*) . . .	120	0	30.0	0	0	25	0
Pear nectar:							
canned, 6 fl. oz. . . .	112	.2	29.6	<.1	0	7	1.1
(*Libby's*), 8 fl. oz. . .	150	0	38.0	0	0	0	0
(*Libby's/Kern's*), 11.5 fl. oz.	220	0	54.0	0	0	5	0

Food and Measure	cal.	prot. (gms)	carbo. (gms)	fat (gms)	chol. (mgs)	sod. (mgs)	fiber (gms)
Pear nectar *(cont.)*							
(Santa Cruz), 8 fl. oz.	120	0	30.0	0	0	30	0
Pear-passion nectar,							
canned *(Goya)*,							
12 fl. oz.	230	0	57.0	0	0	40	4.0
Peas, see specific							
listings							
Peas, butter, frozen							
(Stilwell), ½ cup	110	7.0	20.0	.5	0	10	4.0
Peas, cream, canned							
(Allens/East Texas							
Fair), ½ cup	100	6.0	17.0	1.0	0	460	5.0
Peas, crowder,							
½ cup:							
canned *(Allens/East*							
Texas Fair/							
Homefolks)	110	6.0	19.0	1.0	0	460	8.0
frozen *(Stilwell)* . . .	120	8.0	22.0	1.0	0	10	4.0
Peas, edible-podded:							
fresh:							
raw, ½ cup	30	2.0	5.4	.1	0	3	1.9
boiled, drained,							
½ cup	34	2.6	5.6	.2	0	3	2.2
sugar snap							
(Frieda's), 1 oz.	15	1.0	3.4	.1	0	n.a.	n.a.
frozen:							
boiled, drained,							
½ cup	42	2.8	7.2	.3	0	4	2.4
sugar snap *(Green*							
Giant), ¾ cup . .	35	2.0	7.0	0	0	0	3.0
sugar snap *(Green*							
Giant Harvest							
Fresh), ⅔ cup . .	50	3.0	10.0	0	0	95	3.0
Peas, field, ½ cup:							
canned, fresh shell:							
(Sunshine)	120	7.0	21.0	1.0	0	350	6.0
w/snaps *(Allens/East*							
Texas Fair/							
Homefolks) . . .	120	6.0	21.0	1.0	0	300	6.0

Food and Measure	cal.	prot. (gms)	carbo. (gms)	fat (gms)	chol. (mgs)	sod. (mgs)	fiber (gms)
w/snaps (*Goya*),							
½ cup	110	7.0	19.0	.5	0	180	9.0
canned, dry:							
w/bacon (*Trappey's*)	90	6.0	15.0	1.0	0	380	5.0
w/snaps and bacon							
(*Trappey's*) . . .	110	6.0	19.0	1.0	0	380	4.0
frozen, w/snaps							
(*Stilwell*)	110	8.0	20.0	1.0	0	10	4.0
Peas, green, sweet,							
fresh:							
raw:							
in pod, 1 lb.	140	9.3	24.9	.7	0	8	8.8
shelled, ½ cup . . .	58	3.9	10.4	.3	0	3	3.7
boiled, drained, ½ cup	67	4.3	12.5	.2	0	2	4.4
Peas, green, canned,							
½ cup:							
(*Del Monte*)	60	3.0	11.0	0	0	360	4.0
(*Del Monte* No Salt)	60	3.0	11.0	0	0	10	4.0
(*Goya*)	95	6.0	16.0	.9	0	506	5.0
(*Goya* Tender Sweet)	70	4.0	12.0	0	0	390	2.0
(*S&W* Petit Pois/							
Sweet)	70	4.0	12.0	0	0	330	4.0
(*Stokely*)	60	4.0	10.0	0	0	360	3.0
(*Stokely* No Salt) . .	60	4.0	10.0	0	0	20	3.0
early June:							
(*Sun-Vista*)	80	6.0	18.0	0	0	510	5.0
dry (*Crest Top*) . .	100	5.0	20.0	.5	0	300	6.0
early or sweet:							
(*Green Giant*) . . .	60	4.0	11.0	0	0	390	4.0
(*Green Giant* Less							
Sodium)	60	4.0	11.0	0	0	195	4.0
(*Green Giant* Le-							
Sueur)	60	4.0	12.0	0	0	380	3.0
(*Green Giant* Le-							
Sueur Less So-							
dium)	60	4.0	11.0	0	0	190	4.0
very young, small							
(*Del Monte*)	60	3.0	10.0	0	0	360	4.0

Food and Measure	cal.	prot. (gms)	carbo. (gms)	fat (gms)	chol. (mgs)	sod. (mgs)	fiber (gms)
Peas, green, dried,							
(*Goya*), ¼ cup . . .	100	9.0	24.0	0	0	15	9.0
Peas, green, freeze-							
dried, ½ cup:							
(*AlpineAire*)	81	6.0	14.0	.4	0	2	n.a.
(*Mountain House*) . .	80	5.0	12.0	1.0	0	65	5.0
Peas, green, frozen,							
⅔ cup, except as							
noted:							
(*Seabrook*)	70	5.0	12.0	.5	0	105	4.0
(*Stilwell*)	70	5.0	12.0	0	0	100	4.0
baby, early (*Green Gi-*							
ant Harvest Fresh							
LeSueur)	70	4.0	13.0	0	0	220	4.0
early June (*Green Gi-*							
ant LeSueur)	60	5.0	11.0	0	0	150	5.0
sweet:							
(*Green Giant*) . . .	70	4.0	13.0	0	0	135	4.0
(*Green Giant Har-*							
vest Fresh) . . .	60	4.0	12.0	0	0	200	4.0
baby (*Green Giant*							
LeSueur)	60	5.0	11.0	0	0	150	5.0
butter sauce, ¾ cup:							
baby, early (*Green*							
Giant LeSueur)	100	5.0	16.0	2.0	<5	370	4.0
sweet (*Green Giant*)	100	4.0	16.0	2.0	<5	400	5.0
Peas, green, combi-							
nations, ½ cup, ex-							
cept as noted:							
canned:							
w/mushrooms and							
onions (*Green Gi-*							
ant LeSueur) . .	60	4.0	11.0	0	0	380	2.0
w/pearl onions							
(*Green Giant*) . .	60	4.0	11.0	0	0	520	4.0
w/pearl onions							
(*S&W*)	40	3.0	11.0	0	0	530	3.0
canned, and carrots:							
(*Del Monte*)	60	2.0	11.0	0	0	360	2.0

Food and Measure	cal.	prot. (gms)	carbo. (gms)	fat (gms)	chol. (mgs)	sod. (mgs)	fiber (gms)
(*Goya*)	60	3.0	9.0	0	0	380	2.0
(*Green Giant*) . . .	50	2.0	11.0	0	0	410	3.0
(*S&W*)	50	3.0	10.0	0	0	330	3.0
(*Stokely*)	60	3.0	10.0	0	0	370	3.0
(*Stokely* No Salt/ Sugar)	50	3.0	9.0	0	0	20	3.0
frozen:							
and carrots (*Stilwell*)	50	3.0	9.0	0	0	70	3.0
w/mushrooms (*Green Giant Le-Sueur*), ¾ cup . .	60	4.0	10.0	0	0	105	4.0
w/pearl onions (*Green Giant*), ⅔ cup	60	4.0	12.0	0	0	125	4.0
w/pearl onions (*Green Giant Harvest Fresh*) . . .	50	3.0	10.0	0	0	170	3.0
Peas, lady, canned, ½ cup:							
(*Sunshine*)	100	6.0	17.0	1.0	0	460	5.0
w/snaps (*East Texas Fair*)	100	7.0	17.0	1.0	0	420	4.0
Peas, pepper, canned, (*Allens/East Texas Fair/ Homefolks*), ½ cup	120	6.0	22.0	1.0	0	580	6.0
Peas, purple hull, ½ cup:							
canned (*East Texas*)	120	7.0	21.0	1.0	0	350	6.0
frozen (*Stilwell*) . . .	110	7.0	21.0	1.0	0	10	4.0
Peas, split, see "Split peas"							
Peas, sprouted:							
raw, ½ cup	77	5.3	17.0	.4	0	12	n.a.
boiled, drained, 4 oz.	134	8.0	24.8	.6	0	3	3.7
Peas, sugar snap, see "Peas, edible-podded"							

Food and Measure	cal.	prot. (gms)	carbo. (gms)	fat (gms)	chol. (mgs)	sod. (mgs)	fiber (gms)
Peas, sweet, see "Peas, green"							
Peas, white acre, canned (*East Texas Fair*), ½ cup	100	6.0	17.0	1.0	0	460	5.0
Peas and carrots or onions, see "Peas, green, combinations"							
Pecan, shelled:							
chips (*Planters*), 2-oz. pkg.	390	5.0	9.0	40.0	0	230	7.0
halves (*Planters Gold Measure*), 2-oz. pkg.	390	5.0	9.0	40.0	0	230	3.0
halves or pcs.:							
(*Planters*), 1 oz. . .	190	3.0	4.0	20.0	0	115	2.0
(*Paradise/White Swan*), ¼ cup, 1 oz.	200	4.0	5.0	18.0	0	0	3.0
pcs. (*Planters*), 2-oz. pkg.	390	5.0	9.0	40.0	0	230	3.0
dried:							
1 oz.	190	2.2	5.2	19.2	0	<1	2.2
halves, 1 cup . . .	721	8.4	19.7	73.1	0	1	8.2
chopped, 1 cup . .	794	9.2	21.7	80.5	0	1	9.0
dry-roasted, salted, 1 oz.	187	2.3	6.3	18.4	0	221	n.a.
honey-roasted (*Planters*), 1 oz.	180	2.0	9.0	16.0	0	75	2.0
oil-roasted, salted, 1 oz.	195	2.0	4.6	20.2	0	214	n.a.
Pecan filling, see "Pastry filling"							
Pecan flour, 1 oz. . .	93	9.1	14.4	.4	0	tr.	n.a.
Pecan topping, w/syrup (*Smucker's*), 2 tbsp.	190	1.0	22.0	11.0	0	0	0
Pectin, see "Fruit pectin"							

Food and Measure	cal.	prot. (gms)	carbo. (gms)	fat (gms)	chol. (mgs)	sod. (mgs)	fiber (gms)
Penne, plain, see "Pasta"							
Penne dishes, mix, dry, except as noted:							
Alfredo (*Knorr*), ¾ cup	280	11.0	44.0	6.0	60	890	2.0
herb and butter (*Noodle Roni*), 1 cup*	430	10.0	44.0	24.0	5	780	2.0
herb and garlic (*Golden Saute*), ½ pkg.	230	8.0	44.0	3.0	5	810	2.0
w/sun-dried tomato Parmesan (*Knorr*), ½ cup	270	9.0	51.0	3.0	<5	530	3.0
Penne entree, canned, in meat sauce (*Franco-American*), 1 cup	240	8.0	40.0	5.0	10	1100	3.0
Penne entree, frozen, 1 pkg.:							
w/sausage (*The Budget Gourmet* Light & Healthy)	330	17.0	49.0	8.0	10	530	6.0
spicy, and ricotta (*Weight Watchers*)	280	12.0	45.0	6.0	5	370	5.0
w/sun-dried tomato (*Weight Watchers*)	290	13.0	40.0	9.0	10	560	5.0
Pepper, seasoning:							
black:							
ground, 1 tsp. . . .	6	.3	1.7	.1	0	1	.7
whole, 1 tsp. . . .	8	.3	1.9	0	0	1	.8
chili, 1 tsp.	9	.3	1.2	.3	0	<1	.7
red or cayenne, 1 tsp.	6	.2	1.0	.3	0	1	.7
white:							
1 tsp.	7	.3	1.7	.1	0	0	.2
(*McCormick*), ¼ tsp.	2	.1	.4	0	0	0	.1
(*Tone's*), ¼ tsp. . . .	0	0	0	0	0	0	0

Food and Measure	cal.	prot. (gms)	carbo. (gms)	fat (gms)	chol. (mgs)	sod. (mgs)	fiber (gms)
Pepper, banana, hot or mild (*Vlasic*), 1 oz.	5	0	1.0	0	0	480	0
Pepper, bell, see "Pepper, sweet"							
Pepper, cherry:							
(*Trappey's*), 2 pcs.	10	0	2.0	0	0	260	<1.0
hot (*Hebrew National*), 1⅓ pcs. . . .	25	0	4.0	0	0	800	0
hot (*Progresso*), 1 pc.	15	0	3.0	0	0	250	0
hot or mild (*Vlasic*), 1 oz.	10	0	2.0	0	0	480	0
marinated, drained (*Progresso*), 2 tbsp.	30	0	2.0	2.0	0	30	1.0
Pepper, chili, raw, green and red, w/out seeds:							
1 medium, 1.6 oz. . . .	18	.9	4.3	.1	0	3	.7
chopped, ½ cup . . .	30	1.5	7.1	.2	0	5	1.1
Pepper, chili, in jars:							
chopped, w/liquid ½ cup	17	.6	4.2	.1	0	n.a.	1.3
green, whole:							
(*Chi-Chi's*), ¾ chili	10	0	1.0	0	0	5	0
(*Old El Paso*), 1 chili	10	0	2.0	0	0	230	1.0
(*Rosarita*), 1.2 oz.	5	0	1.0	0	0	75	<1.0
green, chopped (*Old El Paso*), 2 tbsp.	5	0	1.0	0	0	110	1.0
green, diced, 2 tbsp.:							
(*Chi-Chi's*)	10	0	1.0	0	0	5	0
(*Pancho Villa*) . . .	5	0	1.0	0	0	110	1.0
(*Rosarita*)	5	0	1.5	0	0	85	<1.0
yellow, hot (*Del Monte*), 4 pcs., 1 oz.	10	0	3.0	0	0	610	<1.0
Pepper, chili, relish, pickle (*Patak's*), 1 tbsp.	45	0	1.0	4.0	0	590	<1.0

Food and Measure	cal.	prot. (gms)	carbo. (gms)	fat (gms)	chol. (mgs)	sod. (mgs)	fiber (gms)
Pepper, chilpotle							
spice sauce (*Del*							
Monte), 2 tbsp. . .	20	<1.0	4.0	.5	0	430	1.0
Pepper, jalapeño:							
whole:							
(*Del Monte*), .7 oz.	3	0	<1.0	0	0	230	<1.0
(*Goya*), 2 pcs.	10	0	2.0	0	0	320	0
(*Rosarita*), 1.2 oz.	10	<1.0	1.5	0	0	430	1.0
(*Trappey's*), 2 pcs.	10	0	3.0	0	0	700	<1.0
peeled (*Old El*							
Paso), 3 pcs.,							
1.1 oz.	10	0	1.0	0	0	200	1.0
or wheels (*Chi-*							
Chi's)	10	0	1.0	0	0	110	0
diced, 1.1 oz.:							
(*La Victoria*)	10	0	2.0	0	0	290	0
(*Rosarita*)	5	0	1.0	0	0	120	<1.0
hot (*Vlasic*)	10	0	2.0	0	0	490	0
marinated (*La Victo-*							
ria), 1.1 oz.	10	0	2.0	0	0	290	<1.0
nacho, sliced, 1.1 oz.:							
(*La Victoria*)	0	0	<1.0	0	0	370	<1.0
(*Rosarita*)	5	0	1.0	0	0	450	<1.0
pickled:							
(*La Victoria*), 1.1 oz.	10	0	2.0	0	0	115	<1.0
(*Old El Paso*),							
2 pcs.	5	0	1.0	0	0	380	0
whole (*Del Monte*),							
1.1 oz., 2–3 pcs.	5	0	1.0	0	0	560	<1.0
sliced (*Del Monte*),							
1 oz., 2 tbsp. . .	5	0	1.0	0	0	440	<1.0
sliced (*Old El Paso*),							
1.1 oz., 2 tbsp.	15	0	3.0	0	0	400	1.0
nacho, sliced (*Del*							
Monte), 1 oz.,							
2 tbsp.	5	0	1.0	0	0	340	<1.0
Pepper, nacho, pick-							
led (*Goya*), 14 slices	10	0	2.0	0	0	280	0

Food and Measure	cal.	prot. (gms)	carbo. (gms)	fat (gms)	chol. (mgs)	sod. (mgs)	fiber (gms)
Pepper, roasted, see "Pepper, sweet, in jars"							
Pepper, stuffed, frozen:							
(*Stouffer's*), 10 oz.	200	9.0	24.0	8.0	25	900	1.0
(*Stouffer's*), ½ of 15½-oz. pkg. . . .	180	8.0	20.0	7.0	20	590	3.0
Pepper, sweet:							
fresh, green and red:							
raw, 1 medium, 3¾″ × 3″	20	.7	4.8	.1	0	1	1.3
raw, chopped, ½ cup	13	.4	3.2	.1	0	1	.9
boiled, drained, 1 medium	20	.7	4.9	.1	0	1	.9
boiled, drained, chopped, ½ cup	19	.6	4.6	.1	0	1	.8
fresh, yellow, raw:							
1 large, 5″ × 3″ . .	50	1.9	11.8	.4	0	3	n.a.
10 strips, 1.8 oz.	14	.5	3.3	.1	0	1	n.a.
in jars, see "Pepper, sweet, in jars" and "Pimiento"							
freeze-dried, 1 tbsp.	1	.1	.3	<.1	0	1	.1
frozen, chopped, 1 oz.	6	.3	1.3	.1	0	1	.5
Pepper, sweet, in jars:							
filet (*Hebrew National/ Rosoff/Shorr's*), 1 oz.	9	0	2.0	0	0	310	0
fried, drained (*Progresso*), 2 tbsp.	60	0	3.0	5.0	0	60	1.0
rings (*Vlasic*), 1 oz.	25	0	6.0	0	0	170	0
roasted:							
(*Progresso*), ½ pc.	10	0	1.0	0	0	60	0
fire, w/garlic, oil (*Paesana*), 2 tbsp.	20	0	2.0	1.0	0	125	0

Food and Measure	cal.	prot. (gms)	carbo. (gms)	fat (gms)	chol. (mgs)	sod. (mgs)	fiber (gms)
Pepper salad:							
(*B&G*), 1 oz.	10	0	3.0	0	0	240	0
drained (*Progresso*),							
2 tbsp.	25	0	1.0	2.0	0	80	1.0
Pepper sauce (see							
also specific list-							
ings), hot, 1 tsp.,							
except as noted:							
(*Durkee RedHot*) . .	0	0	0	0	0	210	0
(*Gebhardt*)	0	0	0	0	0	90	0
(*Goya*)	0	0	0	0	0	125	0
(*Pickapeppa*), 1 tbsp.	18	0	4.0	0	0	95	0
(*Tabasco*)	0	0	0	0	0	30	0
(*Try Me Cajun/Tennes-*							
see Sunshine) . . .	0	0	0	0	0	160	0
(*Try Me* Tiger)	10	0	2.0	0	0	140	0
jalapeño (*Tabasco*) . .	0	0	0	0	0	70	0
garlic (*Tabasco*) . . .	0	0	0	0	0	95	0
hot or original							
(*Hunt's*)	0	0	0	0	0	205	0
in vinegar (*Goya*) . .	0	0	0	0	0	150	0
Pepper steak, see							
"Beef entree"							
Pepper "steak" en-							
tree, vegetarian,							
frozen (*Hain*), 10 oz.	310	26.0	41.0	6.0	0	440	9.0
Peppercorn sauce							
mix (*Knorr*), 2 tsp.	25	1.0	3.0	1.0	0	350	0
Pepperoncini:							
(*Krinos*), ¼ cup . . .	5	0	2.0	0	0	950	0
(*Nalley*), 1 oz.	5	0	1.0	0	0	310	0
(*Progresso* Tuscan),							
3 peppers	10	0	1.0	0	0	330	1.0
(*Zorba*), 5 pcs.,							
1.1 oz.	15	1.0	2.0	0	0	450	0
salad (*Vlasic*), 1 oz.	5	0	1.0	0	0	440	0
Pepperoni:							
(*Boar's Head*), 1 oz.	140	6.0	0	13.0	30	540	0

Food and Measure	cal.	prot. (gms)	carbo. (gms)	fat (gms)	chol. (mgs)	sod. (mgs)	fiber (gms)
Pepperoni *(cont.)*							
(Hormel/Leoni/Rosa							
Grande), 1 oz.	140	5.0	0	13.0	35	470	0
(Oscar Mayer),							
15 slices, 1.1 oz.	140	6.0	0	13.0	25	550	0
(Patrick Cudahy							
3 oz.), 16 slices,							
1.1 oz.	150	6.0	0	14.0	30	530	0
(Patrick Cudahy							
6 oz.), 15 slices,							
1.1 oz.	170	6.0	0	16.0	40	660	0
(Patrick Cudahy							
Stick), 1 oz.	150	6.0	0	13.0	30	580	0
"Pepperoni," vege-							
tarian (*Yves Veggie*							
Cuisine), 3½ slices	78	14.0	5.0	0	0	340	2.0
Pepperoni bagel							
sandwich, frozen							
(*Hormel Quick*							
Meal), 1 pc.	350	15.0	41.0	15.0	45	920	2.0
Perch, meat only:							
raw, 4 oz.	103	22.0	0	1.1	102	70	0
baked, broiled, or mi-							
crowaved, 4 oz. . .	133	28.2	0	1.3	130	90	0
ocean, see "Ocean							
perch"							
Perch entree, frozen,							
battered (*Van de*							
Kamp's), 2 pcs. . .	300	12.0	19.0	20.0	25	480	n.a.
Persimmon, fresh:							
fuyu (*Frieda's*), 1 oz.	22	.2	5.6	.1	0	2	n.a.
hachiya, trimmed							
(*Frieda's*), 1 oz. . .	36	.2	10.1	.1	0	<1	n.a.
Japanese:							
fresh, 1 medium . .	118	1.0	31.2	.3	0	3	6.0
dried, 1 oz.	78	.4	20.0	.2	0	.1	4.1
native, 1 medium,							
1.1 oz.	32	.2	8.4	.1	0	<1	n.a.

Food and Measure	cal.	prot. (gms)	carbo. (gms)	fat (gms)	chol. (mgs)	sod. (mgs)	fiber (gms)
Persimmon, dried:							
(*Sonoma*), 6–8 pcs.	140	1.0	35.0	0	0	10	3.0
Japanese, 1 oz. . . .	78	.4	20.8	.2	0	1	4.1
Pesto sauce, ¼ cup:							
in jars (*Sonoma*) . .	110	3.0	6.0	9.0	2	125	1.0
refrigerated:							
basil (*Contadina*)	310	6.0	6.0	29.0	10	400	3.0
sun-dried tomato							
(*Contadina*) . . .	250	3.0	8.0	23.0	5	510	2.0
Pesto sauce mix:							
(*Knorr*), ⅓ pkg. . . .	15	<1.0	2.0	0	0	470	0
(*Spice Islands*),							
¼ pkg.	15	0	1.0	.5	0	260	0
creamy (*Knorr*),							
⅕ pkg.	30	1.0	3.0	1.0	0	440	0
red bell pepper							
(*Knorr*), ⅓ pkg. . .	30	1.0	6.0	.5	0	690	<1.0
tomato:							
(*Spice Islands*),							
¼ pkg.	15	0	3.0	0	0	320	0
sun-dried (*Knorr*),							
⅓ pkg.	45	2.0	9.0	.5	0	720	1.0
Pheasant, raw:							
meat w/skin, 4 oz. . .	205	25.7	0	10.5	n.a.	45	0
meat only:							
4 oz.	151	26.7	0	4.1	n.a.	42	0
½ breast, 6.4 oz.	243	44.4	0	5.9	n.a.	60	0
1 leg, 3.8 oz. . . .	143	23.8	0	4.6	n.a.	48	0
Phyllo, see "Fillo pastry"							
Picante sauce (see also "Salsa"), 2 tbsp., except as noted:							
(*Pace*)	10	.5	2.0	0	0	209	.5
all varieties:							
(*Del Monte*)	10	0	2.0	0	0	210	0
(*Hunt's* Homestyle)	10	1.0	2.0	0	0	255	0
black bean (*Arthur's*)	15	1.0	3.0	0	0	10	<1.0

Food and Measure	cal.	prot. (gms)	carbo. (gms)	fat (gms)	chol. (mgs)	sod. (mgs)	fiber (gms)
Picante sauce *(cont.)*							
black-eyed pea (*Arthur's*)	15	1.0	3.0	0	0	50	<1.0
garlic, w/corn and honey (*Arthur's*) . .	15	0	3.0	0	0	10	0
hot:							
(*Chi-Chi's*)	10	0	2.0	0	0	270	0
(*Old El Paso*) . . .	10	0	2.0	0	0	160	0
(*Sun-Vista*)	10	0	2.0	0	0	260	0
or mild (*Arthur's*)	10	0	2.0	0	0	10	0
jalapeño, zesty:							
hot (*Rosarita*) . . .	10	0	2.0	0	0	250	<1.0
medium (*Rosarita*)	10	0	2.0	0	0	255	<1.0
mild (*Rosarita*) . .	10	0	2.0	0	0	240	<1.0
medium:							
(*Chi-Chi's*)	10	0	2.0	0	0	200	0
(*Old El Paso*) . . .	10	0	2.0	0	0	140	0
mesquite (*Arthur's*)	10	0	2.0	0	0	10	0
mild:							
(*Chi-Chi's*)	10	0	2.0	0	0	210	0
(*Old El Paso*) . . .	10	0	2.0	0	0	130	0
(*Sun-Vista*)	5	0	2.0	0	0	200	0
Pickle, cucumber, 1 oz., except as noted:							
bread and butter:							
(*Mrs. Fanning's*), 3 slices, 1 oz. . . .	25	0	6.0	0	0	190	0
(*Shorr's*)	12	0	3.0	0	0	220	0
chips (*Claussen*), 4 slices, 1 oz. . . .	20	0	4.0	0	0	170	0
chunks (*Nalley* Banquet)	2	0	6.0	0	0	200	0
midgets (*Vlasic* Milwaukee)	40	0	10.0	0	0	230	0
sandwich (*Claussen*), 2 slices, 1.1 oz.	20	0	5.0	0	0	190	0

Food and Measure	cal.	prot. (gms)	carbo. (gms)	fat (gms)	chol. (mgs)	sod. (mgs)	fiber (gms)
sandwich stackers							
(*Vlasic*)	30	0	7.0	0	0	170	0
slices (*Nalley*) . . .	25	0	6.0	0	0	220	0
chips:							
(*Nalley* Cucumber)	35	0	9.0	0	0	135	0
w/honey (*Pickle*							
Eater's)	25	0	6.0	0	0	0	0
dill:							
(*Nalley* Banquet) . .	5	0	1.0	0	0	290	0
(*Nalley* Country) . .	5	0	1.0	0	0	270	0
(*Nalley* Dilliest) . .	5	0	1.0	0	0	330	0
(*Vlasic* Milwaukee)	5	0	1.0	0	0	260	0
whole or halves (*Del*							
Monte)	5	0	<1.0	0	0	370	<1.0
baby (*Pickle Eater's*)	0	0	0	0	0	310	0
garlic (*Nalley*) . . .	5	0	1.0	0	0	280	0
hamburger chips							
(*Del Monte*) . . .	5	0	0	0	0	300	0
hamburger chips/							
slices (*Claussen*),							
10 slices, 1.1 oz.	5	0	1.0	0	0	420	0
onion (*Nalley* Walla							
Walla)	5	0	1.0	0	0	280	0
tiny (*Nalley* Ban-							
quet)	5	0	1.0	0	0	270	0
dill, kosher:							
(*Claussen*)	5	0	1.0	0	0	330	0
(*Claussen* Mini),							
.8-oz. pc.	5	0	1.0	0	0	300	0
(*Hebrew National*							
Barrel/Hot),							
1 pickle	23	1.0	4.0	0	0	1570	0
(*Pickle Eater's*) . .	0	0	0	0	0	360	0
(*Pickle Eater's* No							
Salt)	0	0	0	0	0	5	0
sandwich stackers							
(*Vlasic*)	5	0	1.0	0	0	210	0
slices (*Claussen*),							
2 slices, 1.1 oz.	5	0	1.0	0	0	390	0

Food and Measure	cal.	prot. (gms)	carbo. (gms)	fat (gms)	chol. (mgs)	sod. (mgs)	fiber (gms)
Pickle, dill, kosher *(cont.)*							
snack chunks							
(*Vlasic*)	5	0	1.0	0	0	220	0
spears (*Claussen*),							
1.2-oz. spear . .	5	0	1.0	0	0	310	0
spears (*Pickle*							
Eater's)	0	0	0	0	0	330	0
spears (*Vlasic*) . . .	5	0	1.0	0	0	310	0
tiny (*Del Monte*) . .	5	0	1.0	0	0	240	<1.0
dill, Polish, spears							
(*Vlasic*)	5	0	1.0	0	0	280	0
kosher:							
(*Shorr's* Deli) . . .	4	0	1.0	0	0	160	0
whole (*Rosoff/*							
Shorr's)	4	0	1.0	0	0	260	0
halves (*Hebrew Na-*							
tional/Rosoff/							
Shorr's)	4	0	1.0	0	0	290	0
spears (*Hebrew Na-*							
tional/Shorr's) . .	4	0	1.0	0	0	260	0
sour (*Claussen* New							
York Deli), ½ pickle	5	0	1.0	0	0	260	0
sour, kosher:							
(*Hebrew National/*							
Rosoff/Shorr's							
New Half Sours)	4	0	1.0	0	0	210	0
garlic (*Hebrew Na-*							
tional/Shorr's) . .	3	0	1.0	0	0	250	0
spears (*Rosoff/*							
Shorr's Half Sour)	4	0	1.0	0	0	200	0
sweet:							
(*Nalley*)	30	0	8.0	0	0	200	0
all varieties:							
(*Del Monte*) . .	40	0	10.0	0	0	210	<1.0
(*Vlasic*)	40	0	10.0	0	0	170	0
gherkins (*Nalley*)	25	0	7.0	0	0	110	0
midgets (*Nalley*) . .	30	0	8.0	0	0	160	0
Pickle dip, dill (*Nal-*							
ley's), 2 tbsp. . . .	70	0	5.0	5.0	15	260	0

Food and Measure	cal.	prot. (gms)	carbo. (gms)	fat (gms)	chol. (mgs)	sod. (mgs)	fiber (gms)
Pickle and pepper loaf (*Boar's Head*), 2 oz.	150	6.0	2.0	13.0	30	500	0
Pickle and pimiento loaf (*Oscar Mayer*), 1-oz. slice	70	3.0	2.0	6.0	20	360	0
Pickle relish, cucumber (see also specific listings), 1 tbsp.:							
dill, chunky (*Nalley*)	0	0	0	0	0	140	0
hamburger:							
(*Del Monte*)	20	0	6.0	0	0	220	<1.0
(*Nalley*)	15	0	3.0	0	0	110	0
hot dog:							
(*Del Monte*)	15	0	4.0	0	0	140	<1.0
(*Nalley*)	15	0	3.0	0	0	120	0
piccalilli, tomato							
(*Pickle Eater's*) . .	10	0	2.0	0	0	75	0
red hot (*Ron's*) . . .	15	0	4.0	0	0	100	0
sweet:							
(*Claussen*)	15	0	3.0	0	0	85	0
(*Del Monte*)	20	0	5.0	0	0	125	0
(*Hebrew National*)	18	0	4.0	0	0	50	0
(*Nalley*)	20	0	4.0	0	0	125	0
honey (*Pickle Eater's*)	15	0	4.0	0	0	90	0
regular or curry flavor (*Vlasic*) . . .	15	0	4.0	0	0	140	0
Pickled vegetables, see "Vegetables mixed, pickled" and specific listings							
Pickling spice (*Tone's*), 1 tsp. . .	10	.3	1.2	.6	n.a.	1	.3
Pico de gallo, see "Salsa"							

Food and Measure	cal.	prot. (gms)	carbo. (gms)	fat (gms)	chol. (mgs)	sod. (mgs)	fiber (gms)
Pie, ⅙ pie, except as noted:							
apple (*Entenmann's* Homestyle)	300	2.0	42.0	14.0	0	300	2.0
coconut custard (*Entenmann's*)	340	7.0	35.0	19.0	135	310	1.0
lemon (*Entenmann's*)	340	3.0	45.0	17.0	45	420	<1.0
Pie, frozen, ⅙ pie, except as noted:							
apple:							
(*Amy's*), 8 oz. . . .	280	4.0	42.0	12.0	n.a.	180	n.a.
(*Banquet*), ⅕ pie	300	3.0	41.0	13.0	5	370	2.0
(*Mrs. Smith's* 8″)	270	2.0	41.0	11.0	0	300	1.0
(*Mrs. Smith's* 9″), ⅛ pie	310	2.0	44.0	14.0	0	370	1.0
(*Mrs. Smith's* 10″), ⅒ pie	280	2.0	43.0	12.0	0	310	1.0
(*Mrs. Smith's* Old Fashioned 9″), ⅛ pie	350	2.0	50.0	16.0	0	400	2.0
(*Mrs. Smith's* Reduced Fat)	250	2.0	43.0	8.0	0	290	1.0
(*Mrs. Smith's* Reduced Fat No Sugar)	210	2.0	32.0	8.0	0	290	2.0
lattice (*Mrs. Smith's*), ⅕ pie	310	2.0	46.0	15.0	0	350	2.0
apple, Dutch:							
(*Mrs. Smith's* 8″)	320	3.0	48.0	13.0	0	260	1.0
(*Mrs. Smith's* 9″), ⅛ pie	350	3.0	52.0	14.0	0	290	1.0
(*Mrs. Smith's* 10″), ⅒ pie	320	3.0	50.0	12.0	0	250	1.0
(*Mrs. Smith's* Old Fashioned), ⅛ pie	310	2.0	49.0	12.0	0	230	2.0
apple-cranberry (*Mrs. Smith's*)	280	2.0	43.0	11.0	0	300	1.0
banana cream:							
(*Banquet*), ⅓ pie	350	3.0	39.0	21.0	<5	290	<1.0

Food and Measure	cal.	prot. (gms)	carbo. (gms)	fat (gms)	chol. (mgs)	sod. (mgs)	fiber (gms)
(*Mrs. Smith's*),							
¼ pie	280	2.0	37.0	14.0	0	170	1.0
(*Pet-Ritz*), ¼ pie . .	270	3.0	37.0	13.0	5	250	1.0
berry (*Mrs. Smith's*)	280	2.0	43.0	11.0	0	340	0
blackberry (*Mrs.*							
Smith's)	280	2.0	43.0	11.0	0	320	0
blueberry (*Mrs.*							
Smith's)	260	2.0	39.0	11.0	0	320	1.0
Boston cream, see							
"Cake, frozen"							
cherry:							
(*Banquet*), ⅕ pie	290	3.0	39.0	14.0	5	310	2.0
(*Mrs. Smith's 8"*)	270	2.0	39.0	11.0	0	320	1.0
(*Mrs. Smith's 9"*),							
⅛ pie	310	3.0	45.0	13.0	0	390	1.0
(*Mrs. Smith's 10"*),							
¹⁄₁₀ pie	280	2.0	44.0	11.0	0	340	1.0
(*Mrs. Smith's* Old							
Fashioned 9"),							
⅛ pie	320	3.0	48.0	13.0	0	350	1.0
(*Mrs. Smith's* Re-							
duced Fat 8") . .	250	2.0	44.0	8.0	0	310	1.0
(*Mrs. Smith's* Re-							
duced Fat No							
Sugar 8")	220	3.0	35.0	8.0	0	310	1.0
lattice (*Mrs.*							
Smith's), ⅕ pie	320	3.0	47.0	13.0	0	340	1.0
chocolate cream:							
(*Banquet*), ⅓ pie	360	3.0	43.0	20.0	<5	240	3.0
(*Mrs. Smith's*),							
¼ pie	330	3.0	42.0	17.0	0	200	1.0
(*Pet-Ritz*), ¼ pie . .	290	3.0	39.0	13.0	5	270	2.0
(*Sara Lee*), ⅕ pie	500	4.0	49.0	32.0	<5	440	2.0
French silk (*Mrs.*							
Smith's), ⅕ pie	410	3.0	55.0	11.0	5	250	1.0
coconut cream:							
(*Banquet*), ⅓ pie	350	3.0	39.0	20	<5	250	2.0
(*Mrs. Smith's*),							
¼ pie	340	2.0	40.0	19.0	0	260	0

Food and Measure	cal.	prot. (gms)	carbo. (gms)	fat (gms)	chol. (mgs)	sod. (mgs)	fiber (gms)
Pie, frozen, coconut cream *(cont.)*							
(*Pet-Ritz*), ¼ pie . .	270	3.0	37.0	13.0	5	250	1.0
coconut custard,							
(*Mrs. Smith's*),							
⅕ pie	280	7.0	35.0	12.0	75	350	0
fudge vanilla cream							
(*Pet-Ritz*), ¼ pie . .	300	3.0	40.0	15.0	5	190	1.0
lemon cream:							
(*Banquet*), ⅓ pie	360	3.0	43.0	20.0	<5	240	2.0
(*Mrs. Smith's*),							
¼ pie	300	2.0	40.0	19.0	0	160	0
(*Pet-Ritz*), ¼ pie . .	270	3.0	37.0	13.0	5	250	1.0
lemon meringue:							
(*Mrs. Smith's*),							
⅕ pie	302	2.0	55.0	8.2	66	218	0
(*Sara Lee* Home-							
style)	350	2.0	59.0	11.0	0	460	5.0
mince/mincemeat:							
(*Banquet*), ⅕ pie	310	3.0	46.0	13.0	10	430	2.0
(*Mrs. Smith's*) . . .	300	2.0	48.0	11.0	0	400	2.0
peach:							
(*Banquet*), ⅕ pie	260	3.0	36.0	12.0	5	340	2.0
(*Mrs. Smith's 8"*)	260	2.0	38.0	11.0	0	310	1.0
(*Mrs. Smith's 9"*),							
⅛ pie	310	3.0	46.0	13.0	0	350	1.0
peanut butter choco-							
late cream (*Pet-*							
Ritz), ¼ pie	300	3.0	37.0	15.0	5	180	2.0
pecan:							
(*Mrs. Smith's 8"*)	520	5.0	73.0	23.0	70	450	1.0
(*Mrs. Smith's 10"*),							
⅛ pie	500	5.0	68.0	23.0	60	460	1.0
pumpkin:							
(*Banquet*), ⅕ pie	250	4.0	40.0	8.0	20	340	3.0
hearty (*Mrs. Smith's*							
8"), ⅕ pie	250	4.0	42.0	8.0	50	320	2.0
hearty (*Mrs. Smith's*							
9"), ⅛ pie	240	5.0	39.0	7.0	45	300	2.0

Food and Measure	cal.	prot. (gms)	carbo. (gms)	fat (gms)	chol. (mgs)	sod. (mgs)	fiber (gms)
pumpkin cream (*Pet-Ritz*), ¼ pie	270	3.0	37.0	13.0	5	250	1.0
pumpkin custard:							
(*Mrs. Smith's 8"*), ⅕ pie	270	5.0	44.0	8.0	45	350	1.0
(*Mrs. Smith's 9"*), ⅛ pie	240	5.0	39.0	8.0	40	310	1.0
(*Mrs. Smith's 10"*), ⅒ pie	250	5.0	42.0	8.0	50	330	1.0
raspberry, red (*Mrs. Smith's*)	280	2.0	43.0	11.0	0	320	0
strawberry (*Mrs. Smith's*), ⅕ pie . .	280	2.0	45.0	11.0	0	190	1.0
strawberry-rhubarb (*Mrs. Smith's*) . . .	280	2.0	44.0	11.0	0	380	0
Pie, mix (*Jell-O*), ⅙ pie*:							
chocolate silk	310	5.0	38.0	16.0	5	490	<1.0
coconut cream	330	4.0	37.0	19.0	5	410	1.0
Pie, snack, 1 pie, except as noted:							
(*Tastykake Tastyklair*)	410	6.0	53.0	20.0	85	320	2.0
apple:							
(*Aunt Fanny's*), 3½ oz.	400	3.0	53.0	20.0	25	390	1.0
(*Aunt Fanny's*), 4 oz.	460	3.0	61.0	23.0	30	440	1.0
(*Drake's*), 2 pies, 4 oz.	400	4.0	60.0	16.0	0	240	4.0
(*Hostess*)	410	3.0	60.0	19.0	15	370	2.0
(*McMillin's*), 3½ oz.	390	3.0	48.0	21.0	25	330	1.0
(*McMillin's*), 4 oz.	460	3.0	61.0	23.0	30	440	1.0
(*Pet-Ritz*)	430	4.0	58.0	20.0	30	370	2.0
(*Tastykake*)	290	3.0	45.0	12.0	0	320	2.0
French (*Hostess*)	410	3.0	60.0	19.0	15	370	2.0
French (*Tastykake*)	360	3.0	61.0	12.0	0	350	3.0
banana cream (*Aunt Fanny's*)	400	3.0	50.0	21.0	25	350	1.0

Food and Measure	cal.	prot. (gms)	carbo. (gms)	fat (gms)	chol. (mgs)	sod. (mgs)	fiber (gms)
Pie, snack *(cont.)*							
berry:							
(*Aunt Fanny's*),							
3½ oz.	380	4.0	48.0	19.0	25	330	2.0
(*Aunt Fanny's*),							
4 oz.	430	5.0	55.0	22.0	25	380	2.0
(*McMillin's*), 3½ oz.	390	3.0	48.0	20.0	25	330	2.0
(*McMillin's*), 4 oz.	440	3.0	55.0	23.0	25	380	2.0
blackberry or blue-							
berry (*Hostess*) . .	400	4.0	59.0	17.0	15	340	2.0
blueberry:							
(*Pet-Ritz*)	450	4.0	61.0	21.0	30	370	2.0
(*Tastykake*)	320	2.0	54.0	11.0	0	330	3.0
Boston creme:							
(*Aunt Fanny's*),							
3½ oz.	370	3.0	48.0	19.0	20	320	1.0
(*Aunt Fanny's*),							
4 oz.	440	3.0	56.0	22.0	25	340	1.0
(*McMillin's*), 3½ oz.	370	3.0	48.0	19.0	25	320	1.0
(*McMillin's*), 4 oz.	440	3.0	56.0	22.0	25	340	1.0
cherry:							
(*Aunt Fanny's*),							
3½ oz.	350	3.0	48.0	19.0	25	320	4.0
(*Aunt Fanny's*),							
4 oz.	400	3.0	55.0	22.0	30	370	6.0
(*Drake's*), 2 pies,							
4 oz.	420	4.0	60.0	18.0	0	250	4.0
(*Hostess*)	430	4.0	62.0	19.0	15	350	1.0
(*McMillin's*), 3½ oz.	380	3.0	46.0	22.0	25	270	4.0
(*McMillin's*), 4 oz.	430	3.0	53.0	25.0	30	310	4.0
(*Pet-Ritz*)	450	4.0	56.0	23.0	30	300	1.0
(*Tastykake*)	320	3.0	51.0	12.0	0	350	3.0
chocolate creme:							
(*Aunt Fanny's*),							
3½ oz.	390	3.0	46.0	23.0	25	450	3.0
(*Aunt Fanny's*),							
4 oz.	450	3.0	53.0	26.0	30	510	3.0
chocolate pudding:							
(*McMillin's*), 3½ oz.	380	3.0	45.0	21.0	25	330	2.0

Food and Measure	cal.	prot. (gms)	carbo. (gms)	fat (gms)	chol. (mgs)	sod. (mgs)	fiber (gms)
(*McMillin's*), 4 oz.	450	3.0	53.0	26.0	30	510	3.0
coconut creme:							
(*Aunt Fanny's*),							
3½ oz.	390	3.0	49.0	20.0	25	300	2.0
(*Aunt Fanny's*),							
4 oz.	440	3.0	56.0	23.0	25	340	2.0
(*Tastykake*)	390	5.0	47.0	20.0	60	540	3.0
coconut pudding:							
(*McMillin's*), 3½ oz.	380	3.0	45.0	21.0	25	330	2.0
(*McMillin's*), 4 oz.	440	3.0	56.0	22.0	25	340	2.0
lemon:							
(*Hostess*)	420	4.0	58.0	20.0	30	360	1.0
(*McMillin's*), 3½ oz.	360	3.0	47.0	19.0	25	440	2.0
(*McMillin's*), 4 oz.	410	3.0	54.0	22.0	25	500	2.0
(*Pet-Ritz*)	450	4.0	61.0	21.0	30	340	1.0
(*Tastykake*)	320	3.0	50.0	12.0	40	330	2.0
lemon creme:							
(*Aunt Fanny's*),							
3½ oz.	360	3.0	47.0	19.0	25	440	2.0
(*Aunt Fanny's*),							
4 oz.	420	3.0	54.0	22.0	30	510	2.0
marshmallow:							
banana (*Little Debbie*)	320	3.0	54.0	11.0	0	190	0
chocolate (*Little Debbie*)	320	3.0	53.0	11.0	0	190	1.0
oatmeal creme (*Little Debbie*)	300	3.0	48.0	12.0	0	330	1.0
peach:							
(*Aunt Fanny's*),							
3½ oz.	380	3.0	46.0	19.0	25	270	2.0
(*Aunt Fanny's*),							
4 oz.	430	3.0	53.0	22.0	30	310	2.0
(*Hostess*)	400	4.0	59.0	18.0	15	340	2.0
(*McMillin's*), 3½ oz.	370	4.0	50.0	19.0	25	310	1.0
(*McMillin's*), 4 oz.	420	4.0	57.0	22.0	30	350	1.0
(*Tastykake*)	300	3.0	47.0	11.0	0	330	2.0
peanut butter cream							
(*McMillin's*)	450	3.0	53.0	26.0	30	510	3.0

Food and Measure	cal.	prot. (gms)	carbo. (gms)	fat (gms)	chol. (mgs)	sod. (mgs)	fiber (gms)
Pie, snack *(cont.)*							
pineapple:							
(*Hostess*)	400	5.0	60.0	16.0	15	350	2.0
(*Tastykake*)	290	3.0	45.0	12.0	20	310	1.0
cheese (*Tastykake*)	320	4.0	50.0	12.0	20	410	1.0
pumpkin:							
(*Aunt Fanny's*) . . .	420	3.0	56.0	21.0	20	410	2.0
(*McMillin's*)	420	3.0	56.0	21.0	20	410	2.0
(*Tastykake*)	330	4.0	47.0	14.0	25	560	4.0
raisin creme (*Little*							
Debbie)	270	2.0	44.0	11.0	0	220	0
strawberry:							
(*Aunt Fanny's*),							
3½ oz.	370	3.0	49.0	18.0	20	260	2.0
(*Aunt Fanny's*),							
4 oz.	420	3.0	56.0	21.0	20	300	2.0
(*Hostess*)	390	4.0	56.0	18.0	15	340	2.0
(*McMillin's*), 3½ oz.	370	3.0	49.0	18.0	20	260	2.0
(*McMillin's*), 4 oz.	420	3.0	56.0	20.0	20	300	2.0
(*Tastykake*)	310	2.0	50.0	12.0	0	300	1.0
vanilla creme:							
(*Aunt Fanny's*),							
3½ oz.	350	3.0	44.0	18.0	25	310	1.0
(*Aunt Fanny's*),							
4 oz.	400	3.0	50.0	21.0	25	350	1.0
vanilla pudding:							
(*McMillin's*), 3½ oz.	360	3.0	44.0	19.0	25	310	1.0
(*McMillin's*), 4 oz.	400	3.0	50.0	21.0	25	350	1.0
Pie crust:							
chocolate cookie:							
(*Ready Crust*),							
⅛ crust	110	1.0	14.0	5.0	0	100	<1.0
(*Oreo*), ⅙ crust . .	140	1.0	18.0	7.0	0	180	<1.0
cookie crumbs:							
(*Nilla*), 2 tbsp.	70	1.0	13.0	2.5	<5	55	<1.0
(*Oreo*), 2 tbsp.	80	1.0	13.0	3.0	0	140	1.0
graham:							
(*Honey Maid*),							
⅙ crust	140	1.0	18.0	7.0	0	125	<1.0

Food and Measure	cal.	prot. (gms)	carbo. (gms)	fat (gms)	chol. (mgs)	sod. (mgs)	fiber (gms)
mini (*Ready Crust*), .8-oz. crust . . .	120	1.0	15.0	6.0	0	150	<1.0
graham crumbs:							
(*Honey Maid*), 2 tbsp.	70	1.0	13.0	1.5	0	90	<1.0
(*Sunshine*), 2 tbsp.	80	2.0	13.0	2.0	0	150	<1.0
shortbread (*Ready Crust* 9"), ⅛ crust	100	1.0	15.0	4.5	0	95	<1.0
vanilla cookie (*Nilla*), ⅙ crust	140	1.0	20.0	8.0	<5	65	0
Pie crust, frozen or refrigerated (see also "Pastry shell"), ⅛ crust, except as noted:							
(*Oronoque*)	90	1.0	7.0	6.0	0	80	0
(*Oronoque*), ¼ of 6" crust	110	2.0	9.0	7.0	0	105	0
(*Pet-Ritz* 9")	80	1.0	9.0	5.0	5	60	0
(*Pet-Ritz* 9⅝")	120	2.0	13.0	7.0	5	90	0
(*Pillsbury*)	110	<1.0	12.0	7.0	5	140	0
deep dish:							
(*Oronoque* 9") . . .	100	2.0	8.0	7.0	0	95	0
(*Oronoque* 10") . .	130	2.0	10.0	8.0	0	120	0
(*Pet-Ritz*)	100	1.0	10.0	6.0	5	70	0
graham:							
(*Oronoque*)	110	1.0	13.0	6.0	0	120	0
(*Pet Ritz*)	110	1.0	13.0	6.0	0	120	0
vegetable shortening:							
(*Pet-Ritz*)	90	1.0	8.0	6.0	0	60	0
deep dish (*Pet-Ritz*)	100	1.0	9.0	7.0	0	65	0
Pie crust mix:							
(*Betty Crocker*), ⅛ of 9" crust	110	1.0	9.0	8.0	0	150	0
(*Flako*), ¼ cup dry	130	2.0	13.0	8.0	5	170	1.0
(*Pillsbury*), ⅛ of 9" crust	100	1.0	10.0	6.0	0	150	0

Food and Measure	cal.	prot. (gms)	carbo. (gms)	fat (gms)	chol. (mgs)	sod. (mgs)	fiber (gms)
Pie filling (see also "Pastry filling"), canned, ⅓ cup, except as noted:							
apple:							
(*Lucky Leaf/Lucky Leaf* Premium)	90	0	22.0	0	0	40	2.0
(*Lucky Leaf* Lite)	60	0	15.0	0	0	10	1.0
(*Musselman's* 21 oz.)	90	0	22.0	0	0	40	2.0
(*Musselman's* 24 oz.)	100	0	25.0	0	0	20	1.0
apricot (*Lucky Leaf*)	90	0	22.0	0	0	55	1.0
blackberry (*Lucky Leaf*)	90	0	21.0	0	0	45	3.0
blueberry:							
(*Lucky Leaf*)	100	0	26.0	0	0	25	1.0
(*Lucky Leaf* Lite)	60	0	14.0	0	0	15	1.0
(*Lucky Leaf* Premium)	100	0	24.0	0	0	45	1.0
(*Musselman's*) . . .	100	0	26.0	0	0	10	1.0
cherry:							
(*Lucky Leaf/Musselman's*)	100	0	24.0	0	0	40	1.0
(*Lucky Leaf/Musselman's* Lite) . .	60	0	14.0	0	0	10	1.0
dark sweet (*Lucky Leaf/Musselman's*)	110	0	26.0	0	0	15	1.0
coconut creme (*Lucky Leaf*)	110	1.0	25.0	0	0	140	3.0
lemon:							
(*Lucky Leaf/Musselman's* 22 oz.)	130	0	31.0	0	0	150	0
(*Musselman's* 25 oz.)	130	0	32.0	0	0	140	0
creme (*Lucky Leaf*)	130	0	31.0	0	0	220	0
mincemeat:							
(*Lucky Leaf*)	140	0	33.0	0	0	95	2.0
(*None Such*)	190	0	45.0	.5	0	230	0

Food and Measure	cal.	prot. (gms)	carbo. (gms)	fat (gms)	chol. (mgs)	sod. (mgs)	fiber (gms)
(*S&W*), ¼ cup . .	180	<1.0	43.0	2.5	0	210	4.0
w/brandy and rum							
(*None Such*) . . .	200	0	47.0	1.0	0	250	0
condensed (*None*							
Such), 4 tsp. . .	150	0	36.0	.5	0	230	1.0
peach (*Lucky Leaf*)	80	0	21.0	0	0	30	1.0
pineapple (*Lucky Leaf/*							
Musselman's) . . .	100	0	26.0	0	0	25	1.0
pumpkin, mix:							
(*Libby's*), ½ cup . .	100	<1.0	25.0	0	0	150	2.0
(*Stokely*)	100	0	24.0	0	0	290	2.0
raisin (*Lucky Leaf*)	100	0	25.0	0	0	75	1.0
strawberry (*Lucky*							
Leaf/Musselman's)	80	0	21.0	0	0	50	1.0
strawberry-rhubarb							
(*Lucky Leaf*)	90	0	23.0	0	0	35	1.0
Pie filling mix, see "Pudding mix"							
Pie glaze, see "Glaze, fruit"							
Pierogi, frozen or re-frigerated:							
potato cheese (*Empire* Kosher), 4 oz. . . .	214	11.0	38.0	4.0	35	260	2.0
potato onion:							
(*Empire* Kosher),							
4 oz.	165	10.0	36.0	1.0	35	220	2.0
(*Giorgio*), 3 pcs. . .	230	6.0	42.0	3.0	0	380	3.0
Pigeon peas, ½ cup, except as noted:							
fresh:							
raw	105	5.5	18.4	1.3	0	4	3.2
boiled, drained . . .	86	4.6	15.0	1.1	0	3	2.5
dried:							
(*Goya*), ¼ cup . . .	140	8.0	24.0	.5	0	10	3.0
boiled	102	5.7	19.5	.3	0	5	3.9
canned:							
dried (*El Jib*) . . .	80	5.0	18.0	0	0	490	0
green (*Tupi*)	70	4.0	14.0	0	0	390	4.0

Food and Measure	cal.	prot. (gms)	carbo. (gms)	fat (gms)	chol. (mgs)	sod. (mgs)	fiber (gms)
Pig's feet:							
simmered, 4 oz. . . .	220	21.8	0	14.1	113	n.a.	0
pickled:							
cured, 1 oz.	58	3.8	<.1	4.6	26	n.a.	0
(*Hormel*), 2 oz. . .	80	7.0	0	6.0	45	530	0
Pignola nuts, see "Pine nuts"							
Pike:							
northern, meat only:							
raw, 4 oz.	100	21.8	0	.8	44	44	0
baked, broiled, or							
microwaved, 4 oz.	128	28.0	0	1.0	57	56	0
walleye, meat only,							
raw, 4 oz.	105	21.7	0	1.4	98	58	0
baked, broiled, or							
microwaved, 4 oz.	135	27.8	0	1.8	125	74	0
Pili nuts, dried:							
shelled, 1 oz.	204	3.1	1.1	22.6	0	4	<1.0
shelled, 1 cup	863	13.0	4.8	95.5	0	4	3.4
Pimiento, drained:							
(*Goya*), ¼ pepper . .	0	0	1.0	0	0	40	0
(*S&W*), 2¼ oz. . . .	20	1.0	3.0	0	0	180	0
Pina colada mixer:							
bottled (*Holland House/Mr. & Mrs. "T"*), 4.5 fl. oz. . .	180	0	43.0	0	0	130	0
canned (*Goya*), ⅓ cup	120	.7	20.0	4.0	0	30	0
frozen* (*Bacardi*), 8 fl. oz.	190	<1.0	33.0	6.0	0	25	0
mix (*Bar-Tenders*), 1.2-oz. pkt.	140	0	31.0	0	0	45	0
Pine nuts, dried:							
pignolia:							
1 oz.	146	6.8	4.0	14.4	0	1	1.3
1 tbsp.	51	2.4	1.4	5.1	0	<1	.5
(*Krinos*), .5 oz. . .	90	5.0	0	7.5	0	5	1.0
(*Progresso*), 1 oz.	170	10.0	2.0	13.0	0	0	0
pinyon:							
1 oz.	161	3.3	5.5	17.3	0	20	3.0

Food and Measure	cal.	prot. (gms)	carbo. (gms)	fat (gms)	chol. (mgs)	sod. (mgs)	fiber (gms)
10 kernels	6	.1	.2	.6	0	1	.1
Pineapple, ½ cup, except as noted:							
fresh:							
baby, trimmed (*Frieda's Sugar-loaf*), 1 oz.	14	.1	3.9	.1	0	<1	n.a.
diced	39	.3	9.6	.3	0	<1	.9
sliced (*Dole*), 2 slices	90	1.0	21.0	1.0	0	10	2.0
canned, juice:							
all varieties, except sliced (*Del Monte*)	70	0	17.0	0	0	10	1.0
crushed (*Dole*) . . .	70	1.0	17.0	0	0	10	1.0
sliced (*Del Monte*), 2 slices	60	0	16.0	0	0	10	1.0
sliced (*Dole*), 4 oz., 2 slices	60	0	15.0	0	0	10	1.0
tidbits (*Del Monte* Snack), 3.5-oz. cup . . .	60	0	17.0	0	0	10	1.0
tidbits or chunks (*Dole*)	60	0	15.0	0	0	10	1.0
canned, in light syrup:							
(*Del Monte* Snack), 3.5-oz. cup . . .	70	0	17.0	0	0	10	<1.0
all varieties, except sliced (*Dole*) . . .	80	1.0	20.0	0	0	10	1.0
sliced (*Dole*), 4 oz., 3½ slices	60	0	16.0	0	0	10	1.0
w/mandarin orange (*Dole*)	80	0	19.0	<1.0	0	10	1.0
canned, in heavy syrup:							
4 oz.	88	.4	22.9	.1	0	1	.8
all varieties, except sliced (*Dole*) . . .	90	1.0	24.0	0	0	10	1.0
chunks, tidbits, or crushed	100	.5	25.8	.1	0	2	.9

Food and Measure	cal.	prot. (gms)	carbo. (gms)	fat (gms)	chol. (mgs)	sod. (mgs)	fiber (gms)
Pineapple, canned, in heavy syrup *(cont.)*							
crushed or chunks							
(*Del Monte*) . . .	90	0	24.0	0	0	10	1.0
sliced (*Del Monte*),							
2 slices	90	0	23.0	0	0	10	1.0
sliced (*Dole*),							
2 slices	90	1.0	23.0	0	0	10	1.0
sliced (*S&W*) . . .	90	0	23.0	0	0	10	1.0
canned, in extra heavy							
syrup:							
crushed (*Dole*) . . .	110	0	29.0	0	0	10	1.0
cubes (*Dole*)	200	1.0	50.0	0	0	10	1.0
dried (*Sonoma*),							
1.4 oz.	140	0	30.0	2.0	0	30	2.0
frozen, chunks							
(*Goya*), ⅓ pkg. . .	70	1.0	16.0	0	0	10	2.0
frozen, sweetened,							
chunks	104	.5	27.1	.1	0	2	1.3
Pineapple, candied:							
(*Paradise/White*							
Swan), 6 pcs., 1 oz.	90	0	22.0	0	0	10	0
assorted (*Paradise/*							
White Swan),							
2 tbsp., 1 oz. . . .	90	0	22.0	0	0	15	1.0
green (*Paradise/White*							
Swan), 7 pcs., 1 oz.	90	0	22.0	0	0	15	1.0
red (*Paradise/White*							
Swan), 8 pcs.,							
1.1 oz.	100	0	24.0	0	0	15	1.0
slices, natural or color							
(*S&W* Glace),							
2.2 oz.	180	0	46.0	0	0	40	0
wedges, natural or							
color (*S&W* Glace),							
5 pcs., 1 oz.	80	0	21.0	0	0	20	0
Pineapple drink:							
(*Tropicana* Punch,							
16 oz.), 8 fl. oz. . .	120	0	31.0	0	0	15	0

Food and Measure	cal.	prot. (gms)	carbo. (gms)	fat (gms)	chol. (mgs)	sod. (mgs)	fiber (gms)
(*Tropicana* Punch), 10 fl. oz.	160	0	40.0	0	0	20	0
Pineapple drink blends, 8 fl. oz., except as noted:							
coconut:							
(*Farmer's Market*)	120	0	29.0	0	0	15	0
nectar (*Kern's*) . . .	200	<1.0	36.0	6.0	0	40	2.0
nectar (*Kern's*), 11.5 fl. oz.	290	1.0	52.0	8.0	0	55	3.0
grapefruit, pink:							
(*Dole*), 6 fl. oz. . .	100	0	25.0	0	0	15	0
(*Dole*)	130	1.0	32.0	0	0	20	0
guava, nectar (*Goya*), 12 fl. oz.	230	2.0	55.0	0	0	45	5.0
passion fruit, nectar (*Goya*), 12 fl. oz.	220	0	55.0	0	0	20	4.0
Pineapple juice, 8 fl. oz., except as noted:							
(*Del Monte*), 6 fl. oz.	80	<1.0	20.0	0	0	5	0
(*Del Monte*)	130	1.0	32.0	0	0	10	1.0
(*Del Monte* Not from Concentrate)	110	1.0	29.0	0	0	15	2.0
(*Dole* Canned)	120	1.0	29.0	0	0	20	0
(*Dole* Chilled)	130	2.0	29.0	0	0	20	0
(*Goya*), 12 fl. oz. . .	190	2.0	46.0	0	0	35	1.0
(*Minute Maid*)	130	0	32.0	0	0	25	0
(*S&W*), 6 fl. oz. . . .	90	0	23.0	0	0	10	2.0
(*S&W*)	110	0	29.0	0	0	15	2.0
(*S&W*), 12 fl. oz. . .	180	1.0	45.0	0	0	20	3.0
frozen* (*Dole*)	130	1.0	30.0	0	0	20	0
Pineapple juice blends, 8 fl. oz., except as noted:							
coconut (*R.W. Knudsen*)	130	0	32.0	0	0	50	0
grapefruit:							
(*Dole*), 6 fl. oz. . .	100	1.0	24.0	0	0	15	0

Food and Measure	cal.	prot. (gms)	carbo. (gms)	fat (gms)	chol. (mgs)	sod. (mgs)	fiber (gms)
Pineapple juice blends, grapefruit *(cont.)*							
frozen* *(Dole)* . . .	130	1.0	29.0	0	0	20	0
orange:							
(Dole)	120	2.0	27.0	0	0	20	0
frozen* *(Dole)* . . .	120	1.0	29.0	0	0	20	0
orange-banana:							
(Dole)	130	2.0	29.0	0	0	20	0
(Dole), 10 fl. oz. . .	160	1.0	40.0	0	0	25	0
orange-berry *(Dole)*	130	1.0	32.0	0	0	20	0
orange-guava *(Dole)*	120	1.0	29.0	0	0	20	0
orange-strawberry							
(Dole)	130	1.0	32.0	0	0	20	0
passion fruit–banana:							
(Dole)	120	2.0	29.0	0	0	20	0
(Dole), 10 fl. oz. . .	160	1.0	39.0	0	0	25	0
Pineapple topping,							
2 tbsp.:							
(Kraft)	110	0	28.0	0	0	15	0
(Smucker's)	110	0	28.0	0	0	0	0
Pink beans:							
boiled, ½ cup	125	7.6	23.5	.4	0	2	4.5
canned, ½ cup:							
(Goya)	120	7.0	20.0	.5	0	500	7.0
in tomato sauce							
(Goya Guisadas)	100	6.0	17.0	1.0	0	550	6.0
Pinquito beans,							
canned							
(S&W), ½ cup . . .	80	6.0	20.0	.5	0	480	6.0
Pinto beans:							
dry *(Arrowhead Mills)*,							
¼ cup	150	10.0	27.0	.5	0	0	8.0
dry *(Goya)*, ¼ cup	60	7.0	22.0	0	0	15	14.0
boiled, ½ cup	117	7.0	21.8	.4	0	1	7.3
canned, ½ cup:							
w/liquid	93	5.5	17.5	.4	0	499	4.2
(Allens East Texas							
Fair/Brown							
Beauty)	110	5.0	20.0	.5	0	290	7.0
(Eden Organic) . .	90	5.0	17.0	.5	0	15	6.0

Food and Measure	cal.	prot. (gms)	carbo. (gms)	fat (gms)	chol. (mgs)	sod. (mgs)	fiber (gms)
(*Eden* Organic Jars)	120	7.0	22.0	0	0	340	6.0
(*Gebhardt*)	90	6.5	17.5	1.0	0	505	7.0
(*Goya*)	80	6.0	18.0	1.0	0	360	8.0
(*Green Giant/Joan of Arc*)	110	6.0	20.0	.5	0	280	5.0
(*Old El Paso*) . . .	110	6.0	19.0	.5	0	420	7.0
(*Progresso*)	110	7.0	18.0	1.0	0	250	7.0
(*Stokely*)	110	6.0	19.0	.5	0	350	3.0
(*Sun-Vista*)	80	3.0	12.0	.5	0	530	3.0
w/bacon (*Trappey's*)	120	6.0	20.0	1.0	0	270	7.0
w/bacon (*Trappey's* Jalapinto)	120	6.0	22.0	1.0	0	540	8.0
spiced, see "Chili beans"							
in tomato sauce (*Goya* Guisadas) . .	100	5.0	18.0	1.0	0	530	5.0
Pinto beans, sprouted, boiled, drained, 4 oz. . . .	25	2.1	4.6	.4	0	58	<2.0
Pistachio nut, shelled, except as noted:							
dried:							
in shell (*Dole*), 1 oz.	90	3.0	3.0	7.0	0	250	n.a.
1 oz.	164	5.8	7.1	13.7	0	2	3.1
(*Dole*), 1 oz.	163	6.0	7.0	14.0	0	n.a.	n.a.
(*Sonoma*), ¼ cup	190	6.0	9.0	14.0	0	220	3.0
dry-roasted, in shell (*Planters*), ½ cup, 1 oz. edible nuts . .	160	5.0	7.0	14.0	0	180	3.0
dry-roasted:							
1 oz.	172	4.2	7.8	15.0	0	2	3.1
1 cup	776	19.1	35.2	67.6	0	8	13.8
(*Planters*), 1 oz. . .	160	5.0	7.0	14.0	0	220	3.0
(*Planters Munch 'N Go Singles*), 2-oz. pkg.	330	11.0	6.0	29.0	0	450	6.0
Pita, see "Bread"							
Pitanga:							
1 medium, .3 oz. . .	2	.1	.5	<.1	0	<1	<1.0

Food and Measure	cal.	prot. (gms)	carbo. (gms)	fat (gms)	chol. (mgs)	sod. (mgs)	fiber (gms)
Pitanga *(cont.)*							
½ cup	29	.7	6.5	.3	0	3	<1.0
Pizza, frozen, 1 pie, except as noted:							
artichoke heart (*Wolf-gang Puck*), ½ pie	340	15.0	34.0	17.0	25	450	3.0
bacon burger (*Totino's Party*), ½ pie . . .	370	15.0	33.0	20.0	15	880	2.0
Canadian bacon:							
(*Tombstone* Original 12"), ¼ pie . . .	360	20.0	36.0	15.0	40	920	2.0
(*Totino's Party*), ½ pie	320	14.0	33.0	15.0	10	900	2.0
(*Jeno's Crisp 'n Tasty*)	430	17.0	49.0	18.0	10	1150	2.0
cheese:							
(*Celentano* Thick Crust), ½ pie . .	390	18.0	62.0	12.0	25	840	8.0
(*Celeste* Large), ¼ pie	320	14.0	32.0	16.0	25	590	3.0
(*Celeste* for One)	540	23.0	60.0	25.0	45	1090	4.0
(*Empire* Kosher 3 Pack)	210	10.0	23.0	9.0	20	630	7.0
(*Empire* Kosher 10 oz.), ½ pie . .	340	18.0	38.0	13.0	30	970	2.0
(*Jeno's Crisp 'n Tasty*)	450	19.0	51.0	19.0	20	870	2.0
(*Jeno's* Microwave)	240	10.0	25.0	11.0	15	530	1.0
(*Swanson Fun Feast*)	350	14.0	57.0	9.0	15	490	7.0
(*Tombstone For One* ½ Less Fat) . . .	360	23.0	45.0	10.0	15	920	3.0
(*Totino's* Micro-wave)	240	10.0	25.0	11.0	15	530	1.0
(*Totino's Party*), ½ pie	320	15.0	33.0	14.0	20	630	2.0
(*Totino's Party* Fam-ily Size), ⅓ pie	360	16.0	38.0	16.0	20	720	2.0

Food and Measure	cal.	prot. (gms)	carbo. (gms)	fat (gms)	chol. (mgs)	sod. (mgs)	fiber (gms)
cheese, extra:							
(*Marie Callender's*),							
½ pie	410	15.0	30.0	25.0	25	630	2.0
(*Tombstone* Original							
9″), ½ pie	420	20.0	42.0	19.0	30	730	3.0
(*Tombstone* Original							
12″), ¼ pie . . .	370	18.0	36.0	17.0	30	680	2.0
(*Tombstone* For							
One)	540	27.0	41.0	30.0	45	910	3.0
(*Weight Watchers*)	390	23.0	49.0	12.0	35	590	6.0
cheese, three:							
(*Pappalo's* Deep							
Dish), ¼ pie . . .	370	19.0	46.0	12.0	25	670	2.0
(*Pappalo's* Deep							
Dish for One) . .	540	30.0	61.0	20.0	45	1000	3.0
(*Pappalo's* for One)	500	29.0	50.0	20.0	45	960	3.0
(*Pappalo's* 9″),							
½ pie	400	21.0	44.0	15.0	35	760	2.0
(*Pappalo's* 12″),							
¼ pie	340	19.0	39.0	12.0	30	770	2.0
(*Totino's* Select),							
⅓ pie	300	14.0	29.0	14.0	20	590	1.0
Italian (*Tombstone*							
ThinCrust), ¼ pie	380	20.0	25.0	22.0	45	730	2.0
cheese, four:							
(*Celeste* for One)	540	25.0	47.0	30.0	50	1040	4.0
(*Tombstone* Special							
Order 12″), ⅕ pie	400	20.0	37.0	19.0	40	760	2.0
(*Wolfgang Puck*),							
½ pie	360	17.0	40.0	15.0	25	530	5.0
hot and zesty (*Ce-*							
leste for One) . .	530	24.0	50.0	27.0	50	1090	4.0
zesty (*Celeste*							
Large), ¼ pie . .	330	14.0	34.0	16.0	30	610	3.0
cheese, two:							
w/Canadian bacon							
(*Totino's* Select),							
⅓ pie	310	17.0	30.0	14.0	25	790	1.0

Food and Measure	cal.	prot. (gms)	carbo. (gms)	fat (gms)	chol. (mgs)	sod. (mgs)	fiber (gms)
Pizza, frozen, cheese, two *(cont.)*							
w/pepperoni (*Totino's* Select), ⅓ pie	360	16.0	30.0	20.0	35	820	1.0
w/sausage (*Totino's* Select), ⅓ pie . .	360	17.0	31.0	19.0	30	760	2.0
chicken and broccoli (*Marie Callender's*), ½ pie	350	19.0	34.0	15.0	35	610	2.0
combination:							
(*Jeno's* Microwave)	310	11.0	25.0	18.0	15	720	1.0
(*Jeno's Crisp 'n Tasty*)	520	17.0	49.0	28.0	25	1120	3.0
(*Totino's* Microwave)	310	11.0	25.0	18.0	15	720	1.0
(*Totino's Party*), ½ pie	390	15.0	34.0	21.0	20	910	2.0
(*Totino's Party* Family), ¼ pie	300	12.0	28.0	16.0	15	740	1.0
(*Weight Watchers*)	380	23.0	47.0	11.0	40	550	6.0
deluxe:							
(*Celeste* Large), ¼ pie	350	14.0	35.0	18.0	20	880	4.0
(*Celeste* for One)	540	21.0	53.0	29.0	25	1320	6.0
(*Marie Callender's*), ½ pie	380	14.0	30.0	23.0	20	690	3.0
(*Tombstone* Original 9"), ⅓ pie	320	15.0	28.0	16.0	30	620	2.0
(*Tombstone* Original 12"), ¼ pie . . .	320	15.0	29.0	16.0	30	640	2.0
hamburger:							
(*Jeno's Crisp 'n Tasty*)	480	19.0	49.0	23.0	25	1100	3.0
(*Tombstone* Original 9"), ⅓ pie	310	14.0	28.0	16.0	30	620	2.0
(*Tombstone* Original 12"), ⅕ pie . . .	320	15.0	29.0	16.0	30	660	2.0
(*Totino's Party*), ½ pie	350	15.0	33.0	18.0	20	860	2.0

Food and Measure	cal.	prot. (gms)	carbo. (gms)	fat (gms)	chol. (mgs)	sod. (mgs)	fiber (gms)
Italiano, zesty (*To-tino's Party*), ½ pie	390	15.0	35.0	21.0	20	900	2.0
w/meat:							
(*Celeste* Suprema for One)	580	25.0	56.0	31.0	30	1480	7.0
(*Celeste* Suprema, Large), ⅕ pie . .	290	13.0	27.0	16.0	15	770	3.0
meat, five (*Marie Cal-lender's*), ½ pie . .	330	16.0	36.0	14.0	25	770	3.0
meat, four:							
(*Tombstone Special Order 9"*), ⅓ pie	400	19.0	35.0	20.0	45	910	2.0
(*Tombstone Special Order 12"*), ⅙ pie	350	17.0	31.0	18.0	40	810	2.0
combo, Italian (*Tombstone* Thin-Crust), ¼ pie . .	410	20.0	25.0	25.0	50	940	2.0
meat, three:							
(*Jeno's Crisp 'n Tasty*)	500	18.0	48.0	26.0	25	1180	2.0
(*Totino's Party*), ½ pie	360	15.0	33.0	19.0	15	910	2.0
Mexican style, su-preme taco (*Tomb-stone* ThinCrust), ¼ pie	380	16.0	26.0	23.0	50	850	2.0
Mexican style, zesty:							
(*Totino's* Micro-wave)	280	10.0	25.0	16.0	15	560	2.0
(*Totino's Party*), ½ pie	370	15.0	34.0	19.0	15	750	2.0
pepperoni:							
(*Celeste* Large), ¼ pie	350	13.0	33.0	20.0	20	990	3.0
(*Celeste* Pizza for One)	520	19.0	53.0	27.0	25	1280	4.0
(*Hormel Quick Meal*)	380	18.0	47.0	14.0	35	1150	2.0
(*Jeno's* Microwave)	280	10.0	25.0	16.0	15	710	1.0

Food and Measure	cal.	prot. (gms)	carbo. (gms)	fat (gms)	chol. (mgs)	sod. (mgs)	fiber (gms)
Pizza, frozen, pepperoni *(cont.)*							
(*Jeno's Crisp 'n Tasty*)	500	17.0	49.0	26.0	25	1170	2.0
(*Marie Callender's*), ½ pie	440	14.0	30.0	29.0	30	770	3.0
(*Pappalo's* Deep Dish), ⅕ pie . . .	340	17.0	37.0	14.0	30	720	2.0
(*Pappalo's* Deep Dish for One) . .	600	30.0	62.0	26.0	55	1300	3.0
(*Pappalo's* for One)	570	30.0	52.0	27.0	60	1280	3.0
(*Pappalo's* 9"), ½ pie	440	21.0	40.0	19.0	40	950	2.0
(*Pappalo's* 12"), ¼ pie	380	18.0	38.0	17.0	40	840	2.0
(*Tombstone* Original 9"), ⅓ pie	340	15.0	28.0	19.0	30	740	2.0
(*Tombstone* Original 12"), ⅕ pie . . .	340	15.0	29.0	18.0	35	750	2.0
(*Tombstone* For One)	540	25.0	41.0	35.0	50	1170	3.0
(*Tombstone* For One ½ Less Fat) . . .	400	26.0	45.0	13.0	35	1040	4.0
(*Tombstone* Special Order 9"), ⅓ pie	400	19.0	35.0	21.0	45	880	2.0
(*Tombstone* Special Order 12"), ⅙ pie	360	16.0	31.0	19.0	40	790	2.0
(*Totino's* Micro- wave)	280	10.0	25.0	16.0	15	710	1.0
(*Totino's Party*), ½ pie	380	14.0	33.0	21.0	20	920	2.0
(*Totino's Party* Fam- ily), ⅓ pie	410	15.0	37.0	22.0	20	1000	2.0
(*Weight Watchers*)	390	23.0	46.0	12.0	45	650	4.0
double cheese (*Tombstone* Double Top), ⅙ pie	350	19.0	25.0	20.0	45	850	2.0
Italian (*Tombstone* ThinCrust), ¼ pie	420	20.0	25.0	27.0	55	950	2.0

Food and Measure	cal.	prot. (gms)	carbo. (gms)	fat (gms)	chol. (mgs)	sod. (mgs)	fiber (gms)
sausage:							
(*Celeste* for One)	530	23.0	52.0	27.0	25	1400	5.0
(*Jeno's* Microwave)	280	10.0	25.0	16.0	10	650	1.0
(*Jeno's Crisp 'n Tasty*)	510	17.0	49.0	27.0	20	1070	3.0
(*Pappalo's* Deep Dish), ⅕ pie . . .	330	16.0	36.0	13.0	25	600	2.0
(*Pappalo's* 9"), ½ pie	420	20.0	45.0	18.0	35	800	2.0
(*Pappalo's* 12"), ¼ pie	370	18.0	38.0	16.0	30	710	2.0
(*Tombstone* Original 9"), ⅓ pie	310	14.0	28.0	16.0	30	610	2.0
(*Tombstone* Original 12"), ⅕ pie . . .	320	15.0	29.0	26.0	30	650	2.0
(*Totino's* Microwave)	280	10.0	25.0	16.0	10	650	1.0
(*Totino's Party*), ½ pie	380	15.0	34.0	20.0	15	870	2.0
(*Totino's Party* Family), ¼ pie	300	12.0	28.0	16.0	10	720	2.0
double cheese (*Tombstone Double Top*), ⅙ pie	350	20.0	25.0	19.0	40	740	2.0
Italian (*Tombstone For One*)	560	25.0	40.0	33.0	55	1130	3.0
Italian (*Tombstone* ThinCrust), ¼ pie	400	19.0	25.0	24.0	50	880	2.0
sausage, three:							
(*Tombstone Special Order* 9"), ⅓ pie	390	19.0	35.0	19.0	40	830	2.0
(*Tombstone Special Order* 12"), ⅙ pie	340	16.0	31.0	17.0	35	740	2.0
sausage/mushroom (*Tombstone* Original 12"), ⅕ pie	320	15.0	29.0	16.0	30	630	2.0

Food and Measure	cal.	prot. (gms)	carbo. (gms)	fat (gms)	chol. (mgs)	sod. (mgs)	fiber (gms)
Pizza, frozen *(cont.)*							
sausage/pepperoni:							
(*Marie Callender's*),							
½ pie	430	15.0	29.0	28.0	30	730	3.0
(*Pappalo's* Deep							
Dish), ⅕ pie . . .	330	16.0	36.0	14.0	25	650	2.0
(*Pappalo's* Deep							
Dish for One) . .	610	30.0	61.0	27.0	50	1180	3.0
(*Pappalo's* for One)	570	30.0	51.0	27.0	55	1170	3.0
(*Pappalo's* 9"),							
½ pie	430	21.0	44.0	19.0	35	870	2.0
(*Pappalo's* 12"),							
¼ pie	380	18.0	39.0	17.0	35	780	2.0
(*Tombstone* Original							
9"), ⅓ pie	360	16.0	28.0	21.0	35	820	2.0
(*Tombstone* Original							
12"), ⅕ pie . . .	340	16.0	29.0	18.0	35	740	2.0
(*Tombstone For*							
One)	590	25.0	40.0	37.0	45	1200	3.0
(*Totino's* Select),							
⅓ pie	360	17.0	30.0	19.0	30	760	2.0
double cheese							
(*Tombstone*							
Double Top),							
⅙ pie	360	20.0	25.0	20.0	45	800	2.0
supreme:							
(*Jeno's Crisp 'n*							
Tasty)	520	17.0	49.0	28.0	25	1120	3.0
(*Pappalo's* Deep							
Dish), ⅕ pie . . .	340	17.0	37.0	14.0	25	680	2.0
(*Pappalo's* Deep							
Dish for One) . .	610	30.0	62.0	27.0	50	1230	4.0
(*Pappalo's* for One)	560	29.0	50.0	27.0	55	1170	3.0
(*Pappalo's* 9"),							
⅓ pie	290	14.0	30.0	13.0	25	610	2.0
(*Pappalo's* 12"),							
¼ pie	380	18.0	40.0	16.0	30	790	2.0
(*Tombstone* Original							
12"), ⅕ pie . . .	330	15.0	29.0	17.0	35	720	2.0

Food and Measure	cal.	prot. (gms)	carbo. (gms)	fat (gms)	chol. (mgs)	sod. (mgs)	fiber (gms)
(*Tombstone* Light), ⅕ pie	270	25.0	30.0	9.0	20	710	2.0
Italian (*Tombstone* ThinCrust), ¼ pie	400	18.0	26.0	24.0	45	880	2.0
(*Tombstone For One*)	570	24.0	41.0	34.0	50	1130	3.0
(*Tombstone For One* ½ Less Fat) . . .	400	27.0	45.0	13.0	35	1090	4.0
(*Totino's* Micro-wave)	290	10.0	25.0	17.0	15	680	2.0
(*Totino's Party*), ½ pie	380	15.0	34.0	20.0	20	890	2.0
(*Totino's* Select), ⅓ pie	340	16.0	29.0	18.0	30	770	2.0
super (*Tombstone Special Order 9"*), ⅓ pie	400	19.0	36.0	21.0	45	900	2.0
super (*Tombstone Special Order 12"*), ⅙ pie . . .	350	17.0	31.0	18.0	40	800	2.0
tomato and mozzarella (*Marie Callender's*), ½ pie	350	14.0	40.0	15.0	20	600	3.0
vegetable:							
(*Celeste* for One)	480	20.0	52.0	23.0	5	1270	5.0
(*Tombstone* Light), ⅕ pie	240	25.0	31.0	7.0	10	500	3.0
(*Tombstone For One* ½ Less Fat) . . .	360	272.0	46.0	10.0	15	730	5.0
primavera (*Marie Callender's*), ½ pie	350	14.0	40.0	15	20	630	2.0
Pizza, bagel (*Empire Kosher*), 2-oz. pc.	150	7.0	15.0	5.0	15	390	0
Pizza, croissant, fro-zen (*Pepperidge Farm*):							
cheese, 1 pc.	390	12.0	39.0	20.0	90	770	6.0
deluxe, 1 pc.	450	14.0	40.0	27.0	85	910	7.0

Food and Measure	cal.	prot. (gms)	carbo. (gms)	fat (gms)	chol. (mgs)	sod. (mgs)	fiber (gms)
Pizza, croissant *(cont.)*							
pepperoni, 1 pc. . . .	420	15.0	39.0	23.0	90	810	5.0
Pizza, English muffin							
(*Empire* Kosher),							
2-oz. pc.	130	7.0	15.0	5.0	15	390	1.0
Pizza, French bread,							
frozen, 1 pc. or							
½ pkg., except as							
noted:							
bacon cheddar							
(*Stouffer's*)	440	16.0	44.0	22.0	30	940	4.0
cheese:							
(*Healthy Choice*) . .	310	20.0	49.0	4.0	10	470	6.0
(*Lean Cuisine*),							
6 oz.	350	22.0	48.0	8.0	20	400	4.0
(*Stouffer's*)	350	15.0	42.0	14.0	15	660	3.0
double (*Stouffer's*)	420	19.0	44.0	19.0	30	790	5.0
cheeseburger							
(*Stouffer's*)	440	21.0	31.0	26.0	55	1110	5.0
deluxe:							
(*Lean Cuisine*),							
6⅛ oz.	330	23.0	45.0	6.0	30	560	5.0
(*Stouffer's*)	440	19.0	42.0	22.0	35	980	5.0
pepperoni:							
(*Healthy Choice*) . .	360	22.0	48.0	9.0	25	580	5.0
(*Lean Cuisine*),							
5¼ oz.	330	20.0	46.0	7.0	25	590	4.0
(*Stouffer's*)	420	18.0	42.0	20.0	35	930	3.0
pepperoni and mush-							
room (*Stouffer's*)	430	17.0	43.0	21.0	30	1000	3.0
sausage:							
(*Healthy Choice*) . .	330	20.0	52.0	4.0	20	470	5.0
(*Stouffer's*)	420	19.0	41.0	20.0	35	900	4.0
sausage and pepper-							
oni (*Stouffer's*) . .	490	22.0	45.0	25.0	40	1130	4.0
supreme (*Healthy*							
Choice)	340	22.0	49.0	6.0	25	510	5.0
vegetable deluxe							
(*Stouffer's*)	400	18.0	43.0	17.0	25	830	5.0

Food and Measure	cal.	prot. (gms)	carbo. (gms)	fat (gms)	chol. (mgs)	sod. (mgs)	fiber (gms)
white (*Stouffer's*) . .	490	17.0	43.0	28.0	25	760	5.0
Pizza, Italian bread, frozen (*Celeste*), 1 pc.:							
cheese, four	300	15.0	32.0	12.0	25	820	3.0
chicken, zesty	260	17.0	34.0	8.0	20	960	3.0
deluxe	290	16.0	36.0	11.0	15	1000	3.0
pepperoni	320	17.0	37.0	13.0	20	1140	3.0
Pizza crust, refriger- ated, ¼ crust:							
(*Pillsbury*)	180	6.0	33.0	2.5	0	390	1.0
(*Totino's*)	180	4.0	25.0	7.0	0	190	1.0
Pizza Hut, 1 slice of medium pie, except as noted:							
Bigfoot, 1 slice:							
cheese	186	10.0	25.0	6.0	16	525	2.0
pepperoni	205	10.0	25.0	7.0	20	589	2.0
pepperoni, mush- room, and sau- sage	214	11.0	25.0	8.0	21	665	2.0
breadsticks, 5 pcs.	750	24.0	129.0	15.0	5	1335	7.5
hand-tossed:							
cheese	235	13.0	29.0	7.0	25	621	2.0
beef	260	15.0	29.0	9.0	26	797	2.0
ham	213	12.0	29.0	5.0	21	657	2.0
Meat Lovers	314	17.0	29.0	11.0	38	958	2.0
pepperoni	238	12.0	29.0	8.0	24	689	2.0
Pepperoni Lovers	306	16.0	30.0	14.0	40	897	2.0
pork topping	268	14.0	29.0	10.0	26	797	2.0
sausage, Italian . .	267	13.0	29.0	11.0	31	737	2.0
supreme	284	16.0	30.0	12.0	30	884	3.0
supreme, super . .	296	16.0	30.0	13.0	34	946	3.0
Veggie Lovers . . .	216	11.0	30.0	6.0	17	632	3.0
pan pizza:							
cheese	261	12.0	28.0	11.0	25	501	2.0
beef	286	14.0	28.0	13.0	26	677	2.0
ham	239	11.0	28.0	21.0	21	537	2.0
Meat Lovers	340	16.0	28.0	18.0	38	838	2.0

Food and Measure	cal.	prot. (gms)	carbo. (gms)	fat (gms)	chol. (mgs)	sod. (mgs)	fiber (gms)
Pizza Hut, pan pizza *(cont.)*							
pepperoni	265	11.0	28.0	12.0	24	569	2.0
Pepperoni Lovers	332	15.0	28.0	17.0	24	777	2.0
pork topping	294	13.0	28.0	14.0	26	677	2.0
sausage, Italian . .	293	12.0	27.0	15.0	31	617	2.0
supreme	311	15.0	28.0	15.0	30	764	3.0
supreme, super . .	323	15.0	28.0	17.0	34	826	3.0
Veggie Lovers . . .	243	10.0	29.0	10.0	17	512	3.0
Personal Pan Pizza:							
pepperoni, 1 pie . .	637	27.0	69.0	28.0	55	1340	5.0
supreme, 1 pie . .	722	33.0	70.0	34.0	66	1760	6.0
Thin 'N Crispy:							
cheese	205	11.0	21.0	8.0	25	534	2.0
beef	229	13.0	21.0	11.0	26	709	2.0
ham	184	10.0	21.0	7.0	22	591	1.0
Meat Lovers	288	15.0	21.0	13.0	39	892	2.0
pepperoni	215	11.0	21.0	10.0	25	627	2.0
Pepperoni Lovers	289	15.0	22.0	16.0	42	862	2.0
pork topping	237	12.0	21.0	12.0	26	709	2.0
sausage, Italian . .	236	11.0	21.0	12.0	31	650	2.0
supreme	257	14.0	21.0	13.0	31	795	2.0
supreme, super . .	270	14.0	22.0	14.0	35	880	2.0
Veggie Lovers . . .	186	9.0	22.0	7.0	17	545	2.0
Pizza nuggets, frozen (*Hormel Quick Meal*), 5 pcs., 2.8 oz.	210	7.0	25.0	9.0	25	600	1.0
Pizza pepper (*Lawry's*), ¼ tsp.	0	0	0	0	0	0	0
Pizza pocket, frozen, 1 pc.:							
(*Amy's*)	290	14.0	38.0	9.0	20	390	3.0
deluxe (*Lean Pockets*)	270	12.0	37.0	8.0	25	680	2.0
pepperoni:							
(*Croissant Pockets*)	350	16.0	39.0	15.0	30	870	3.0
(*Hot Pockets*) . . .	350	13.0	38.0	17.0	30	780	2.0
pepperoni and sausage (*Hot Pockets*)	340	12.0	38.0	16.0	30	630	3.0
sausage (*Hot Pockets*)	340	12.0	37.0	16.0	25	690	2.0

Food and Measure	cal.	prot. (gms)	carbo. (gms)	fat (gms)	chol. (mgs)	sod. (mgs)	fiber (gms)
vegetable (Ken & Robert's Veggie Pockets)	270	9.0	41.0	8.0	0	490	4.0
vegetable, pepperoni style (Amy's) . . .	220	12.0	28.0	7.0	15	490	3.0
Pizza Pops (Totino's), 1 pc.:							
pepperoni	320	13.0	30.0	16.0	25	790	2.0
sausage, Italian . . .	310	13.0	30.0	15.0	20	680	2.0
sausage/pepperoni . .	320	13.0	28.0	17.0	20	680	2.0
supreme	300	11.0	30.0	15.0	25	680	2.0
Pizza rolls, frozen (Totino's), 10 rolls:							
cheese, three	360	15.0	42.0	15.0	35	610	2.0
combination	370	15.0	38.0	17.0	40	410	2.0
hamburger and cheese	350	15.0	40.0	14.0	35	570	2.0
meat, three	340	15.0	37.0	15.0	35	630	2.0
nacho and beef . . .	340	13.0	37.0	16.0	40	730	2.0
pepperoni and cheese	360	15.0	37.0	17.0	35	580	2.0
sausage and cheese	350	14.0	39.0	15.0	30	580	2.0
sausage and mushroom	330	13.0	38.0	14.0	30	570	2.0
spicy, Italian style . .	370	15.0	37.0	18.0	40	370	2.0
Pizza sauce, ¼ cup:							
(Contadina)	25	1.0	4.0	.5	0	300	1.0
(Contadina Chunky)	30	1.0	6.0	0	0	280	1.0
(Contadina Pizza Squeeze)	35	1.0	6.0	1.5	0	350	1.0
(Pastorelli Italian Chef)	40	2.0	6.0	1.0	0	310	2.0
(Prince Traditional)	20	1.0	4.0	0	0	250	1.0
(Progresso)	35	1.0	5.0	1.0	0	140	1.0
(Ragu Quick)	40	1.0	5.0	1.5	0	340	1.0
w/cheese:							
Italian (Contadina)	30	1.0	4.0	1.0	0	350	1.0
Italian (Contadina Pizza Squeeze)	40	1.0	6.0	1.5	0	420	1.0

Food and Measure	cal.	prot. (gms)	carbo. (gms)	fat (gms)	chol. (mgs)	sod. (mgs)	fiber (gms)
Pizza sauce, w/cheese *(cont.)*							
three (*Contadina* Chunky)	35	1.0	5.0	.5	0	190	1.0
mushroom (*Contadina* Chunky)	30	1.0	5.0	0	0	290	1.0
pepperoni (*Contadina*)	30	1.0	4.0	1.0	0	360	1.0
Pizza seasoning (*Tone's Presti's*), ¾ tsp.	10	0	1.0	1.0	0	5	0
Pizza stuffed sand-wich, see "Pizza pocket"							
Plantain:							
raw:							
(*Frieda's*), 1 oz. . .	34	.3	8.8	.1	0	1	n.a.
1 medium, 9.7 oz.	218	2.3	57.1	.7	0	7	4.1
sliced, ½ cup . . .	91	1.0	23.6	.3	0	3	1.7
cooked, sliced, ½ cup	89	.6	24.0	.1	0	4	1.8
fried (*Goya* Tostone), 3 pcs.	170	1.0	37.0	2.0	0	0	2.0
Plum:							
fresh:							
Japanese or hybrid, 2⅛" fruit	36	.5	8.6	.4	0	tr.	<1.0
sliced, ½ cup . . .	46	.7	10.7	.5	0	1	1.2
canned, juice:							
½ cup	73	.7	19.1	<.1	0	2	1.3
3 plums and 2 tbsp. liquid	55	.5	14.4	<.1	0	1	1.0
canned, light syrup:							
½ cup	79	.5	20.5	.1	0	25	1.3
3 plums and 2¾ tbsp. liquid	83	.5	21.7	.1	0	26	1.3
canned, heavy syrup:							
½ cup	115	.5	30.0	.1	0	25	1.3
whole (*S&W*), ½ cup	130	0	33.0	0	0	15	2.0
Plum sauce:							
(*Ka-Me*), 2 tbsp. . . .	80	0	19.0	0	0	420	0

Food and Measure	cal.	prot. (gms)	carbo. (gms)	fat (gms)	chol. (mgs)	sod. (mgs)	fiber (gms)
(*La Choy*), 1 tbsp. . . .	25	0	6.0	0	0	5	0
Poi, ½ cup	134	.5	32.7	.2	0	14	.5
Pocket sandwich, see specific listings							
Poke greens, canned (*Allens*), ½ cup . .	35	2.0	5.0	1.0	0	5	3.0
Pokeberry shoots:							
raw, ½ cup	18	2.1	3.0	.3	0	n.a.	1.4
boiled, drained, ½ cup	16	1.9	2.5	.3	0	n.a.	1.2
Polenta, refrigerated, 2 slices, ½″, except as noted:							
(*Frieda's*), 4 oz. . . .	100	3.0	21.0	0	0	440	3.0
(*San Gennaro's*) . . .	70	2.0	15.0	0	0	310	1.0
basil and garlic (*San Gennaro*)	71	2.0	15.0	0	0	310	1.0
sun-dried tomato (*San Gennaro*)	74	2.0	16.0	0	0	310.	1.0
Polenta mix (*Fantastica*), 1 cup*	260	8.0	46.0	5.0	5	550	4.0
Polish sausage (see also "Kielbasa"):							
beef:							
(*Hebrew National*), 3-oz. link	240	12.0	1.0	22.0	50	680	0
(*Hebrew National*), 4-oz. link	330	16.0	1.0	29.0	70	910	0
skinless (*John Morrell*), 2 oz.	180	7.0	3.0	15.0	55	720	0
Pollock, meat only:							
Atlantic:							
raw, 4 oz.	104	22.1	0	1.1	80	98	0
baked, broiled, or microwaved, 4 oz.	134	28.3	0	1.4	103	125	0
walleye:							
raw, 4 oz.	91	19.5	0	.9	81	112	0
baked, broiled, or microwaved, 4 oz.	128	26.7	0	1.3	109	132	0

Food and Measure	cal.	prot. (gms)	carbo. (gms)	fat (gms)	chol. (mgs)	sod. (mgs)	fiber (gms)
Pomegranate:							
9.7-oz. fruit	104	1.5	26.4	.5	0	5	.9
(*Frieda's*), 1 oz. . . .	18	.1	4.6	.1	0	1	n.a.
Pomegranate juice							
(*R.W. Knudsen*),							
8 fl. oz.	150	0	37.0	0	0	10	0
Pompano, Florida,							
meat only:							
raw, 4 oz.	186	21.0	0	10.7	57	74	0
baked, broiled, or mi-							
crowaved, 4 oz. . .	239	26.4	0	13.8	73	86	0
Popcorn, 2 tbsp., ex-							
cept as noted:							
(*Arrowhead Mills*),							
¼ cup, 1¾ oz. . . .	180	6.0	36.0	2.5	0	0	6.0
(*Orville Redenbacher*							
Original or White)	90	3.0	22.0	1.0	0	0	5.0
hot air (*Orville*							
Redenbacher) . . .	90	4.0	23.0	<1.0	0	0	6.0
microwave:							
(*Orville*							
Redenbacher) . .	120	3.0	19.0	6.0	0	350	5.0
(*Redenbudders*							
Movie Theater)	180	2.0	16.0	13.0	0	500	4.0
(*Redenbudders*							
Movie Theater							
Light)	115	3.0	19.0	5.0	0	320	4.5
(*Smart Pop*)	100	3.0	19.5	3.0	0	445	5.0
butter (*Orville*							
Redenbacher) . .	170	2.0	15.0	12.5	0	390	4.0
butter (*Orville*							
Redenbacher							
Light)	120	3.0	19.0	5.5	0	350	4.6
caramel (*Orville*							
Redenbacher) . .	180	1.0	23.0	10.0	0	50	2.0
cheddar (*Orville*							
Redenbacher) . .	140	2.5	16.0	9.0	<5	285	4.0
herb and garlic							
(*Redenbudders*)	180	2.0	16.0	13.0	0	500	4.0

Food and Measure	cal.	prot. (gms)	carbo. (gms)	fat (gms)	chol. (mgs)	sod. (mgs)	fiber (gms)
natural (*Orville* *Redenbacher*) . .	160	2.0	17.5	11.0	0	510	4.0
zesty (*Redenbudders*)	180	2.0	16.0	13.0	0	430	4.0
Popcorn, popped:							
(*Barrel O'Fun* Canola), 3 cups	145	2.0	14.0	9.0	0	255	1.0
(*Barrel O'Fun* Light), 3 cups	110	3.0	22.0	3.0	0	210	3.0
(*Chester's* Triple Mix), 1½ cups	140	1.0	19.0	6.0	0	240	1.0
(*Wise* Choice), 2½ cups	140	3.0	18.0	6.0	0	80	2.0
air-popped, 5 cups:							
white (*Jolly Time*)	100	4.0	24.0	.5	0	0	6.0
yellow (*Jolly Time*)	100	4.0	24.0	.1.0	0	0	6.0
butter/butter flavor:							
(*Borden*), 1-oz. bag	150	2.0	14.0	10.0	0	320	2.0
(*Chester's*), 3 cups	160	2.0	15.0	12.0	0	330	3.0
(*Smartfood*), 3 cups	150	2.0	15.0	9.0	5	240	1.0
(*Smartfood* Reduced Fat), 3⅓ cups . .	130	3.0	21.0	6.0	0	410	4.0
(*Wise* Reduced Fat), 3 cups	130	3.0	19.0	5.0	0	160	3.0
caramel:							
(*Barrel O'Fun* Fat Free), ¾ cup . .	120	1.0	27.0	0	0	255	1.0
(*Chester's*), ¾ cup	130	1.0	27.0	2.0	0	210	1.0
(*Cracker Jack* Fat Free), 1 cup, 1 oz.	110	1.0	27.0	0	0	85	1.0
(*Smart Snackers*), .9 oz.	100	1.0	22.0	1.0	0	45	1.0
(*Wise* Fat Free), 1 cup	110	<1.0	26.0	0	0	85	<1.0
caramel w/peanuts:							
(*Barrel O'Fun*), ⅔ cup	130	3.0	21.0	4.0	0	120	1.0
(*Cracker Jack*), ⅔ cup	120	2.0	23.0	2.5	0	90	1.0

Food and Measure	cal.	prot. (gms)	carbo. (gms)	fat (gms)	chol. (mgs)	sod. (mgs)	fiber (gms)
Popcorn, popped, caramel w/peanuts *(cont.)*							
(*Cracker Jack*),							
1.25-oz. box . . .	150	2.0	29.0	2.5	0	110	1.0
(*Old Dutch*), 1 oz.	128	2.0	23.0	3.0	0	75	1.0
cheddar, white:							
(*Barrel O'Fun*),							
3 cups	185	2.0	13.0	13.0	0	400	1.0
(*Chester's*), 3 cups	190	3.0	17.0	13.0	<5	300	3.0
(*Smartfood*), 2 cups	190	3.0	17.0	12.0	5	310	2.0
(*Smartfood* Reduced							
Fat), 3 cups . . .	140	4.0	19.0	6.0	<5	280	3.0
cheese, 2½ cups:							
(*Barrel O'Fun*) . . .	135	2.0	14.0	13.0	0	300	2.0
(*Barrel O'Fun* Low							
Fat)	140	3.0	20.0	5.0	0	300	2.0
microwave:							
(*Jolly Time*), 4 cups	160	3.0	16.0	10.0	0	160	4.0
(*Jolly Time* Light),							
4 cups	100	<3.0	16.0	4.0	0	100	4.0
nacho (*Pop Secret*),							
1 cup	30	<1.0	3.0	2.0	0	50	<1.0
microwave, butter fla-							
vor:							
(*Chester's*), 5 cups	200	3.0	22.0	12.0	0	300	4.0
(*Jolly Time*), 4 cups	140	3.0	16.0	8.0	0	160	4.0
(*Jolly Time* Light),							
4 cups	80	3.0	16.0	4.0	0	100	<4.0
toffee, butter:							
(*Cracker Jack* Fat							
Free), 1 cup, 1 oz.	110	<1.0	26.0	0	0	95	<1.0
(*Wise* Fat Free),							
1 cup	110	<1.0	26.0	0	0	95	<1.0
w/peanuts (*Cracker							
Jacks*), 1.25-oz.							
box	160	1.0	26.0	6.0	5	200	<1.0
w/pecans and al-							
monds (*Cracker							
Jacks*), 1 oz. . .	130	1.0	19.0	6.0	5	135	<1.0

Food and Measure	cal.	prot. (gms)	carbo. (gms)	fat (gms)	chol. (mgs)	sod. (mgs)	fiber (gms)
toffee crunch							
(*Smartfood*), ¾ cup	130	1.0	28.0	1.0	0	250	1.0
toffee, w/nuts (*Frank-*							
lin), ⅔ cup	140	2.0	24.0	4.0	<5	160	<1.0
Popcorn bar, 1 bar:							
caramel (*Pop Secret*)	80	0	14.0	2.5	0	45	0
chocolate (*Pop Se-*							
cret)	80	0	14.0	2.5	0	45	0
Popcorn cakes:							
(*Mother's*), 1 cake . .	35	1.0	8.0	0	0	0	0
apple cinnamon							
(*Orville Redenbacher*							
Mini), 1.1 oz. . . .	100	2.0	26.0	0	0	40	5.0
butter:							
(*Orville*							
Redenbacher),							
3 cakes	115	4.0	26.0	2.0	0	190	7.0
(*Orville Redenbacher*							
Mini), 1.1 oz. . .	100	3.0	23.0	2.0	0	170	6.0
(*Quaker* Mini),							
6 cakes	50	1.0	12.0	0	0	120	n.a.
caramel:							
(*Orville*							
Redenbacher),							
2 cakes	80	2.0	23.0	0	0	30	4.0
or honey nut							
(*Orville*							
Redenbacher							
Mini), 1.1 oz. . .	100	2.0	26.0	0	0	30	5.0
cheddar, white:							
(*Lundberg* Mini),							
5 cakes	70	1.0	12.0	1.0	0	100	2.0
(*Orville*							
Redenbacher),							
3 cakes	110	4.0	26.0	2.0	0	110	7.0
(*Orville Redenbacher*							
Mini), 1.1 oz. . .	100	3.0	23.0	2.0	0	100	6.0
Popcorn seasoning							
(*Tone's*), ¼ tsp. . .	0	0	0	0	0	630	0

Food and Measure	cal.	prot. (gms)	carbo. (gms)	fat (gms)	chol. (mgs)	sod. (mgs)	fiber (gms)
Poppy seed:							
1 tsp.	15	.5	.7	1.3	0	1	.8
(*McCormick*), ¼ tsp.	4	.2	.2	.3	0	<1	.2
Poppy seed filling,							
see "Pastry filling"							
Porgy, see "Scup"							
Pork, meat only,							
4 oz., except as							
noted:							
leg, see "Ham"							
loin, whole:							
braised, lean w/fat	417	30.8	0	31.6	116	74	0
braised, lean only	310	37.4	0	16.6	119	85	0
broiled, lean w/fat	392	26.7	0	30.9	107	75	0
broiled, lean only	291	31.6	0	17.3	108	85	0
roasted, lean w/fat	362	26.6	0	27.5	102	71	0
roasted, lean only	272	30.5	0	15.8	102	78	0
loin, blade:							
braised, lean w/fat	465	27.2	0	38.7	122	78	0
braised, lean only	355	33.7	0	23.3	128	92	0
broiled, lean w/fat	446	23.4	0	38.4	111	76	0
broiled, lean only	340	28.2	0	24.3	113	87	0
roasted, lean w/fat	413	23.9	0	34.5	102	69	0
roasted, lean only	316	28.0	0	21.9	101	77	0
loin, center:							
braised, lean w/fat	401	33.3	0	28.7	121	58	0
braised, lean only	308	39.4	0	15.5	126	62	0
broiled, lean w/fat	358	31.1	0	25.1	110	79	0
broiled, lean w/fat,							
3.1 oz. (3.7 oz.							
raw chop w/bone)	275	23.9	0	19.2	84	61	0
broiled, lean only	262	36.3	0	11.9	111	88	0
broiled, lean only,							
2.5 oz. (3.7 oz.							
raw chop w/bone							
and fat)	166	23.0	0	7.5	71	56	0
roasted, lean w/fat	346	28.8	0	24.7	103	73	0
roasted, lean only	272	32.3	0	14.8	103	78	0

Food and Measure	cal.	prot. (gms)	carbo. (gms)	fat (gms)	chol. (mgs)	sod. (mgs)	fiber (gms)
loin, center rib:							
braised, lean w/fat	416	32.4	0	30.8	108	54	0
braised, lean only	314	39.1	0	16.4	110	59	0
broiled, lean w/fat	389	27.9	0	29.9	106	69	0
broiled, lean only	293	32.7	0	16.9	107	76	0
roasted, lean w/fat	361	28.1	0	26.8	92	50	0
roasted, lean only	278	32.0	0	15.6	86	52	0
loin, top:							
braised, lean w/fat	432	31.4	0	33.1	108	53	0
braised, lean only	314	39.1	0	16.4	110	59	0
broiled, lean w/fat	408	26.9	0	32.5	105	67	0
broiled, lean only	293	32.7	0	16.9	107	76	0
roasted, lean only	278	32.0	0	15.6	90	52	0
shoulder, whole:							
roasted, lean w/fat	370	25.0	0	29.1	109	77	0
roasted, lean only	277	28.8	0	17.0	110	86	0
shoulder, arm (picnic):							
roasted, lean w/fat	375	25.3	0	29.6	107	79	0
roasted, lean w/fat, diced, 1 cup . . .	463	31.3	0	36.5	132	97	0
roasted, lean only	259	30.3	0	14.3	108	91	0
roasted, lean only, diced, 1 cup . . .	319	37.4	0	17.7	133	112	0
shoulder, Boston blade:							
braised, lean w/fat	421	29.9	0	32.5	126	76	0
braised, lean only	333	35.3	0	19.9	132	85	0
broiled, lean w/fat	397	24.8	0	32.3	117	85	0
broiled, lean only	311	28.5	0	20.9	119	95	0
roasted, lean only	290	27.6	0	19.1	111	83	0
sirloin:							
braised, lean w/fat	399	31.7	0	29.2	120	61	0
braised, lean only	296	38.0	0	14.8	125	67	0
broiled, lean w/fat	375	27.4	0	28.6	110	62	0
broiled, lean w/fat, 3 oz. (3.7 oz. raw chop w/bone) . .	278	20.3	0	21.2	81	46	0
broiled, lean only	276	32.1	0	15.4	111	68	0

Food and Measure	cal.	prot. (gms)	carbo. (gms)	fat (gms)	chol. (mgs)	sod. (mgs)	fiber (gms)
Pork, sirloin *(cont.)*							
broiled, lean only,							
2.4 oz. (3.7 oz.							
raw chop w/bone							
and fat)	165	19.2	0	9.2	67	41	0
roasted, lean w/fat	330	28.4	0	23.1	103	67	0
roasted, lean only	268	31.2	0	14.9	102	70	0
spareribs, lean w/fat,							
braised, 6.3 oz.							
(1 lb. raw w/bone)	703	51.4	0	53.6	214	165	0
tenderloin, lean only,							
roasted	188	32.6	0	5.5	105	76	0
Pork, cured (see also							
"Ham"), 4 oz.:							
arm (picnic), roasted:							
lean w/fat	318	23.2	0	24.2	66	1216	0
lean only	193	28.3	0	8.0	54	1396	0
blade roll, lean w/fat,							
roasted	325	19.6	.4	26.6	76	1103	0
Pork, pickled (see							
also "Pig's feet"),							
2 oz.:							
hocks (*Hormel*) . . .	110	9.0	0	8.0	45	530	0
tidbits (*Hormel*) . . .	100	8.0	0	8.0	45	530	0
Pork, refrigerated:							
loin, center (*John							
Morrell Table Trim*),							
4 oz.	190	19.0	0	13.0	65	65	0
smoked shoulder butt							
(*Oscar Mayer Sweet							
Morsel*), 3 oz. . . .	180	11.0	0	15.0	50	990	0
tenderloin (*John Mor-							
rell Table Trim*),							
4 oz.	120	20.0	0	4.5	65	65	0
Pork batter, frying							
(*House of Tsang*),							
4 tbsp.	140	3.0	32.0	.5	0	1300	0
Pork belly, raw, 1 oz.	147	2.7	0	15.1	20	9	0

Food and Measure	cal.	prot. (gms)	carbo. (gms)	fat (gms)	chol. (mgs)	sod. (mgs)	fiber (gms)
Pork dinner, frozen, barbecue (*Swanson Hungry Man*), 1 pkg.	770	58.0	78.0	38.0	90	1540	9.0
Pork entree, canned, chow mein (*La Choy* Bi-Pack), 1 cup	80	7.0	10.0	2.0	10	1185	1.5
Pork entree, freeze-dried, sweet and sour, w/rice (*Mountain House*), 1 cup	270	10.0	40.0	8.0	25	760	2.0
Pork entree, frozen, 1 pkg.:							
cutlet (*Banquet*) . . .	410	13.0	37.0	24.0	35	940	5.0
ribs, barbecue sauce (*Swanson Fun Feast*)	450	37.0	44.0	24.0	45	1060	3.0
rib-shape patty, barbecue (*Swanson*)	460	34.0	48.0	22.0	45	1060	6.0
sweet and sour (*Chun King*)	450	12.0	86.0	6.0	20	1180	4.0
Pork fat, roasted, 1 oz.	167	2.2	0	17.5	24	177	0
Pork gravy, 1/4 cup:							
(*Franco-American*) . .	45	6.0	3.0	4.0	4	340	1.0
mix*:							
(*Durkee*)	10	.5	3.0	0	0	240	0
(*French's*)	10	0	3.0	.5	0	250	0
Pork lunch meat, 2 oz.:							
(*Hormel Deli Pork Roast*)	70	12.0	1.0	1.5	30	570	0
seasoned (*Boar's Head*)	80	14.0	0	3.0	35	310	0
Pork rind snack, 1/2 oz.:							
(*Old Dutch Bac'n Puffs*)	80	8.0	0	5.0	15	340	0

Food and Measure	cal.	prot. (gms)	carbo. (gms)	fat (gms)	chol. (mgs)	sod. (mgs)	fiber (gms)
Pork rind snack *(cont.)*							
(*Baken-ets*)	80	8.0	<1.0	5.0	20	330	<1.0
(*Baken-ets* Cracklins)	80	7.0	<1.0	6.0	20	550	<1.0
hot and spicy:							
(*Baken-ets*)	80	8.0	<1.0	5.0	20	440	<1.0
(*Baken-ets* Crack-							
lins)	80	7.0	<1.0	5.0	20	370	<1.0
Pork sandwich, fro-							
zen, barbecued							
(*Hormel Quick*							
Meal), 1 pc.	350	15.0	39.0	15.0	60	580	2.0
Pork seasoning mix:							
(*Durkee/French's*							
Roasting Bag),							
1/6 pkg.	25	.5	5.0	0	0	320	0
(*Shake'n Bake* Original							
Recipe), 1/8 pkg. . .	40	1.0	9.0	0	0	320	0
barbecue glaze							
(*Shake'n Bake*),							
1/8 pkg.	35	0	8.0	0	0	250	0
chops (*McCormick*							
Bag 'n Season),							
2 tsp. mix	15	0	4.0	0	0	590	0
extra crispy (*Oven*							
Fry), 1/8 pkg.	60	2.0	11.0	1.5	0	340	0
hot and spicy							
(*Shake'n Bake*),							
1/8 pkg.	45	1.0	8.0	.5	0	220	0
sparerib (*Durkee*							
Roasting Bag),							
1/7 pkg.	25	0	5.0	0	0	430	0
Pork and beans, see							
"Baked beans" and							
specific bean list-							
ings							
Pot pie, see specific							
entree listings							

Food and Measure	cal.	prot. (gms)	carbo. (gms)	fat (gms)	chol. (mgs)	sod. (mgs)	fiber (gms)
Pot roast, see "Beef dinner" and "Beef entree"							
Pot roast seasoning mix, ⅙ pkg.:							
(*Durkee* Roasting Bag)	15	.5	3.0	0	0	350	0
(*French's* Roasting Bag)	20	.5	4.0	0	0	410	0
(*Lawry's*), 1 tsp. . . .	5	0	1.0	0	0	250	0
onion (*French's* Roasting Bag) . . .	25	1.0	4.0	0	0	350	0
sauerbraten (*Knorr*)	35	1.0	5.0	1.0	0	430	0
Potato:							
raw:							
unpeeled, 1 lb. . . .	269	7.1	61.2	.3	0	21	5.4
peeled, 2½″ potato	88	2.3	20.1	.1	0	7	1.8
peeled, diced, ½ cup	59	1.6	13.5	.1	0	5	1.2
baked:							
in skin, 4¾″ × 2⅓″	220	4.7	51.0	.2	0	16	4.8
w/out skin, 4 oz.	105	2.2	24.4	.1	0	6	1.7
w/out skin, ½ cup	57	1.2	13.2	.1	0	3	.9
boiled in skin, baby (*Frieda's*), 4 oz. . .	86	2.4	19.4	.1	0	3	n.a.
boiled in skin, peeled:							
2½″ potato	119	2.5	27.4	.1	0	6	2.4
½ cup	68	1.5	15.7	.1	0	3	1.4
boiled w/out skin:							
2½″ potato	116	2.3	27.0	.1	0	7	2.4
½ cup	67	1.3	15.6	.1	0	4	1.4
microwaved in skin:							
4¾″ × 2⅓″ potato	212	4.9	48.7	.2	0	16	<5.0
peeled, ½ cup . . .	78	1.6	18.2	.1	0	5	1.2
skin only, 2 oz. . .	75	2.5	16.8	.1	0	9	n.a.
mashed, w/whole milk:							
½ cup	81	2.0	18.4	.6	2	318	2.1
w/butter, ½ cup . .	111	2.0	17.5	4.4	13	309	2.1

Food and Measure	cal.	prot. (gms)	carbo. (gms)	fat (gms)	chol. (mgs)	sod. (mgs)	fiber (gms)
Potato, mashed, w/whole milk *(cont.)*							
w/margarine, ½ cup	111	2.0	17.5	4.4	2	309	2.1
Potato, canned:							
w/liquid, 4 oz.	45	1.5	9.8	.2	0	341	1.8
drained, 1.2-oz. potato	21	.5	4.8	.1	0	n.a.	<1.0
whole:							
(*Butterfield/Sunshine*), 5.6 oz.,							
2½ pcs.	90	2.0	20.0	0	0	330	2.0
(*Stokely*), 5½ oz.	80	1.0	12.0	0	0	400	2.0
(*Stokely* No Salt),							
5½ oz.	80	1.0	12.0	0	0	30	2.0
new (*Del Monte*),							
2 medium							
w/liquid	60	1.0	13.0	0	0	360	2.0
new (*S&W*), ½ cup	60	1.0	14.0	0	0	260	1.0
sliced:							
(*Butterfield*), ½ cup	100	2.0	22.0	0	0	390	4.0
(*Del Monte*), ⅔ cup	60	1.0	13.0	0	0	360	2.0
diced (*Butterfield*),							
⅔ cup	100	2.0	22.0	0	0	350	3.0
mashed, ⅓ cup:							
(*Idahoan* Real) . . .	80	2.0	17.0	1.0	0	270	1.0
(*Idahoan* Complete)	100	2.0	19.0	2.0	0	310	2.0
Potato, frozen (see also "Potato dishes, frozen"), 3 oz., except as noted:							
whole (*Stilwell*),							
3 pcs.	50	1.0	13.0	0	0	25	1.0
fried or french-fried:							
(*Ore-Ida* Deep Fries)	160	2.0	22.0	7.0	0	20	2.0
(*Ore-Ida* Deep Fries Crinkle Cuts) . .	160	2.0	23.0	6.0	0	25	2.0
(*Ore-Ida* Shoestrings)	150	2.0	22.0	6.0	0	20	2.0
(*Ore-Ida* Steak Fries)	110	2.0	19.0	3.0	0	20	1.0
(*Ore-Ida* Crispers!)	220	2.0	24.0	13.0	0	460	2.0

Food and Measure	cal.	prot. (gms)	carbo. (gms)	fat (gms)	chol. (mgs)	sod. (mgs)	fiber (gms)
(*Ore-Ida* Crispy Crowns!)	190	2.0	20.0	11.0	0	410	2.0
(*Ore-Ida* Crispy Crunchies!) . . .	160	2.0	20.0	8.0	0	310	2.0
(*Ore-Ida* Fast Fries)	150	2.0	20.0	6.0	0	330	2.0
(*Ore-Ida* Golden Crinkles)	140	2.0	23.0	3.5	0	20	2.0
(*Ore-Ida* Golden Fries)	120	2.0	20.0	3.5	0	20	1.0
(*Ore-Ida* Golden Twirls)	150	2.0	23.0	6.0	0	270	2.0
(*Ore-Ida* Golden Pixie Crinkles) . .	130	2.0	21.0	5.0	0	25	2.0
(*Ore-Ida* Homestyle Wedges with Skin)	110	2.0	19.0	3.0	0	15	2.0
(*Ore-Ida* Snackin' Fries), 5-oz. pkg.	340	4.0	36.0	20.0	0	590	3.0
(*Ore-Ida* Texas Crispers!)	170	2.0	20.0	9.0	0	280	2.0
(*Ore-Ida* Waffle Fries)	150	2.0	21.0	7.0	0	250	2.0
(*Ore-Ida* Zesties) . .	160	2.0	20.0	8.0	0	390	1.0
cottage fries (*Ore-Ida*)	130	2.0	25.0	4.0	0	25	1.0
country fries (*Ore-Ida*)	120	2.0	19.0	3.5	0	280	2.0
crinkle cut (*Empire* Kosher), ½ cup	90	1.0	18.0	1.5	0	20	7.0
ranch flavor (*Ore-Ida* Fast Fries) . .	150	2.0	21.0	7.0	0	430	1.0
zesty (*Ore-Ida* Snackin' Fries), 5-oz. pkg.	340	4.0	34.0	21.0	0	500	4.0
hash brown:							
(*Ore-Ida* Golden Patties), 1 pc.	160	2.0	17.0	9.0	0	180	2.0
(*Ore-Ida* Microwave), 4-oz. pkg.	220	1.0	26.0	12.0	0	290	1.0

Food and Measure	cal.	prot. (gms)	carbo. (gms)	fat (gms)	chol. (mgs)	sod. (mgs)	fiber (gms)
Potato, frozen, hash brown *(cont.)*							
w/cheddar (*Ore-Ida Cheddar Browns*), 1 pc.	80	3.0	14.0	2.0	5	370	1.0
country (*Ore-Ida*), 1 cup	60	2.0	14.0	0	0	20	1.0
shredded (*Ore-Ida*), 1 pc.	70	2.0	15.0	0	0	25	1.0
Southern style (*Ore-Ida*), ¾ cup . . .	80	2.0	17.0	0	0	30	2.0
toaster (*Ore-Ida*), 2 pcs.	190	2.0	25.0	11.0	0	470	1.0
mashed (*Ore-Ida*), ⅔ cup	90	2.0	16.0	2.5	<5	150	1.0
O'Brien (*Ore-Ida*), ¾ cup	60	1.0	15.0	0	0	20	2.0
puffs:							
(*Hot Tots*)	160	2.0	20.0	7.0	0	370	2.0
(*Tater Tots*)	160	2.0	21.0	8.0	0	300	2.0
(*Tater Tots* Microwave), 4-oz. pkg.	180	2.0	27.0	8.0	0	280	2.0
Potato, mix, dry, ½ cup except as noted:							
(*Betty Crocker Potato Buds*), ⅓ cup . . .	80	2.0	18.0	0	0	20	1.0
au gratin:							
(*Hungry Jack*) . . .	110	2.0	22.0	1.0	0	570	1.0
(*Idahoan*), ⅓ cup	110	2.0	23.0	1.5	0	600	2.0
cheddar and sour cream (*Betty Crocker*), ⅔ cup . .	120	2.0	24.0	1.5	<5	560	1.0
French country (*Good Harvest*), ⅓ cup . .	100	3.0	22.0	1.0	0	210	2.0
Italian, southern (*Good Harvest*), ⅓ cup	110	3.0	23.0	.5	0	140	2.0
mashed:							
(*Barbara's*), ⅓ cup	70	2.0	17.0	0	0	10	1.0

Food and Measure	cal.	prot. (gms)	carbo. (gms)	fat (gms)	chol. (mgs)	sod. (mgs)	fiber (gms)
(*Idahoan* Flakes),							
⅓ cup	80	2.0	18.0	0	0	15	2.0
(*Pillsbury* Idaho),							
2 tbsp.	90	2.0	20.0	0	0	25	2.0
cheddar and bacon							
(*Hungry Jack*) . .	110	2.0	22.0	1.0	0	500	2.0
cheese (*Hungry*							
Jack), ⅓ cup . .	80	2.0	17.0	0	0	45	1.0
scalloped:							
(*Betty Crocker*),							
⅔ cup	100	2.0	21.0	1.0	0	560	1.0
(*Idahoan*), ⅓ cup	110	2.0	23.0	1.5	0	430	3.0
cheesy (*Betty*							
Crocker), ⅔ cup	100	2.0	19.0	2.0	0	500	1.0
cheesy (*Hungry*							
Jack)	110	2.0	22.0	1.5	0	520	1.0
creamy (*Hungry*							
Jack)	110	2.0	22.0	1.5	0	420	2.0
sour cream and chive							
(*Hungry Jack*) . . .	110	2.0	22.0	2.0	<5	460	1.0
vegetable and herb							
(*Good Harvest*),							
⅓ cup	110	3.0	22.0	.5	0	230	2.0
Western (*Idahoan*),							
¼ cup	100	2.0	20.0	1.0	0	380	3.0
Potato, stuffed, see "Potato dishes, frozen"							
Potato, sweet, see "Sweet potato"							
Potato chips and crisps, 1 oz.:							
(*Barbara's* Regular/ Ripple)	150	2.0	15.0	10.0	0	180	1.0
(*Barbara's* No Salt)	150	2.0	15.0	10.0	0	20	1.0
(*Barrel O'Fun*)	150	2.0	15.0	9.0	0	160	0
(*Barrel O'Fun* Ripple)	150	2.0	16.0	8.0	0	160	0
(*Borden* Lightly Salted)	150	2.0	14.0	10.0	0	85	1.0

Food and Measure	cal.	prot. (gms)	carbo. (gms)	fat (gms)	chol. (mgs)	sod. (mgs)	fiber (gms)
Potato chips and crisps *(cont.)*							
(*Kettle* Chips)	150	2.0	15.0	9.0	0	110	1.0
(*Kettle* Crisps)	110	3.0	22.0	1.5	0	135	2.0
(*Lay's*)	150	2.0	15.0	10.0	0	120	1.0
(*Lay's* Baked)	110	2.0	23.0	1.5	0	150	2.0
(*Lay's* Wavy)	160	2.0	15.0	10.0	0	120	1.0
(*Mr. Phipps* Crisps)	120	2.0	20.0	4.5	0	220	1.0
(*Munchos*)	150	1.0	18.0	10.0	0	270	1.0
(*New York Deli*) . . .	150	2.0	14.0	10.0	0	170	1.0
(*No Fries* Original) . .	110	2.0	24.0	0	0	230	1.0
(*Old Dutch*)	150	2.0	16.0	9.0	0	160	1.0
(*Old Dutch Ripl*) . . .	150	2.0	16.0	9.0	0	150	1.0
(*Ridgies* Flat or Cur-lie)	150	2.0	14.0	10.0	0	170	1.0
(*Ridgies* Super Crispy)	150	2.0	14.0	10.0	0	220	1.0
(*Ruffles*)	150	2.0	14.0	10.0	0	125	1.0
(*Ruffles* Reduced Fat)	140	2.0	18.0	6.7	0	130	1.0
(*Wise* Ripple)	150	2.0	14.0	10.0	0	220	1.0
barbecue:							
(*Barbara's*)	160	2.0	16.0	10.0	0	230	1.0
(*Barrel O'Fun*) . . .	145	2.0	16.0	8.0	0	250	0
(*Borden*)	160	2.0	15.0	10.0	0	210	1.0
(*Lay's* Baked) . . .	110	2.0	23.0	1.5	0	220	2.0
(*Lay's* Hickory) . .	150	1.0	15.0	10.0	0	220	1.0
(*Lay's* KC Master-piece)	150	2.0	15.0	9.0	0	270	1.0
(*Mr. Phipps* Crisps)	130	2.0	21.0	4.0	0	270	1.0
(*No Fries*)	110	2.0	24.0	0	0	140	1.0
(*Munchos*)	160	1.0	15.0	10.0	0	250	1.0
(*Old Dutch*)	150	2.0	15.0	9.0	0	300	1.0
(*Old Dutch Ripl*) . .	150	2.0	16.0	9.0	0	180	<1.0
barbecue, mesquite:							
(*Krunchers!*)	140	2.0	16.0	8.0	0	200	1.0
(*Old Dutch* Kettle)	130	2.0	19.0	6.0	0	230	2.0
(*Ruffles* KC Master-piece)	150	1.0	15.0	9.0	0	120	1.0
Caribbean flavor (*Borden* Calypso)	160	2.0	15.0	10.0	0	130	1.0

Food and Measure	cal.	prot. (gms)	carbo. (gms)	fat (gms)	chol. (mgs)	sod. (mgs)	fiber (gms)
cheddar:							
(*Health Valley* Puffs)	110	2.0	21.0	3.0	<5	260	1.0
New York, w/herbs							
(*Kettle* Chips) . .	150	2.0	15.0	9.0	0	190	1.0
cheddar/sour cream:							
(*Barrel O'Fun* Ripple)	150	2.0	15.0	9.0	0	270	0
(*Old Dutch*)	160	2.0	16.0	9.0	0	190	1.0
(*Old Dutch Ripl*) . .	150	2.0	15.0	9.0	0	190	1.0
(*Ruffles*)	160	1.0	15.0	10.0	0	230	1.0
(*Wise*)	150	2.0	14.0	10.0	0	220	1.0
(*Wise* Super Crispy)	160	2.0	15.0	10.0	0	220	1.0
Dijon, golden (*Ruffles*)	150	1.0	16.0	9.0	0	190	1.0
dill pickle (*Old Dutch*)	140	2.0	16.0	8.0	<5	330	1.0
honey barbecue (*Kettle* Crisps)	110	3.0	22.0	1.5	0	160	2.0
honey Dijon (*Kettle* Chips)	150	2.0	16.0	8.0	0	150	1.0
hot:							
(*Barrel O'Fun*) . . .	150	2.0	15.0	9.0	0	230	0
(*Lay's* Flamin') . . .	150	1.0	15.0	10.0	0	180	1.0
jalapeño:							
(*Krunchers!*)	140	2.0	16.0	8.0	0	210	1.0
jack (*Kettle* Chips)	140	2.0	15.0	9.0	0	160	1.0
and cheddar (*Old Dutch*)	130	2.0	17.0	6.0	0	190	1.0
onion, French:							
(*Old Dutch Ripl*) . .	150	2.0	15.0	10.0	0	180	1.0
(*Ruffles*)	150	2.0	15.0	10.0	0	180	1.0
onion and garlic:							
(*Barrel O'Fun*) . . .	140	2.0	14.0	9.0	0	150	0
(*Borden*)	150	2.0	14.0	10.0	0	310	1.0
(*Lay's*)	150	2.0	16.0	9.0	0	200	1.0
(*Old Dutch*)	140	2.0	16.0	8.0	<5	420	1.0
pesto (*Kettle* Crisps)	110	3.0	22.0	1.5	0	140	2.0
ranch:							
(*Lay's Hidden Valley* Wavy)	160	2.0	14.0	11.0	0	150	1.0
(*Ruffles*)	150	2.0	15.0	9.0	0	280	1.0

Food and Measure	cal.	prot. (gms)	carbo. (gms)	fat (gms)	chol. (mgs)	sod. (mgs)	fiber (gms)
Potato chips and crisps, ranch *(cont.)*							
puffs (*Health Valley*)	110	2.0	21.0	2.5	0	260	1.0
salsa:							
and cheese (*Lay's*)	160	2.0	19.0	9.0	0	180	1.0
w/mesquite (*Kettle*							
Chips)	140	2.0	15.0	8.0	0	160	1.0
salt and sour (*Barrel*							
O'Fun)	150	2.0	15.0	10.0	0	220	0
salt and vinegar:							
(*Borden*)	150	2.0	14.0	10.0	0	290	1.0
(*Kettle* Chips) . . .	150	2.0	15.0	8.0	0	180	1.0
(*Lay's*)	160	2.0	15.0	10.0	0	340	1.0
(*Old Dutch*)	130	1.0	18.0	6.0	0	360	1.0
sour cream/onion:							
(*Barrel O'Fun*) . . .	150	2.0	15.0	9.0	0	230	0
(*Borden*)	150	2.0	14.0	10.0	0	210	1.0
(*Lay's*)	160	2.0	15.0	9.0	0	180	1.0
(*Lay's* Baked) . . .	110	2.0	23.0	1.5	0	170	1.0
(*Mr. Phipps* Crisps)	130	1.0	21.0	4.0	0	210	1.0
(*Old Dutch*)	150	2.0	17.0	9.0	<5	220	1.0
(*Ruffles* Reduced							
Fat)	130	3.0	18.0	6.0	0	200	1.0
yogurt and green on-							
ion:							
(*Barbara's*)	150	2.0	15.0	9.0	0	240	<1.0
(*Barbara's* No Salt)	150	2.0	15.0	9.0	0	20	<1.0
(*Kettle* Chips) . . .	150	2.0	15.0	8.0	0	170	1.0
Potato dishes,							
canned:							
au gratin, and bacon							
(*Hormel*), 7½ oz.	250	8.0	23.0	14.0	25	840	2.0
scalloped, and ham:							
(*Hormel*), 7½ oz.	260	7.0	20.0	16.0	35	920	2.0
(*Nalley*), 7½ oz. . .	210	8.0	27.0	7.0	15	800	3.0
sliced, and beef (*Dinty*							
Moore), 7½ oz. . .	230	10.0	28.0	9.0	25	1050	4.0

Food and Measure	cal.	prot. (gms)	carbo. (gms)	fat (gms)	chol. (mgs)	sod. (mgs)	fiber (gms)
Potato dishes, fro- **zen**, 1 pkg., except as noted:							
(*Goya* Rellenos de Papa), 2 pcs. . . .	280	11.0	36.0	10.0	20	800	5.0
(*Goya* Rellenos de Papa Cocktail), 6 pcs.	260	10.0	33.0	9.0	15	730	5.0
au gratin (*Stouffer's* Side Dish), 4.6 oz.	130	4.0	15.0	6.0	15	590	1.0
baked, 5 oz.:							
butter flavor (*Ore-Ida* Twice Baked)	200	4.0	26.0	8.0	0	360	5.0
cheddar (*Ore-Ida* Twice Baked) . .	190	5.0	26.0	8.0	<5	450	3.0
sour cream/chive (*Ore-Ida* Twice Baked)	190	4.0	27.0	7.0	0	360	3.0
baked, broccoli/ cheese:							
(*The Budget Gour- met* Light & Healthy)	270	11.0	38.0	8.0	25	580	5.0
(*Ore-Ida* Twice Baked)	150	6.0	25.0	4.0	10	410	2.0
(*Weight Watchers*)	250	12.0	35.0	7.0	10	590	6.0
cheddar (*Lean Cui- sine Lunch Ex- press*)	220	12.0	30.0	6.0	15	580	5.0
cheddar/cheddared:							
(*The Budget Gour- met* Side Dish), 5.5 oz.	260	8.0	21.0	9.0	40	740	4.0
(*Lean Cuisine* Deluxe)	230	13.0	32.0	6.0	20	570	6.0
and broccoli (*The Budget Gourmet* Side Dish), 5.25 oz.	170	7.0	17.0	8.0	25	440	2.0

Food and Measure	cal.	prot. (gms)	carbo. (gms)	fat (gms)	chol. (mgs)	sod. (mgs)	fiber (gms)
Potato dishes, frozen, cheddar/cheddared *(cont.)*							
pocket (*Ken & Robert's Veggie Pockets*), 1 pc.	260	6.0	42.0	8.0	0	370	2.0
scalloped:							
(*Stouffer's* Side Dish), 4.6 oz. . .	140	4.0	17.0	6.0	<5	450	2.0
and ham (*Swanson*)	290	18.0	29.0	12.0	45	1020	4.0
three cheese (*The Budget Gourmet* Side Dish), 6.1 oz.	230	8.0	22.0	12.0	35	530	3.0
Potato entree, see "Potato dishes"							
Potato flour, 1 cup	628	14.3	143.0	1.4	0	61	10.9
Potato pancake, frozen:							
(*Empire* Kosher), 2-oz. cake	80	1.0	15.0	2.0	0	200	8.0
mini (*Empire* Kosher), 2 cakes, 2 oz. . . .	90	1.0	16.0	2.5	0	160	6.0
Potato pancake mix (*Knorr*), 2 tbsp. . .	80	2.0	18.0	0	0	420	2.0
Potato seasoning, 1 tbsp.:							
cheddar, savory (*Lipton Recipe Secrets*)	60	1.0	1.0	5.0	5	420	0
garlic herb (*Lipton Recipe Secrets*) . .	50	0	2.0	5.0	5	290	0
onion, California (*Lipton Recipe Secrets*)	60	0	2.0	5.0	5	340	0
Potato seasoning mix:							
(*Potato Shakers*), 3 tsp.	25	<1.0	5.0	.5	<5	550	0
cheddar (*Shake 'n Bake Perfect Potatoes*), ⅙ pkg. . . .	30	2.0	2.0	2.0	5	380	0

Food and Measure	cal.	prot. (gms)	carbo. (gms)	fat (gms)	chol. (mgs)	sod. (mgs)	fiber (gms)
herb garlic (*Shake'n Bake Perfect Potatoes*), ⅙ pkg. . . .	20	0	5.0	0	0	370	0
Potato salad seasoning (*Tone's*), 1 tsp.	5	.2	.3	.2	0	1498	.1
Potato sticks:							
1 oz.	148	1.9	15.1	9.8	0	71	<2.0
(*Butterfield*), 1.7 oz.	250	3.0	26.0	15.0	1	150	3.0
(*Butterfield*), ⅔ cup	150	2.0	16.0	9.0	0	90	2.0
(*Pik-Nik* Fabulous Fries), 1 oz.	150	2.0	16.0	9.0	0	120	1.0
hot (*Chester's* Fries Flamin'), 1 oz. . . .	140	2.0	17.0	7.0	0	240	<1.0
ketchup (*Pik-Nik* Ket'n Fries), ⅔ cup . . .	160	2.0	17.0	10.0	0	160	1.0
shoestring:							
(*French's*), ¾ cup	180	2.0	16.0	12.0	n.a.	190	1.0
(*Pik-Nik*), 1.75-oz. can	280	2.0	26.0	18.0	0	180	2.0
(*Pik-Nik*), ⅔ cup . .	160	1.0	15.0	10.0	0	105	1.0
(*Pik-Nik* Less Salt), ¾ cup, 1.1 oz.	165	2.0	16.0	12.0	0	60	1.0
BBQ (*Pik-Nik*), ⅔ cup	180	2.0	18.0	12.0	0	240	2.0
sour cream/cheddar (*Pik-Nik*), ⅔ cup	180	2.0	17.0	13.0	0	130	2.0
Poultry, see specific listings							
Poultry seasoning, 1 tsp.	5	.1	1.0	.1	0	tr.	.2
Pout, ocean, meat only:							
raw, 4 oz.	90	18.9	0	1.0	59	69	0
baked, broiled, or microwaved, 4 oz. . .	116	24.2	0	1.3	76	88	0
Preserves, see "Jam and preserves"							

Food and Measure	cal.	prot. (gms)	carbo. (gms)	fat (gms)	chol. (mgs)	sod. (mgs)	fiber (gms)
Pretzels:							
(*Barbara's* Honey-sweet), 1 oz.	100	4.0	21.0	1.0	0	135	3.0
(*Barrel O'Fun* Minis), 1 oz.	105	3.0	22.0	0	0	300	.5
(*Borden* Tiny Thins/Mini)	100	3.0	23.0	0	0	540	<1.0
(*Borden* Thins/Ultra Thins)	100	3.0	22.0	0	0	630	<1.0
(*Little Debbie*), 1.2 oz.	140	3.0	28.0	0	0	600	1.0
(*Mister Salty* Mini), 1 oz.	110	3.0	22.0	2.0	0	440	1.0
(*Old Dutch*), 1⅛-oz. bag	125	3.0	24.0	2.0	0	280	<1.0
(*Pepperidge Farm* Goldfish), 45 pcs., 1.1 oz.	120	3.0	22.0	2.5	0	430	<1.0
(*Quinlan* Beer), 2 pcs., 1 oz.	110	2.0	21.0	2.0	0	420	1.0
(*Quinlan* Nuggets), 1.1-oz. bag	130	3.0	24.0	2.0	0	310	<1.0
(*Quinlan* Party Thins), 1 oz.	110	2.0	22.0	2.0	0	550	1.0
(*Quinlan* Sticks), 1 oz.	110	3.0	22.0	1.0	0	570	<1.0
(*Quinlan* Thin), 1.5-oz. bag	160	3.0	33.0	1.5	0	990	1.0
(*Quinlan* Tiny Thins/Mini), 1-oz. bag . .	110	2.0	22.0	2.0	0	550	1.0
(*Quinlan* Ultra Thin), 8 pieces, 1 oz. . . .	110	2.0	22.0	1.0	0	760	<1.0
bagel shaped (*Manischewitz*), 4 pcs., 1 oz.	110	3.0	22.0	0	0	260	1.0
Bavarian, 1 oz.:							
(*Barbara's*)	100	5.0	20.0	1.5	0	170	3.0
(*Barbara's* No Salt)	100	5.0	20.0	1.5	0	20	3.0
(*Rold Gold*)	110	3.0	21.0	2.0	0	440	1.0

Food and Measure	cal.	prot. (gms)	carbo. (gms)	fat (gms)	chol. (mgs)	sod. (mgs)	fiber (gms)
cheddar:							
(*Combos*), 1 oz. . .	130	3.0	18.0	5.0	0	310	0
(*Combos*), 1.8-oz.							
bag	240	5.0	33.0	9.0	5	560	1.0
cheese (*Handi-*							
Snacks), 1.1-oz. pc.	110	4.0	11.0	6.0	15	420	<1.0
chips, 1 oz.:							
(*Mr. Phipps*)	120	2.0	21.0	2.5	0	630	<1.0
(*Mr. Phipps* Fat							
Free)	100	2.0	22.0	0	0	630	<1.0
(*Mr. Phipps* Lower							
Sodium)	120	2.0	21.0	2.5	0	410	<1.0
(*Mr. Salty*)	110	2.0	21.0	2.5	0	620	<1.0
(*Mr. Salty* Fat Free)	100	2.0	22.0	0	0	620	1.0
Dutch (*Mister Salty*),							
2 pcs., 1.1 oz. . . .	120	3.0	25.0	1.0	0	580	1.0
hard, plain, 1 oz. . .	108	2.6	22.5	1.0	0	486	.8
honey mustard-onion:							
(*Old Dutch*), 1.1 oz.	140	2.0	21.0	5.0	0	240	1.0
(*Old Dutch*), 2-oz.							
bag	260	4.0	40.0	9.0	0	450	2.0
mini, 1 oz.:							
(*Barbara's*)	100	5.0	21.0	1.5	0	290	4.0
(*Barbara's* No Salt)	100	5.0	21.0	1.5	0	30	4.0
mustard:							
(*Combos*), 1 oz. . .	130	2.0	19.0	4.0	0	270	1.0
(*Combos*), 1.8-oz.							
bag	230	4.0	35.0	8.0	0	500	1.0
nacho:							
(*Combos*), 1 oz. . .	130	3.0	19.0	5.0	0	320	1.0
(*Combos*), 1.8-oz.							
bag	230	5.0	34.0	8.0	0	580	1.0
9-grain (*Barbara's*),							
1 oz.	100	4.0	21.0	1.5	0	180	3.0
oat bran nuggets							
(*Smart Snackers*),							
1½ oz.	170	4.0	33.0	2.5	0	250	3.0

Food and Measure	cal.	prot. (gms)	carbo. (gms)	fat (gms)	chol. (mgs)	sod. (mgs)	fiber (gms)
Pretzels *(cont.)*							
pizza:							
(Combos), 1 oz. . . .	130	3.0	19.0	4.0	0	290	1.0
(Combos), 1.8-oz.							
bag	230	5.0	35.0	8.0	0	520	1.0
rods, 3 pcs.:							
(Old Dutch), 1.2 oz.	130	4.0	26.0	1.5	0	440	<1.0
(Rold Gold), 1 oz.	110	3.0	22.0	1.5	0	370	1.0
soft:							
(Superpretzel),							
2.3-oz. pc.	170	6.0	37.0	0	0	140	2.0
(Superpretzel Added							
Salt), 2.3-oz. pc.	170	6.0	37.0	0	0	930	2.0
bites *(Superpretzel)*,							
4 pcs., 1½ oz. . . .	110	4.0	23.0	0	0	95	<1.0
bites *(Superpretzel*							
Added Salt),							
4 pcs., 1½ oz. . . .	110	4.0	23.0	0	0	880	<1.0
cinnamon raisin							
(Superpretzel),							
2 pcs., 2 oz.	190	5.0	40.0	1.5	0	240	1.0
soft, cheese-filled:							
cheddar or pizza							
(Superpretzel							
Softstix), 2 pcs.,							
1.8 oz.	140	5.0	24.0	2.5	10	250	1.0
nacho *(Superpretzel*							
Softstix), 2 pcs.,							
1.8 oz.	140	4.0	24.0	2.5	10	270	1.0
sourdough:							
(Quinlan), 1 pc. . .	80	2.0	18.0	0	0	470	<1.0
(Quinlan No Salt),							
1 pc.	80	2.0	18.0	0	0	60	<1.0
Bavarian or twists							
(Barbara's),							
1.1 oz.	110	3.0	24.0	0	0	260	1.0
hard *(Rold Gold)*,							
1 oz.	110	2.0	23.0	0	0	370	1.0

Food and Measure	cal.	prot. (gms)	carbo. (gms)	fat (gms)	chol. (mgs)	sod. (mgs)	fiber (gms)
sticks, 1 oz.:							
(*Bachman Stix*) . .	100	2.0	20.0	1.0	0	1460	1.0
(*Mister Salty* Fat Free)	110	3.0	23.0	0	0	370	1.0
(*Old Dutch*)	110	3.0	22.0	1.5	0	280	<1.0
(*Quinlan*)	100	3.0	22.0	0	0	570	<1.0
(*Rold Gold* Fat Free)	110	3.0	23.0	0	0	530	1.0
sticks, sesame (*Barbara's*), 1.1 oz. . .	110	5.0	21.0	2.5	0	420	4.0
thins:							
(*Old Dutch* Fat Free), 1.1 oz. . .	110	3.0	24.0	0	0	280	<1.0
(*Quinlan*)	120	2.0	22.0	2.0	0	0	<1.0
(*Rold Gold*), 1 oz.	110	3.0	22.0	1.0	0	510	1.0
(*Rold Gold* Fat Free), 1 oz. . . .	110	2.0	23.0	0	0	520	1.0
twists:							
(*Old Dutch*), 1 oz.	110	3.0	22.0	1.5	0	260	<1.0
(*Mister Salty*), 1 oz.	110	3.0	23.0	0	0	380	1.0
(*Planters*), 1 oz. . .	100	3.0	23.0	.5	0	420	1.0
(*Planters*), 1½-oz. bag	160	4.0	35.0	1.0	0	640	1.0
tiny (*Rold Gold* Fat Free), 1 oz. . . .	100	3.0	23.0	0	0	420	1.0
Prickly pear:							
1 medium, 4.8 oz. . .	42	.8	9.9	.5	0	6	3.7
(*Frieda's*), 3½ oz. . .	42	.5	10.9	.1	0	2	n.a.
Prosciutto (*Primissimo*), 2 oz.	210	11.0	0	18.0	50	1100	0
Prune:							
canned, in heavy syrup:							
pitted, 4 oz.	119	1.0	31.5	.2	0	3	4.3
½ cup	123	1.0	32.5	.2	0	3	4.4
5 pcs., 2 tbsp. liquid	90	.8	23.9	.2	0	2	3.3
(*Sonoma*), 3–4 pcs., 1.4 oz.	110	1.0	26.0	0	0	5	2.0

Food and Measure	cal.	prot. (gms)	carbo. (gms)	fat (gms)	chol. (mgs)	sod. (mgs)	fiber (gms)
Prune, canned, in heavy syrup *(cont.)*							
stewed (*S&W*),							
8 pcs., 4.9 oz. . . .	210	2.0	52.0	0	0	15	4.0
dehydrated:							
uncooked, ½ cup	224	2.4	58.8	.5	0	4	n.a.
cooked, ½ cup . .	158	1.7	41.6	.3	0	3	n.a.
dried:							
(*Del Monte*), ¼ cup	120	1.0	29.0	0	0	5	3.0
(*Dole*), 2 oz.	140	1.0	36.0	1.0	0	<10	n.a.
w/pits, ½ cup . . .	193	2.1	50.5	.4	0	3	5.7
pitted, 10 prunes	201	2.2	52.7	.4	0	3	6.0
pitted (*Sonoma*),							
¼ cup	120	1.0	29.0	0	0	5	3.0
dried, stewed, w/pits,							
unsweetened, ½ cup	113	1.2	29.8	.2	0	2	7.0
Prune juice, 8 fl. oz.:							
(*Del Monte*)	170	1.0	43.0	0	0	20	1.0
(*Goya*)	180	0	40.0	0	0	25	0
(*Lucky Leaf/Mus-*							
selman's)	160	0	40.0	0	0	25	0
(*R.W. Knudsen*) . . .	170	1.0	45.0	0	0	20	0
(*S&W*)	180	2.0	41.0	0	0	10	1.0
Pudding, 4 oz., ex-							
cept as noted:							
banana:							
(*Del Monte* Snack),							
3.5-oz. cup . . .	120	1.0	22.0	3.0	0	130	0
(*Hunt's Snack Pack*)	160	2.0	25.0	6.0	0	165	0
(*Jell-O* Snack) . . .	170	3.0	25.0	7.0	0	170	0
nondairy (*Imagine*)	150	1.0	30.0	3.0	0	40	0
butterscotch:							
(*Del Monte* Snack),							
3.5-oz. cup . . .	120	1.0	22.0	3.0	0	130	0
(*Hunt's Snack Pack*)	150	2.0	24.0	6.0	0	210	0
(*Rich's*), 3 oz. . . .	140	2.0	19.0	6.0	0	110	0
(*Swiss Miss*)	160	2.0	24.0	6.0	0	180	0
nondairy (*Imagine*)	150	1.0	31.0	3.0	0	45	0

Food and Measure	cal.	prot. (gms)	carbo. (gms)	fat (gms)	chol. (mgs)	sod. (mgs)	fiber (gms)
chocolate:							
(*Del Monte* Snack),							
3.5-oz. cup . . .	130	2.0	23.0	4.0	0	110	0
(*Del Monte* Snack Fat Free),							
3.5-oz. cup . . .	90	2.0	20.0	0	0	150	0
(*Hunt's Snack Pack*)	170	2.0	25.0	6.0	0	175	0
(*Hunt's Snack Pack* Fat Free)	100	2.0	21.0	0	0	210	0
(*Jell-O* Snack) . . .	160	3.0	28.0	5.0	0	190	0
(*Jell-O Free* Snack)	100	3.0	23.0	0	0	190	0
(*Rich's*), 3 oz. . . .	140	2.0	19.0	7.0	0	125	0
(*Swiss Miss*)	170	3.0	26.0	6.0	0	180	0
or chocolate fudge (*Swiss Miss* Fat Free)	100	2.0	23.0	0	0	150	0
nondairy (*Imagine*)	170	1.0	36.0	3.0	0	65	1.0
chocolate fudge:							
(*Del Monte* Snack), 3.5-oz. cup . . .	130	2.0	24.0	4.0	0	115	0
(*Hunt's Snack Pack*)	170	2.0	26.0	6.0	0	190	0
(*Swiss Miss*)	175	3.0	28.0	6.0	0	210	0
parfait (*Swiss Miss*)	160	3.0	25.0	0	0	200	0
chocolate marshmallow (*Hunt's Snack Pack*)	155	2.0	23.0	6.0	0	125	0
chocolate vanilla parfait (*Swiss Miss*)	160	3.0	25.0	6.0	0	200	0
chocolate swirl:							
caramel (*Hunt's Snack Pack*) . . .	170	2.0	26.0	6.0	0	175	0
caramel (*Swiss Miss*)	170	2.0	26.0	6.0	0	180	0
caramel or vanilla (*Jell-O* Snack) . .	160	3.0	27.0	5.0	0	180	0
caramel or vanilla (*Jell-O Free* Snack)	100	3.0	23.0	0	0	210	0

Food and Measure	cal.	prot. (gms)	carbo. (gms)	fat (gms)	chol. (mgs)	sod. (mgs)	fiber (gms)
Pudding, chocolate swirl *(cont.)*							
milk (*Hunt's Snack Pack*)	160	2.0	26.0	6.0	0	165	0
vanilla (*Swiss Miss*)	170	3.0	26.0	6.0	0	160	0
lemon:							
(*Hunt's Snack Pack*)	160	0	33.0	3.5	0	100	0
nondairy (*Imagine*)	150	1.0	33.0	3.0	0	50	1.0
S'mores swirl (*Hunt's Snack Pack*)	150	1.0	25.0	6.0	0	130	0
tapioca:							
(*Del Monte* Snack), 3.5-oz. cup . . .	120	2.0	21.0	3.0	0	100	0
(*Hunt's Snack Pack*)	150	2.0	23.0	6.0	0	130	0
(*Hunt's Snack Pack* Fat Free)	95	2.0	21.0	0	0	185	0
(*Jell-O* Snack) . . .	140	0	26.0	4.0	0	160	0
(*Swiss Miss*)	140	2.0	24.0	4.0	0	180	0
(*Swiss Miss* Fat Free)	100	2.0	22.0	0	0	150	0
vanilla:							
(*Del Monte* Snack), 3.5-oz. cup . . .	120	1.0	22.0	3.0	0	130	0
(*Del Monte* Snack Fat Free), 3.5-oz. cup . . .	90	2.0	20.0	0	0	140	0
(*Hunt's Snack Pack*)	160	2.0	25.0	6.0	0	170	0
(*Hunt's Snack Pack* Fat Free)	95	2.0	21.0	0	0	170	0
(*Jell-O* Snack) . . .	160	3.0	25.0	5.0	0	170	0
(*Jell-O Free* Snack)	100	2.0	23.0	0	0	240	0
(*Rich's*), 3 oz. . . .	140	2.0	19.0	6.0	0	110	0
(*Swiss Miss*)	160	2.0	24.0	6.0	0	180	0
(*Swiss Miss* Fat Free)	100	2.0	22.0	0	0	160	0
vanilla chocolate parfait:							
(*Swiss Miss*)	160	3.0	25.0	6.0	0	200	0

Food and Measure	cal.	prot. (gms)	carbo. (gms)	fat (gms)	chol. (mgs)	sod. (mgs)	fiber (gms)
(*Swiss Miss* Fat							
Free)	100	2.0	23.0	0	0	170	0
vanilla-chocolate swirl:							
(*Jell-O* Snack) . . .	170	3.0	26.0	5.0	0	180	0
(*Jell-O Free* Snack)	100	3.0	23.0	0	0	220	0
Pudding mix,							
½ cup*, except as							
noted:							
banana (*Jell-O* Sugar/							
Fat Free)	70	4.0	12.0	0	0	410	0
banana cream:							
(*Jell-O*)	140	4.0	26.0	2.5	10	240	0
(*Jell-O* Instant) . .	150	4.0	29.0	2.5	10	410	0
butter pecan (*Jell-O*							
Instant)	160	4.0	29.0	3.0	10	410	0
butterscotch:							
(*Jell-O*)	160	4.0	26.0	2.5	10	190	0
(*Jell-O* Instant) . .	150	4.0	29.0	2.5	10	450	0
(*Jell-O* Sugar/Fat							
Free)	70	4.0	12.0	0	0	400	0
chocolate:							
(*D-Zerta*)	60	5.0	11.0	0	0	65	<1.0
(*Jell-O*)	150	5.0	28.0	2.5	10	170	<1.0
(*Jell-O* Instant) . .	160	4.0	31.0	2.5	10	470	<1.0
(*Jell-O* Sugar Free)	80	4.0	11.0	2.5	10	170	<1.0
(*Jell-O* Sugar/Fat							
Free)	80	5.0	14.0	0	0	390	<1.0
(*My*T*Fine*)	90	0	22.0	0	0	140	<1.0
milk (*Jell-O*)	150	5.0	28.0	2.5	10	170	<1.0
milk (*Jell-O* Instant)	160	5.0	31.0	3.0	10	470	<1.0
chocolate fudge:							
(*Jell-O*)	150	5.0	28.0	2.5	10	170	1.0
(*Jell-O* Instant) . .	160	5.0	31.0	3.0	10	460	<1.0
(*Jell-O* Sugar/Fat							
Free)	80	5.0	14.0	0	0	390	<1.0
chocolate mousse,							
dry:							
dark (*Alsa*), 2 tbsp.	80	0	8.0	4.0	0	40	0

Food and Measure	cal.	prot. (gms)	carbo. (gms)	fat (gms)	chol. (mgs)	sod. (mgs)	fiber (gms)
Pudding mix, chocolate mousse *(cont.)*							
milk (*Alsa*), 2 tbsp.	80	0	10.0	4.0	0	40	0
white (*Alsa*), 2 tbsp.	70	0	8.0	3.5	0	40	0
coconut cream:							
(*Jell-O*)	150	4.0	24.0	2.5	10	210	<1.0
(*Jell-O* Instant) . .	160	4.0	27.0	4.5	10	320	<1.0
custard:							
(*Jell-O Americana*)	140	5.0	25.0	2.5	10	190	0
tropical (*Goya* Tem-							
bleque)	100	0	23.0	1.0	0	55	1.0
flan:							
(*Alsa* Creme Cara-							
mel), 1⅓ tbsp.							
mix, 1 tbsp. cara-							
mel	110	0	27.0	0	5	15	0
(*Goya*)	100	0	23.0	.5	0	110	1.0
(*Jell-O*)	140	4.0	26.0	2.5	10	65	0
w/caramel (*Goya*)	190	0	21.0	.5	0	130	1.0
lemon:							
(*Jell-O*)	140	1.0	29.0	2.0	75	75	0
(*Jell-O* Instant) . .	150	4.0	29.0	2.5	10	360	0
pistachio:							
(*Jell-O* Instant) . .	160	4.0	29.0	3.0	10	410	0
(*Jell-O* Sugar/Fat							
Free)	70	4.0	12.0	0	0	380	0
rice, see "Rice pud-							
ding mix"							
tapioca (*Jell-O Ameri-*							
cana)	140	4.0	26.0	2.5	10	170	0
vanilla:							
(*Jell-O*)	140	4.0	26.0	2.5	10	200	0
(*Jell-O* Instant) . .	160	4.0	29.0	2.5	10	410	0
(*Jell-O* Sugar Free)	80	4.0	11.0	2.5	10	170	0
(*Jell-O* Sugar/Fat							
Free)	70	4.0	12.0	0	0	400	0
French (*Jell-O* In-							
stant)	150	4.0	29.0	2.5	10	410	0

Food and Measure	cal.	prot. (gms)	carbo. (gms)	fat (gms)	chol. (mgs)	sod. (mgs)	fiber (gms)
Pummelo:							
1 medium, 5½" . . .	228	4.6	58.6	.2	0	7	6.1
sections, ½ cup . . .	36	.7	9.1	<.1	0	1	1.0
(*Frieda's*), 3.5 oz. . .	38	.8	9.6	<.1	0	1	n.a.
Pumpkin, ½ cup:							
fresh, pulp:							
raw, 1" cubes . . .	15	.6	3.8	.1	0	1	1.0
boiled, drained,							
mashed	24	.9	6.0	.1	0	2	1.0
canned:							
w/or w/out winter							
squash	41	1.3	9.9	.3	0	6	3.4
(*Libby's*)	60	2.0	15.0	.5	0	5	4.0
(*Stokely*)	50	1.0	10.0	0	0	0	4.0
pie mix, see "Pie							
filling"							
Pumpkin butter							
(*Smucker's*), 1 tbsp.	45	0	11.0	0	0	25	0
Pumpkin flower:							
raw, ½ cup	3	.2	.5	<.1	0	1	<1.0
boiled, drained, ½ cup	10	.7	2.2	.1	0	4	.6
Pumpkin leaf:							
raw, ½ cup	4	.6	.5	.1	0	2	<1.0
boiled, drained, ½ cup	7	1.0	1.2	.1	0	3	.9
Pumpkin pie spice,							
1 tsp.	6	.1	1.2	.2	0	1	.3
Pumpkin seed:							
roasted, in shell:							
1 oz. or 85 seeds	127	5.3	15.3	5.5	0	5	n.a.
1 cup	285	11.9	34.4	12.4	0	12	n.a.
salted, 1 oz.	127	5.3	15.3	5.5	0	163	n.a.
roasted, shelled:							
1 oz.	148	9.4	3.8	12.0	0	5	1.8
salted, 1 oz.	148	9.4	3.8	12.0	0	163	1.8
dried, shelled, 1 oz.							
or 142 kernels . . .	154	7.0	5.1	13.0	0	5	n.a.
tamari-roasted, spicy							
(*Eden*), 1 oz.	170	11.0	5.0	11.0	0	80	3.0

Food and Measure	cal.	prot. (gms)	carbo. (gms)	fat (gms)	chol. (mgs)	sod. (mgs)	fiber (gms)
Punch, see "Citrus drink," "Fruit drink blends," "Fruit juice blends" and specific fruit listings							
Purslane, ½ cup:							
raw	4	.3	.7	<.1	0	10	<1.0
boiled, drained	10	.9	2.1	.1	0	26	<1.0

Q

Food and Measure	cal.	prot. (gms)	carbo. (gms)	fat (gms)	chol. (mgs)	sod. (mgs)	fiber (gms)
Quail, raw:							
meat w/skin:							
1 quail, 3.8 oz.							
(4.3 oz. w/bone)	210	21.4	0	13.1	n.a.	58	0
1 oz.	54	5.6	0	3.4	n.a.	15	0
meat only:							
1 quail, 3.2 oz.							
(4.3 oz. w/bone							
and skin)	123	20.0	0	4.2	n.a.	47	0
1 oz.	38	6.2	0	1.3	n.a.	14	0
breast meat only:							
1 breast, 2 oz. . . .	69	12.7	0	1.8	n.a.	31	0
1 oz.	35	6.4	0	.8	n.a.	16	0
Quince:							
1 medium, 5.3 oz. . . .	53	.4	14.1	.1	0	4	1.7
peeled, seeded, 1 oz.	16	.1	4.3	<.1	0	1	.5
pineapple, pulp							
(*Frieda's*), 3.5 oz.	57	.4	15.3	.1	0	4	n.a.
Quinoa:							
(*Eden*), ¼ cup	170	6.0	31.0	2.5	0	0	3.0
black and white							
(*Frieda's*), 2 oz. dry							
or ½ cup cooked	218	7.8	37.9	3.9	9	<30	n.a.
Quinoa seeds (*Arrow-*							
head Mills), ¼ cup	140	5.0	25.0	2.0	0	0	4.0

R

Food and Measure	cal.	prot. (gms)	carbo. (gms)	fat (gms)	chol. (mgs)	sod. (mgs)	fiber (gms)
Rabbit, meat only:							
domesticated:							
roasted, 4 oz. . . .	223	33.0	0	9.1	93	53	0
stewed, 4 oz. . . .	234	34.5	0	9.5	98	42	0
stewed, diced,							
1 cup	288	42.5	0	11.8	120	52	0
wild, stewed:							
4 oz.	196	37.4	0	4.0	139	51	0
diced, 1 cup	242	46.2	0	4.9	172	63	0
Radiatore entree,							
vegetarian, frozen							
(*Hain* Bolognese),							
10 oz.	290	17.0	52.0	2.5	0	470	5.0
Radicchio, fresh:							
trimmed, 1 oz.	7	.4	1.3	.1	0	6	n.a.
1 medium leaf, .3 oz.	2	.1	.4	<.1	0	2	n.a.
shredded, ½ cup . .	5	.3	.9	.1	0	4	n.a.
Radish:							
10 medium, ¾"–1"	7	.3	1.6	.2	0	11	.7
sliced, ½ cup	10	.4	2.1	.3	0	14	.9
Radish, black, 1 oz.	5	.3	1.0	<.1	0	5	n.a.
Radish, Oriental:							
raw, 1 medium, 7"	62	2.0	13.9	.3	0	71	5.4
raw, sliced, ½ cup	8	.3	1.8	<.1	0	9	.7
boiled, drained, sliced,							
½ cup	13	.5	2.5	.2	0	10	1.2
dried, 1 oz.	77	2.2	18.0	.2	0	79	2.4
Radish, white-icicle:							
1 medium, .6 oz. . .	2	.2	.5	<.1	0	3	n.a.
sliced, ½ cup	7	.6	1.3	.1	0	8	n.a.

Food and Measure	cal.	prot. (gms)	carbo. (gms)	fat (gms)	chol. (mgs)	sod. (mgs)	fiber (gms)
Radish sprouts (*Jonathan's*), 1 cup . . .	57	3.0	3.0	2.0	0	5	2.0
Rainbow baking morsels (*Nestlé*), 1 tbsp.	70	0	10.0	3.0	0	0	1.0
Raisin, ¼ cup, except as noted:							
monukka/Thompson (*Sonoma*)	130	1.0	31.0	0	0	10	2.0
golden seedless:							
not packed	110	1.3	28.9	.2	0	5	1.5
(*Del Monte*)	120	1.0	33.0	0	0	20	5.0
(*Dole*), ½ cup . . .	250	3.0	66.0	0	0	25	n.a.
(*S&W*)	130	1.0	31.0	0	0	10	2.0
(*Sun•Maid*)	130	1.0	31.0	0	0	10	2.0
muscat (*Sun•Maid*)	130	1.0	31.0	.5	0	10	2.0
seeded, not packed	107	.9	28.5	.2	0	11	2.5
seedless:							
not packed	109	1.2	28.7	.2	0	5	1.5
(*Del Monte*)	120	1.0	33.0	0	0	20	5.0
(*Del Monte*), 1.5-oz. box	130	1.0	36.0	0	0	20	5.0
(*Dole*), ½ cup . . .	250	3.0	66.0	0	0	25	n.a.
(*S&W*)	130	1.0	31.0	0	0	10	2.0
(*Sun•Maid*)	130	1.0	31.0	0	0	10	2.0
chocolate or yogurt coated, see "Candy"							
Raisin sauce (*Reese*), ¼ cup	150	0	36.0	0	0	55	n.a.
Ranch dip, 2 tbsp:							
(*Heluva* Good Classic)	60	1.0	2.0	5.0	20	180	0
(*Heluva* Good Fat Free)	25	1.0	3.0	0	0	230	0
(*Kraft*)	60	1.0	3.0	4.0	0	210	0
(*Marie's* Creamy) . .	190	1.0	3.0	20.0	15	170	0
(*Marie's* Homestyle)	150	2.0	3.0	15.0	15	140	0
(*Nalley*)	110	1.0	2.0	11.0	10	240	0
(*Old Dutch*)	50	1.0	3.0	4.5	10	260	0
(*Ruffles*)	70	1.0	4.0	6.0	0	300	0

Food and Measure	cal.	prot. (gms)	carbo. (gms)	fat (gms)	chol. (mgs)	sod. (mgs)	fiber (gms)
Ranch dip *(cont.)*							
(*Ruffles* Low Fat) . .	40	2.0	6.0	1.0	0	230	<1.0
bacon (*Marie's*) . . .	150	2.0	3.0	16.0	15	200	0
peppercorn (*Marie's*							
Fat Free)	35	0	7.0	0	0	260	1.0
vegetable (*Bernstein's*)	120	0	2.0	11.0	0	250	0
Ranch dip mix,							
cracked pepper							
(*Knorr*), ½ tsp. . .	5	0	1.0	0	0	100	0
Raspberry, red:							
1 pint	154	2.8	36.1	1.7	0	<1	21.2
½ cup	31	.6	7.1	.3	0	<1	4.2
frozen:							
sweetened, ½ cup	129	.9	32.7	.2	0	1	5.5
unsweetened (*Big*							
Valley), ⅔ cup . .	60	1.0	12.0	0	0	0	2.0
Raspberry drink,							
8 fl. oz.:							
(*Farmer's Market*) . .	120	0	30.0	0	0	0	0
hibiscus (*R.W. Knud-*							
sen)	90	0	23.0	0	0	40	0
lemon (*Santa Cruz*)	120	0	29.0	0	0	35	0
Raspberry juice,							
8 fl. oz.:							
(*Heinke's*)	120	0	30.0	0	0	25	0
blend (*Dole* Country)	140	1.0	34.0	0	0	30	0
cranberry (*Apple &*							
Eve)	120	1.0	30.0	0	0	20	0
peach (*R.W. Knudsen*)	120	0	31.0	0	0	25	0
Raspberry nectar,							
8 fl. oz.:							
(*R.W. Knudsen*) . . .	120	0	30.0	0	0	25	0
(*Santa Cruz*)	100	0	26.0	0	0	35	0
Raspberry syrup:							
(*Fox's No Cal*),							
2 tbsp.	0	0	0	0	0	40	0
(*R.W. Knudsen*),							
¼ cup	150	0	38.0	0	0	0	0

Food and Measure	cal.	prot. (gms)	carbo. (gms)	fat (gms)	chol. (mgs)	sod. (mgs)	fiber (gms)
Ravioli, frozen or re-frigerated:							
(*Monterey Pasta Company* Mediterra-nean), 3 oz.	250	11.0	35.0	7.0	15	190	2.0
cheddar-roasted garlic (*Monterey Pasta Company*), 3 oz. . .	240	11.0	33.0	7.0	25	120	2.0
cheese:							
(*Amy's*), 9.5 oz. . .	340	15.0	44.0	12.0	20	580	6.0
(*Celentano*), ½ of 13-oz. pkg. . . .	400	21.0	61.0	9.0	100	390	11.0
(*Celentano* Great Choice), ½ of 13-oz. pkg. . . .	360	12.0	69.0	4.0	35	700	1.0
(*Stouffer's*), 9⅜ oz.	360	15.0	43.0	14.0	60	700	7.0
four (*Contadina*), 1 cup	280	13.0	31.0	12.0	85	350	2.0
four (*Contadina* Light), 1 cup . .	240	13.0	35.0	5.0	60	340	2.0
mini (*Celentano*), 4 oz.	270	13.0	42.0	6.0	30	150	2.0
mini, round (*Celentano*), 4 oz.	270	13.0	42.0	6.0	30	150	2.0
crab, snow (*Monterey Pasta Company*), 3 oz.	230	10.0	41.0	2.5	10	150	2.0
garden vegetable (*Contadina* Light), 1 cup	240	12.0	36.0	5.0	55	320	2.0
garlic basil cheese (*Monterey Pasta Company*), 3 oz. . .	240	12.0	34.0	6.0	20	100	2.0
gorgonzola roasted walnut (*Monterey Pasta Company*), 3 oz.	240	12.0	33.0	7.0	20	160	2.0

Food and Measure	cal.	prot. (gms)	carbo. (gms)	fat (gms)	chol. (mgs)	sod. (mgs)	fiber (gms)
Ravioli *(cont.)*							
Monterey Jack, smoked (*Monterey Pasta Company*), 3 oz.	240	11.0	33.0	7.0	20	150	2.0
parsley (*Putney*), 1 cup	250	11.0	39.0	5.0	35	290	<1.0
tofu (*Tofutti*), 1 cup	320	15.0	54.0	5.0	0	440	2.0
Ravioli entree, canned, 1 cup, except as noted:							
beef, tomato sauce:							
(*Franco-American*)	250	9.0	40.0	6.0	15	1160	3.0
(*Hunt's* Homestyle)	220	10.0	31.5	7.5	15	1115	4.0
(*Libby's*), 7¾ oz.	230	11.0	29.0	9.0	15	1040	7.0
(*Nalley*)	280	11.0	40.0	9.0	15	1240	7.0
(*Progresso*)	260	9.0	45.0	5.0	5	940	4.0
(*Top Shelf*), 10 oz.	300	20.0	35.0	9.0	45	800	4.0
w/meat (*Chef Boyardee*)	230	9.0	37.0	5.0	20	1150	4.0
w/meat (*Franco-American*)	300	15.0	42.0	10.0	25	1160	3.0
mini, w/meat (*Franco-American*)	270	12.0	36.0	8.0	15	1160	3.0
mini w/meat (*Chef Boyardee* Bowl), 7½ oz.	180	7.0	34.0	2.0	10	650	3.0
cheese, tomato sauce:							
(*Chef Boyardee*) . .	210	7.0	44.0	0	<5	860	4.0
(*Progresso*)	220	7.0	43.0	2.0	<5	930	4.0
w/cheese (*Chef Boyardee* Bowl), 7½ oz.	170	6.0	35.0	0	<5	790	2.0
w/meat (*Chef Boyardee* Bowl), 7½ oz.	190	8.0	33.0	3.0	15	800	3.0
mini (*Kid's Kitchen*), 7½ oz.	240	10.0	35.0	7.0	20	920	3.0

Food and Measure	cal.	prot. (gms)	carbo. (gms)	fat (gms)	chol. (mgs)	sod. (mgs)	fiber (gms)
tomato sauce (*Hormel* Micro Cup), 7½ oz.	270	9.0	34.0	11.0	25	990	2.0
Ravioli entree, frozen, cheese, 1 pkg.:							
(*The Budget Gourmet* Light & Healthy) . .	310	12.0	36.0	13.0	45	720	3.0
(*Kid Cuisine* Raptor)	320	7.0	63.0	4.5	10	780	6.0
(*Swanson Fun Feast* Roaring)	440	15.0	73.0	10.0	25	540	8.0
cheese (*Lean Cuisine*)	240	11.0	34.0	7.0	50	590	4.0
Florentine (*Smart Ones*)	190	8.0	37.0	2.0	5	420	5.0
in marinara sauce (*Marie Callender's*)	370	14.0	47.0	14.0	35	520	4.0
parmigiana (*Healthy Choice*)	250	11.0	44.0	4.0	20	290	6.0
Red beans (see also "Kidney beans" and "Mexican beans"), dried:							
(*Goya* Dominican), ¼ cup	160	8.0	32.0	0	0	0	12.0
canned, ½ cup:							
(*Allens*)	160	6.0	19.0	.5	0	310	9.0
(*Green Giant/Joan of Arc*)	100	6.0	19.0	.5	0	350	6.0
(*Stokely*)	110	6.0	19.0	.5	0	350	3.0
(*Van Camp's*) . . .	90	6.0	20.0	0	0	560	5.0
small (*Hunt's*) . . .	90	6.0	19.0	.5	0	715	4.0
Red snapper, see "Snapper"							
Redfish, see "Ocean perch"							
Refried beans, canned, ½ cup:							
(*Allens*)	150	7.0	24.0	2.5	0	360	11.0
(*Chi-Chi's*)	130	5.0	16.0	6.0	0	570	4.0
(*Chi-Chi's* Fat Free)	80	5.0	14.0	0	0	620	3.0
(*Gebhardt*)	110	6.0	20.0	3.0	<5	500	6.0

Food and Measure	cal.	prot. (gms)	carbo. (gms)	fat (gms)	chol. (mgs)	sod. (mgs)	fiber (gms)
Refried beans *(cont.)*							
(*Gebhardt* No Fat) . .	90	7.0	19.5	0	0	480	6.0
(*Goya*)	110	7.0	20.0	.5	0	330	3.0
(*Las Palmas*)	110	6.0	17.0	2.0	<5	500	5.0
(*Las Palmas* No Fat)	110	6.0	19.0	0	0	470	6.0
(*Old El Paso*)	110	6.0	17.0	2.0	<5	500	5.0
(*Old El Paso* Fat Free)	110	6.0	20.0	0	0	480	6.0
(*Rosarita*)	125	7.5	22.5	2.5	0	585	8.0
(*Rosarita* No Fat) . .	110	9.0	22.5	0	0	600	8.0
bacon (*Rosarita*) . . .	115	8.0	19.0	3.0	<5	490	8.0
black beans:							
(*Las Palmas*) . . .	120	6.0	18.0	2.0	0	340	6.0
(*Old El Paso*) . . .	120	6.0	18.0	2.0	0	340	6.0
(*Rosarito* Low Fat)	105	7.5	22.5	<1.0	0	570	7.5
w/cheese:							
(*Old El Paso*) . . .	130	7.0	18.0	3.5	5	500	6.0
nacho (*Rosarita*) . .	135	8.0	24.0	3.0	<5	705	8.0
w/green chilies:							
(*Old El Paso*) . . .	110	6.0	19.0	.5	<5	720	6.0
(*Rosarita*)	110	6.0	20.0	3.0	<5	495	6.5
and lime (*Rosarita* No Fat)	100	7.5	22.0	0	0	565	7.5
w/jalapeño (*Gebhardt*)	105	7.0	19.0	3.0	<5	380	6.5
w/onion (*Rosarita*) . .	115	6.5	21.0	3.0	<5	510	6.0
w/salsa, zesty (*Rosarita* No Fat)	100	6.5	22.0	0	0	555	7.5
w/sausage (*Old El Paso*)	200	7.0	14.0	13.0	10	360	8.0
spicy:							
(*Old El Paso*) . . .	140	6.0	22.0	3.0	<5	560	6.0
(*Rosarita*)	120	7.0	22.0	2.5	0	575	6.0
vegetarian:							
(*Chi-Chi's*)	80	5.0	14.0	0	0	620	3.0
(*Gebhardt*)	120	8.0	20.0	2.5	0	550	6.5
(*Old El Paso*) . . .	100	6.0	16.0	1.0	0	490	6.0
(*Rosarita*)	120	7.5	23.5	2.0	0	560	6.0
Refried beans, mix,							
(*Fantastic*), ½ cup*	160	9.0	29.0	1.0	0	320	11.0

Food and Measure	cal.	prot. (gms)	carbo. (gms)	fat (gms)	chol. (mgs)	sod. (mgs)	fiber (gms)
Relish, see "Pickle relish" and specific listings							
Remoulade sauce							
(*Zararain's*), ¼ cup	80	2.0	9.0	8.0	0	780	1.0
Rennet (*Junket*),							
1 tablet	1	0	0	0	0	165	0
Rhubarb:							
fresh:							
diced, ½ cup . . .	13	.6	2.8	.1	0	2	1.1
regular or hothouse							
(*Frieda's*), 1 oz.	5	.2	1.0	<.1	0	1	n.a.
frozen:							
(*Stilwell*), 1 cup . .	30	1.0	5.0	.5	0	0	2.0
cooked, sweetened,							
½ cup	139	.5	37.4	.1	0	2	2.4
Rice, dry, ¼ cup, except as noted:							
Arborio:							
(*Fantastic Foods*)	210	4.0	45.0	0	0	0	1.0
(*Frieda's*)	210	4.0	45.0	0	0	0	1.0
brown (*Lundberg Nutra-Farmed*)	160	5.0	33.0	1.5	0	0	3.0
white (*Lundberg Nutra-Farmed*) . . .	160	4.0	35.0	1.0	0	0	4.0
basmati, brown:							
(*Arrowhead Mills*)	150	3.0	33.0	1.0	0	0	2.0
(*Fantastic Foods*)	170	3.0	36.0	1.5	0	0	1.0
(*Lundberg* Organic)	160	4.0	34.0	1.5	0	0	2.0
(*Lundberg Nutra-Farmed*/Royal) . .	170	4.0	38.0	2.0	0	0	2.0
basmati, white:							
(*Casbah*)	158	3.0	36.0	0	0	0	1.0
(*Fantastic Foods*)	180	3.0	38.0	0	0	0	1.0
(*Lundberg* Organic)	180	4.0	38.0	.5	0	0	1.0
(*Lundberg Nutra-Farmed*)	180	4.0	41.0	.5	0	0	0

Food and Measure	cal.	prot. (gms)	carbo. (gms)	fat (gms)	chol. (mgs)	sod. (mgs)	fiber (gms)
Rice *(cont.)*							
blends:							
(*Lundberg Country-* wild)	150	3.0	35.0	1.5	0	0	3.0
(*Lundberg Jubilee*)	170	4.0	39.0	1.5	0	0	3.0
(*Lundberg Wild* Blend)	150	4.0	35.0	1.5	0	0	3.0
field (*Lundberg Ja-* ponica)	170	5.0	38.0	2.0	0	0	3.0
brown:							
(*Carolina/Mahatma/* River)	150	3.0	32.0	1.0	0	0	1.0
(*Lundberg Wehani*)	170	3.0	38.0	1.5	0	0	3.0
(*Success*), ½ cup	150	4.0	33.0	1.0	0	5	2.0
brown, long grain:							
(*Arrowhead Mills*)	150	3.0	33.0	1.0	0	0	2.0
(*Lundberg Nutra-* Farmed/Organic)	170	2.0	37.0	2.0	0	0	3.0
(*S&W*)	150	3.0	32.0	1.0	0	0	1.0
(*Uncle Ben's* Whole Grain)	170	5.0	35.0	1.5	0	0	2.0
(*Uncle Ben's* In- stant), ½ cup . .	190	4.0	42.0	1.5	0	20	2.0
brown, medium grain:							
(*Arrowhead Mills*)	160	3.0	35.0	1.0	0	0	2.0
(*Arrowhead Mills* Quick)	150	3.0	32.0	1.0	0	0	2.0
brown, quick (*Lund-* berg)	150	3.0	32.0	1.5	0	0	2.0
brown, short grain:							
(*Arrowhead Mills*)	170	4.0	36.0	1.0	0	0	2.0
(*Lundberg Nutra-* Farmed/Organic)	170	3.0	40.0	1.5	0	0	3.0
brown, precooked (*S&W* Quick), ½ cup	150	4.0	33.0	1.0	0	5	2.0
glutinous or sweet . .	171	3.2	37.8	.3	0	3	1.3
(*Goya* Fancy Blue Rose)	170	3.0	37.0	0	0	0	0

Food and Measure	cal.	prot. (gms)	carbo. (gms)	fat (gms)	chol. (mgs)	sod. (mgs)	fiber (gms)
(*Goya* Valencia) . . .	170	4.0	37.0	0	0	0	0
jasmine:							
(*Fantastic Foods*)	170	3.0	38.0	0	0	0	1.0
brown (*Fantastic*							
Foods)	170	3.0	36.0	1.5	0	0	1.0
sushi (*Lundberg* Or-							
ganic)	160	3.0	36.0	0	0	0	1.0
white, long grain:							
(*Canilla*)	160	3.0	35.0	0	0	0	0
(*Carolina*)	150	3.0	35.0	1.0	0	0	1.0
(*Mahatma*)	150	3.0	35.0	0	0	0	0
(*River/Water Maid*)	160	3.0	37.0	0	0	0	<1.0
(*Success*), ½ cup	190	4.0	44.0	0	0	5	<1.0
extra (*Goya*)	160	3.0	35.0	0	0	0	0
instant (*Carolina*)	160	4.0	36.0	0	0	0	1.0
instant (*Mahatma*)	160	4.0	36.0	0	0	5	1.0
instant (*Minute*),							
½ cup	170	4.0	37.0	0	0	5	0
instant (*Minute* Pre-							
mium), ½ cup . .	170	3.0	36.0	0	0	5	0
instant (*Minute* Boil-							
in Bag), ½ cup	190	4.0	42.0	0	0	10	0
instant (*Uncle*							
Ben's), ½ cup . .	190	3.0	43.0	.5	0	15	1.0
parboiled (*Uncle*							
Ben's Converted)	170	4.0	38.0	0	0	0	0
Rice, wild, see "Wild							
rice"							
Rice beverage, see							
" 'Milk,' nondairy"							
Rice bran, crude,							
1 cup	262	11.1	41.2	17.3	0	4	18.0
Rice cake (see also							
"Popcorn cakes"),							
1 cake, except as							
noted:							
plain (*Mother's* Mini							
Unsalted), 7 cakes	60	1.0	12.0	0	0	0	0

Food and Measure	cal.	prot. (gms)	carbo. (gms)	fat (gms)	chol. (mgs)	sod. (mgs)	fiber (gms)
Rice cake *(cont.)*							
all varieties:							
(*Lundberg*)	60	1.0	14.0	0	0	120	2.0
(*Lundberg* Unsalted)	60	1.0	14.0	0	0	0	2.0
(*Pritikin*)	35	1.0	7.0	0	0	20	0
(*Pritikin* Unsalted)	35	1.0	7.0	0	0	0	0
bars (*Health Valley* Crisp Fat Free)	110	1.0	26.0	0	0	5	1.0
except cheddar (*Quaker* Mini), 5 cakes	50	1.0	12.0	0	0	25	0
except plain (*Mother's* Mini), 5 cakes	50	1.0	12.0	0	0	40	0
apple:							
cinnamon (*Crispy Cakes*)	35	1.0	7.0	<1.0	0	60	n.a.
cinnamon (*Quaker*)	50	1.0	11.0	0	0	0	0
crisp (*Pritikin* Mini), 5 cakes	50	1.0	12.0	0	0	20	0
brown:							
(*Lundberg* Mini), 5 cakes	60	1.0	14.0	0	0	115	2.0
toasted (*Crispy Cakes*)	30	1.0	7.0	<1.0	0	15	n.a.
butter-flavored corn (*Mother's*)	35	1.0	7.0	0	0	0	0
caramel nut (*Pritikin* Mini), 5 cakes . . .	50	1.0	12.0	0	0	45	0
cheese:							
cheddar (*Crispy Cakes*)	35	1.0	7.0	<1.0	0	50	n.a.
cheddar, white (*Quaker*)	40	1.0	8.0	0	0	100	0
cheddar, white (*Quaker* Mini), 6 cakes	50	1.0	11.0	0	0	120	0
nacho (*Lundberg* Mini), 5 cakes . .	60	1.0	13.0	.5	0	115	2.0

Food and Measure	cal.	prot. (gms)	carbo. (gms)	fat (gms)	chol. (mgs)	sod. (mgs)	fiber (gms)
nacho corn (*Quaker*)	40	1.0	8.0	0	0	80	0
cinnamon crunch (*Quaker*)	50	1.0	11.0	0	0	25	0
dill, creamy (*Lundberg Mini*), 5 cakes . . .	60	1.0	13.0	1.0	0	55	2.0
multigrain (*Mother's*)	35	1.0	7.0	0	0	30	0
pizza or ranch (*Crispy Cakes*)	30	1.0	7.0	<1.0	0	50	n.a.
vegetable, garden (*Crispy Cakes*) . . .	35	1.0	7.0	<1.0	0	45	n.a.
wheat:							
(*Mother's*)	35	1.0	7.0	0	0	0	0
(*Quaker*)	35	1.0	7.0	0	0	45	0
Rice dishes, canned:							
Chinese fried (*La Choy*), 1 cup	240	5.0	53.0	1.0	0	1020	2.0
Mexican (*Old El Paso*), ½ cup . . .	410	8.0	90.0	2.0	0	1350	3.0
Spanish, 1 cup:							
(*Old El Paso*) . . .	130	3.0	28.0	1.0	0	1340	2.0
(*Van Camp's*) . . .	180	3.0	37.0	3.0	0	1290	3.0
Rice dishes, freeze-dried, wild, pilaf, w/almonds (*AlpineAire*), 1⅓ cups	291	10.0	89.0	6.0	0	1233	n.a.
Rice dishes, frozen (see also "Rice entree, frozen" and specific listings):							
Oriental, w/vegetables (*The Budget Gourmet*), 5.75 oz. . . .	220	5.0	25.0	12.0	15	560	2.0
pilaf, w/green beans (*The Budget Gourmet*), 5.62 oz. . . .	230	5.0	28.0	12.0	10	570	1.0

Food and Measure	cal.	prot. (gms)	carbo. (gms)	fat (gms)	chol. (mgs)	sod. (mgs)	fiber (gms)
Rice dishes, mix,							
2 oz. dry[1], except as noted:							
and beans:							
black (*Carolina/Mahatma*)	200	8.0	39.0	1.5	0	850	6.0
black (*Goya*)	160	5.0	34.0	0	0	570	3.0
black, Mediterranean, pilaf (*Near East*)	270	7.0	52.0	5.0	0	990	5.0
black, savory (*Good Harvest*), ⅓ cup	160	6.0	31.0	2.0	0	320	4.0
black, spicy (*Spice Islands* Quick), 1 pkg.	180	8.0	35.0	1.0	0	430	4.0
Cajun (*Lipton* Rice & Sauce), ½ pkg.	260	7.0	53.0	1.0	0	540	7.0
Cajun (*Rice-A-Roni*), 1 cup*	280	8.0	52.0	5.0	0	1220	3.0
pinto (*Mahatma*) . .	190	6.0	40.0	.5	0	280	4.0
red (*Carolina/Mahatma*)	190	6.0	40.0	1.0	0	790	6.0
red (*Goya*)	160	5.0	35.0	0	0	610	3.0
red (*Rice-A-Roni*), 1 cup*	280	8.0	51.0	7.0	0	1200	5.0
red, pilaf (*Near East*)	220	7.0	41.0	3.5	0	730	4.0
red, spicy (*Good Harvest*), ⅓ cup	160	5.0	32.0	1.0	0	280	3.0
red, spicy (*Spice Islands* Quick Meal), 1 pkg.	180	6.0	35.0	1.5	0	520	6.0
Spanish (*Fantastic Only A Pinch Cup*), 2.2 oz. . .	210	9.0	49.0	1.5	0	140	8.0
tomato herb, pilaf (*Near East*) . . .	270	7.0	52.0	5.0	0	945	5.0

[1] *Yield is approximately 1 cup prepared.*

Food and Measure	cal.	prot. (gms)	carbo. (gms)	fat (gms)	chol. (mgs)	sod. (mgs)	fiber (gms)
vegetables, garden,							
pilaf (*Near East*)	270	7.0	52.0	5.0	0	1120	5.0
beef/beef favor:							
(*Country Inn*) . . .	200	5.0	43.0	1.5	0	860	1.0
(*Golden Saute*),							
⅓ pkg.	230	6.0	43.0	4.0	0	930	1.0
(*Lipton* Rice &							
Sauce), ½ pkg.	230	7.0	48.0	1.0	0	940	2.0
(*Rice-A-Roni*),							
1 cup*	320	7.0	51.0	10.0	0	1170	3.0
(*Rice-A-Roni* Less							
Salt), 1 cup* . .	280	7.0	53.0	5.0	0	750	3.0
(*Success*)	190	5.0	43.0	.5	0	920	2.0
broccoli (*Lipton*							
Rice & Sauce),							
½ pkg.	230	6.0	46.0	1.0	0	940	2.0
and mushroom							
(*Rice-A-Roni*),							
1 cup*	290	7.0	51.0	7.0	0	1170	3.0
pilaf (*Near East*) . .	220	5.0	42.0	4.5	0	850	1.0
broccoli:							
Alfredo (*Lipton* Rice							
& Sauce), ½ pkg.	250	7.0	44.0	4.5	10	860	1.0
cheese (*Mahatma*)	200	5.0	41.0	1.5	5	620	2.0
cheese (*Rice-A-Roni*							
Fast), 1 cup* . .	300	6.0	41.0	12.0	5	730	1.0
cheese (*Success*)	210	4.0	40.0	4.5	25	840	1.0
broccoli au gratin:							
(*Country Inn*) . . .	200	6.0	41.0	2.0	5	830	2.0
(*Rice-A-Roni*),							
1 cup*	370	8.0	47.0	17.0	5	890	2.0
(*Rice-A-Roni* Less							
Salt), 1 cup* . .	320	8.0	49.0	11.0	5	590	2.0
(*Savory Classics*),							
1 cup*	390	9.0	47.0	5.0	10	840	2.0
brown and wild:							
(*Success*)	190	6.0	40.0	1.0	0	830	3.0
herb (*Arrowhead*							
Quick), ¼ pkg.	140	4.0	28.0	1.0	0	220	3.0

Food and Measure	cal.	prot. (gms)	carbo. (gms)	fat (gms)	chol. (mgs)	sod. (mgs)	fiber (gms)
Rice dishes, mix *(cont.)*							
Cajun (*Lipton* Rice and Sauce), ½ pkg.	230	6.0	49.0	1.0	0	930	2.0
cheddar, white, w/herbs (*Rice-A-Roni*), 1 cup*	340	7.0	49.0	14.0	5	980	1.0
cheddar broccoli (*Lipton* Rice & Sauce), ½ pkg.	250	6.0	48.0	3.0	<5	940	1.0
cheese (*Country Inn*)	210	5.0	41.0	2.5	5	810	1.0
chicken/chicken flavor:							
(*Country Inn*) . . .	200	5.0	42.0	1.0	0	990	1.0
(*Golden Saute*), ⅓ pkg.	240	6.0	44.0	5.0	0	920	1.0
(*Lipton* Rice & Sauce), ½ pkg.	240	7.0	48.0	2.0	<5	900	1.0
(*Rice-A-Roni*), 1 cup*	320	7.0	51.0	10.0	0	110	1.0
(*Rice-A-Roni* Less Salt), 1 cup* . .	280	7.0	53.0	5.0	0	690	2.0
(*Rice-A-Roni* Fast), 1 cup*	250	6.0	41.0	7.0	5	920	1.0
(*Savory Classics*), 1 cup*	300	8.0	52.0	8.0	5	1400	2.0
(*Success* Classic)	150	4.0	32.0	1.0	0	720	1.0
creamy (*Lipton* Rice & Sauce), ½ pkg.	260	7.0	46.0	5.0	0	770	2.0
pilaf (*Eastern Traditons*)	200	6.0	41.0	1.0	0	690	1.0
pilaf (*Knorr*), ⅓ cup	210	5.0	45.0	1.0	0	1000	2.0
pilaf (*Lundberg* Quick Country)	220	5.0	47.0	3.0	0	370	4.0
pilaf (*Near East*) . .	220	5.0	42.0	4.5	0	940	1.0
pilaf (*Spice Islands* Quick), 1 pkg. . . .	180	4.0	38.0	1.0	0	570	<1.0
pilaf, w/wild rice, Mediterranean (*Near East*) . . .	220	5.0	43.0	4.0	0	910	1.0

Food and Measure	cal.	prot. (gms)	carbo. (gms)	fat (gms)	chol. (mgs)	sod. (mgs)	fiber (gms)
chicken and broccoli:							
(Country Inn) . . .	200	5.0	43.0	1.5	0	860	1.0
(Golden Saute),							
½ pkg.	260	6.0	47.0	4.5	0	800	2.0
(Lipton Rice &							
Sauce), ½ pkg.	250	6.0	48.0	2.0	<5	940	2.0
(Rice-A-Roni),							
1 cup*	290	7.0	51.0	7.0	0	1410	2.0
chicken and mushrooms							
(Rice-A-Roni), 1 cup*	360	8.0	52.0	14.0	5	1480	2.0
chicken w/vegetables:							
(Country Inn) . . .	200	5.0	42.0	2.0	5	640	1.0
(Rice-A-Roni),							
1 cup*	290	6.0	52.0	7.0	0	1470	2.0
chicken and wild rice:							
(Country Inn) . . .	190	5.0	41.0	1.0	0	800	1.0
almond (Savory							
Classics), 1 cup*	310	7.0	53.0	9.0	0	1320	2.0
chili (Lundberg One							
Step)	180	6.0	42.0	1.0	0	420	5.0
curry:							
(Lundberg One							
Step)	160	5.0	38.0	1.5	0	400	5.0
pilaf (Near East) . .	220	5.0	42.0	4.0	0	660	1.0
fried:							
(Golden Saute),							
½ pkg.	240	5.0	47.0	1.0	0	900	1.0
(Rice-A-Roni),							
1 cup*	320	6.0	52.0	11.0	0	1590	2.0
garlic basil (Lundberg							
One Step)	160	6.0	37.0	1.0	0	480	5.0
gumbo (Mahatma) . .	160	3.0	31.0	2.5	0	720	1.0
herb, savory (Golden							
Saute), ⅓ pkg. . . .	240	6.0	43.0	4.5	0	900	1.0
herb and butter:							
(Golden Saute),							
⅓ pkg.	240	6.0	42.0	5.0	<5	870	1.0
(Lipton Rice &							
Sauce), ½ pkg.	240	5.0	43.0	4.0	10	920	1.0

Food and Measure	cal.	prot. (gms)	carbo. (gms)	fat (gms)	chol. (mgs)	sod. (mgs)	fiber (gms)
Rice dishes, mix, herb and butter *(cont.)*							
(*Rice-A-Roni*),							
1 cup*	310	6.0	53.0	9.0	5	1160	1.0
jambalaya (*Mahatma*)	190	4.0	43.0	1.0	0	700	<1.0
long grain and wild:							
(*Lipton* Rice &							
Sauce Original),							
½ pkg.	250	7.0	51.0	1.0	0	890	2.0
(*Mahatma*)	190	5.0	41.0	.5	0	710	2.0
(*Rice-A-Roni*),							
1 cup*	240	5.0	43.0	6.0	0	1170	1.0
(*Uncle Ben's* Fast)	190	6.0	41.0	1.0	5	840	1.0
(*Uncle Ben's* Origi-							
nal)	190	6.0	41.0	.5	0	620	1.0
butter and herb							
(*Uncle Ben's*) . .	200	5.0	40.0	2.0	5	770	1.0
chicken w/almonds							
(*Rice-A-Roni*),							
1 cup*	290	7.0	51.0	9.0	0	1240	3.0
chicken and herb							
(*Uncle Ben's*) . .	200	7.0	40.0	1.5	0	410	1.0
mushroom and herb							
(*Lipton* Rice &							
Sauce), ½ pkg.	250	6.0	50.0	1.5	0	550	1.0
pilaf (*Near East*) . .	220	6.0	42.0	4.5	0	810	2.0
pilaf (*Rice-A-Roni*),							
1 cup*	240	5.0	43.0	6.0	0	920	1.0
vegetable herb (*Un-*							
cle Ben's)	200	6.0	40.0	1.5	0	740	1.0
medley (*Lipton* Rice &							
Sauce), ½ pkg. . .	240	7.0	46.0	2.0	<5	810	2.0
Mexican:							
(*Goya*)	160	3.0	37.0	0	0	325	0
(*Pritikin*)	200	6.0	43.0	2.0	0	105	4.0
(*Savory Classics* Fi-							
esta), 1 cup* . .	310	8.0	55.0	7.0	0	1640	3.0
mushroom:							
(*Lipton* Rice &							
Sauce), ½ pkg.	220	6.0	45.0	1.0	0	890	1.0

Food and Measure	cal.	prot. (gms)	carbo. (gms)	fat (gms)	chol. (mgs)	sod. (mgs)	fiber (gms)
brown (*Uncle Ben's*)	190	6.0	40.0	1.5	0	600	2.0
onion mushroom							
(*Golden Saute*),							
⅓ pkg.	240	6.0	45.0	4.0	0	850	2.0
Oriental:							
(*Golden Saute*),							
⅓ pkg.	240	6.0	43.0	4.5	0	910	1.0
(*Lipton* Rice &							
Sauce), ½ pkg.	240	7.0	48.0	2.0	<5	900	1.0
(*Pritikin*)	190	6.0	43.0	1.5	0	260	4.0
(*Rice-A-Roni*),							
1 cup*	290	6.0	53.0	6.0	0	1090	2.0
(*Rice-A-Roni* Fast),							
1 cup*	290	6.0	43.0	11.0	0	930	1.0
(*Savory Classics*),							
1 cup*	290	5.0	43.0	12.0	0	870	2.0
and vegetables							
(*Spice Islands*							
Quick), 1 pkg. . .	180	4.0	39.0	1.5	0	590	1.0
pilaf (see also specific							
listings):							
(*Casbah*), 1 oz. . .	100	3.0	22.0	0	0	220	<1.0
(*Country Inn*) . . .	200	4.0	44.0	.5	0	680	1.0
(*Eastern Traditions*)	190	5.0	43.0	0	0	760	0
(*Eastern Traditions*							
Harvest)	190	6.0	40.0	1.0	0	770	2.0
(*Knorr* Original),							
⅓ cup	220	5.0	47.0	.5	0	900	2.0
(*Lipton* Rice &							
Sauce), ½ pkg.	230	6.0	46.0	1.0	0	850	1.0
(*Mahatma*)	190	5.0	43.0	0	0	820	<1.0
(*Near East*)	220	6.0	42.0	4.5	0	870	1.0
(*Rice-A-Roni*),							
1 cup*	310	6.0	53.0	9.0	0	1100	1.0
(*Success*)	200	5.0	44.0	0	0	630	2.0
almond, toasted							
(*Near East*) . . .	230	5.0	41.0	6.0	0	730	2.0
brown rice (*Near*							
East)	220	6.0	41.0	5.0	0	710	2.0

Food and Measure	cal.	prot. (gms)	carbo. (gms)	fat (gms)	chol. (mgs)	sod. (mgs)	fiber (gms)
Rice dishes, mix, pilaf *(cont.)*							
brown rice, w/miso (*Fantastic Foods*)	250	7.0	55.0	3.0	0	570	1.0
garden (*Savory Classics*), 1 cup*	240	6.0	41.0	6.0	0	1230	2.0
garlic herb (*Lundberg* Quick) . . .	210	5.0	47.0	2.5	0	510	4.0
lemon herb, w/jasmine rice (*Knorr*), ⅓ cup	270	5.0	56.0	2.0	0	770	2.0
Mediterranean (*Good Harvest*), ⅓ cup	160	4.0	32.0	2.0	0	330	2.0
mushroom, savory (*Lundberg* Quick)	190	4.0	41.0	2.5	0	590	4.0
nutted (*Casbah*), 1 oz.	110	2.0	20.0	0	0	290	<1.0
three grain (*Fantastic Foods*)	240	7.0	49.0	2.0	0	570	8.0
primavera (*Goya*)	160	5.0	35.0	0	0	405	1.0
risotto:							
(*Rice-A-Roni*), 1 cup*	310	6.0	51.0	9.0	0	1530	2.0
broccoli au gratin (*Knorr*), ⅓ cup	260	6.0	54.0	2.5	5	920	1.0
chicken (*Lipton* Rice & Sauce), ½ pkg.	230	7.0	44.0	2.0	5	740	1.0
garlic primavera (*Lundberg*), ¼ cup	140	4.0	29.0	1.0	0	520	1.0
Italian herb (*Lundberg*), ¼ cup . .	140	4.0	28.0	1.0	0	530	1.0
Milanese (*Knorr*), ⅓ cup	280	6.0	61.0	1.0	0	1060	2.0
mushroom (*Knorr*), ⅓ cup	300	7.0	66.0	1.0	0	1140	2.0
onion herb (*Knorr*), ⅓ cup	310	7.0	66.0	1.0	0	1340	2.0

Food and Measure	cal.	prot. (gms)	carbo. (gms)	fat (gms)	chol. (mgs)	sod. (mgs)	fiber (gms)
Parmesan, creamy (*Lundberg*), ¼ cup	140	5.0	27.0	1.5	0	490	1.0
primavera (*Knorr*), ⅓ cup	290	6.0	61.0	1.0	0	1070	2.0
tomato basil (*Lundberg*), ¼ cup . .	140	4.0	30.0	1.0	0	630	1.0
tomato-wild mushroom (*Good Harvest*), ⅓ cup . .	160	3.0	31.0	.5	0	340	1.0
Spanish:							
(*Country Inn*) . . .	200	5.0	43.0	1.0	0	750	2.0
(*Golden Saute*), ½ pkg.	250	6.0	46.0	4.5	0	910	2.0
(*Good Harvest*), ⅓ cup	160	5.0	32.0	1.0	0	390	4.0
(*Lipton* Rice & Sauce), ½ pkg.	240	6.0	49.0	1.0	0	940	2.0
(*Mahatma*)	180	4.0	42.0	.5	0	760	2.0
(*Rice-A-Roni*), 1 cup*	270	7.0	46.0	8.0	0	1210	3.0
(*Success*)	190	5.0	43.0	.5	0	780	1.0
brown (*Arrowhead Mills* Quick), ¼ pkg.	150	4.0	30.0	1.0	0	250	2.0
brown rice pilaf (*Fantastic Foods*)	240	7.0	55.0	2.0	0	650	2.0
pilaf (*Casbah*), 1 oz.	100	2.0	22.0	0	0	310	<1.0
pilaf (*Knorr*), ⅓ cup	230	5.0	50.0	1.0	0	1120	2.0
pilaf (*Near East*) . .	230	5.0	42.0	6.0	0	990	1.0
pilaf, brown (*Lundberg* Quick Fiesta)	190	5.0	43.0	2.0	0	750	3.0
Stroganoff (*Rice-A-Roni*), 1 cup*	360	8.0	50.0	14.0	5	1040	1.0
vegetable: country (*Spice Islands* Quick), 1 pkg.	180	5.0	38.0	1.0	0	570	2.0

Food and Measure	cal.	prot. (gms)	carbo. (gms)	fat (gms)	chol. (mgs)	sod. (mgs)	fiber (gms)
Rice dishes, mix, vegetable *(cont.)*							
herb (*Arrowhead Mills* Quick), ¼ pkg.	150	4.0	30.0	1.0	0	160	3.0
wild:							
and bean (*Good Harvest*), ⅓ cup	160	5.0	31.0	1.5	0	310	3.0
and vegetables (*Spice Islands* Quick), 1 pkg. . . .	170	1.0	35.0	1.0	0	530	1.0
yellow:							
(*Goya*)	170	4.0	37.0	0	0	546	1.0
saffron (*Carolina/ Mahatma*)	190	4.0	43.0	0	0	970	<1.0
Rice entree, frozen							
(see also "Rice dishes, frozen"), 1 pkg.:							
and beans, Santa Fe (*Weight Watchers*)	290	12.0	41.0	9.0	5	670	10.0
and broccoli (*Green Giant*)	320	8.0	15.0	12.0	5	1000	2.0
and chicken, stir-fry (*Lean Cuisine*) . . .	280	11.0	39.0	9.0	15	590	3.0
fried:							
w/chicken (*Chun King*)	270	9.0	44.0	6.0	25	1330	4.0
w/pork (*Chun King*)	290	11.0	48.0	6.0	25	1310	5.0
Mexican, w/chicken (*Lean Cuisine*) . . .	270	10.0	39.0	8.0	20	590	3.0
pilaf Florentine (*Weight Watchers*)	290	9.0	47.0	7.0	5	550	6.0
risotto, w/cheese and mushrooms (*Weight Watchers*)	290	11.0	44.0	8.0	20	540	4.0
and vegetables:							
(*Green Giant* Medley)	240	6.0	15.0	3.0	5	880	3.0

Food and Measure	cal.	prot. (gms)	carbo. (gms)	fat (gms)	chol. (mgs)	sod. (mgs)	fiber (gms)
Hunan style (*Weight Watchers*)	250	7.0	39.0	7.0	5	690	8.0
Oriental (*Green Giant* International)	180	7.0	37.0	.5	0	980	4.0
pilaf (*Green Giant*)	230	6.0	15.0	3.0	5	1020	3.0
white and wild (*Green Giant*) . .	250	6.0	15.0	5.0	0	1000	3.0
paella (*Weight Watchers*)	280	7.0	48.0	7.0	5	680	5.0
Peking style (*Weight Watchers*)	270	7.0	48.0	6.0	5	640	3.0
Rice flour:							
(*Goya*), 3 tbsp: . . .	120	2.0	26.0	.5	0	0	0
brown, 1 cup	574	11.4	120.8	4.4	0	12	7.3
brown (*Arrowhead Mills*), ¼ cup . . .	120	3.0	27.0	1.0	0	0	2.0
white, 1 cup	578	9.4	126.6	2.2	0	1	3.9
white (*Arrowhead Mills*), ¼ cup . . .	160	5.0	33.0	.5	0	0	1.0
Rice pudding mix:							
(*Goya*), ½ cup* . . .	90	1.0	20.0	1.0	0	100	1.0
(*Jell-O Americana*), ½ cup*	160	5.0	30.0	2.5	10	160	0
cinnamon and raisin (*Uncle Ben's*), 1.5 oz.	160	2.0	37.0	1.0	0	180	0
cinnamon raisin or honey almond (*Lundberg* Elegant), ½ cup	70	2.0	15.0	.5	0	0	1.0
coconut (*Lundberg* Elegant), ½ cup . . .	70	0	13.0	2.0	0	0	1.0
Rice seasoning mix:							
fried (*Durkee*), ¼ pkg.	15	1.0	2.0	0	0	840	0
Mexican (*Lawry's*), 1½ tbsp.	40	<1.0	9.0	0	0	840	0
Rice syrup (*Lundberg Nutra-Farmed*/Organic), ¼ cup . . .	170	0	42.0	0	0	5	0

Food and Measure	cal.	prot. (gms)	carbo. (gms)	fat (gms)	chol. (mgs)	sod. (mgs)	fiber (gms)
Rigatoni, canned, Italian garden sauce (*Hunt's* Homestyle), 1 cup	165	6.5	28.0	5.0	0	830	4.0
Rigatoni dishes, mix, cheddar and broccoli (*Noodle Roni*), 1 cup*	400	12.0	48.0	19.0	10	920	2.0
Rigatoni entree, frozen:							
(*Lean Cuisine*), 9 oz.	180	10.0	25.0	4.0	20	560	4.0
cream sauce, w/broccoli, chicken (*The Budget Gourmet* Light & Healthy), 10.8 oz.	310	17.0	5.0	6.0	15	670	5.0
parmigiana:							
(*Marie Callender's*), 7.5 oz.	300	12.0	32.0	14.0	25	650	3.0
(*Marie Callender's* Multi-Serve), 8 oz.	320	14.0	15.0	32.0	25	670	4.0
Risotto, see "Rice dishes, mix"							
Rockfish, meat only:							
raw, 4 oz.	107	21.3	0	1.8	39	68	0
baked, broiled, or microwaved, 4 oz. . .	137	27.3	0	2.3	50	87	0
Roe (see also "Caviar"):							
raw, 1 oz.	40	6.3	.4	1.8	106	n.a.	0
raw, 1 tbsp.	22	3.6	.2	1.0	60	n.a.	0
baked, broiled, or microwaved, 4 oz. . .	231	32.5	2.2	9.3	543	n.a.	0
Roll (see also "Biscuit" and "Bun, sweet"), 1 roll, except as noted:							
(*Arnold Francisco 3"*)	90	3.0	18.0	1.0	0	200	1.0

Food and Measure	cal.	prot. (gms)	carbo. (gms)	fat (gms)	chol. (mgs)	sod. (mgs)	fiber (gms)
(*Arnold Bran'nola* Buns)	130	6.0	27.0	1.5	0	210	3.0
assorted (*Brownberry* Hearth)	120	4.0	22.0	1.5	0	220	1.0
brown and serve:							
(*Pepperidge Farm* Hearth), 3 rolls	150	5.0	28.0	2.0	0	300	2.0
(*Roman Meal*), 2 rolls	140	5.0	26.0	2.0	0	290	2.0
club (*Pepperidge Farm*)	120	5.0	22.0	1.5	0	240	2.0
French (*Pepperidge Farm* 3)	240	10.0	45.0	2.5	0	490	3.0
French (*Pepperidge Farm* 2), ½ roll	180	8.0	34.0	2.0	0	400	2.0
sourdough (*Arnold Francisco*)	80	3.0	17.0	1.0	0	180	1.0
crescent, butter (*Pepperidge Farm* Heat & Serve)	110	3.0	13.0	5.0	15	160	1.0
croissant, see "Croissant"							
dinner:							
(*Arnold* 12 Pack)	110	4.0	19.0	2.5	0	140	1.0
(*Arnold* 24 Pack)	110	3.0	20.0	2.0	0	150	<1.0
(*Arnold August Bros.*)	90	3.0	18.0	2.0	0	180	1.0
(*Arnold Bran'nola*)	70	3.0	13.0	1.0	0	95	1.0
(*Brownberry Francisco Intl.*)	120	3.0	26.0	1.0	0	220	1.0
(*Pepperidge Farm* Country Style), 3 rolls	150	9.0	22.0	3.0	0	230	1.0
(*Roman Meal*), 2 rolls	150	6.0	27.0	2.5	0	285	2.0
all varieties (*Awrey's*), 2 rolls, 1.6 oz.	110	3.0	19.0	2.0	0	210	<1.0

Food and Measure	cal.	prot. (gms)	carbo. (gms)	fat (gms)	chol. (mgs)	sod. (mgs)	fiber (gms)
Roll, dinner *(cont.)*							
finger, poppy or sesame (*Pepperidge Farm*), 3 rolls	150	7.0	20.0	4.5	5	230	1.0
parker house (*Pepperidge Farm*), 3 rolls	150	7.0	20.0	4.5	5	230	1.0
potato (*Arnold*), 2 rolls	110	4.0	21.0	1.5	0	125	1.0
potato (*Pepperidge Farm* Deli Classic)	80	3.0	12.0	2.5	5	110	1.0
sesame seed (*Arnold*), 2 rolls . .	110	4.0	19.0	2.5	0	140	<1.0
wheat (*Arnold August Bros.*) . . .	100	4.0	19.0	2.0	0	160	1.0
white (*Arnold August Bros.*) . . .	90	3.0	19.0	1.0	0	190	1.0
egg, twist (*Arnold Levy* Old Country)	170	5.0	30.0	4.0	5	240	1.0
French:							
(*Arnold* 6″)	160	6.0	35.0	1.5	0	320	2.0
(*Brownberry Francisco Intl.* 6″) . .	170	5.0	35.0	1.0	0	260	1.0
(*Pepperidge Farm*)	100	4.0	19.0	1.0	0	230	1.0
mini (*Arnold Francisco*)	110	4.0	22.0	1.0	0	200	<1.0
7 grain (*Pepperidge Farm* 9)	80	4.0	19.0	2.0	0	270	2.0
sourdough (*Pepperidge Farm*)	100	4.0	18.0	1.0	0	240	1.0
golden twist (*Pepperidge Farm* Heat & Serve)	110	2.0	13.0	4.0	<5	160	1.0
hamburger:							
(*Arnold* 8 Pack) . .	130	4.0	26.0	2.0	0	250	1.0
(*Arnold* 12 Pack)	120	4.0	24.0	2.0	0	200	1.0
(*Arnold August Bros.*)	140	5.0	26.0	2.5	0	210	1.0

Food and Measure	cal.	prot. (gms)	carbo. (gms)	fat (gms)	chol. (mgs)	sod. (mgs)	fiber (gms)
(*Pepperidge Farm*)	130	5.0	22.0	2.5	0	230	1.0
(*Roman Meal*) . . .	120	5.0	22.0	2.0	0	230	2.0
wheat (*Arnold August Bros.*) . . .	130	6.0	25.0	2.0	0	210	2.0
hoagie (see also "sub," below):							
(*Awrey's*)	230	6.0	46.0	1.0	0	340	2.0
(*Pepperidge Farm* Deli Classic) . . .	200	7.0	32.0	4.5	0	340	2.0
multigrain (*Pepperidge Farm*)	200	7.0	32.0	4.5	0	340	2.0
hot dog/frankfurter:							
(*Arnold* 11 oz.) . .	100	3.0	19.0	2.0	0	150	1.0
(*Arnold* 12 oz.) . .	110	4.0	21.0	2.0	0	210	1.0
(*Arnold* 12 Pack)	110	3.0	21.0	2.0	0	180	1.0
(*Arnold Bran'nola*)	110	5.0	21.0	1.5	0	170	2.0
(*Arnold* New England)	110	4.0	21.0	2.0	0	210	1.0
(*Brownberry*) . . .	110	4.0	22.0	2.0	0	210	1.0
(*Pepperidge Farm*)	140	5.0	24.0	2.5	0	270	<1.0
(*Roman Meal*) . . .	110	4.0	20.0	2.0	0	215	2.0
Dijon (*Pepperidge Farm*)	140	6.0	23.0	3.0	0	240	2.0
potato (*Arnold*) . .	120	4.0	23.0	2.0	0	170	1.0
wheat (*Brownberry*)	110	4.0	21.0	2.0	0	180	1.0
Italian (*Arnold Savoni* 8")	280	10.0	56.0	3.5	0	610	3.0
kaiser:							
(*Arnold August Bros.*)	160	6.0	32.0	2.0	0	250	1.0
(*Arnold Francisco* 6")	170	6.0	35.0	2.0	0	290	2.0
(*Arnold Levy* Old Country)	170	5.0	34.0	2.0	0	270	1.0
(*Awrey's*)	190	5.0	37.0	2.0	0	340	1.0
(*Brownberry* Hearth)	150	6.0	30.0	2.5	0	270	1.0
(*Brownberry Francisco*)	170	5.0	35.0	1.0	0	260	1.0

Food and Measure	cal.	prot. (gms)	carbo. (gms)	fat (gms)	chol. (mgs)	sod. (mgs)	fiber (gms)
Roll, kaiser *(cont.)*							
sesame (*Arnold* Sandwich)	140	5.0	25.0	3.5	0	200	1.0
onion:							
(*Arnold* Deli)	170	6.0	35.0	2.0	0	250	2.0
(*Arnold August Bros.*)	160	6.0	33.0	2.0	0	240	2.0
(*Arnold Levy* Old Country)	160	5.0	31.0	3.0	5	210	3.0
party (*Pepperidge Farm* 20), 5 rolls	170	7.0	26.0	4.5	10	240	2.0
potato:							
(*Arnold*)	150	6.0	28.0	2.0	0	170	1.0
sesame (*Arnold*) . .	150	6.0	27.0	3.0	0	170	1.0
sandwich roll/bun:							
(*Pepperidge Farm* Hearty)	230	8.0	39.0	5.0	0	360	2.0
(*Roman Meal*) . . .	185	7.0	35.0	3.0	0	390	3.0
multigrain (*Pepperidge Farm*)	150	6.0	24.0	3.0	0	230	3.0
onion (*Pepperidge Farm*)	150	5.0	26.0	3.0	0	270	1.0
potato (*Brownberry*)	150	6.0	28.0	2.5	0	200	1.0
potato (*Pepperidge Farm*)	160	4.0	28.0	4.0	0	260	<1.0
sesame, soft (*Arnold*)	140	5.0	23.0	3.5	0	190	1.0
sesame seed (*Pepperidge Farm*) . .	140	5.0	23.0	3.0	0	240	1.0
soft (*Arnold* 8 Pack)	140	5.0	24.0	3.0	0	200	<1.0
soft (*Arnold* 12 Pack)	130	4.0	24.0	3.0	0	190	1.0
sourdough (*Pepperidge Farm*)	170	6.0	28.0	3.5	0	290	1.0
wheat (*Brownberry*)	130	5.0	24.0	2.0	0	230	2.0
white (*Brownberry*)	140	6.0	25.0	2.5	0	210	1.0
sesame (*Arnold August Bros.*)	170	6.0	33.0	2.5	0	240	1.0

Food and Measure	cal.	prot. (gms)	carbo. (gms)	fat (gms)	chol. (mgs)	sod. (mgs)	fiber (gms)
sourdough (*Arnold Francisco*)	90	3.0	17.0	1.0	0	180	1.0
steak:							
(*Arnold* Premium)	170	6.0	33.0	2.5	0	360	2.0
(*Arnold August Bros.*)	170	6.0	33.0	2.5	0	360	2.0
(*Arnold Francisco*)	170	6.0	35.0	2.0	0	320	2.0
sub:							
(*Arnold August Bros.*)	170	6.0	33.0	2.5	0	380	2.0
(*Arnold Levy* Old Country)	140	5.0	30.0	1.5	0	250	1.0
super loaf (*Arnold Francisco*), 1 oz.	70	2.0	14.0	.5	0	150	1.0
Roll, frozen or refrigerated:							
(*Rich's* Homestyle), 2 rolls	150	4.0	27.0	3.0	0	280	1.0
butterflake (*Pillsbury*), 1 roll	130	3.0	19.0	5.0	0	530	<1.0
crescent, 2 rolls:							
(*Pillsbury*)	200	4.0	22.0	11.0	0	430	<1.0
cheese (*Pillsbury*) . .	210	4.0	21.0	12.0	<5	600	<1.0
garlic cheese (*Pepperidge Farm*), 1 roll	130	6.0	16.0	5.0	15	280	2.0
Roll, mix, hot:							
(*Dromedary*), 1/16 pkg.	100	4.0	20.0	.5	0	340	1.0
(*Pillsbury*), 1/4 cup . .	110	3.0	21.0	1.0	0	200	<1.0
(*Pillsbury*), 1/15 pkg.*	130	4.0	21.0	3.0	15	220	<1.0
Roll, sweet, see "Bun, sweet"							
Roman beans:							
dry (*Goya*), 1/4 cup	80	8.0	24.0	0	0	15	13.0
canned (*Goya*), 1/4 cup	90	7.0	20.0	<1	0	370	6.0
Roseapple, 1 oz. . .	7	.2	1.6	.1	0	<1	<1.0
Roselle, 1 oz., 1/2 cup	14	.3	3.2	.2	0	2	<1.0
Rosemary, dried:							
1 tsp.	4	.1	.8	.2	0	1	.2
(*McCormick*), 1/4 tsp.	2	0	.3	0	0	<1	.2

Food and Measure	cal.	prot. (gms)	carbo. (gms)	fat (gms)	chol. (mgs)	sod. (mgs)	fiber (gms)
Rotini dishes, mix:							
mushroom sauce							
(*Knorr*), ⅔ cup . .	250	10.0	50.0	1.0	0	710	1.0
primavera (*Lipton*							
Pasta & Sauce),							
½ pkg.	240	8.0	42.0	5.0	10	880	2.0
Roughy, orange,							
meat only:							
raw, 4 oz.	143	16.7	0	8.0	23	72	0
baked, broiled, or mi-							
crowaved, 4 oz. . .	101	21.4	0	1.0	29	92	0
Roy Rogers, 1 serv-							
ing:							
bagel, plain	300	10.0	60.0	2.0	0	520	n.a.
bagel, cinnamon raisin	300	10.0	63.0	1.0	0	490	n.a.
Big Country Breakfast							
Platter:							
w/bacon	740	25.0	61.0	43.0	305	1800	n.a.
w/ham	710	24.0	67.0	39.0	330	2210	n.a.
w/sausage	920	33.0	61.0	60.0	340	2230	n.a.
breakfast biscuit:							
plain	390	6.0	44.0	21.0	0	1000	n.a.
bacon	420	9.0	44.0	23.0	5	1140	n.a.
bacon and egg . . .	470	14.0	44.0	26.0	150	1190	n.a.
Cinnamon 'N' Raisin	370	3.0	48.0	18.0	0	450	n.a.
ham and cheese . .	450	11.0	48.0	24.0	25	1570	n.a.
ham and egg . . .	460	14.0	48.0	23.0	165	1395	n.a.
ham, egg and							
cheese	500	16.0	48.0	27.0	170	1620	n.a.
sausage	510	14.0	44.0	31.0	25	1360	n.a.
sausage and egg	560	18.0	44.0	35.0	170	1400	n.a.
hash rounds	230	3.0	24.0	14.0	0	560	n.a.
pancakes, 3 pcs.:							
plain	280	8.0	56.0	2.0	15	890	n.a.
w/2 strips bacon	350	13.0	56.0	9.0	25	1130	n.a.
w/1 sausage	430	16.0	56.0	16.0	40	1290	n.a.
sourdough, ham, egg							
and cheese	480	20.0	45.0	24.0	185	1440	n.a.

Food and Measure	cal.	prot. (gms)	carbo. (gms)	fat (gms)	chol. (mgs)	sod. (mgs)	fiber (gms)
sandwiches:							
bacon cheeseburger	490	30.0	29.0	28.0	35	800	n.a.
bacon cheeseburger,							
sourdough	730	35.0	43.0	46.0	65	1470	n.a.
cheeseburger . . .	300	13.0	34.0	13.0	25	690	n.a.
cheeseburger, ¼ lb.	470	27.0	42.0	22.0	30	680	n.a.
chicken, grilled . .	340	25.0	32.0	11.0	30	910	n.a.
chicken, grilled,							
sourdough	500	30.0	46.0	21.0	45	1530	n.a.
chicken fillet	500	19.0	49.0	24.0	20	1050	n.a.
Fisherman's Fillet	490	21.0	56.0	21.0	15	1040	n.a.
hamburger	260	11.0	33.0	9.0	20	460	n.a.
hamburger, ¼ lb.	430	25.0	41.0	18.0	25	450	n.a.
roast beef	260	24.0	30.0	4.0	60	700	n.a.
chicken, fried:							
breast	370	29.0	29.0	15.0	75	1190	n.a.
leg	170	13.0	15.0	7.0	45	570	n.a.
thigh	330	19.0	30.0	15.0	60	1000	n.a.
wing	200	10.0	23.0	8.0	30	740	n.a.
¼ *Roy's Roaster:*							
dark meat	490	43.0	2.0	34.0	225	1120	n.a.
dark meat, skin off	190	24.0	1.0	10.0	110	400	n.a.
white meat	500	56.0	3.0	29.0	240	1450	n.a.
white meat, skin off	190	32.0	2.0	6.0	100	700	n.a.
chicken nuggets:							
6 pcs.	290	12.0	20.0	18.0	15	610	n.a.
9 pcs.	460	20.0	32.0	29.0	25	970	n.a.
salads:							
chicken, grilled . .	120	18.0	2.0	4.0	60	520	n.a.
garden	190	12.0	3.0	14.0	40	280	n.a.
side salad	140	1.0	3.0	n.a.	0	20	n.a.
potatoes:							
baked	130	3.0	27.0	1.0	0	65	n.a.
baked, w/margarine	240	3.0	27.0	13.0	0	220	n.a.
baked, w/margarine							
and sour cream	300	4.0	28.0	19.0	15	230	n.a.
fries, regular	350	5.0	49.0	15.0	0	150	n.a.
fries, large	430	6.0	59.0	18.0	0	190	n.a.
mashed, 5 oz. . . .	92	2.0	20.0	n.a.	0	320	n.a.

Food and Measure	cal.	prot. (gms)	carbo. (gms)	fat (gms)	chol. (mgs)	sod. (mgs)	fiber (gms)
***Roy Rogers*, potatoes** *(cont.)*							
gravy for mashed	20	n.a.	3.0	n.a.	0	260	n.a.
sides:							
baked beans, 5 oz.	160	6.0	30.0	2.0	10	560	n.a.
coleslaw, 5 oz.	295	2.0	16.0	25.0	15	430	n.a.
corn bread	310	4.0	35.0	17.0	30	260	n.a.
vanilla frozen yogurt							
cone	180	5.0	29.0	4.0	15	80	n.a.
Rum runner mixer,							
frozen* (*Bacardi*),							
8 fl. oz.	140	0	35.0	0	0	10	0
Rutabaga, ½ cup:							
fresh, cubed:							
raw	25	.8	5.7	.1	0	14	1.8
boiled, drained . . .	33	1.1	7.4	.2	0	17	1.5
fresh, boiled, drained,							
mashed	47	1.6	10.5	.3	0	25	2.2
canned (*Sunshine*)	30	<1.0	7.0	0	0	220	3.0
Rye, whole grain:							
1 cup	567	25.0	117.9	4.2	0	10	24.7
(*Arrowhead Mills*),							
¼ cup	160	6.0	34.0	1.0	0	0	6.0
Rye flakes, rolled (*Ar-*							
rowhead Mills),							
⅓ cup	110	4.0	24.0	.5	0	0	4.0
Rye flour:							
(*Arrowhead Mills*),							
¼ cup	100	5.0	20.0	1.0	0	0	4.0
dark, 1 cup	415	18.0	88.0	3.4	0	2	n.a.
light, 1 cup	374	8.6	81.8	1.4	0	2	14.9
medium, 1 cup . . .	361	9.9	79.0	1.8	0	3	14.9
medium (*Pillsbury*),							
¼ cup	100	3.0	22.0	0	0	0	2.0
Rye-wheat flour							
(*Pillsbury's* Bohemian							
Style), ¼ cup . . .	100	3.0	22.0	0	0	0	2.0

S

Food and Measure	cal.	prot. (gms)	carbo. (gms)	fat (gms)	chol. (mgs)	sod. (mgs)	fiber (gms)
Sablefish, meat only:							
raw, 4 oz.	222	15.2	0	17.4	56	64	0
baked, broiled, or mi-							
crowaved, 4 oz. . . .	284	19.5	0	22.2	71	82	0
smoked, 4 oz.	291	20.0	0	22.8	73	836	0
Safflower kernels,							
dried, 1 oz.	147	4.6	9.7	10.9	0	<1	1.0
Safflower meal, par-							
tially defatted, 1 oz.	97	10.1	13.8	.7	0	n.a.	<3.0
Saffron, 1 tsp.	2	.1	.5	<.1	0	1	0
Sage, ground:							
1 tsp.	2	.1	.4	.1	0	<1	0
(*McCormick*), ¼ tsp.	1	0	.1	0	0	0	.1
Salad blend mix,							
fresh, 3½ oz.:							
Caesar (*Dole Salad-*							
in-a-Minute)	170	3.0	9.0	14.0	5	480	1.0
classic (*Dole*)	25	1.0	4.0	1.0	0	20	1.0
French (*Dole*)	25	1.0	4.0	.5	0	15	1.0
Italian (*Dole*)	25	1.0	3.0	1.0	0	45	1.0
Oriental (*Dole Salad-*							
in-a-Minute)	110	2.0	12.0	7.0	0	290	2.0
spinach (*Dole Salad-*							
in-a-Minute)	180	5.0	19.0	9.0	0	660	3.0
Salad dressing,							
2 tbsp.:							
bacon and tomato:							
(*Kraft*)	140	<1.0	2.0	14.0	<5	260	0
(*Kraft Deliciously*							
Right)	60	<1.0	3.0	5.0	<5	300	0

Food and Measure	cal.	prot. (gms)	carbo. (gms)	fat (gms)	chol. (mgs)	sod. (mgs)	fiber (gms)
Salad dressing *(cont.)*							
balsamic vinegar							
(*S&W* Vintage) . .	35	0	8.0	0	0	460	0
berry vinaigrette							
(*Knott's Berry Farm*)	40	0	7.0	1.5	0	120	0
blue cheese:							
(*Bernstein's* Dress-							
ing/Dip)	180	2.0	0	20.0	10	210	0
(*Bernstein's* Dress-							
ing/Dip Lite) . . .	80	1.0	1.0	8.0	20	220	0
(*Kraft Free*)	50	<1.0	12.0	0	0	340	1.0
(*Kraft Roka*)	90	1.0	5.0	7.0	10	470	0
(*Marie's* Salad Bar							
Reduced Calorie)	100	1.0	7.0	7.0	5	330	1.0
creamy (*Bernstein's*)	110	1.0	2.0	13.0	5	180	0
creamy (*Marie's*							
Low Fat)	30	0	6.0	0	0	340	0
vinaigrette (*Herb*							
Magic)	160	2.0	0	17.0	5	450	0
blue cheese, chunky:							
(*Marie's*)	180	1.0	3.0	19.0	15	170	0
(*Marie's* Reduced							
Calorie)	100	1.0	7.0	7.0	10	260	0
(*Seven Seas*) . . .	90	1.0	5.0	7.0	10	470	0
(*Wish-Bone*)	170	<1.0	2.0	17.0	10	280	0
(*Wish-Bone* Free)	35	1.0	7.0	0	0	310	0
(*Wish-Bone* Lite)	80	1.0	2.0	7.0	0	380	0
Caesar:							
(*Bernstein's* Dress-							
ing/Dip)	100	1.0	1.0	10.0	15	190	0
(*Bernstein's* Extra							
Rich)	110	1.0	2.0	11.0	10	340	0
(*Kraft*)	130	<1.0	2.0	13.0	<5	370	0
(*Kraft Deliciously*							
Right)	60	<1.0	2.0	5.0	<5	560	0
(*Salad Celebrations*)	10	0	1.0	0	0	390	0
cheese, 3 (*Salad*							
Celebrations) . .	40	0	5.0	2.0	10	190	0

Food and Measure	cal.	prot. (gms)	carbo. (gms)	fat (gms)	chol. (mgs)	sod. (mgs)	fiber (gms)
creamy (*Seven Seas*)	140	<1.0	1.0	15.0	10	300	0
creamy (*Seven Seas Viva*)	120	<1.0	2.0	12.0	0	500	0
creamy, w/cracked pepper (*Lawry's*)	130	0	1.0	14.0	30	230	0
garlic, roasted (*Knott's Berry Farm*)	140	<1.0	2.0	15.0	0	260	0
olive oil (*Wish-Bone*)	100	0	2.0	9.5	0	400	0
olive oil (*Wish-Bone* Lite)	60	<1.0	2.0	5.0	<5	380	0
ranch (*Kraft*)	140	<1.0	1.0	15.0	10	300	0
cheese (*Bernstein's* Fantastico!)	110	1.0	2.0	11.0	5	410	0
chicken salad, Oriental (*Knott's Berry Farm*)	130	<1.0	4.0	12.0	0	220	0
citrus vinaigrette (*Knott's Berry Farm*)	40	0	8.0	1.0	0	120	0
coleslaw:							
(*Kraft*)	150	0	8.0	12.0	25	420	0
(*Marie's*)	150	0	6.0	13.0	10	210	0
cucumber, creamy (*Herb Magic*) . . .	15	0	4.0	0	0	270	0
Dijon vinaigrette:							
(*Wish-Bone* Lite)	60	0	3.0	5.0	0	400	0
balsamic (*Pritikin*)	30	0	6.0	0	0	125	0
dill, creamy (*Nasoya Vegi-Dressing*) . . .	60	0	3.0	5.0	0	135	0
French:							
(*Kraft*)	120	0	4.0	12.0	0	260	0
(*Kraft Catalina*) . .	140	0	8.0	11.0	0	390	0
(*Kraft Deliciously Right*)	50	0	6.0	3.0	0	260	0
(*Kraft Deliciously Right Catalina*)	80	0	9.0	4.0	0	400	0
(*Kraft Free*)	50	0	12.0	0	0	300	<1.0
(*Kraft Free Catalina*)	45	0	11.0	0	0	360	<1.0

Food and Measure	cal.	prot. (gms)	carbo. (gms)	fat (gms)	chol. (mgs)	sod. (mgs)	fiber (gms)
Salad dressing, French *(cont.)*							
(*Nally*)	110	0	6.0	9.0	0	240	0
(*Nally* Fat Free) . .	40	1.0	8.0	0	0	470	0
(*Salad Celebrations*)	40	0	9.0	0	0	200	0
(*Wish-Bone*)	120	0	5.0	11.0	0	170	0
herbal, creamy							
(*Bernstein's*) . . .	130	0	8.0	11.0	0	260	0
w/honey (*Kraft Cata-*							
lina)	140	0	8.0	12.0	0	310	0
honey (*Pritikin*) . .	40	0	11.0	0	0	135	0
style (*Pritikin*) . . .	35	0	8.0	0	0	130	0
style (*Wish-Bone*							
Lite)	100	0	5.0	8.0	<5	250	0
sweet 'n spicy							
(*Wish-Bone*) . . .	130	0	6.0	12.0	0	330	0
sweet 'n spicy							
(*Wish-Bone* Fat							
Free)	30	0	7.0	0	0	220	0
tangy (*Marie's*) . .	130	0	8.0	11.0	0	260	0
vinaigrette, true							
(*Herb Magic*) . .	170	0	<1.0	19.0	<5	430	0
fruit salad (*Knott's*							
Berry Farm)	70	0	8.0	4.0	0	125	0
fruit vinaigrette							
(*Knott's Berry Farm*)	45	0	9.0	1.0	0	120	0
garden, zesty (*Kraft*							
Salsa)	70	0	1.0	6.0	0	280	<1.0
garlic:							
creamy (*Kraft*) . . .	110	0	2.0	11.0	0	350	0
roasted, creamy							
(*Wish-Bone*) . . .	140	0	3.0	13.0	0	240	0
roasted, creamy							
(*Wish-Bone* Free)	40	0	9.0	0	0	280	0
green goddess (*Seven*							
Seas)	120	0	1.0	13.0	0	260	0
herb:							
garden (*Nasoya*							
Vegi-Dressing) . .	60	0	3.0	5.0	0	135	0

Food and Measure	cal.	prot. (gms)	carbo. (gms)	fat (gms)	chol. (mgs)	sod. (mgs)	fiber (gms)
vinaigrette, zesty							
(*Marie's* Free) . .	30	0	7.0	0	0	250	0
herbs and spices							
(*Seven Seas*) . . .	120	0	1.0	12.0	0	320	0
honey Dijon:							
(*Kraft*)	150	0	4.0	15.0	0	200	0
(*Kraft* Free)	50	<1.0	11.0	0	0	330	<1.0
(*Pritikin*)	45	0	11.0	0	0	130	0
(*Salad Celebrations*)	45	0	11.0	0	0	150	0
(*Wish-Bone*)	130	<1.0	9.0	10.0	0	390	0
(*Wish-Bone* Free)	45	1.0	10.0	0	0	270	0
viniagrette, zesty							
(*Marie's* Free) . .	50	0	11.0	0	0	125	0
honey mustard:							
(*Bernstein's* Dress-							
ing/Dip)	130	0	7.0	12.0	5	100	0
(*Knott's Berry Farm*)	130	0	4.0	13.0	0	100	0
(*Marie's*)	160	0	8.0	15.0	5	160	<1.0
(*Nally*)	130	0	7.0	12.0	5	100	0
Italian:							
(*Bernstein's*)	140	0	1.0	16.0	0	230	0
(*Bernstein's* Re-							
duced Calorie) . .	25	0	3.0	1.5	0	310	0
(*Bernstein's* Restau-							
rant)	80	1.0	12.0	4.0	0	390	0
(*Bernstein's* Wine							
Country)	110	0	2.0	11.0	0	250	0
(*Herb Magic*) . . .	10	0	2.0	0	0	400	0
(*Kraft Deliciously*							
Right)	70	0	3.0	7.0	0	240	0
(*Kraft* Free)	10	0	2.0	0	0	290	0
(*Kraft* House) . . .	120	0	3.0	12.0	<5	240	0
(*Kraft* Oil/Fat Free)	5	0	2.0	0	0	450	0
(*Kraft* Presto) . . .	140	0	2.0	15.0	0	290	0
(*Ott's* Zesty)	90	0	1.0	10.0	0	210	0
(*Pritikin*)	20	0	5.0	0	0	115	0
(*Salad Celebrations*)	10	0	2.0	0	0	360	0
(*Seven Seas* Free)	10	0	2.0	0	0	480	0
(*Seven Seas Viva*)	110	0	2.0	11.0	0	580	0

Food and Measure	cal.	prot. (gms)	carbo. (gms)	fat (gms)	chol. (mgs)	sod. (mgs)	fiber (gms)
Salad dressing, Italian *(cont.)*							
(*Seven Seas Viva* Reduced Calorie)	45	0	2.0	4.0	0	390	0
(*Wish-Bone*)	100	0	3.0	9.0	0	590	0
(*Wish-Bone* Classic House)	140	0	2.0	14.0	<5	360	0
(*Wish-Bone* Free)	15	0	2.0	0	0	280	0
(*Wish-Bone* Lite)	15	0	2.0	.5	0	380	0
(*Wish-Bone* Robusto)	100	0	4.0	10.0	0	610	0
cheese, 2 (*Seven Seas*)	70	0	3.0	7.0	0	240	0
cheese and garlic (*Bernstein's*) . . .	110	1.0	2.0	11.0	0	340	0
creamy (*Kraft*) . . .	110	0	3.0	11.0	0	230	0
creamy (*Kraft Deliciously Right*) . .	50	0	3.0	5.0	0	250	0
creamy (*Nasoya Vegi-Dressing*) . .	60	0	3.0	5.0	0	170	0
creamy (*Salad Celebrations*)	30	0	7.0	0	0	360	0
creamy (*Seven Seas*)	110	0	2.0	12.0	0	510	0
creamy (*Seven Seas* Reduced Calorie)	60	0	2.0	5.0	0	490	0
creamy (*Wish-Bone*)	100	0	3.0	10.0	0	310	0
creamy (*Wish-Bone* Lite)	60	0	7.0	3.5	<5	240	0
garlic, creamy (*Marie's*)	180	0	3.0	19.0	5	220	0
garlic, creamy (*Marie's* Reduced Calorie)	90	.5	6.0	7.0	5	240	1.0
herb, creamy (*Marie's* Low Fat)	30	0	7.0	0	0	340	0
herb and garlic, creamy (*Bernstein's*)	130	1.0	3.0	13.0	5	280	0

Food and Measure	cal.	prot. (gms)	carbo. (gms)	fat (gms)	chol. (mgs)	sod. (mgs)	fiber (gms)
olive oil (*Seven Seas* Reduced Calorie)	50	0	2.0	5.0	0	450	0
olive oil (*Wish-Bone*)	70	0	4.0	6.0	0	400	0
vinaigrette, zesty (*Marie's* Free) . .	35	0	8.0	0	0	280	0
zesty (*Kraft*)	110	0	2.0	11.0	0	530	0
mango–key lime vinegar (*S&W* Vintage Lite)	30	0	7.0	0	0	390	0
mayonnaise type, see "Mayonnaise"							
olive oil vinaigrette (*Wish-Bone*)	60	0	4.0	5.0	0	250	0
Oriental rice wine vinegar (*S&W* Vintage Lite)	30	0	8.0	0	0	280	0
(*Ott's* Famous Original)	80	0	9.0	6.0	0	210	0
(*Ott's* Famous Free)	35	0	9.0	0	0	310	0
(*Ott's* Famous Reduced Calorie) . . .	60	0	8.0	3.0	0	210	0
Parmesan, creamy (*Marie's* Low Fat)	35	0	7.0	0	0	280	0
peppercorn, ground (*Knott's Berry Farm*)	160	<1.0	1.0	17.0	0	210	0
poppyseed:							
(*Herb Magic*) . . .	170	0	8.0	15.0	5	330	0
(*Knott's Berry Farm*)	120	0	10.0	9.0	0	190	0
(*Marie's*)	150	0	8.0	12.0	10	200	0
(*Ott's* Free)	45	0	12.0	0	0	210	0
(*Ott's* Reduced Calorie)	90	0	9.0	7.0	0	210	0
potato salad:							
(*Best Foods/Hellmann's One Step*)	160	0	2.0	17.0	5	370	0

Food and Measure	cal.	prot. (gms)	carbo. (gms)	fat (gms)	chol. (mgs)	sod. (mgs)	fiber (gms)
Salad dressing, potato salad *(cont.)*							
(*Best Foods/Hell-mann's One Step* ⅓ Less Fat) . . .	110	0	4.0	11.0	5	440	0
ranch:							
(*Bernstein's* Dress-ing/Dip)	110	0	1.0	12.0	10	200	0
(*Bernstein's* Dress-ing/Dip Lite) . . .	70	0	2.0	6.0	10	210	0
(*Herb Magic*) . . .	15	<1.0	4.0	0	0	270	0
(*Kraft*)	170	0	2.0	18.0	5	270	0
(*Kraft Deliciously Right*)	110	0	2.0	11.0	10	310	0
(*Kraft Free*)	50	<1.0	11.0	0	0	310	<1.0
(*Kraft Salsa*)	130	0	1.0	13.0	10	320	0
(*Marie's* Salad Bar Reduced Calorie)	90	1.0	7.0	7.0	5	390	<1.0
(*Nalley*)	100	0	6.0	8.0	10	250	0
(*Ott's* Buttermilk)	140	0	1.0	15.0	0	120	0
(*Salad Celebrations*)	35	0	7.0	0	0	270	0
(*Seven Seas*) . . .	150	0	2.0	16.0	5	250	0
(*Seven Seas* Re-duced Calorie) . .	100	0	5.0	9.0	0	320	0
(*Seven Seas Free*)	50	<1.0	12.0	0	0	330	1.0
(*Wish-Bone*)	160	0	1.0	17.0	10	210	0
(*Wish-Bone* Free)	40	0	9.0	0	0	270	0
(*Wish-Bone* Lite)	100	0	5.0	8.0	5	240	0
buttermilk (*Kraft*)	150	0	2.0	16.0	<5	230	0
buttermilk (*Marie's*)	180	0	4.0	18.0	15	230	0
creamy (*Marie's* Re-duced Calorie) . .	100	.5	7.0	8.0	10	280	<1.0
cucumber (*Kraft*)	150	0	2.0	15.0	0	220	0
cucumber (*Kraft De-liciously Right*)	60	0	2.0	5.0	0	450	0
Parmesan (*Marie's*)	180	1.0	2.0	14.0	10	140	<1.0
Parmesan garlic (*Bernstein's*) . . .	110	1.0	3.0	11.0	5	330	0
peppercorn (*Kraft*)	170	<1.0	1.0	18.0	10	340	0

Food and Measure	cal.	prot. (gms)	carbo. (gms)	fat (gms)	chol. (mgs)	sod. (mgs)	fiber (gms)
peppercorn (*Kraft* Free)	50	<1.0	11.0	0	0	360	<1.0
sour cream and on-ion (*Kraft*)	170	0	1.0	18.0	10	240	0
zesty (*Marie's* Low Fat)	30	0	7.0	0	0	310	0
raspberry blush vine-gar (*S&W* Vintage Lite)	40	0	10.0	0	0	410	0
raspberry vinaigrette: (*Knott's Berry Farm* Low Fat)	50	0	8.0	2.0	0	110	0
(*Pritikin*)	45	0	11.0	0	0	70	0
zesty (*Marie's* Free)	35	0	8.0	0	0	35	0
red wine vinaigrette, zesty (*Marie's* Free)	40	0	10.0	0	0	300	0
red wine vinegar: (*Kraft Free*)	15	0	3.0	0	0	400	0
(*Seven Seas Free*)	15	0	3.0	0	0	400	0
w/herbs (*S&W* Vin-tage Lite)	40	0	8.0	0	0	440	0
and oil (*Seven Seas*)	110	0	2.0	11.0	0	510	0
and oil (*Seven Seas* Reduced Calorie)	60	0	2.0	5.0	0	310	0
Roquefort (*Bernstein's* Dressing/Dip) . . .	140	1.0	1.0	15.0	20	210	0
Russian: (*Kraft*)	130	0	10.0	10.0	0	280	0
(*Salad Celebrations*)	45	0	8.0	1.5	10	190	0
(*Seven Seas Viva*)	150	0	3.0	16.0	0	230	0
(*Wish-Bone*)	110	0	15.0	6.0	0	350	0
salsa and sour cream (*Bernstein's* Dress-ing/Dip)	90	0	2.0	9.0	15	160	0
Santa Fe (*Wish-Bone*)	150	0	3.0	15.0	5	220	0
sesame garlic (*Nasoya* Vegi-Dressing*) . . .	60	0	3.0	5.0	0	125	0
Sierra (*Wish-Bone*)	150	0	2.0	16.0	0	260	0

Food and Measure	cal.	prot. (gms)	carbo. (gms)	fat (gms)	chol. (mgs)	sod. (mgs)	fiber (gms)
Salad dressing *(cont.)*							
sour cream and dill							
(*Marie's*)	190	1.0	3.0	20.0	15	160	0
sweet and sour:							
(*Herb Magic*) . . .	35	0	9.0	0	0	240	0
(*Old Dutch*)	50	0	13.0	0	0	480	0
Thousand Island:							
(*Bernstein's* Dress-							
ing/Dip)	120	0	4.0	11.0	15	180	0
(*Herb Magic*) . . .	15	0	4.0	0	0	170	0
(*Kraft*)	110	0	5.0	10.0	10	310	0
(*Kraft Deliciously*							
Right)	70	0	8.0	4.0	5	320	0
(*Kraft Free*)	45	0	11.0	0	0	300	1.0
(*Marie's*)	240	0	7.0	23.0	20	320	0
(*Marie's* Salad Bar)	170	0	6.0	16.0	10	250	<1.0
(*Nalley*)	120	0	4.0	11.0	15	180	0
(*Nasoya Vegi-Dress-*							
ing)	60	0	6.0	4.0	0	140	0
(*Salad Celebrations*)	45	0	8.0	1.5	10	190	0
(*Wish-Bone*)	130	0	7.0	12.0	10	340	0
(*Wish-Bone* Free)	35	0	8.0	0	0	290	0
(*Wish-Bone* Lite)	80	0	7.0	5.0	10	250	0
w/bacon (*Kraft*) . .	120	0	5.0	12.0	0	190	0
tomato, sun-dried,							
vinaigrette (*Knotts*							
Berry Farm)	100	<1.0	3.0	9.0	0	230	0
tuna salad (*Best*							
Foods/Hellmann's							
One Step)	140	0	4.0	14.0	5	270	0
vinaigrette (see also							
specific listings)							
(*Herb Magic*) . . .	10	0	3.0	0	0	270	0
white wine vinaigrette,							
zesty (*Marie's* Free)	40	0	10.0	0	0	310	0
white wine vinegar w/							
herbs (*S&W* Vintage							
Lite)	40	0	10.0	0	0	450	0

Food and Measure	cal.	prot. (gms)	carbo. (gms)	fat (gms)	chol. (mgs)	sod. (mgs)	fiber (gms)
Salad dressing mix, 2 tbsp.*, except as noted:							
buttermilk:							
(*Tone's*), ½ tsp. . . .	5	0	1.0	0	0	200	0
farm (*Good Seasons*)	120	1.0	2.0	12.0	10	260	0
Caesar, gourmet (*Good Seasons*) . .	150	0	3.0	16.0	0	300	0
cheese garlic (*Good Seasons*)	140	0	1.0	16.0	0	330	0
garlic and herbs (*Good Seasons*) . .	140	0	1.0	15.0	0	340	0
herb, zesty (*Good Seasons* Free) . . .	10	0	2.0	0	0	260	0
honey mustard:							
(*Good Seasons*) . .	150	0	3.0	15.0	0	240	0
(*Good Seasons* Free)	20	0	5.0	0	0	280	0
Italian:							
(*Good Seasons*) . .	140	0	1.0	15.0	0	320	0
(*Good Seasons* Free)	10	0	3.0	0	0	290	0
(*Good Seasons* Reduced Calorie) . .	50	0	2.0	5.0	0	280	0
creamy (*Good Seasons* Free)	20	<1.0	3.0	0	0	280	0
mild (*Good Seasons*)	150	0	2.0	15.0	0	370	0
zesty (*Good Seasons*)	140	0	1.0	15.0	0	220	0
zesty (*Good Seasons* Reduced Calorie)	50	0	2.0	5.0	0	260	0
Mexican spice (*Good Seasons*)	140	0	2.0	15.0	0	310	0
Oriental sesame (*Good Seasons*) . .	150	0	3.0	15.0	0	310	0

Food and Measure	cal.	prot. (gms)	carbo. (gms)	fat (gms)	chol. (mgs)	sod. (mgs)	fiber (gms)
Salad dressing mix *(cont.)*							
ranch:							
(*Good Seasons*) . .	120	1.0	2.0	12.0	10	220	0
(*Good Seasons* Reduced Calorie) . .	60	1.0	3.0	5.0	0	240	0
Salad seasoning (*McCormick*), ½ tsp.	0	0	0	0	0	100	0
Salad toppers (see also "Croutons"), 1 tbsp.:							
bacon cheddar or Caesar mix (*Pepperidge Farm*)	35	1.0	4.0	2.0	0	85	0
cinnamon raisin (*Pepperidge Farm*) . . .	35	1.0	4.0	2.0	0	15	0
garlic Italian (*Pepperidge Farm*)	35	1.0	4.0	1.5	0	70	0
Salami, 2 oz., except as noted:							
beef:							
(*Boar's Head* Chub)	120	10.0	0	9.0	25	470	0
(*Hebrew National*)	170	8.0	0	14.0	40	420	0
(*Hebrew National* Lean)	90	9.0	1.0	6.0	30	340	0
(*Hebrew National* Reduced Fat) . .	110	8.0	0	8.0	30	380	0
(*Oscar Mayer* Machiach), 2 slices, 1.6 oz.	120	6.0	1.0	10.0	30	510	0
beer (*Oscar Mayer*), 2 slices, 1.6 oz. . .	110	6.0	1.0	9.0	30	580	0
cooked (*Boar's Head*)	130	8.0	0	11.0	40	550	0
cotto, 2 slices, 1.6 oz.:							
(*Oscar Mayer*) . . .	110	6.0	0	9.0	35	500	0
beef (*Oscar Mayer*)	90	6.0	1.0	7.0	35	590	0
dry or hard, 1 oz.:							
(*Boar's Head*) . . .	110	6.0	<1.0	9.0	25	490	0
(*Hormel Homeland/ Sandwich Maker*)	110	5.0	0	10.0	35	450	0

Food and Measure	cal.	prot. (gms)	carbo. (gms)	fat (gms)	chol. (mgs)	sod. (mgs)	fiber (gms)
(*Oscar Mayer*),							
3 slices	100	6.0	0	9.0	25	510	0
Genoa:							
(*Boar's Head*) . . .	180	12.0	1.0	14.0	55	970	0
(*Di Lusso*), 1 oz.	120	6.0	0	8.0	25	500	0
(*Hormel Pillow*							
Pack), 1 oz. . . .	120	5.0	1.0	10.0	25	510	0
(*Hormel Sandwich*							
Maker), 1 oz. . .	120	5.0	0	11.0	35	430	0
(*Oscar Mayer*), 1 oz.	100	5.0	0	9.0	25	490	0
(*San Remo Brand*),							
1 oz.	120	6.0	0	9.0	30	470	0
"Salami," vegetar-							
ian, frozen:							
roll (*Worthington*),							
3 slices	130	12.0	2.0	8.0	0	930	2.0
sliced (*Worthington*),							
⅜″ slice	120	12.0	2.0	8.0	0	900	2.0
Salisbury steak, see							
"Beef dinner" and							
"Beef entree"							
Salmon, fresh, meat							
only, 4 oz.:							
Atlantic, farmed:							
raw	207	22.6	0	12.3	67	66	0
baked, broiled, or							
microwaved . . .	234	25.0	0	14.0	71	69	0
Atlantic, wild:							
raw	161	22.5	0	7.2	62	50	0
baked, broiled, or							
microwaved . . .	206	28.8	0	9.2	81	64	0
Chinook:							
raw	204	22.8	0	11.9	75	53	0
baked, broiled, or							
microwaved . . .	262	29.2	0	15.2	96	68	0
chum:							
raw	136	22.8	0	4.3	84	112	0
baked, broiled, or							
microwaved . . .	175	29.3	0	5.5	108	73	0

Food and Measure	cal.	prot. (gms)	carbo. (gms)	fat (gms)	chol. (mgs)	sod. (mgs)	fiber (gms)
Salmon *(cont.)*							
coho, farmed:							
raw	182	24.1	0	8.7	58	53	0
baked, broiled, or							
microwaved . . .	202	27.6	0	9.3	71	59	0
coho, wild:							
raw	165	25.0	0	6.7	51	53	0
baked, broiled, or							
microwaved . . .	158	26.6	0	4.9	62	66	0
boiled, poached, or							
steamed	209	31.0	0	8.5	65	60	0
pink:							
raw	132	22.6	0	3.9	59	76	0
baked, broiled, or							
microwaved . . .	169	29.0	0	5.0	76	98	0
sockeye:							
raw	191	24.2	0	9.7	70	53	0
baked, broiled, or							
microwaved . . .	245	31.0	0	12.4	99	75	0
smoked, see "Salmon,							
smoked"							
Salmon, canned:							
chum:							
drained, 4 oz. . . .	160	24.3	0	6.2	44	552	0
(*Peter Pan*), ¼ cup	90	13.0	0	4.0	40	270	0
coho (*Peter Pan*),							
¼ cup	90	12.0	0	5.0	40	270	0
king (*Peter Pan*),							
¼ cup	140	12.0	0	10.0	40	270	0
Norwegian fillet							
(*Abelvaer*), 3 oz. . .	170	16.0	0	12.0	42	460	0
pink, skinless fillet:							
(*Bumble Bee*),							
¼ cup	70	14.0	0	2.0	40	220	0
(*Chicken of the*							
Sea), 2 oz.	60	10.0	0	2.0	20	280	0
(*Libby's*), ¼ cup . .	90	12.0	0	5.0	40	270	0
(*Libby's*), ⅓ cup . .	70	14.0	0	2.0	40	190	0
(*Peter Pan*), ¼ cup	90	12.0	0	5.0	40	270	0

Food and Measure	cal.	prot. (gms)	carbo. (gms)	fat (gms)	chol. (mgs)	sod. (mgs)	fiber (gms)
red:							
(*Libby's*), ¼ cup . .	110	13.0	0	7.0	40	270	0
(*Peter Pan*), ¼ cup	110	13.0	0	7.0	40	270	0
blueback (*Rubin-*							
stein's), ¼ cup	110	13.0	0	7.0	40	270	0
red, sockeye:							
(*S&W*), 3¾-oz. can	190	22.0	0	11.0	70	460	0
(*S&W*), ¼ cup . .	110	13.0	0	7.0	40	270	0
Salmon, frozen,							
4 oz.:							
chum, fillet or steak							
(*Peter Pan*)	130	23.0	0	4.0	85	55	0
coho, fillet (*Peter*							
Pan)	160	24.0	0	7.0	45	50	0
Salmon, refrigerated,							
boneless, skinless:							
burger (*Salmon Chef*),							
3-oz. burger	80	17.0	0	.5	10	65	0
cuts, 5-oz. pc.:							
(*Salmon Chef*) . . .	110	29.0	0	1.0	20	85	0
dill-sorrel-chive							
marinade (*Salmon*							
Chef)	140	27.0	1.0	5.0	20	115	0
kabob, 3.3 oz.:							
(*Salmon Chef*) . . .	100	18.0	4.0	.5	10	250	0
in teriyaki sesame							
marinade (*Salmon*							
Chef)	110	29.0	0	1.0	20	85	0
loin, 2 pcs., 4 oz.:							
(*Salmon Chef*) . . .	110	23.0	0	.5	15	70	0
in chili-cilantro mar-							
inade (*Salmon*							
Chef)	130	22.0	0	4.0	15	90	0
tenderloin, 6-oz. pc.:							
(*Salmon Chef*) . . .	110	33.0	0	1.0	25	100	0
sweet pepper–sage							
marinade (*Salmon*							
Chef)	160	33.0	1.0	6.0	25	120	0

Food and Measure	cal.	prot. (gms)	carbo. (gms)	fat (gms)	chol. (mgs)	sod. (mgs)	fiber (gms)
Salmon, smoked:							
Chinook:							
4 oz.	133	20.7	0	4.9	26	889	0
lox, 4 oz.	133	20.7	0	4.9	26	2268	0
lox:							
(*Vita*), 2 oz.	50	11.0	<1.0	1.0	20	800	0
(*Vita*), 3-oz. pkg.	80	16.0	1.0	1.5	35	1200	0
Nova, natural:							
(*Vita*), 2 oz.	50	11.0	<1.0	1.0	20	650	0
(*Vita*), 3-oz. pkg.	80	16.0	1.0	1.5	35	960	0
Nova, w/color:							
(*Vita*), 2 oz.	50	11.0	<1.0	1.0	20	580	0
(*Vita*), 3-oz. pkg.	80	16.0	1.0	1.5	35	870	0
Salmon, smoked, spread:							
(*Vita*), ¼ cup, 2 oz.	180	5.0	29.0	5.0	30	430	0
cream cheese (*Vita*), ¼ cup, 2 oz.	180	4.0	2.0	17.0	50	220	0
Salsa, 2 tbsp., except as noted:							
(*Del Monte* Mexicana)	5	0	2.0	0	0	200	1.0
(*Del Monte* Taquera)	5	0	2.0	0	0	220	1.0
(*Goya*)	10	1.0	2.0	0	0	150	0
(*Kaukauna* Extra Chunky)	14	<1.0	3.0	<1.0	0	170	0
(*La Victoria* Ranchera)	10	0	2.0	0	0	170	0
(*La Victoria* Victoria)	5	0	1.0	0	0	160	0
(*Marie's* Tomato) . .	10	0	2.0	0	0	250	0
(*Pace* Thick & Chunky)	10	.5	2.0	0	0	212	0
all varieties:							
(*Del Monte* Traditional/Thick & Chunky/Fire Roasted)	10	0	2.0	0	0	210	0
(*Hunt's* Alfresco Homestyle) . . .	10	0	2.0	0	0	200	0
(*Hunt's* Homestyle)	30	1.0	6.0	0	0	235	1.0

Food and Measure	cal.	prot. (gms)	carbo. (gms)	fat (gms)	chol. (mgs)	sod. (mgs)	fiber (gms)
(*Old El Paso* Chunky)	15	1.0	3.0	0	0	230	1.0
(*Old El Paso* Home-style)	5	0	1.0	0	0	110	0
(*Progresso*)	10	0	2.0	0	0	170	<1.0
(*Tostitos*)	15	<1.0	3.0	0	0	230	1.0
cheese, see "Cheese dip" w/chipolte or cilantro (*S&W* Ready-Cut), ¼ cup	20	<1.0	4.0	0	0	190	<1.0
garlic:							
(*Del Monte*)	10	0	2.0	0	0	210	0
roasted (*Marie's*)	10	0	2.0	0	0	230	0
green:							
(*Goya*)	10	0	2.0	0	0	240	0
(*La Victoria* Jalapeña)	10	0	1.0	0	0	180	<1.0
green chili:							
(*La Victoria*)	10	0	1.0	0	0	170	0
medium (*Old El Paso*)	10	0	2.0	0	0	110	<1.0
hot:							
(*Chi-Chi's*)	10	0	1.0	0	0	160	0
(*Guiltless Gourmet*)	10	0	2.0	0	0	140	0
(*La Victoria* Thick N Chunky)	10	0	1.0	0	0	135	0
(*Las Palmas* Mexi-cana)	10	0	2.0	0	0	75	0
(*Old El Paso* Thick 'n Chunky)	10	0	2.0	0	0	130	0
(*Sun-Vista*)	5	0	2.0	0	0	170	<1.0
or mild (*Heluva* Good Thick & Chunky)	10	1.0	2.0	0	0	180	0
medium:							
(*Chi-Chi's*)	10	0	1.0	0	0	140	0
(*La Victoria* Suprema)	5	0	1.0	0	0	180	0

Food and Measure	cal.	prot. (gms)	carbo. (gms)	fat (gms)	chol. (mgs)	sod. (mgs)	fiber (gms)
Salsa, medium *(cont.)*							
(*Las Palmas* Mexi-cana)	10	0	2.0	0	0	85	0
(*Porino's*)	10	0	2.0	0	0	125	1.0
(*Rosarita*)	10	0	2.0	0	0	245	<1.0
(*Rosarita* Extra Chunky)	10	0	1.0	0	0	230	<1.0
or mild (*La Victoria* Thick N Chunky)	10	0	1.0	0	0	160	0
or mild (*Old El Paso* Thick 'n Chunky)	10	0	2.0	0	0	140	0
or mild (*S&W* Ready-Cut), ¼ cup	20	1.0	4.0	0	0	190	1.0
mild:							
(*Chi-Chi's*)	10	0	1.0	0	0	150	0
(*La Victoria* Suprema)	10	0	2.0	0	0	180	0
(*Las Palmas* Mexi-cana)	10	0	1.0	0	0	90	0
(*Rosarita* Tradi-tional)	10	0	<1.0	0	0	235	<1.0
(*Sun-Vista*)	5	0	0	0	0	210	0
picante (see also "Pi-cante sauce"):							
(*Old Dutch*)	10	0	2.0	0	0	200	0
(*Old El Paso*) . . .	10	0	2.0	0	0	230	0
medium (*La Victoria* Suprema)	10	0	1.0	0	0	150	0
mild (*La Victoria* Suprema)	10	0	1.0	0	0	180	0
pico de gallo:							
(*Chi-Chi's*)	10	0	2.0	0	0	170	0
(*Old El Paso*) . . .	5	0	2.0	0	0	260	<1.0
red (*La Victoria* Jalapeña)	10	0	2.0	0	0	150	1.0
roasted (*Rosarita*) . .	10	0	2.0	0	0	190	<1.0
taco, see "Taco sauce"							

Food and Measure	cal.	prot. (gms)	carbo. (gms)	fat (gms)	chol. (mgs)	sod. (mgs)	fiber (gms)
tomatillo, green							
(*Rosarita*)	10	0	2.0	0	0	235	<1.0
verde:							
(*Del Monte*)	10	0	2.0	0	0	280	<1.0
(*Old El Paso*) . . .	10	0	2.0	0	0	95	0
medium or mild							
(*Chi-Chi's*)	15	0	3.0	0	0	180	0
Salsa seasoning							
(*Lawry's*), ½ tsp.	5	0	1.0	0	0	90	0
Salsify:							
raw, untrimmed, 1 lb.	325	13.0	73.4	.8	0	79	13.0
raw, sliced, ½ cup	55	2.2	12.5	.1	0	13	2.2
boiled, drained, sliced,							
½ cup	46	1.9	10.5	.1	0	11	2.1
Salt (see also specific							
listings), ¼ tsp.:							
(*McCormick Season-*							
All)	0	0	0	0	0	340	0
(*Morton Lite*)	0	0	0	0	0	290	0
iodized or noniodized							
(*Morton*)	0	0	0	0	0	590	0
kosher (*Morton*) . . .	0	0	0	0	0	450	0
seasoned:							
(*House of Tsang*							
Hong King) . . .	0	0	0	0	0	170	0
(*Lawry's*)	0	0	0	0	0	380	0
(*Morton*)	0	0	0	0	0	325	0
(*Morton Nature's*							
Seasons)	<1	0	0	0	0	350	0
red pepper							
(*Lawry's*)	0	0	0	0	0	330	0
Salt, substitute:							
(*Morton*), ¼ tsp. . .	0	0	0	0	0	610	0
seasoned:							
(*Lawry's* Salt Free),							
¼ tsp.	0	0	0	0	0	0	0
(*Morton*), 1 tsp. . . .	2	0	.5	0	0	<1	0
Salt pork, raw, 1 oz.	212	1.4	0	22.8	25	404	0

Food and Measure	cal.	prot. (gms)	carbo. (gms)	fat (gms)	chol. (mgs)	sod. (mgs)	fiber (gms)
Sandwich, see specific listings							
Sandwich dressing (*Vlasic Sandwich Zesters*), 2 tbsp.:							
bell pepper salsa . .	15	0	4.0	0	0	210	0
garden onion	15	0	4.0	0	0	250	0
Italian tomato	10	0	3.0	0	0	240	0
jalapeño salsa	15	0	4.0	0	0	230	0
mushroom and onion	10	0	3.0	0	0	170	0
Sandwich sauce, ¼ cup, except as noted:							
(*Durkee Famous*), 1 tbsp.	60	.5	2.0	6.0	15	330	0
(*Manwich* Original)	30	1.0	6.0	.5	0	365	1.0
(*Manwich* Bold) . . .	60	.5	13.0	1.0	0	800	1.0
(*Manwich* Thick & Chunky)	45	1.5	8.5	.5	0	735	1.0
barbecue (*Manwich*)	60	1.0	14.0	0	0	890	1.0
Mexican (*Manwich*)	25	1.0	5.0	0	0	550	1.0
Sloppy Joe:							
(*Del Monte* Original)	50	1.0	11.0	0	0	620	0
(*Green Giant*) . . .	50	2.0	11.0	0	0	420	2.0
(*Heinz*), ½ cup . .	70	3.0	14.0	.5	0	770	2.0
(*Hormel Not-So-Sloppy Joe Sauce*)	70	1.0	15.0	0	0	720	1.0
(*Libby's*), ⅓ cup . .	45	1.0	10.0	0	0	430	1.0
hickory flavor (*Del Monte*)	60	1.0	14.0	0	0	660	0
w/meat (*Green Giant*)	200	14.0	11.0	11.0	15	470	2.0
taco, see "Taco sauce"							
Sandwich sauce seasoning mix, Sloppy Joe (*Lawry's*), 1 tsp.	15	<1.0	3.0	0	0	370	0

Food and Measure	cal.	prot. (gms)	carbo. (gms)	fat (gms)	chol. (mgs)	sod. (mgs)	fiber (gms)
Sandwich spread (see also "Sandwich sauce" and specific listings):							
(*Blue Plate*), 1 tbsp.	75	0	3.0	7.0	5	105	0
(*Hellmann's*), 1 tbsp.	50	0	3.0	5.0	<5	170	0
(*Kraft* Spread & Burger Sauce), 1 tbsp.	50	0	3.0	5.0	<5	100	0
(*Loma Linda*), ¼ cup	80	4.0	7.0	4.5	0	260	3.0
Sapodilla:							
1 medium, 3″ × 2½″	140	.7	33.9	1.9	0	20	9.0
½ cup	100	.5	24.1	1.3	0	15	6.4
Sapote:							
1 medium, 11.2 oz.	301	4.8	76.0	1.4	0	21	5.9
trimmed, 1 oz.	38	.6	9.6	.2	0	3	.7
white (*Frieda's*), 1 oz.	35	.5	9.0	.2	0	n.a.	n.a.
Sardine, fresh, see "Herring"							
Sardine, canned:							
Atlantic, in oil:							
drained, 2 oz. . . .	118	14.8	0	6.5	81	286	0
2 medium, 3″ long	50	5.9	0	2.8	34	121	0
in lemon (*Goya*), ¼ cup	120	10.0	0	9.0	20	300	0
in mustard sauce (*Underwood*), 3¾-oz. can	180	17.0	2.0	12.0	105	820	1.0
in olive oil, drained:							
(*Goya*), ¼ cup . . .	130	13.0	0	9.0	20	20	0
Norway brisling, (*S&W*), 3¾-oz. can	160	10.0	0	13.0	60	190	0
skinless, boneless (*Granadaisa*), ¼ cup	120	13.0	0	7.0	24	280	0
skinless, boneless (*S&W*), 3¾-oz. can	100	12.0	0	6.0	20	250	0

Food and Measure	cal.	prot. (gms)	carbo. (gms)	fat (gms)	chol. (mgs)	sod. (mgs)	fiber (gms)
Sardine, canned *(cont.)*							
small *(Goya*							
Sardinilla), ¼ cup	120	11.0	0	9.0	20	300	0
in soy oil, drained:							
skinless, boneless							
(King Oscar),							
3 pcs.	120	13.0	0	7.0	20	350	0
(Underwood), 3 oz.	220	18.0	1.0	16.0	100	310	0
spiced *(Goya)*, ¼ cup	120	12.0	0	9.0	20	280	0
in tomato sauce:							
(Goya), ¼ cup . . .	130	12.0	1.0	9.0	20	300	0
(Goya Oval), ¼ cup	80	10.0	1.0	4.0	36	170	1.0
(Goya Tinapa),							
2 pcs.	50	8.0	2.0	.5	45	15	2.0
(Del Monte), 2 oz.,							
½ fish, w/sauce	80	10.0	1.0	4.0	35	170	<1.0
(Underwood),							
3¾ oz.	180	16.0	4.0	11.0	115	960	1.0
Pacific, 2 oz.	101	9.3	n.a.	6.8	35	235	<1.0
Sauce, see specific							
listings							
Sauerkraut, 2 tbsp.,							
except as noted:							
(Boar's Head)	5	0	1.0	0	0	180	1.0
(Claussen), ¼ cup . .	5	0	1.0	0	0	210	1.0
(Del Monte)	0	0	<1.0	0	0	150	<1.0
(Eden Organic),							
½ cup	25	2.0	4.0	0	0	580	3.0
(Frank's/Snowfloss)	5	<1.0	1.0	0	0	180	<1.0
(Hebrew National) . .	5	0	1.0	0	0	180	1.0
(Hebrew National),							
½ cup	25	0	4.0	0	0	800	0
(Hebrew National/							
Shorr's New),							
½ cup	50	1.0	11.0	1.0	0	550	0
(Pickle Eater's Kozmic							
Kraut)	0	0	1.0	0	0	180	0
(Pickle Eater's Re-							
duced Sodium) . .	0	0	.6	0	0	134	0

Food and Measure	cal.	prot. (gms)	carbo. (gms)	fat (gms)	chol. (mgs)	sod. (mgs)	fiber (gms)
(*Rosoff* Home Style),							
½ cup	50	1.0	11.0	1.0	0	550	0
(*S&W* 14 oz.)	5	0	2.0	0	0	180	0
(*S&W* 22 oz.)	5	0	2.0	0	0	220	0
(*Stokely*)	5	0	1.0	0	0	190	1.0
(*Stokely*), ½ cup . . .	25	0	5.0	0	0	740	3.0
Bavarian style:							
(*Del Monte*)	15	0	4.0	0	0	120	0
(*Frank's/Snowfloss*)	15	<1.0	3.0	0	0	170	<1.0
(*Stokely*)	10	0	2.0	0	0	220	1.0
(*Stokely*), ½ cup . .	35	1.0	7.0	0	0	860	3.0
sweet and sour:							
(*Stokely*)	20	0	5.0	0	0	210	1.0
(*Stokely*), ½ cup . .	80	0	18.0	0	0	850	3.0
Sauerkraut juice:							
(*S&W*), 10-oz. can	35	2.0	7.0	0	0	1950	0
(*Stokely*), 8 fl. oz. . .	20	1.0	4.0	0	0	1720	0
Sausage (see also specific listings), cooked, 2 links, except as noted:							
(*Hormel Special Recipe*), 1 link	111	3.0	0	11.0	18	180	0
(*Hormel Special Recipe*), 1 patty	178	5.0	0	17.0	29	255	0
beef:							
(*Jones Dairy Farm* Golden Brown)	170	7.0	1.0	15.0	40	410	0
roll (*Jones Dairy Farm* All Natural), 2 oz.	170	12.0	0	13.0	55	510	0
smoked (*Oscar Mayer* Smokies), 1 link	120	5.0	1.0	1.0	30	420	0
brown and serve:							
(*Little Sizzlers*), 3 links	230	8.0	1.0	22.0	45	670	0
(*Little Sizzlers*), 2 patties	190	7.0	1.0	18.0	40	560	0

Food and Measure	cal.	prot. (gms)	carbo. (gms)	fat (gms)	chol. (mgs)	sod. (mgs)	fiber (gms)
Sausage, brown and serve *(cont.)*							
beef, smoked (*Jones Dairy Farm*)	180	6.0	1.0	17.0	35	360	0
light (*Jones Dairy Farm*)	110	7.0	1.0	9.0	30	280	0
pork (*Jones Dairy Farm*)	190	5.0	1.0	18.0	35	280	0
pork and bacon (*Jones Dairy Farm*)	180	6.0	1.0	17.0	35	420	0
cheese, smoked: (*Oscar Mayer* Smokies), 1 link . . .	130	6.0	1.0	12.0	30	450	0
(*Oscar Mayer* Little Smokies), 6 links	180	7.0	1.0	16.0	35	600	0
dinner, 1 link or patty: (*Jones Dairy Farm*)	210	9.0	1.0	19.0	40	439	0
(*Jones Dairy Farm All Natural*) . . .	130	6.0	1.0	14.0	35	310	0
Italian (*Jones Dairy Farm*)	140	10.0	1.0	16.0	40	410	0
sandwich patty (*Jones Dairy Farm*)	140	5.0	1.0	16.0	30	260	0
Italian, pork, 1 oz. . . .	92	5.7	.4	7.3	22	261	0
pickled, smoked or hot (*Hormel*), 6 links	140	8.0	1.0	11.0	40	380	0
pork: fresh, .5 oz. (1 oz. raw link)	48	2.6	.1	4.1	11	168	0
(*Jones Dairy Farm All Natural Light*)	130	8.0	1.0	11.0	20	420	0
(*Jones Dairy Farm All Natural Little Links*), 3 links . .	190	8.0	1.0	17.0	45	420	0
(*Little Sizzlers*), 3 links	180	8.0	0	20.0	45	570	0

Food and Measure	cal.	prot. (gms)	carbo. (gms)	fat (gms)	chol. (mgs)	sod. (mgs)	fiber (gms)
(*Oscar Mayer*) . . .	170	9.0	1.0	15.0	40	410	0
hot and spicy (*Little Sizzlers*), 3 links	180	8.0	0	20.0	45	570	0
light (*Jones Dairy Farm* Golden Brown)	110	7.0	1.0	9.0	30	230	0
maple (*Jones Dairy Farm* Golden Brown)	190	5.0	1.0	18.0	35	260	0
mild or milk (*Jones Dairy Farm* Golden Brown)	190	6.0	1.0	18.0	35	300	0
spicy (*Jones Dairy Farm* Golden Brown)	190	6.0	1.0	18.0	35	300	0
pork, patty: (*Jones Dairy Farm* All Natural), 1 patty	130	5.0	0	12.0	30	250	0
(*Jones Dairy Farm* Golden Brown), 1 patty	150	5.0	1.0	14.0	30	240	0
(*Little Sizzlers*), 2 patties	210	10.0	0	23.0	50	680	0
pork roll, regular or hot (*Jones Dairy Farm* All Natural), 2 oz.	230	9.0	1.0	21.0	50	430	0
smoked: (*Boar's Head*), 4.5 oz.	400	17.0	2.0	36.0	75	1050	0
(*John Morrell* Bun Size), 1 link . . .	270	10.0	4.0	23.0	80	1100	0
(*John Morrell* Bun Size Less Fat), 1 link	180	10.0	9.0	12.0	75	1180	0
(*Light & Lean 97* Dinner Link), 1 link	60	8.0	2.0	2.0	20	640	0

Food and Measure	cal.	prot. (gms)	carbo. (gms)	fat (gms)	chol. (mgs)	sod. (mgs)	fiber (gms)
Sausage, smoked *(cont.)*							
(*Oscar Mayer* Little Smokies), 6 links	170	7.0	1.0	16.0	35	580	0
(*Oscar Mayer* Smokie Links), 1 link	130	5.0	1.0	12.0	25	430	0
hot (*Boar's Head*), 3.2 oz.	280	12.0	1.0	25.0	55	740	0
Sausage, canned (*Diana* Salchichas), 3 links	130	5.0	1.0	12.0	55	340	0
"Sausage," vegetarian:							
.9-oz. link	64	4.6	2.5	4.5	0	222	.7
1.3-oz. patty	97	7.0	3.7	6.9	0	337	1.1
canned:							
(*Loma Linda* Little Links), 2 links . .	90	8.0	2.0	6.0	0	230	2.0
(*Worthington* Saucettes*), 1 link	90	6.0	1.0	6.0	0	200	1.0
frozen:							
(*Green Giant* Breakfast), 3 links . . .	110	12.0	5.0	5.0	0	340	4.0
(*Green Giant* Breakfast), 2 patties . .	100	10.0	5.0	4.0	0	280	3.0
(*Morningstar Farms* Breakfast), 2 links	60	8.0	2.0	2.5	0	340	2.0
(*Morningstar Farms* Breakfast), 1 patty	70	8.0	2.0	3.0	0	270	2.0
(*Worthington* Prosage Links), 2 links	60	8.0	2.0	2.5	0	340	2.0
(*Worthington* Prosage Patties), 1 patty	100	9.0	3.0	3.0	0	300	2.0
ground (*Worthington* Vegetarian), ½ cup	110	11.0	3.0	6.0	0	330	3.0

Food and Measure	cal.	prot. (gms)	carbo. (gms)	fat (gms)	chol. (mgs)	sod. (mgs)	fiber (gms)
roll (*Worthington Prosage*), ⅝" slice	140	10.0	2.0	10.0	0	390	0
mix* (*Fantastic Nature's Sausage*), 1 patty	65	6.0	7.0	1.5	0	240	2.0
Sausage biscuit, frozen, 1 pc.:							
(*Hormel Quick Meal*)	350	9.0	30.0	22.0	45	840	1.0
(*Weight Watchers*) . .	230	11.0	20.0	11.0	25	660	2.0
w/cheese (*Hormel Quick Meal*)	410	13.0	30.0	26.0	65	950	1.0
w/egg (*Hormel Quick Meal*)	390	12.0	31.0	24.0	120	830	1.0
w/egg, cheese (*Swanson Great Starts*)	490	46.0	36.0	30.0	145	1110	3.0
Sausage gravy mix (*Durkee/French's*), ¼ cup*	35	1.0	5.0	2.0	0	570	0
Sausage hash, canned (*Mary Kitchen*), 1 cup . .	410	21.0	29.0	23.0	75	1060	4.0
Sausage seasoning, pork (*Tone's*), 1 tsp.	12	.4	2.7	.3	0	1	.7
Sausage stick, 1 pc., except as noted:							
(*Tombstone* Snappy Sticks)	110	4.0	<1.0	10.0	20	260	0
beef:							
(*Boar's Head*), .6 oz.	100	3.0	2.0	9.0	20	240	0
(*Old Dutch*), 1 oz.	110	6.0	1.0	9.0	20	340	0
(*Rustlers Roundup* Jerky)	30	2.0	1.0	2.0	10	140	<1.0
(*Tombstone* Jerky)	35	6.0	<1.0	0	15	310	0
(*Tombstone* Stick)	110	3.0	0	10.0	20	270	0
hot (*Rustlers Roundup*)	40	2.0	1.0	3.0	10	140	<1.0

Food and Measure	cal.	prot. (gms)	carbo. (gms)	fat (gms)	chol. (mgs)	sod. (mgs)	fiber (gms)
Sausage stick *(cont.)*							
smoked:							
mild or spicy (*Slim Jim*), 1.4-oz. box	210	9.0	2.0	19.0	25	570	1.0
(*Rustlers Roundup Steak Stick*) . . .	60	8.0	1.0	2.0	20	580	0
spicy (*Rustlers Roundup*)	50	2.0	<1.0	4.0	10	140	<1.0
summer sausage (*Old Dutch*), 1 oz. . . .	110	7.0	0	10.0	20	370	0
Savory, ground:							
1 tsp.	4	.1	1.0	.1	0	<1	<1.0
(*McCormick*), ¼ tsp.	2	0	.4	0	0	<1	.2
summer (*Tone's*), 1 tsp.	4	.1	1.0	.1	0	1	<1.0
Scallion, see "Onion, green"							
Scallop, meat only:							
raw, 4 oz.	100	19.0	2.7	.9	38	183	0
raw, 2 large or 5 small, 1.1 oz. . . .	26	5.0	.7	.2	10	48	0
Scallop, fried, frozen, (*Mrs. Paul's*), 12 pcs.	200	12.0	20.0	8.0	10	360	1.0
"Scallop," vegetarian, from surimi, 4 oz.	112	14.5	12.1	.5	25	902	0
canned:							
(*Loma Linda Tender Bits*), 6 pcs.	110	11.0	7.0	4.5	0	440	3.0
(*Worthington Vegetable Skallops*), ½ cup	90	15	3.0	1.5	0	410	3.0
Scallop squash, ½ cup:							
raw, sliced	12	.8	2.5	.1	0	1	1.2
boiled, drained, sliced	14	.9	3.0	.2	0	1	1.1
boiled, drained, mashed	19	1.2	4.0	.2	0	1	1.4

Food and Measure	cal.	prot. (gms)	carbo. (gms)	fat (gms)	chol. (mgs)	sod. (mgs)	fiber (gms)
Scrapple (*Jones Dairy Farm*), 2 oz.	120	5.0	7.0	8.0	30	280	0
Scrod, fresh, see "Cod, Atlantic"							
Scup, meat only:							
raw, 4 oz.	119	21.4	0	3.1	n.a.	48	0
baked, broiled, or microwaved, 4 oz. . .	153	27.5	0	4.0	n.a.	61	0
Sea bass, meat only:							
raw, 4 oz.	110	20.9	0	2.3	47	77	0
baked, broiled, or microwaved, 4 oz. . .	141	26.8	0	2.9	60	99	0
Sea trout, meat only:							
raw, 4 oz.	118	19.0	0	4.1	94	66	0
baked, broiled, or microwaved, 4 oz. . .	151	24.3	0	5.3	120	84	0
Seafood, see specific listings							
Seafood sauce (see also specific listings), cocktail, ¼ cup, except as noted:							
(*Bookbinder's* Restaurant Style)	70	1.0	15.0	1.5	0	1000	1.0
(*Crosse & Blackwell*)	110	1.0	25.0	0	0	770	0
(*Del Monte*)	100	1.0	24.0	0	0	910	0
(*Heinz*)	60	1.0	14.0	0	0	680	1.0
(*Heluva Good*)	40	0	10.0	0	0	410	0
(*Maull's*), 2 tbsp. . .	45	0	10.0	0	0	280	0
(*Nalley*)	65	1.0	15.0	0	0	470	0
(*Sauceworks*)	60	1.0	13.0	.5	0	800	<1.0
(*S&W*), 1 tsp.	20	0	5.0	0	0	220	0
hot and spicy (*Bookbinder's*)	70	1.0	15.0	1.5	0	1040	1.0
Seafood seasoning, see "Fish seasoning and coating mix"							

Food and Measure	cal.	prot. (gms)	carbo. (gms)	fat (gms)	chol. (mgs)	sod. (mgs)	fiber (gms)
Seasoning (see also specific listings), ¼ tsp.:							
(*Ac'cent*), ⅛ tsp. . . .	0	0	0	0	0	160	0
(*Sa-son* con Ajo Cebolla)	0	0	0	0	0	140	0
(*Sa-son* con Azafran)	0	0	0	0	0	125	0
(*Sa-son* con Culantro)	0	0	0	0	0	170	0
(*Sa-son Ac'cent*) . .	0	0	0	0	0	150	0
Seasoning and coating mix (see also specific listings), ⅛ pkt.:							
country (*Shake'n Bake*)	35	0	5.0	2.0	0	240	0
glaze, honey mustard (*Shake'n Bake*) . .	45	0	9.0	1.0	0	290	0
glaze, tangy honey (*Shake'n Bake*) . .	45	0	10.0	1.0	0	280	0
Italian herb (*Shake'n Bake*)	40	1.0	7.0	.5	0	300	0
Seaweed:							
agar:							
raw, 1 oz.	7	.2	1.9	tr.	0	3	.1
dried, 1 oz.	87	1.8	22.9	.1	0	29	2.2
flakes or bar (*Eden*), 1 tbsp.	10	0	2.0	0	0	10	2.0
arame (*Eden*), ½ cup	30	1.0	7.0	0	0	120	7.0
hiziki (*Eden*), ½ cup	30	<1.0	6.0	0	0	160	6.0
Irish moss, raw, 1 oz.	14	.4	3.5	<.1	0	19	.4
kelp, raw, 1 oz. . . .	12	.5	2.7	.2	0	66	.4
kombu (*Eden*), ½ of 7″ pc.	10	0	2.0	0	0	90	1.0
laver, raw, 1 oz. . . .	10	1.6	1.4	.1	0	1	4.1
nori (*Eden*), 1 sheet	10	1.0	1.0	0	0	5	1.0
spirulina, 1 oz.:							
raw	8	1.7	.7	.1	0	28	n.a.
dried	82	16.3	6.8	2.2	0	297	1.0

Food and Measure	cal.	prot. (gms)	carbo. (gms)	fat (gms)	chol. (mgs)	sod. (mgs)	fiber (gms)
wakame:							
raw, 1 oz.	13	.9	2.6	.2	0	247	.1
(*Eden*), ½ cup . . .	25	2.0	4.0	0	0	660	4.0
flakes (*Eden*),							
½ cup	25	2.0	4.0	0	0	720	2.0
Seitan mix (*Arrow-*							
head Mills), ⅓ cup	150	21.0	14.0	1.0	0	20	2.0
Semolina, whole							
grain, 1 cup	602	21.2	121.6	1.8	0	2	6.5
Semolina flour, mix							
(*Arrowhead Mills*),							
½ cup	240	9.0	50.0	1.0	0	0	4.0
Sesame butter							
(*Roaster Fresh*),							
1 oz.	168	5.0	6.0	15.0	0	3	0
Sesame flour, 1 oz.:							
high fat	149	8.7	7.6	10.5	0	12	1.8
partially defatted . . .	109	11.5	10.0	3.4	0	12	1.7
low fat	95	14.2	10.1	.5	0	11	1.4
Sesame meal, par-							
tially defatted, 1 oz.	161	4.8	7.4	13.6	0	11	1.1
Sesame paste (see							
also "Tahini"), from							
whole seeds,							
1 tbsp.	95	2.9	4.1	8.1	0	2	.9
Sesame seasoning:							
(*Eden*), ½ tsp.	10	0	0	.5	0	40	<1.0
garlic or seaweed							
(*Eden*), ½ tsp. . . .	10	0	0	.5	0	35	<1.0
Sesame seeds:							
raw (*McCormick*),							
¼ tsp.	2	0	.4	0	0	<1	.2
whole:							
brown (*Arrowhead*							
Mills), ¼ cup . .	200	7.0	8.0	20.0	0	20	5.0
roasted, toasted,							
1 oz.	161	4.8	7.3	13.6	0	3	4.0

Food and Measure	cal.	prot. (gms)	carbo. (gms)	fat (gms)	chol. (mgs)	sod. (mgs)	fiber (gms)
Sesame seeds *(cont.)*							
kernels, decorticated:							
(*Arrowhead Mills*),							
¼ cup	210	7.0	5.0	20.0	0	0	5.0
dried, 1 tsp.	16	.7	.3	1.5	0	1	<1.0
toasted, 1 oz. . . .	161	4.8	7.4	13.6	0	11	4.8
Sesbania flower:							
raw, 1 cup	5	.3	1.4	<.1	0	3	n.a.
steamed, ½ cup . . .	11	.6	2.7	<.1	0	6	n.a.
Shad, meat only:							
raw, 4 oz.	223	19.2	0	15.6	n.a.	58	0
baked, broiled, or mi-							
crowaved, 4 oz. . .	286	24.6	0	20.0	n.a.	74	0
Shallot:							
fresh or stored:							
peeled, 1 oz.	20	.7	4.8	<.1	0	3	<1.0
chopped, 1 tbsp.	7	.3	1.7	<.1	0	1	<1.0
freeze-dried: 1 tbsp.	3	.1	.7	tr.	0	1	<1.0
(*McCormick*), ¼ tsp.	<1	0	.1	0	0	0	0
Shark, meat only,							
raw, 4 oz.	148	23.8	0	5.1	58	90	0
Sheepshead, meat							
only:							
raw, 4 oz.	123	22.9	0	2.7	n.a.	81	0
baked, broiled, or mi-							
crowaved, 4 oz. . .	143	29.5	0	1.8	n.a.	83	0
Shellie beans,							
canned:							
w/liquid, ½ cup . . .	37	2.1	7.6	.2	0	408	4.1
(*Stokely*), ½ cup . . .	45	2.0	8.0	0	0	400	3.0
Shells, pasta, mix,							
white cheddar (*Noo-*							
dle Roni), 1 cup*	390	12.0	48.0	17.0	15	1150	2.0
Shells, pasta,							
stuffed, w/out							
sauce, frozen:							
(*Celentano*), 4 shells	330	17.0	32.0	15.0	70	500	7.0
(*Celentano* Value							
Pack), 3 shells . . .	240	13.0	23.0	11.0	50	370	5.0

Food and Measure	cal.	prot. (gms)	carbo. (gms)	fat (gms)	chol. (mgs)	sod. (mgs)	fiber (gms)
Shells, pasta, stuffed, entree, frozen, 1 pkg., except as noted:							
(*Celentano*)	400	23.0	34.0	20.0	90	840	n.a.
(*Celentano*), ½ of 14-oz. pkg.	300	14.0	30.0	14.0	50	720	8.0
(*Celentano* Great Choice)	250	16.0	41.0	2.5	15	650	5.0
(*Celentano* Value Pack), 3 shells, 8 oz.	340	16.0	35.0	15.0	60	820	n.a.
broccoli (*Celentano* Great Choice) . . .	190	12.0	31.0	4.0	15	520	4.0
Florentine (*Celentano*)	240	14.0	32.0	6.0	0	630	5.0
marinara (*Healthy Choice*)	370	25.0	59.0	4.0	25	390	5.0
Sherbet (see also "Ice" and "Sorbet"), ½ cup, except as noted:							
orange:							
½ cup	132	1.1	29.2	1.9	5	44	<.5
(*Carnation* Cup), 3 fl. oz.	90	1.0	19.0	1.0	5	20	0
(*Carnation* Plastic), 5 fl. oz.	150	1.0	32.0	1.5	5	30	0
pink lemonade (*Edy's*)	130	1.0	27.0	1.5	4	30	0
strawberry kiwi (*Edy's*)	120	1.0	27.0	1.5	4	25	0
Swiss orange (*Edy's*)	150	1.5	30.0	3.0	5	50	0
tangerine (*Edy's*) . .	130	1.0	28.0	2.0	4	25	0
tropical (*Edy's*) . . .	130	1.0	27.0	2.0	4	25	0
Shortening, 1 tbsp.:							
lard or vegetable oil	115	0	0	12.8	n.a.	0	0
vegetable, regular/butter flavor (*Crisco*)	110	0	0	12.0	0	0	0
Shrimp, meat only:							
raw, 4 oz.	120	23.0	1.0	2.0	173	168	0

Food and Measure	cal.	prot. (gms)	carbo. (gms)	fat (gms)	chol. (mgs)	sod. (mgs)	fiber (gms)
Shrimp *(cont.)*							
raw, 4 large, 1 oz. . . .	30	5.7	.3	.5	43	42	0
boiled or steamed:							
4 oz.	112	23.7	n.a.	1.2	221	254	0
4 large	22	4.6	n.a.	.2	43	49	0
Shrimp, canned:							
drained, 1 cup	154	29.6	1.3	2.5	222	216	0
deveined, small/me-dium (*S&W*),							
¼ cup	45	10.0	0	0	115	650	0
all sizes (*Goya*), 2 oz.	44	10.0	0	0	113	650	0
"Shrimp," imitation:							
from surimi, 4 oz. . . .	115	14.1	10.4	1.7	41	800	0
frozen, jumbo (*Captain Jac Shrimp Tasties*), 3 pcs., 3 oz.	80	6.0	14.0	0	5	250	1.0
Shrimp cocktail:							
(*Sau-Sea*), 4-oz. jar	100	8.0	17.0	0	85	1010	3.0
(*Sau-Sea*), 6-oz. jar	150	11.0	26.0	0	120	1510	4.0
(*Vita*), 4-oz. jar . . .	110	8.0	20.0	0	85	710	3.0
Shrimp dinner, frozen, Mariner (*The Budget Gourmet Light & Healthy*), 11 oz.	260	12.0	39.0	6.0	60	540	5.0
Shrimp entree, canned, chow mein *La Choy* Bi-Pack), 1 cup	55	3.0	10.0	1.0	10	950	2.0
Shrimp entree, freeze-dried, 1½ cups:							
Alfredo (*AlpineAire*)	300	18.0	44.0	3.0	n.a.	641	n.a.
Newburg (*AlpineAire*)	318	16.0	49.0	6.0	n.a.	538	n.a.
Shrimp entree, frozen:							
beer batter (*Gorton's*), 6 pcs.	250	9.0	19.0	15.0	70	630	n.a.

Food and Measure	cal.	prot. (gms)	carbo. (gms)	fat (gms)	chol. (mgs)	sod. (mgs)	fiber (gms)
breaded:							
(*Gorton's*), 6 pcs.	230	10.0	18.0	13.0	80	550	n.a.
(*Mrs. Paul's*), 1 pkg.	350	25.0	32.0	16.0	95	720	2.0
(*Van de Kamp's*),							
7 pcs.	240	13.0	26.0	10.0	50	520	2.0
butterfly (*Van de*							
Kamp's), 7 pcs.	280	12.0	28.0	14.0	55	580	2.0
w/pasta (*Marie Cal-*							
lender's), 1 cup	300	11.0	27.0	12.0	30	470	3.0
scampi (*Gorton's*),							
6 pcs.	250	9.0	18.0	16.0	70	4210	n.a.
marinara, 1 pkg.:							
(*Healthy Choice*) . .	220	10.0	44.0	.5	50	220	5.0
(*Smart Ones*) . . .	200	8.0	37.0	2.0	40	590	4.0
popcorn, breaded:							
(*Gorton's*), 1 cup	260	9.0	21.0	16.0	60	600	n.a.
(*Van de Kamp's*),							
4 oz.	270	11.0	28.0	13.0	35	610	1.0
garlic and herb							
(*Gorton's*), 3.5 oz.	270	11.0	26.0	13.0	100	500	n.a.
and vegetables							
(*Healthy Choice*),							
12.5 oz.	270	15.0	46.0	3.0	35	540	5.0
Shrimp entree mix,							
creole (*Luzianne*),							
⅕ pkg.	150	3.0	34.0	.5	<5	810	<1.0
Shrimp sauce (*Crosse*							
& Blackwell), ¼ cup	110	1.0	25.0	0	0	790	0
Shrimp spice (*Tone's*							
Craboil), 1 tsp. . .	10	.3	1.2	.6	1	1	.3
Sizzler, 1 serving:							
hot entrees:							
hamburger on bun,							
w/lettuce, tomato	626	45.0	36.0	33.0	142	335	1.0
chicken breast,							
5 oz.:							
hibachi, w/pineapple	193	28.0	13.0	3.0	65	686	1.0
lemon-herb	140	27.0	0	3.0	65	380	0
Santa Fe	150	30.0	0	3.0	65	350	0

Food and Measure	cal.	prot. (gms)	carbo. (gms)	fat (gms)	chol. (mgs)	sod. (mgs)	fiber (gms)
***Sizzler,* hot entrees** *(cont.)*							
Malibu chicken patty	310	23.0	11.0	19.0	75	588	0
salmon, 8 oz. . . .	247	32.0	0	12.0	41	232	0
shrimp, broiled,							
5 oz.	150	23.0	0	6.0	218	377	0
shrimp, fried, 4 pcs.	223	18.0	35.0	2.0	118	706	2.0
shrimp, mini, 4 oz.	152	13.0	24.0	1.0	80	480	1.0
shrimp scampi,							
5 oz.	143	27.0	0	3.0	150	386	0
steak, Dakota							
Ranch:							
6 oz.	316	30.0	0	20.0	101	253	0
8 oz.	421	37.0	0	27.0	135	337	0
9.5 oz.	500	47.0	0	32.0	160	400	0
swordfish, 8 oz. . . .	315	45.0	0	14.0	89	331	0
side dishes:							
cheese toast	273	6.0	16.0	21.0	5	494	1.0
french fries, 4 oz.	358	5.0	45.0	12.0	0	245	4.0
potato, baked, pulp	105	2.0	24.0	0	0	6	2.0
rice pilaf, 6 oz. . .	256	4.0	47.0	5.0	0	866	1.0
sauces, 1½ oz.:							
buttery dipping . .	330	0	0	37.0	0	0	0
cocktail sauce . . .	40	0	8.0	0	0	396	0
hibachi sauce . . .	57	0	11.0	0	0	707	0
Malibu sauce . . .	283	0	0	31.0	28	354	0
sour dressing . . .	89	0	0	9.0	0	44	0
tartar sauce	170	0	6.0	17.0	5	453	0
hot bar:							
chicken wings, 1 oz.	73	4.0	4.0	4.0	20	135	0
focaccia bread,							
2 pcs.	108	2.0	9.0	7.0	1	134	0
marinara sauce,							
1 oz.	13	0	3.0	0	0	90	0
meatballs, 4	157	9.0	5.0	11.0	30	461	1.0
nacho sauce, 2 oz.	120	5.0	3.0	10.0	30	600	0
pasta, fettuccine,							
2 oz.	80	3.0	15.0	1.0	5	5	0
pasta, spaghetti,							
2 oz.	80	3.0	16.0	0	0	1	1.0

Food and Measure	cal.	prot. (gms)	carbo. (gms)	fat (gms)	chol. (mgs)	sod. (mgs)	fiber (gms)
potato skins, 2 oz.	160	2.0	22.0	8.0	0	463	3.0
refried beans,							
¼ cup	62	4.0	11.0	1.0	5	272	3.0
saltines, 2 pcs. . .	25	1.0	4.0	1.0	1	74	0
taco filling, 2 oz.	103	2.0	3.0	9.0	16	232	1.0
taco shells, 1 pc.	50	1.0	7.0	2.0	0	20	1.0
hot bar, soup, 4 oz.:							
broccoli cheese . .	139	3.0	10.0	9.0	8	355	0
chicken noodle soup	31	2.0	4.0	1.0	7	495	0
clam chowder . . .	118	3.0	11.0	6.0	6	511	0
minestrone soup . .	36	1.0	7.0	0	1	443	2.0
vegetable sirloin . .	60	6.0	6.0	2.0	10	364	0
salads, prepared,							
2 oz.:							
carrot and raisin . .	130	1.0	10.0	10.0	3	104	1.0
Chinese chicken . .	54	4.0	6.0	2.0	10	119	1.0
jicama, spicy	16	0	4.0	0	0	28	0
Mediterranean							
Minted Fruit . . .	29	1.0	7.0	0	0	11	0
Mexican Fiesta . . .	54	2.0	10.0	1.0	0	99	1.0
pasta, seafood Louis	64	3.0	9.0	2.0	17	139	1.0
potato, old-fash-							
ioned	84	1.0	10.0	5.0	3	231	1.0
potato, red herb . .	121	1.0	9.0	9.0	9	271	1.0
seafood Louis . . .	56	3.0	4.0	3.0	7	255	0
teriyaki beef	49	4.0	5.0	2.0	7	136	1.0
tuna pasta	133	6.0	6.0	10.0	10	188	0
dressings, 1 oz.:							
blue cheese	111	1.0	1.0	12.0	8	168	0
guacamole	42	0	2.0	4.0	0	425	0
honey mustard . .	160	0	4.0	16.0	10	110	0
Italian, lite	14	0	2.0	0	0	350	0
Parmesan, Italian	100	0	2.0	10.0	0	450	0
ranch	120	0	2.0	12.0	10	240	0
ranch, lite	90	0	4.0	8.0	10	270	0
rice vinegar, Japa-							
nese	10	0	2.0	0	0	172	0
salsa	7	0	2.0	0	0	156	0
sour dressing . . .	60	0	0	6.0	0	30	0

Food and Measure	cal.	prot. (gms)	carbo. (gms)	fat (gms)	chol. (mgs)	sod. (mgs)	fiber (gms)
Sizzler, dressings, 1 oz. *(cont.)*							
Thousand Island . .	143	0	3.0	15.0	11	125	0
Sloppy Joe entree,							
frozen (*Swanson*							
Fun Feast), 1 pkg.	290	15.0	41.0	10.0	70	530	3.0
Sloppy Joe sauce,							
see "Sandwich							
sauce"							
Smelt, rainbow, meat							
only:							
raw, 4 oz.	110	20.0	0	2.8	80	68	0
baked, broiled, or mi-							
crowaved, 4 oz. . .	141	25.6	0	3.5	102	87	0
Snack bar (see also							
"Cookie" and "Gra-							
nola and Cereal							
bar"), 1 bar:							
(*Little Debbie Star*							
Crunch)	280	2.0	44.0	11.0	0	150	1.0
blueberry:							
(*Little Debbie Fruit*							
Boosters)	190	2.0	41.0	3.0	0	110	1.0
(*Sweet Rewards*)	120	1.0	29.0	0	0	80	0
brownie:							
(*Sweet Rewards*)	90	2.0	22.0	0	0	90	1.0
(*Sweet Success*							
Chewy)	120	2.0	23.0	4.0	<5	35	3.0
chocolate chip (*Sweet*							
Success Chewy) . .	120	2.0	23.0	4.0	<5	40	3.0
chocolate raspberry or							
peanut butter							
(*Sweet Success*							
Chewy)	120	2.0	23.0	4.0	<5	35	3.0
fig (*Little Debbie*							
Figaroos)	180	2.0	45.0	0	0	160	2.0
strawberry:							
(*Little Debbie Fruit*							
Boosters)	190	2.0	42.0	3.0	0	130	1.0
(*Sweet Rewards*)	120	1.0	29.0	0	0	80	<+>"

Food and Measure	cal.	prot. (gms)	carbo. (gms)	fat (gms)	chol. (mgs)	sod. (mgs)	fiber (gms)
Snack chips and crisps (see also specific listings), 1 oz., except as noted:							
(*Zings* Chips), 1.8-oz. bag	240	3.0	34.0	11.0	0	420	2.0
apple cinnamon (*Crunchwells Crumpet Chips*)	110	4.0	21.0	1.0	0	230	n.a.
cheddar (*Old Dutch Multicrisps*)	130	2.1	20.0	4.6	1	179	1.0
hot and spicy (*Eden Wasabi*), 1.1 oz. . .	130	<1.0	24.0	4.0	0	260	0
mixed (*Terra* Chips)	140	1.0	18.0	7.0	0	70	2.0
onion:							
(*Funyons*)	140	2.0	18.0	7.0	0	250	<1.0
French (*Old Dutch Multicrisps*) . . .	128	2.1	21.0	4.0	1	190	1.2
Parmesan garlic (*Crunchwells Crumpet Chips*)	100	4.0	20.0	1.0	0	310	n.a.
raspberry (*Crunchwells Crumpet Chips*)	110	4.0	21.0	1.0	0	210	n.a.
spicy barbecue (*Crunchwells Crumpet Chips*)	100	4.0	20.0	1.0	0	560	n.a.
Snack mix:							
(*Cheez-It*), ½ cup . .	140	4.0	19.0	5.0	0	270	1.0
(*Chex Mix*), ⅔ cup	130	3.0	22.0	3.5	0	280	1.0
(*Chex Mix* Bold n' Zesty), ½ cup . . .	150	3.0	17.0	7.0	0	390	5.0
(*Old Dutch* Party Mix), ⅔ cup	150	3.0	19.0	7.0	0	248	1.0
(*Pepperidge Farm* Light Season), ½ cup	170	4.0	22.0	8.0	<5	400	1.0

Food and Measure	cal.	prot. (gms)	carbo. (gms)	fat (gms)	chol. (mgs)	sod. (mgs)	fiber (gms)
Snack mix *(cont.)*							
(*Pepperidge Farm*							
Goldfish), ½ cup	170	5.0	21.0	8.0	5	360	2.0
cheddar:							
(*Chex Mix*), ⅔ cup	140	3.0	24.0	4.5	0	250	2.0
zesty (*Pepperidge*							
Farm Goldfish),							
½ cup	180	1.0	19.0	10.0	<5	390	1.0
honey mustard and							
onion (*Pepperidge*							
Farm), ½ cup . . .	180	4.0	19.0	10.0	<5	390	1.0
nutty, extra (*Pepper-*							
idge Farm), ½ cup	180	5.0	20.0	9.0	25	330	2.0
Snail, sea, see							
"Whelk"							
Snapper, meat only:							
raw, 4 oz.	113	23.3	0	1.5	42	73	0
baked, broiled, or mi-							
crowaved, 4 oz. . .	145	3.0	0	2.0	53	65	0
Snow peas, see							
"Peas, edible-pod-							
ded"							
Snow pea sprouts							
(*Jonathan's*), 1 cup	40	3.0	8.0	0	0	0	3.0
Soft drinks, carbon-							
ated, 12 fl. oz., ex-							
cept as noted:							
all varieties:							
(*R.W. Knudsen*							
Spritzer Light) . .	110	0	28.0	0	0	15	0
(*R.W. Knudsen Fruit*							
TeaZer)	110	0	26.0	0	0	20	0
sparkling (*Santa*							
Cruz)	150	1.0	38.0	0	0	70	0
apple:							
(*R.W. Knudsen*							
Spritzer)	160	0	42.0	0	0	25	0
(*Welch's* Sparkling)	200	0	56.0	0	0	26	0

Food and Measure	cal.	prot. (gms)	carbo. (gms)	fat (gms)	chol. (mgs)	sod. (mgs)	fiber (gms)
spiced (*Natural Brew*)	170	0	42.0	0	0	18	0
amaretto almond (*After the Fall* Spritzer)	150	1.0	36.0	0	0	25	0
berry (*After the Fall* Berrymeister Spritzer)	160	1.0	40.0	0	0	25	0
birch beer (*Canada Dry*), 8 fl. oz. . . .	110	0	27.0	0	0	40	0
boysenberry (*R.W. Knudsen* Spritzer)	160	0	42.0	0	0	25	0
cafe mocha (*Natural Brew*)	150	0	34.0	0	0	0	0
(*Canada Dry* Cactus Cooler), 8 fl. oz. . .	110	0	27.0	0	0	40	0
(*Canada Dry Hi-Spot*), 8 fl. oz.	110	0	28.0	0	0	50	0
cherry:							
(*After the Fall* American Pie Spritzer)	150	1.0	35.0	0	0	20	0
(*Crush*)	200	<1.0	52.0	<1.0	0	80	0
(*Sundrop*)	180	<1.0	46.0	<1.0	0	70	0
(*Sunkist*), 8 fl. oz.	140	0	35.0	0	0	35	0
amaretto (*Natural Brew*)	160	0	40.0	0	0	20	0
black (*After the Fall* Spritzer)	170	0	42.0	0	0	20	0
black (*Canada Dry*), 8 fl. oz.	130	0	32.0	0	0	40	0
black (*R.W. Knudsen* Spritzer) . . .	170	0	42.0	0	0	20	0
black (*Shasta*) . . .	170	0	41.0	0	0	45	0
French (*Snapple*), 8 fl. oz.	120	0	29.0	0	0	0	0
spice (*Slice*)	150	0	39.0	0	0	35	0
wild (*Canada Dry*), 8 fl. oz.	110	0	28.0	0	0	40	0
cherry-lime:							
(*Spree*)	170	0	45.0	0	0	45	0

Food and Measure	cal.	prot. (gms)	carbo. (gms)	fat (gms)	chol. (mgs)	sod. (mgs)	fiber (gms)
Soft drinks, cherry-lime *(cont.)*							
rickey (*Snapple*),							
8 fl. oz.	110	0	27.0	0	0	0	0
chocolate, see "Choc-							
olate drink"							
citrus, 8 fl. oz.:							
(*Canada Dry* Half &							
Half)	110	0	27.0	0	0	25	0
(*Sunkist*)	100	0	25.0	0	0	35	0
club soda:							
(*Canada Dry*),							
8 fl. oz.	0	0	0	0	0	60	0
(*Schweppes*),							
8 fl. oz.	0	0	0	0	0	70	0
(*Shasta*)	0	0	0	0	0	90	0
cola:							
(*Canada Dry* Ja-							
maica), 8 fl. oz.	110	0	27.0	0	0	10	0
(*Coca-Cola* Classic),							
8 fl. oz.	100	0	27.0	0	0	35	0
(*Juice Fizz* Cooler),							
8 fl. oz.	110	0	28.0	0	0	25	0
(*Pepsi/Crystal Pepsi*)	150	0	41.0	0	0	35	0
(*Shasta*)	170	0	42.0	0	0	45	0
(*Slice*)	160	0	43.0	0	0	35	0
(*Spree*)	170	0	42.0	0	0	45	0
cola, cherry:							
(*R.W. Knudsen*							
Spritzer)	170	1.0	42.0	0	0	20	0
(*Shasta*)	160	0	43.0	0	0	45	0
wild (*Pepsi*)	160	0	43.0	0	0	35	0
cola, ginseng (*Natural*							
Brew)	170	0	42.0	0	0	18	0
collins mixer:							
(*Canada Dry*),							
8 fl. oz.	100	0	21.0	0	0	15	0
(*Schweppes*),							
8 fl. oz.	100	0	25.0	0	0	55	0

Food and Measure	cal.	prot. (gms)	carbo. (gms)	fat (gms)	chol. (mgs)	sod. (mgs)	fiber (gms)
cranberry:							
(*After the Fall* Tart							
'n Sweet Spritzer)	170	1.0	40.0	0	0	15	0
(*R.W. Knudsen*							
Spritzer)	190	1.0	45.0	0	0	65	0
(*Shasta*)	180	0	44.0	0	0	45	0
cran-orange (*After the*							
Fall Tart 'n Sweet							
Spritzer)	170	1.0	40.0	0	0	15	0
cran-raspberry (*After*							
the Fall Tart 'n							
Sweet Spritzer) . .	160	1.0	40.0	0	0	15	0
cream/creme:							
(*A&W*), 8 fl. oz. . .	110	0	28.0	0	0	30	0
(*Hires*)	180	<1.0	48.0	<1.0	0	80	0
(*IBC*)	180	0	42.0	0	0	30	0
(*Mug*)	170	0	48.0	0	0	65	0
(*Shasta*)	190	0	47.0	0	0	45	0
vanilla (*Canada*							
Dry), 8 fl. oz. . .	120	0	30.0	0	0	40	0
vanilla (*Crush*) . . .	180	<1.0	44.0	<1.0	0	80	0
vanilla (*Natural*							
Brew)	170	0	42.0	0	0	18	0
vanilla (*R.W. Knud-*							
sen Spritzer) . . .	160	0	35.0	0	0	20	0
vanilla (*Snapple*),							
8 fl. oz.	130	0	33.0	0	0	0	0
(*Doc Shasta*)	160	0	39.0	0	0	45	0
(*Dr. Pepper*)	160	0	40.0	0	0	55	0
(*Dr. Slice*)	140	0	39.0	0	0	35	0
fruit punch/blend:							
(*Canada Dry* Tahi-							
tian), 8 fl. oz. . .	150	0	36.0	0	0	45	0
(*Juice Fizz*), 8 fl. oz.	130	0	32.0	0	0	25	0
(*Juice Fizz* Maui							
Magic/Wild Red),							
8 fl. oz.	120	0	30.0	0	0	25	0
(*Shasta*)	200	0	50.0	0	0	45	0
(*Slice*)	190	0	50.0	0	0	55	0

Food and Measure	cal.	prot. (gms)	carbo. (gms)	fat (gms)	chol. (mgs)	sod. (mgs)	fiber (gms)
Soft drinks, fruit punch/blend *(cont.)*							
(*Sunkist*), 8 fl. oz.	130	0	33.0	0	0	35	0
(*Welch's* Sparkling)	210	0	53.0	0	0	28	0
ginger ale:							
(*After the Fall* Nantucket)	140	1.0	35.0	0	0	25	0
(*Canada Dry*), 8 fl. oz.	90	0	25.0	0	0	15	0
(*Canada Dry* Golden), 8 fl. oz.	100	0	24.0	0	0	10	0
(*Natural Brew* Outrageous)	170	0	42.0	0	0	18	0
(*R.W. Knudsen* Spritzer)	160	1.0	40.0	0	0	25	0
(*Schweppes*), 8 fl. oz.	90	0	22.0	0	0	50	0
(*Shasta*)	130	0	32.0	0	0	45	0
cherry (*Canada Dry*), 8 fl. oz. . .	100	0	27.0	0	0	25	0
cranberry (*After the Fall*)	140	1.0	35.0	0	0	65	0
cranberry or lemon (*Canada Dry*), 8 fl. oz.	90	0	25.0	0	0	15	0
grape, dry (*Schweppes*), 8 fl. oz. . .	100	0	25.0	0	0	50	0
raspberry (*After the Fall*)	150	1.0	36.0	0	0	25	0
raspberry (*Schweppes*), 8 fl. oz. . .	100	0	26.0	0	0	50	0
ginger beer:							
(*Goya*)	190	0	27.0	0	0	30	0
(*Schweppes*), 8 fl. oz.	100	0	25.0	0	0	90	0
grape:							
(*After the Fall* Concord Spritzer) . .	180	1.0	45.0	0	0	15	0
(*Canada Dry* Concord), 8 fl. oz. . .	120	0	29.0	0	0	45	0

Food and Measure	cal.	prot. (gms)	carbo. (gms)	fat (gms)	chol. (mgs)	sod. (mgs)	fiber (gms)
(*Crush*)	200	<1.0	52.0	<1.0	0	80	0
(*Juice Fizz* Purple Thunder), 8 fl. oz.	130	0	34.0	0	0	25	0
(*R.W. Knudsen* Spritzer)	170	1.0	41.0	0	0	30	0
(*Schweppes*), 8 fl. oz.	130	0	33.0	0	0	55	0
(*Shasta*)	190	0	48.0	0	0	45	0
(*Slice*)	190	0	51.0	0	0	70	0
(*Welch's* Sparkling)	200	0	51.0	0	0	38	0
grapefruit:							
(*Schweppes*), 8 fl. oz.	110	0	27.0	0	0	75	0
(*Shasta* Ruby Red)	190	0	47.0	0	0	45	0
(*Spree*)	170	0	41.0	0	0	45	0
(*Wink*), 8 fl. oz. . .	130	0	31.0	0	0	35	0
(*Wink* Diet), 8 fl. oz.	5	0	1.0	0	0	95	0
kiwi-lime (*R.W. Knudsen* Spritzer)	160	1.0	40.0	0	0	25	0
kiwi-strawberry:							
(*After the Fall* Spritzer)	170	1.0	40.0	0	0	15	0
(*Shasta*)	170	0	43.0	0	0	45	0
(*Snapple*), 8 fl. oz.	130	0	33.0	0	0	5	0
lemon:							
bitter (*Schweppes*), 8 fl. oz.	110	0	26.0	0	0	45	0
sour (*Canada Dry*), 8 fl. oz.	100	0	21.0	0	0	15	0
sour (*Schweppes*), 8 fl. oz.	110	0	26.0	0	0	25	0
spicy (*After the Fall* Spritzer)	150	0	37.0	0	0	35	0
lemonade:							
(*Country Time*), 8 fl. oz.	120	0	26.0	0	0	15	0
(*Sunkist*), 8 fl. oz.	120	0	30.0	0	0	35	0
Jamaica (*R.W. Knudsen* Spritzer)	170	0	41.0	0	0	25	0

Food and Measure	cal.	prot. (gms)	carbo. (gms)	fat (gms)	chol. (mgs)	sod. (mgs)	fiber (gms)
Soft drinks, lemonade *(cont.)*							
tangerine, kiwi berry							
or raspberry							
(*Country Time*),							
8 fl. oz.	110	0	27.0	0	0	60	0
lemon-lime:							
(*R.W. Knudsen*							
Spritzer)	170	1.0	41.0	0	0	25	0
(*Schweppes*),							
8 fl. oz.	100	0	25.0	0	0	75	0
(*Slice*)	150	0	40.0	0	0	55	0
(*Spree*)	170	0	42.0	0	0	45	0
lime:							
(*After the Fall* Carib-							
bean Spritzer) . .	170	2.0	42.0	0	0	25	0
(*Canada Dry* Island),							
8 fl. oz.	140	0	33.0	0	0	15	0
lime-lemon (*Shasta*							
Twist), 12 fl. oz. . .	150	0	38.0	0	0	55	0
mandarin-lime:							
(*R.W. Knudsen*							
Spritzer)	170	0	42.0	0	0	20	0
(*Spree*)	170	0	42.0	0	0	45	0
mandarin-pineapple							
(*After the Fall*							
Spritzer)	150	1.0	37.0	0	0	25	0
mango:							
(*After the Fall* Ha-							
waiian Spritzer)	180	0	45.0	0	0	20	0
(*R.W. Knudsen* Fan-							
dango Spritzer)	190	1.0	45.0	0	0	30	0
mango ginger (*After*							
the Fall Spritzer) . .	150	1.0	38.0	0	0	25	0
(*Mountain Dew*) . . .	170	0	46.0	0	0	70	0
orange:							
(*After the Fall* Icicle							
Spritzer)	170	1.0	42.0	0	0	25	0
(*After the Fall*							
Zudachi Spritzer)	160	1.0	40.0	0	0	35	0

Food and Measure	cal.	prot. (gms)	carbo. (gms)	fat (gms)	chol. (mgs)	sod. (mgs)	fiber (gms)
(*Canada Dry* Sun-ripe), 8 fl. oz. . .	140	0	35.0	0	0	45	0
(*Crush*)	200	<1.0	52.0	<1.0	0	80	0
(*Orangina*), 10 fl. oz.	120	<1.0	28.0	.5	0	115	0
(*Shasta*)	200	0	49.0	0	0	45	0
(*Sunkist*), 8 fl. oz.	140	0	35.0	0	0	40	0
(*Welch's* Sparkling)	200	0	51.0	0	0	25	0
mandarin (*Slice*) . .	190	0	51.0	0	0	55	0
orange passion fruit (*R.W. Knudsen* Spritzer)	160	0	40.0	0	0	25	0
passion fruit (*Snapple*), 8 fl. oz.	120	0	29.0	0	0	0	0
peach:							
(*Canada Dry*), 8 fl. oz.	120	0	30.0	0	0	40	0
(*R.W. Knudsen* Spritzer)	160	2.0	37.0	0	0	35	0
(*Shasta*)	170	0	43.0	0	0	45	0
(*Snapple* Melba), 8 fl. oz.	120	0	31.0	0	0	4	0
(*Sunkist*), 8 fl. oz.	120	0	30.0	0	0	40	0
(*Welch's* Sparkling)	220	0	52.0	0	0	10	0
peach vanilla (*After the Fall* Spritzer) . .	170	0	42.0	0	0	35	0
pear (*Kristian Regale* Swedish Sparkler), 8 fl. oz.	100	0	26.0	0	0	15	0
pineapple:							
(*Canada Dry*), 8 fl. oz.	110	0	26.0	0	0	40	0
(*Crush*)	200	<1.0	52.0	<1.0	0	80	0
(*Shasta*)	200	0	51.0	0	0	45	0
(*Slice*)	190	0	51.0	0	0	70	0
(*Sunkist*), 8 fl. oz.	140	0	35.0	0	0	35	0
(*Welch's* Sparkling)	210	0	53.0	0	0	52	0
pineapple-orange (*Shasta*)	180	0	46.0	0	0	45	0

Food and Measure	cal.	prot. (gms)	carbo. (gms)	fat (gms)	chol. (mgs)	sod. (mgs)	fiber (gms)
Soft drinks *(cont.)*							
raspberry:							
(*After the Fall* Spritzer)	170	0	42.0	0	0	25	0
(*Snapple* Royal), 8 fl. oz.	120	0	31.0	0	0	0	0
creme (*Shasta*) . .	170	0	44.0	0	0	45	0
red (*R.W. Knudsen* Spritzer)	170	0	42.0	0	0	25	0
red:							
(*Shasta*)	170	0	43.0	0	0	45	0
(*Slice*)	190	0	51.0	0	0	55	0
root beer:							
(*A&W*), 8 fl. oz. . .	110	0	20.0	0	0	35	0
(*Hires*)	180	<1.0	46.0	<1.0	0	110	0
(*IBC*)	168	0	42.0	0	0	16	0
(*Mug*)	160	0	43.0	0	0	65	0
(*Shasta*)	170	0	42.0	0	0	45	0
(*Snapple* Tru), 8 fl. oz.	110	0	29.0	0	0	0	0
(*Spree*)	170	0	42.0	0	0	45	0
seltzer, all flavors:							
(*Canada Dry*) . . .	0	0	0	0	0	10	0
except raspberry (*Schweppes*) . .	0	0	0	0	0	10	0
raspberry (*Schweppes*)	0	0	0	0	0	0	0
(*7Up*)	160	0	39.0	0	0	75	0
(*7Up* Cherry)	160	0	39.0	0	0	35	0
sour mixer (*Canada Dry*), 8 fl. oz. . . .	90	0	22.0	0	0	25	0
spritzer, see specific soda listings							
strawberry:							
(*After the Fall* Twist O' Spritzer) . . .	150	0	37.0	0	0	25	0
(*Canada Dry* California), 8 fl. oz. . .	110	0	27.0	0	0	45	0
(*Crush*)	180	<1.0	46.0	<1.0	0	80	0

Food and Measure	cal.	prot. (gms)	carbo. (gms)	fat (gms)	chol. (mgs)	sod. (mgs)	fiber (gms)
(*R.W. Knudsen* Spritzer)	170	0	42.0	0	0	25	0
(*Shasta*)	190	0	46.0	0	0	45	0
(*Slice*)	170	0	47.0	0	0	55	0
(*Sunkist*), 8 fl. oz.	140	0	34.0	0	0	35	0
(*Welch's* Sparkling)	200	0	51.0	0	0	26	0
peach (*Shasta*) . .	170	0	42.0	0	0	45	0
strawberry vanilla (*After the Fall* Spritzer)	160	0	42.0	0	0	25	0
(*Sundrop*)	200	<1.0	46.0	<1.0	0	70	0
tangerine spritzer:							
(*After the Fall*) . . .	170	2.0	40.0	0	0	35	0
(*R.W. Knudsen*) . .	170	2.0	39.0	0	0	35	0
tonic:							
(*Canada Dry*), 8 fl. oz.	100	0	24.0	0	0	15	0
(*Schweppes*), 8 fl. oz.	90	0	22.0	0	0	45	0
(*Shasta*)	170	0	42.0	0	0	45	0
w/fruit flavors (*Schweppes*), 8 fl. oz.	90	0	20.0	0	0	25	0
w/lime (*Canada Dry*), 8 fl. oz. . .	100	0	24.0	0	0	20	0
vanilla, see "cream," above							
vanilla bean (*After the Fall* Spritzer)	170	0	42.0	0	0	25	0
vichy (*Canada Dry*), 8 fl. oz.	0	0	0	0	0	490	0
Sole:							
fresh, see "Flatfish"							
frozen (*Van de Kamp's* Natural), 4 oz.	110	23.0	0	1.5	50	125	0
Sole entree, frozen: breaded, 1 fillet:							
(*Mrs. Paul's* Premium)	250	20.0	22.0	13.0	40	510	2.0

Food and Measure	cal.	prot. (gms)	carbo. (gms)	fat (gms)	chol. (mgs)	sod. (mgs)	fiber (gms)
Sole entree *(cont.)*							
(*Van de Kamp's* Light)	220	14.0	17.0	11.0	40	410	n.a.
Sopressata (*Boar's Head Cinghiale* Mini), 1 oz.	100	8.0	<1.0	8.0	15	540	0
Sorbet (see also "Ice" and "Sherbet"), ½ cup:							
(*Ben & Jerry's Doonesbury*)	130	0	33.0	0	0	15	<1.0
chocolate:							
(*Häagen-Dazs*) . . .	130	2.0	30.0	0	0	80	2.0
(*Tofutti*)	90	1.0	16.0	0	0	108	1.0
coffee (*Tofutti*)	80	0	19.0	0	0	85	0
and cream:							
orange (*Häagen-Dazs*)	200	2.0	27.0	9.0	60	45	0
raspberry (*Häagen-Dazs*)	190	3.0	23.0	9.0	60	45	<1.0
lemon:							
(*Häagen-Dazs* Zesty)	120	0	31.0	0	0	5	<1.0
(*Tofutti*)	90	0	22.0	0	0	33	0
lemonade, pink (*Ben & Jerry's*)	120	0	30.0	0	0	15	0
mocha (*Ben & Jerry's*)	140	1.0	33.0	0	0	10	1.0
orange-peach-mango (*Tofutti*)	90	0	21.0	0	0	2	0
peach (*Häagen-Dazs* Orchard)	140	<1.0	35.0	0	0	0	<1.0
pina colada (*Ben & Jerry's*)	140	0	33.0	0	0	20	<1.0
purple passion (*Ben & Jerry's*)	120	0	33.0	0	0	15	0
raspberry (*Häagen-Dazs*)	120	0	29.0	0	0	5	1.0
raspberry (*Tofutti*) . .	80	0	21.0	0	0	2	0
strawberry:							
(*Häagen-Dazs*) . . .	130	0	33.0	0	0	0	1.0

Food and Measure	cal.	prot. (gms)	carbo. (gms)	fat (gms)	chol. (mgs)	sod. (mgs)	fiber (gms)
(*Tofutti*)	80	0	19.0	0	0	1	0
kiwi (*Ben & Jerry's*)	100	0	25.0	0	0	15	0
Sorbet bar, 1 bar:							
berry, wild (*Häagen-Dazs*)	90	0	22.0	0	0	5.0	<1.0
chocolate (*Häagen-Dazs*)	80	1.0	20.0	0	0	50	1. 0
Sorbet-yogurt bar, chocolate and cherry (*Häagen-Dazs* Sorbet 'n Yogurt), 1 bar	100	3.0	21.0	0	0	40	<1.0
Sorghum, whole-grain, 1 cup	650	21.7	143.3	6.3	0	n.a.	n.a.
Sorghum syrup:							
½ cup	479	0	123.7	0	0	13	0
1 tbsp.	61	0	15.7	0	0	2	0
Sorrel, see "Dock"							
Soup, canned, ready-to-serve, 1 cup, except as noted:							
bean:							
(*Grandma Brown's*)	190	9.0	31.0	3.5	0	700	10.0
black (*Goya*)	210	12.0	34.0	2.5	0	1400	10.0
black (*Progresso*)	170	8.0	30.0	1.5	<5	730	10.0
black, w/bacon (*Old El Paso*)	160	11.0	26.0	1.5	5	960	7.0
black, and vegetable (*Health Valley*) . .	110	11.0	24.0	0	0	220	12.0
salsa (*Campbell's* Home Cookin'*)	160	2.0	31.0	1.0	0	730	7.0
bean w/bacon and ham (*Campbell's* Microwave), 1 cont.	180	9.0	26.0	6.0	10	750	7.0
bean and ham:							
(*Campbell's* Chunky)	190	3.0	29.0	2.0	15	880	9.0
(*Campbell's* Chunky), 10¾ oz.	240	5.0	37.0	3.0	20	1130	11.0

Food and Measure	cal.	prot. (gms)	carbo. (gms)	fat (gms)	chol. (mgs)	sod. (mgs)	fiber (gms)
Soup, canned, ready-to-serve, bean and ham *(cont.)*							
(*Campbell's* Chunky Ham 'n Bean), 10¾ oz.	270	15.0	34.0	10.0	25	1160	8.0
(*Campbell's* Home Cookin')	180	2.0	33.0	1.5	5	720	9.0
(*Campbell's* Home Cookin'), 10¾ oz.	230	3.0	41.0	2.0	5	890	11.0
(*Healthy Choice*) . .	185	10.0	34.0	2.0	5	465	10.0
(*Progresso*)	160	10.0	25.0	2.0	10	870	8.0
beans and rice:							
creole (*Campbell's* Chunky)	210	12.0	27.0	8.0	15	720	6.0
creole (*Campbell's* Chunky), 10¾ oz.	260	15.0	33.0	10.0	15	890	7.0
beef:							
barley (*Progresso*)	130	10.0	13.0	4.0	25	780	3.0
barley (*Progresso* Healthy Classics)	140	11.0	20.0	2.0	20	490	3.0
broth (*Health Valley*)	20	5.0	0	0	0	160	0
broth (*Swanson*) . .	20	2.0	2.0	1.0	<5	820	0
chunky (*Campbell's* Microwave), 1 cont.	210	8.0	24.0	5.0	35	1120	3.0
hearty (*Old El Paso*)	120	10.0	14.0	2.5	25	690	0
minestrone (*Progresso*) . . .	140	12.0	14.0	4.0	25	850	3.0
noodle (*Progresso*)	140	13.0	15.0	3.5	30	950	1.0
pasta (*Campbell's* Chunky)	150	5.0	18.0	3.0	20	970	2.0
pasta (*Campbell's* Chunky), 10¾ oz.	190	6.0	23.0	4.0	20	1200	3.0
potato (*Healthy Choice*)	120	10.0	8.0	2.0	10	635	2.5
Stroganoff (*Campbell's* Chunky), 10¾ oz.	310	25.0	28.0	16.0	45	1180	4.0

Food and Measure	cal.	prot. (gms)	carbo. (gms)	fat (gms)	chol. (mgs)	sod. (mgs)	fiber (gms)
beef vegetable:							
(*Progresso* Healthy Classics)	150	10.0	25.0	1.5	15	410	6.0
country (*Campbell's* Chunky)	160	6.0	18.0	4.0	25	900	3.0
country (*Campbell's* Chunky), 10¾ oz.	200	8.0	22.0	5.0	30	1130	4.0
and rotini (*Progresso* Pasta Soup)	120	11.0	10.0	3.5	20	830	3.0
borscht (*Gold's*) . . .	70	1.0	16.0	0	0	780	1.0
broccoli:							
carotene (*Health Valley*)	70	6.0	16.0	0	0	240	7.0
cream of (*Progresso* Healthy Classics)	90	2.0	13.0	3.0	<5	580	2.0
and shells (*Progresso* Pasta Soup)	70	3.0	14.0	1.0	<5	720	3.0
broccoli cheese (*Campbell's* Chunky)	200	18.0	14.0	12.0	25	1120	1.0
chicken:							
(*Campbell's* Chunky Old Fashioned)	130	5.0	12.0	3.0	20	950	3.0
(*Campbell's* Chunky Old Fashioned), 10¾ oz.	160	8.0	19.0	5.0	25	1180	3.0
(*Progresso* Chickarina)	120	8.0	10.0	5.0	20	710	1.0
barley (*Progresso*)	110	10.0	14.0	2.5	15	720	3.0
hearty (*Healthy Choice*)	130	8.5	20.0	2.5	20	460	1.5
hearty (*Progresso*), 10½ oz.	120	13.0	10.0	2.5	25	1070	0
minestrone (*Progresso*) . . .	120	10.0	12.0	3.5	20	790	2.0
chicken, cream of:							
(*Campbell's* Home Cookin')	210	28.0	8.0	18.0	15	1170	2.0

Food and Measure	cal.	prot. (gms)	carbo. (gms)	fat (gms)	chol. (mgs)	sod. (mgs)	fiber (gms)
Soup, canned, ready-to-serve, chicken, cream of *(cont.)*							
(*Campbell's* Home Cookin'), 10¾ oz.	260	34.0	11.0	22.0	20	1460	3.0
(*Progresso*)	170	8.0	11.0	10.0	35	880	0
w/mushrooms (*Healthy Choice*)	125	7.0	20.0	2.0	10	420	1.0
w/vegetables (*Healthy Choice*)	125	7.0	21.0	2.0	10	385	1.0
chicken broth:							
(*Campbell's* Low Sodium), 10¾ oz.	40	3.0	2.0	2.0	5	140	0
(*Campbell's Healthy Request*)	20	0	1.0	0	0	480	0
(*College Inn*)	25	1.0	1.0	1.5	<5	1050	0
(*College Inn* Less Sodium)	25	1.0	1.0	1.5	<5	640	0
(*Health Valley*) . . .	30	6.0	0	0	0	170	0
(*Pritikin*)	15	2.0	1.0	0	0	60	0
(*Progresso*)	20	2.0	1.0	.5	5	860	0
(*Swanson*)	30	3.0	1.0	2.0	0	1000	0
(*Swanson* Natural Goodness)	15	0	1.0	0	0	560	0
chicken chowder:							
corn (*Campbell's Healthy Request*)	140	5.0	22.0	3.0	15	480	2.0
mushroom (*Campbell's* Chunky) . .	210	18.0	15.0	12.0	10	970	3.0
chicken noodle:							
(*Campbell's* Chunky Classic)	130	5.0	16.0	3.0	20	1050	2.0
(*Campbell's* Chunky Classic), 10¾ oz.	160	5.0	20.0	3.5	25	1310	3.0
(*Campbell's* Home Cookin')	100	5.0	11.0	3.5	15	980	1.0
(*Campbell's* Home Cookin'), 10¾ oz.	120	6.0	14.0	4.0	20	1220	2.0
(*Campbell's* Low Sodium), 10¾ oz.	170	8.0	18.0	5.0	50	120	2.0

Food and Measure	cal.	prot. (gms)	carbo. (gms)	fat (gms)	chol. (mgs)	sod. (mgs)	fiber (gms)
(*Campbell's* Micro- wave), 1 cont. . .	90	6.0	10.0	4.0	20	850	1.0
(*Healthy Choice* Old Fashioned)	140	9.0	20.0	3.0	10	400	<1.0
(*Progresso*)	80	9.0	8.0	2.0	20	730	1.0
(*Progresso*), 10½ oz.	110	11.0	10.0	2.5	25	910	1.0
(*Progresso* Healthy Classics)	80	7.0	10.0	2.0	10	480	1.0
(*Weight Watchers*), 10½ oz.	150	9.0	25.0	2.0	30	740	4.0
chunky (*Campbell's* Microwave), 1 cont.	160	7.0	17.0	5.0	35	1060	3.0
creamy (*Campbell's* Chunky)	210	26.0	12.0	17.0	20	1020	1.0
creamy (*Campbell's* Chunky), 10¾ oz.	270	31.0	14.0	20.0	25	1270	1.0
hearty (*Campbell's* Healthy Request)	160	5.0	25.0	3.0	20	480	2.0
hearty (*Old El Paso*)	110	9.0	10.0	3.0	25	720	0
w/mushroom (*Campbell's* Chunky)	120	5.0	10.0	3.5	25	930	1.0
chicken pasta:							
(*Healthy Choice*) . .	120	7.0	17.5	3.0	10	495	1.5
(*Pritikin*)	100	6.0	18.0	1.0	5	160	1.0
penne, spicy (*Progresso* Pasta Soup)	120	8.0	13.0	4.0	20	680	0
chicken rice:							
(*Campbell's* Chunky)	140	5.0	18.0	3.0	25	840	2.0
(*Campbell's* Home Cookin')	110	2.0	17.0	1.5	15	910	2.0
(*Campbell's* Home Cookin'), 10¾ oz.	140	3.0	21.0	2.0	20	1130	2.0
(*Campbell's* Micro- wave), 1 cont. . .	120	4.0	20.0	2.5	10	1130	2.0

Food and Measure	cal.	prot. (gms)	carbo. (gms)	fat (gms)	chol. (mgs)	sod. (mgs)	fiber (gms)
Soup, canned, ready-to-serve, chicken rice *(cont.)*							
(*Campbell's Healthy*							
Request)	100	3.0	15.0	2.0	40	480	1.0
(*Old El Paso*) . . .	90	8.0	10.0	2.5	15	680	0
(*Pritikin*)	80	5.0	13.0	1.0	5	250	2.0
(*Weight Watchers*),							
10½ oz.	110	6.0	17.0	1.5	10	720	4.0
w/rice (*Campbell's*							
Microwave),							
1 cont.	90	6.0	12.0	4.0	10	820	1.0
w/rice (*Healthy*							
Choice)	110	7.0	15.0	3.0	6	425	<1.0
w/vegetables							
(*Progresso*) . . .	110	7.0	12.0	3.0	15	750	<1.0
w/vegetables							
(*Progresso*),							
10½ oz.	130	9.0	15.0	4.0	20	940	<1.0
w/vegetables							
(*Progresso*							
Healthy Classics)	90	7.0	12.0	1.5	10	450	1.0
wild rice							
(*Progresso*) . . .	100	6.0	15.0	2.0	15	820	2.0
chicken and rotini							
(*Progresso* Pasta							
Soup)	90	10.0	8.0	2.0	20	860	0
chicken vegetable:							
(*Campbell's* Chunky)	90	2.0	13.0	1.0	10	870	3.0
(*Campbell's* Home							
Cookin')	130	5.0	20.0	3.5	10	820	3.0
(*Campbell's* Home							
Cookin'), 10¾ oz.	170	6.0	24.0	4.0	10	1020	4.0
(*Old El Paso*) . . .	110	9.0	13.0	2.5	15	620	0
(*Progresso* Home-							
style)	100	9.0	10.0	2.5	15	680	1.0
hearty (*Campbell's*							
Healthy Request)	120	3.0	18.0	2.0	20	480	3.0
nuggets (*Campbell's*							
Chunky)	150	8.0	19.0	5.0	15	830	3.0

Food and Measure	cal.	prot. (gms)	carbo. (gms)	fat (gms)	chol. (mgs)	sod. (mgs)	fiber (gms)
nuggets (*Campbell's* Chunky), 10¾ oz.	190	11.0	24.0	7.0	15	1030	4.0
and penne (*Progresso* Pasta Soup)	100	7.0	11.0	2.5	10	780	3.0
chili beef w/beans:							
(*Campbell's* Chunky)	230	9.0	30.0	6.0	15	850	7.0
(*Campbell's* Chunky), 10¾ oz.	300	11.0	38.0	7.0	10	1080	9.0
(*Campbell's* Micro- wave), 1 cont. . .	180	8.0	28.0	5.0	10	790	7.0
(*Healthy Choice*) . .	165	14.0	30.0	1.0	10	385	5.0
clam chowder, Man- hattan:							
(*Bookbinder's*), ½ cup	80	6.0	12.0	.5	0	1140	2.0
(*Campbell's* Chunky)	130	6.0	20.0	4.0	5	900	3.0
(*Campbell's* Chunky), 10¾ oz.	170	6.0	25.0	4.0	5	1120	4.0
(*Progresso*)	110	12.0	11.0	2.0	10	710	3.0
clam chowder, New England:							
(*Bookbinder's*), ½ cup	120	6.0	16.0	3.0	<5	1190	2.0
(*Campbell's* Chunky)	240	23.0	21.0	15.0	10	980	2.0
(*Campbell's* Chunky), 10¾ oz.	300	28.0	26.0	18.0	15	1210	3.0
(*Campbell's* Home Cookin')	210	25.0	12.0	16.0	5	1120	2.0
(*Campbell's* Micro- wave), 1 cont. . .	200	22.0	14.0	14.0	15	950	3.0
(*Campbell's Healthy Request*)	120	5.0	17.0	3.0	15	480	1.0
(*Healthy Choice*) . .	125	6.0	23.0	1.0	10	480	2.0
(*Progresso*)	180	6.0	17.0	10.0	15	850	2.0
(*Progresso*), 10½ oz.	220	7.0	21.0	3.5	20	1050	2.0
(*Progresso* Healthy Classics)	120	5.0	20.0	2.0	5	530	1.0

Food and Measure	cal.	prot. (gms)	carbo. (gms)	fat (gms)	chol. (mgs)	sod. (mgs)	fiber (gms)
Soup, canned, ready-to-serve, clam chowder, New England *(cont.)*							
chunky (*Campbell's* Microwave), 1 cont.	290	26.0	26.0	17.0	20	1150	3.0
clam rotini chowder (*Progresso* Pasta Soup)	200	7.0	21.0	9.0	10	800	0
corn, country, and vegetable (*Health Valley*)	70	5.0	17.0	0	0	135	7.0
corn chowder:							
(*Campbell's* Chunky)	250	23.0	18.0	15.0	25	870	3.0
(*Campbell's* Chunky), 10¾ oz.	310	29.0	22.0	19.0	30	1080	4.0
(*Progresso*)	180	5.0	20.0	10.0	10	780	2.0
chicken (*Healthy Choice*)	175	8.0	30.0	3.0	10	465	2.0
crab bisque (*Book-binder's*), ½ cup . .	120	5.0	10.0	7.0	25	920	<1.0
egg flower (*Rice Road*)	90	2.0	15.0	2.5	15	1000	1.0
escarole, in chicken broth (*Progresso*)	25	2.0	2.0	1.0	<5	980	0
garlic pasta (*Progresso* Healthy Classics)	100	4.0	18.0	1.5	<5	450	3.0
gazpacho	57	8.7	.8	2.2	0	1183	<2.0
hot and sour (*Rice Road*)	90	3.0	15.0	3.0	0	1340	2.0
Italian, carotene (*Health Valley* Fat Free)	80	7.0	19.0	0	0	240	6.0
lentil:							
(*Healthy Choice*) . .	145	8.5	28.0	1.0	<5	420	5.0
(*Pritikin*)	130	10.0	24.0	.5	0	280	8.0
(*Progresso*)	140	9.0	22.0	2.0	0	750	7.0
(*Progresso*), 10½ oz.	170	11.0	27.0	2.5	0	930	8.0

Food and Measure	cal.	prot. (gms)	carbo. (gms)	fat (gms)	chol. (mgs)	sod. (mgs)	fiber (gms)
(*Progresso* Healthy Classics)	130	8.0	20.0	1.5	0	440	6.0
and carrots (*Health Valley* Fat Free)	90	10.0	25.0	0	0	220	14.0
hearty (*Campbell's* Home Cookin')	130	1.0	24.0	.5	0	860	5.0
hearty (*Campbell's* Home Cookin'), 10¾ oz.	190	5.0	33.0	3.0	0	1070	6.0
w/sausage (*Progresso*) . . .	170	8.0	19.0	7.0	15	780	5.0
and shells (*Progresso* Pasta Soup)	130	7.0	22.0	1.5	0	840	4.0
lobster bisque (*Book-binder's*), ½ cup . .	90	4.0	10.0	4.0	25	710	<1.0
macaroni and bean (*Progresso*)	160	7.0	23.0	4.0	<5	800	6.0
meatballs and pasta pearls (*Progresso* Pasta Soup)	140	7.0	13.0	7.0	15	700	0
minestrone:							
(*Campbell's* Chunky)	140	8.0	22.0	5.0	5	800	2.0
(*Healthy Choice*) . .	110	6.0	23.0	1.0	<5	390	3.0
(*Pritikin*)	90	5.0	19.0	1.0	0	330	3.0
(*Progresso*)	130	6.0	22.0	2.5	0	960	5.0
(*Progresso*), 10½ oz.	170	7.0	27.0	3.5	0	1190	6.0
(*Progresso* Healthy Classics)	120	5.0	20.0	2.5	0	510	1.0
(*Weight Watchers*), 10½ oz.	130	5.0	23.0	2.0	5	760	6.0
hearty (*Campbell's* Healthy Request*)	120	3.0	24.0	2.0	<5	480	3.0
Italian (*Health Valley*)	80	8.0	21.0	0	0	210	11.0
shells (*Progresso* Pasta Soup) . . .	120	5.0	20.0	1.5	0	700	4.0

Food and Measure	cal.	prot. (gms)	carbo. (gms)	fat (gms)	chol. (mgs)	sod. (mgs)	fiber (gms)
Soup, canned, ready-to-serve, minestrone *(cont.)*							
Tuscany (*Campbell's* Home Cookin'*)	160	11.0	21.0	7.0	5	880	5.0
Tuscany (*Campbell's* Home Cookin'*), 10¾ oz.	200	12.0	26.0	8.0	5	1100	6.0
zesty (*Progresso*)	150	6.0	17.0	6.0	10	790	4.0
mushroom, cream of:							
(*Campbell's* Home Cookin'*)	170	20.0	9.0	13.0	15	970	3.0
(*Campbell's* Home Cookin'*), 10¾ oz.	210	26.0	12.0	17.0	20	1210	3.0
(*Campbell's* Low Sodium), 10¾ oz.	200	22.0	18.0	14.0	20	65	3.0
(*Healthy Choice*) . .	75	4.0	14.0	1.0	<5	450	<1.0
(*Progresso*)	140	3.0	12.0	8.0	20	920	1.0
mushroom rice (*Campbell's* Home Cookin'*)	80	1.0	16.0	.5	0	820	2.0
Oriental broth (*Swanson*)	15	1.0	3.0	0	0	1070	0
oyster stew (*Bookbinder's*), ½ can . .	90	4.0	8.0	5.0	15	240	0
pasta:							
Bolognese (*Health Valley Healthy Pasta*)	70	5.0	17.0	0	0	135	7.0
cacciatore (*Health Valley Healthy Pasta*)	90	6.0	19.0	0	0	210	4.0
Chinese (*Rice Road*)	70	1.0	12.0	2.0	0	1260	1.0
fagioli (*Health Valley Healthy Pasta*) . .	80	6.0	17.0	0	0	250	4.0
primavera (*Health Valley Healthy Pasta*)	80	8.0	21.0	0	0	210	11.0
Romano (*Health Valley Healthy Pasta*)	140	10.0	32.0	0	0	250	13.0

Food and Measure	cal.	prot. (gms)	carbo. (gms)	fat (gms)	chol. (mgs)	sod. (mgs)	fiber (gms)
pea, split:							
(*Campbell's* Low							
Sodium), 10¾ oz.	240	6.0	38.0	4.0	5	50	5.0
(*Grandma Brown's*)	210	12.0	31.0	4.0	0	520	6.0
(*Pritikin*)	140	11.0	29.0	.5	0	290	10.0
(*Progresso* Healthy							
Classics)	180	10.0	30.0	2.5	<5	420	5.0
and carrots (*Health*							
Valley)	110	8.0	17.0	0	0	230	4.0
green (*Progresso*)	170	10.0	25.0	3.0	5	870	5.0
pea, split, w/ham:							
(*Campbell's* Chunky)	190	5.0	27.0	3.0	20	1120	3.0
(*Campbell's*							
Chunky), 10¾ oz.	240	5.0	33.0	3.5	20	1400	4.0
(*Campbell's* Home							
Cookin')	170	2.0	30.0	1.5	5	880	6.0
(*Campbell's* Home							
Cookin'), 10¾ oz.	210	3.0	37.0	2.0	5	1100	8.0
(*Campbell's Healthy*							
Request)	170	3.0	28.0	2.0	10	480	4.0
(*Healthy Choice*) . .	155	11.0	25.5	2.0	10	400	2.5
(*Progresso*)	160	9.0	20.0	4.0	15	830	5.0
penne:							
hearty, chicken							
broth (*Progresso*							
Pasta Soup) . . .	70	5.0	12.0	1.0	<5	930	0
zesty (*Campbell's*							
Healthy Request)	90	1.0	17.0	.5	5	470	2.0
pepper steak:							
(*Campbell's* Chunky)	140	4.0	18.0	2.5	20	830	3.0
(*Campbell's*							
Chunky), 10¾ oz.	180	5.0	22.0	3.5	25	1040	3.0
potato ham chowder							
(*Campbell's*							
Chunky), 10¾ oz.	270	28.0	20.0	18.0	25	1050	3.0
seafood bisque (*Book-*							
binder's), ½ cup . .	140	7.0	9.0	8.0	25	1010	<1.0
shrimp bisque (*Book-*							
binder's), ½ cup . .	120	6.0	9.0	7.0	50	840	<1.0

Food and Measure	cal.	prot. (gms)	carbo. (gms)	fat (gms)	chol. (mgs)	sod. (mgs)	fiber (gms)
Soup, canned, ready-to-serve *(cont.)*							
sirloin burger:							
chunky (*Campbell's* Microwave),							
1 cont.	210	12.0	24.0	8.0	15	1090	5.0
w/vegetable (*Campbell's* Chunky) . .	190	14.0	20.0	9.0	20	930	4.0
snapper (*Bookbinder's*), ½ cup . .	110	4.0	11.0	6.0	15	550	<1.0
steak and potato:							
(*Campbell's* Chunky)	160	6.0	20.0	4.0	20	890	3.0
(*Campbell's* Chunky), 10¾ oz.	200	8.0	24.0	5.0	25	1110	4.0
tomato:							
(*Campbell's* Low Sodium), 10¾ oz.	170	9.0	28.0	6.0	10	60	2.0
(*Progresso*)	90	3.0	15.0	2.0	0	990	4.0
beef and rotini (*Progresso*) . . .	140	11.0	15.0	4.5	15	750	2.0
garden (*Campbell's* Home Cookin'), 10¾ oz.	150	6.0	27.0	4.0	5	900	4.0
garden (*Healthy Choice*)	105	5.0	21.0	2.0	<5	425	3.0
hearty, rotini (*Progresso* Pasta Soup)	90	4.0	16.0	1.0	5	820	3.0
tortellini (*Progresso* Pasta Soup) . . .	120	5.0	13.0	5.0	10	910	2.0
vegetable (*Campbell's Healthy Request*)	120	3.0	22.0	2.0	5	480	3.0
vegetable (*Health Valley*)	80	6.0	17.0	0	0	240	5.0
vegetable, garden (*Progresso Healthy Classics*)	100	3.0	19.0	1.0	0	480	4.0

Food and Measure	cal.	prot. (gms)	carbo. (gms)	fat (gms)	chol. (mgs)	sod. (mgs)	fiber (gms)
tortellini:							
in chicken broth							
(*Progresso*) . . .	80	4.0	10.0	2.0	5	750	2.0
creamy (*Progresso*)	210	5.0	15.0	15.0	30	830	0
turkey w/wild rice:							
(*Healthy Choice*) . .	100	5.5	13.5	2.5	<5	355	1.0
vegetable (*Camp-bell's Healthy Re-quest*)	120	4.0	17.0	2.5	15	480	2.0
vegetable:							
(*Campbell's* Chunky)	130	5.0	22.0	3.0	0	870	4.0
(*Campbell's* Chunky), 10¾ oz.	160	6.0	28.0	4.0	0	1090	5.0
(*Campbell's* Micro-wave), 1 cont. . .	100	3.0	17.0	2.0	0	850	2.0
(*Campbell's Healthy Request*)	120	1.0	22.0	.5	5	460	4.0
(*Progresso*)	90	4.0	15.0	2.0	<5	850	3.0
(*Progresso* Healthy Classics)	80	4.0	13.0	1.5	5	470	1.0
(*Weight Watchers*), 10½ oz.	130	4.0	27.0	1.0	0	680	6.0
barley (*Health Valley* Fat Free)	90	6.0	19.0	0	0	210	4.0
carotene (*Health Valley* Fat Free)	70	5.0	17.0	0	0	240	6.0
country (*Campbell's* Home Cookin'*)	110	2.0	19.0	1.0	5	760	2.0
country (*Campbell's* Home Cookin'*), 10¾ oz.	130	3.0	26.0	2.0	5	940	2.0
country (*Healthy Choice*)	105	4.0	23.0	<1.0	<5	430	2.5
5 bean (*Health Val-ley*)	140	10.0	32.0	0	0	250	13.0
14 garden (*Health Valley* Fat Free)	80	6.0	17.0	0	0	250	4.0
garden (*Healthy Choice*)	130	8.5	26.0	1.0	0	405	3.0

Food and Measure	cal.	prot. (gms)	carbo. (gms)	fat (gms)	chol. (mgs)	sod. (mgs)	fiber (gms)
Soup, canned, ready-to-serve, vegetable *(cont.)*							
garden (*Old El Paso*)	110	5.0	17.0	2.5	<5	710	0
harborside (*Campbell's* Home Cookin')	80	2.0	13.0	1.5	5	770	2.0
hearty (*Campbell's Healthy Request*)	100	2.0	20.0	1.0	0	470	2.0
hearty (*Pritikin*) . .	90	4.0	20.0	.5	0	290	3.0
hearty, w/pasta (*Campbell's* Chunky)	130	5.0	21.0	3.0	0	1080	3.0
hearty, w/rotini (*Progresso* Pasta Soup)	110	4.0	20.0	1.0	0	720	3.0
Italian (*Campbell's* Home Cookin')	100	6.0	14.0	4.0	5	860	2.0
Italian (*Campbell's* Home Cookin'), 10¾ oz.	130	8.0	17.0	5.0	5	1070	3.0
Mediterranean (*Campbell's* Chunky)	140	8.0	21.0	5.0	5	850	1.0
Southwestern (*Campbell's* Home Cookin')	130	4.0	24.0	2.5	0	750	4.0
Southwestern (*Campbell's Healthy Request*)	140	2.0	28.0	1.0	0	480	5.0
vegetarian (*Pritikin*)	100	4.0	23.0	0	0	290	3.0
vegetable beef:							
(*Campbell's* Chunky)	150	8.0	17.0	5.0	15	870	3.0
(*Campbell's* Chunky), 10¾ oz.	180	9.0	20.0	6.0	20	1090	4.0
(*Campbell's* Home Cookin')	120	3.0	18.0	2.0	5	1010	3.0
(*Campbell's* Home Cookin'), 10¾ oz.	150	4.0	22.0	2.5	10	1260	4.0

Food and Measure	cal.	prot. (gms)	carbo. (gms)	fat (gms)	chol. (mgs)	sod. (mgs)	fiber (gms)
(*Campbell's* Low Sodium), 10¾ oz.	160	7.0	19.0	4.5	80	95	4.0
(*Campbell's* Micro-wave), 1 cont. . . .	90	3.0	13.0	2.0	10	780	2.0
(*Healthy Choice*) . .	130	10.5	22.0	1.0	<5	420	2.0
hearty (*Campbell's Healthy Request*)	140	4.0	20.0	2.5	20	480	3.0
vegetable broth:							
(*Pritikin*)	10	1.0	2.0	0	0	290	0
(*Swanson*)	20	2.0	3.0	1.0	0	1000	0
Soup, canned, condensed (see also "Soup, canned, semi-condensed"), undiluted, ½ cup:							
asparagus, cream of (*Campbell's*)	110	11.0	9.0	7.0	<5	910	1.0
bean:							
w/bacon (*Campbell's*)	180	8.0	25.0	5.0	<5	890	7.0
w/bacon (*Campbell's Healthy Request*)	150	3.0	26.0	2.0	5	480	7.0
black (*Campbell's*)	120	3.0	19.0	2.0	0	1030	5.0
beef:							
broth, double rich (*Campbell's*) . . .	15	0	1.0	0	<5	900	0
consomme (*Campbell's*)	25	0	2.0	0	5	820	0
noodle (*Campbell's*)	70	4.0	8.0	2.5	15	920	1.0
w/vegetables, barley (*Campbell's*) . . .	80	3.0	11.0	2.0	15	920	2.0
broccoli:							
cream of (*Campbell's*)	100	9.0	9.0	6.0	5	770	1.0
cream of (*Campbell's Healthy Request*)	70	3.0	9.0	2.0	5	480	1.0
cheese (*Campbell's*)	110	11.0	7.0	9.0	10	860	2.0

Food and Measure	cal.	prot. (gms)	carbo. (gms)	fat (gms)	chol. (mgs)	sod. (mgs)	fiber (gms)
Soup, canned, condensed *(cont.)*							
celery, cream of:							
(*Campbell's*)	110	11.0	9.0	7.0	<5	900	1.0
(*Campbell's* Reduced Fat)	80	5.0	11.0	3.5	5	900	1.0
(*Campbell's Healthy Request*)	70	3.0	11.0	2.0	5	480	1.0
cheese:							
cheddar (*Campbell's*)	130	12.0	11.0	8.0	20	1080	1.0
nacho (*Campbell's*)	140	12.0	11.0	8.0	15	810	2.0
chicken:							
alphabet, w/vegetables (*Campbell's*)	80	3.0	11.0	2.0	10	880	1.0
broth (*Campbell's*)	30	3.0	2.0	2.0	<5	770	0
cream of (*Campbell's*)	130	12.0	11.0	8.0	10	890	1.0
cream of (*Campbell's* Reduced Fat)	80	6.0	9.0	4.0	15	950	1.0
cream of (*Campbell's Healthy Request*)	70	3.0	12.0	2.0	15	480	0
cream of, and broccoli (*Campbell's*)	120	12.0	9.0	8.0	15	860	1.0
cream of, and broccoli (*Campbell's Healthy Request*)	80	4.0	10.0	2.5	5	480	1.0
dumplings (*Campbell's*)	80	5.0	10.0	3.0	25	1050	2.0
gumbo (*Campbell's*)	60	3.0	9.0	1.5	10	990	1.0
mushroom, creamy (*Campbell's*) . . .	130	14.0	9.0	9.0	15	1000	1.0
noodle (*Campbell's*)	60	3.0	8.0	2.0	15	980	1.0
noodle (*Campbell's Healthy Request*)	70	3.0	9.0	2.0	15	480	0
noodle, creamy (*Campbell's*) . . .	130	11.0	12.0	7.0	15	880	2.0

Food and Measure	cal.	prot. (gms)	carbo. (gms)	fat (gms)	chol. (mgs)	sod. (mgs)	fiber (gms)
noodlé (*Campbell's* Homestyle) . . .	70	4.0	9.0	2.5	20	970	1.0
noodle O's (*Campbell's*)	80	5.0	10.0	3.0	15	980	1.0
w/rice (*Campbell's*)	70	4.0	9.0	2.5	<5	830	0
w/rice (*Campbell's Healthy Request*)	60	4.0	10.0	2.5	5	480	<1.0
and stars (*Campbell's*)	70	3.0	9.0	2.0	0	1010	1.0
vegetable (*Campbell's*)	80	3.0	12.0	2.0	10	940	2.0
vegetable (*Campbell's Healthy Request*)	80	3.0	12.0	2.0	5	480	1.0
vegetable, Southwestern (*Campbell's*)	110	2.0	18.0	1.5	10	900	4.0
wild rice (*Campbell's*)	70	3.0	9.0	2.0	10	900	1.0
wonton (*Campbell's*)	45	2.0	5.0	1.0	15	940	1.0
chili beef w/beans (*Campbell's*)	170	8.0	24.0	5.0	15	910	4.0
clam chowder:							
Manhattan (*Campbell's*)	60	1.0	12.0	.5	<5	910	2.0
New England (*Campbell's*) . . .	100	4.0	15.0	2.5	<5	980	1.0
New England (*Doxsee*)	90	1.0	18.0	2.0	0	600	2.0
corn, golden (*Campbell's*)	120	5.0	20.0	3.5	<5	730	2.0
minestrone:							
(*Campbell's*)	100	3.0	16.0	2.0	0	960	4.0
(*Campbell's Healthy Request*)	90	2.0	17.0	1.0	0	480	2.0
mushroom:							
beefy (*Campbell's*)	70	5.0	6.0	3.0	5	1000	2.0
cream of (*Campbell's*)	110	11.0	9.0	7.0	<5	870	1.0

Food and Measure	cal.	prot. (gms)	carbo. (gms)	fat (gms)	chol. (mgs)	sod. (mgs)	fiber (gms)
Soup, canned, condensed, mushroom *(cont.)*							
cream of (*Campbell's* Reduced Fat)	70	5.0	10.0	3.5	5	940	1.0
cream of (*Campbell's Healthy Request*)	70	4.0	10.0	2.5	10	480	.0
golden (*Campbell's*)	80	5.0	10.0	3.0	5	930	1.0
noodle:							
curly, chicken broth (*Campbell's*) . . .	80	4.0	12.0	2.5	15	840	1.0
double, chicken broth (*Campbell's*)	100	4.0	15.0	2.5	15	810	2.0
and ground beef (*Campbell's*) . . .	100	6.0	11.0	4.0	25	900	2.0
onion:							
creamy (*Campbell's*)	110	9.0	13.0	6.0	20	910	1.0
French, w/beef stock (*Campbell's*) . . .	70	4.0	10.0	2.5	<5	980	1.0
oyster stew (*Campbell's*)	90	9.0	6.0	6.0	20	940	0
pea:							
green (*Campbell's*)	180	5.0	29.0	3.0	5	890	5.0
split, w/ham and bacon (*Campbell's*)	180	5.0	28.0	3.5	<5	860	5.0
pepper, cream of Mexican (*Campbell's*)	110	11.0	10.0	7.0	<5	860	2.0
pepperpot (*Campbell's*)	100	8.0	9.0	5.0	15	1020	1.0
potato, cream of (*Campbell's*)	100	5.0	14.0	3.0	10	890	1.0
Scotch broth (*Campbell's*)	80	5.0	9.0	3.0	10	870	1.0
shrimp, cream of (*Campbell's*)	100	11.0	8.0	7.0	20	890	1.0
tomato:							
(*Campbell's*)	100	3.0	18.0	2.0	0	730	2.0

Food and Measure	cal.	prot. (gms)	carbo. (gms)	fat (gms)	chol. (mgs)	sod. (mgs)	fiber (gms)
(Campbell's Healthy Request)	90	3.0	18.0	2.0	0	460	1.0
bisque *(Campbell's)*	130	5.0	24.0	3.0	5	900	2.0
cream of *(Campbell's* Homestyle)	110	4.0	21.0	2.5	5	860	1.0
fiesta *(Campbell's)*	70	0	16.0	0	0	860	1.0
Italian, w/basil, oregano *(Campbell's)*	100	1.0	23.0	.5	0	820	2.0
rice *(Campbell's* Old Fashioned)	120	3.0	23.0	2.0	5	790	1.0
turkey:							
noodle *(Campbell's)*	80	4.0	10.0	2.5	15	970	1.0
vegetable *(Campbell's)*	80	4.0	11.0	2.5	10	840	2.0
vegetable:							
(Campbell's)	80	2.0	14.0	1.5	<5	920	2.0
(Campbell's Homestyle)	70	3.0	10.0	2.0	0	970	2.0
(Campbell's Old Fashioned)	70	4.0	10.0	2.5	<5	950	2.0
(Campbell's Healthy Request)	90	2.0	16.0	1.0	5	480	2.0
beef *(Campbell's)*	80	3.0	10.0	2.0	10	810	2.0
beef *(Campbell's Healthy Request)*	80	3.0	11.0	2.0	5	480	2.0
California style *(Campbell's)* . . .	60	2.0	10.0	1.0	0	850	2.0
hearty *(Campbell's Healthy Request)*	90	2.0	16.0	1.0	5	480	2.0
hearty, w/pasta *(Campbell's)* . . .	90	2.0	18.0	1.0	0	830	2.0
vegetarian *(Campbell's)*	70	2.0	14.0	1.0	0	770	2.0

Food and Measure	cal.	prot. (gms)	carbo. (gms)	fat (gms)	chol. (mgs)	sod. (mgs)	fiber (gms)
Soup, canned, semi-condensed, undiluted, ⅔ cup:							
bacon, lettuce, tomato w/chicken broth (*Pepperidge Farm*)	130	11.0	14.0	7.0	5	1130	1.0
black bean w/sherry (*Pepperidge Farm*)	120	4.0	19.0	2.5	0	1050	4.0
broccoli, cream of (*Pepperidge Farm*)	90	7.0	11.0	4.5	5	940	2.0
chicken curry (*Pepperidge Farm*) . . .	170	12.0	16.0	8.0	25	1030	2.0
chicken w/rice:							
(*Pepperidge Farm*)	80	5.0	8.0	3.5	15	960	1.0
w/bacon and ham (*Campbell's*) . . .	150	6.0	22.0	4.0	15	1050	1.0
clam chowder:							
Manhattan (*Pepperidge Farm*)	80	3.0	12.0	2.0	<5	860	2.0
New England (*Pepperidge Farm*) . .	160	12.0	13.0	8.0	20	1160	1.0
consommé Madrilene (*Pepperidge Farm*)	50	1.0	6.0	.5	0	910	0
corn chowder (*Pepperidge Farm*) . . .	140	12.0	14.0	8.0	10	1050	2.0
crab (*Pepperidge Farm*)	80	3.0	9.0	2.0	10	1150	2.0
gazpacho (*Pepperidge Farm*)	70	3.0	12.0	2.0	0	1050	2.0
hunter's, w/turkey, beef (*Pepperidge Farm*)	130	9.0	9.0	6.0	15	1150	2.0
lobster bisque (*Pepperidge Farm*) . . .	160	17.0	12.0	11.0	40	1090	1.0
minestrone (*Pepperidge Farm*)	100	6.0	12.0	4.0	<5	870	3.0
mushroom, shiitake (*Pepperidge Farm*)	80	5.0	10.0	3.0	<5	1100	2.0

Food and Measure	cal.	prot. (gms)	carbo. (gms)	fat (gms)	chol. (mgs)	sod. (mgs)	fiber (gms)
onion, French (*Pepperidge Farm*) . . .	50	2.0	7.0	1.0	<5	1080	1.0
oyster stew (*Pepperidge Farm*)	160	15.0	12.0	10.0	30	1040	1.0
pea, green, w/ham (*Pepperidge Farm*)	210	9.0	28.0	6.0	10	1100	4.0
vichyssoise (*Pepperidge Farm*)	120	12.0	11.0	8.0	15	950	2.0
watercress (*Pepperidge Farm*)	80	5.0	11.0	3.5	<5	930	2.0
Soup, frozen (*Tabatchnik*), 7.5 oz.:							
barley mushroom . .	70	2.0	13.0	0	0	540	3.0
barley mushroom, no salt	70	2.0	13.0	0	0	98	3.0
bean, Yankee	160	10.0	27.0	1.5	0	570	11.0
broccoli, cream of . .	90	3.0	12.0	4.0	5	740	3.0
cabbage	60	1.0	14.0	0	0	160	2.0
cheddar vegetable, Wisconsin	140	4.0	12.0	9.0	13	930	1.0
chicken w/noodles:							
and dumplings . . .	70	1.0	13.0	2.0	20	830	1.0
and vegetables . . .	35	2.0	6.0	0	0	850	0
corn chowder	150	3.0	22.0	6.0	5	650	1.0
lentil, Tuscany	140	8.0	25.0	0	0	460	7.0
minestrone	150	9.0	27.0	1.0	0	550	10.0
pea	180	12.0	31.0	1.5	0	520	11.0
pea, no salt	180	12.0	31.0	1.5	0	79	11.0
potato:							
New England	150	4.0	21.0	6.0	9	540	2.0
old-fashioned . . .	70	2.0	16.0	.0	0	540	2.0
spinach, cream of . .	90	3.0	11.0	4.0	5	630	2.0
vegetable	110	5.0	20.0	1.0	0	580	4.0
vegetable, no salt . .	110	5.0	20.0	1.0	0	77	4.0

Food and Measure	cal.	prot. (gms)	carbo. (gms)	fat (gms)	chol. (mgs)	sod. (mgs)	fiber (gms)
Soup mix (see also "Bouillon" and "Soup base, mix"), dry, 1 pkg., except as noted:							
barley:							
better (*Aunt Patsy's Pantry*), 2 tbsp.	90	4.0	17.0	.5	0	360	4.0
chowder (*Buckeye Burgoo*), ⅛ pkg.	125	5.0	25.0	1.0	0	500	4.0
vegetable, hearty (*Fantastic* Cup)	150	6.0	29.0	.5	0	470	6.0
bean:							
(*Bean Cuisine* Bouillabaisse), 1 serving	99	6.0	18.0	<1.0	0	5	5.0
black (*Aunt Patsy's Pantry*), ⅙ pkg.	190	12.0	36.0	1.0	0	260	7.0
black (*Bean Cuisine* Island), 1 serving	126	7.0	24.0	<1.0	0	7	8.0
black (*Knorr* Cup)	190	10.0	36.0	1.0	0	590	9.0
black (*Smart Soup*)	190	10.0	32.0	1.5	0	560	13.0
black, hearty (*Fantastic Jumpin'* Cup)	210	12.0	39.0	1.0	0	470	8.0
black, Santa Fe (*Campbell's Soupsations*)	250	2.0	48.0	1.5	<5	1080	6.0
black, spicy, w/ couscous (*Health Valley*), ⅓ cup . .	130	6.0	29.0	0	0	280	5.0
black, zesty, w/rice (*Health Valley*), ⅓ cup	100	5.0	22.0	0	0	280	4.0
5, hearty (*Fantastic* Cup)	230	12.0	43.0	1.0	0	480	10.0
many (*Buckeye*), ⅛ pkg.	160	10.0	30.0	1.0	0	330	6.0

Food and Measure	cal.	prot. (gms)	carbo. (gms)	fat (gms)	chol. (mgs)	sod. (mgs)	fiber (gms)
many (*Buckeye Northwest Bean*), ⅛ pkg.	200	12.0	35.0	1.0	0	530	5.0
many (*Buckeye*), 3 tbsp.	110	7.0	20.0	.5	0	220	4.0
navy (*Knorr* Cup)	130	7.0	26.0	.5	0	660	5.0
navy (*Aunt Patsy's Pantry*), 3 tbsp.	120	8.0	21.0	0	0	160	2.0
pasta, see "pasta and bean," below							
rice, see "rice and beans," below							
white (*Bean Cuisine* Provençale), 1 serving	103	6.0	19.0	<1.0	0	7	6.0
bean and ham (*Hormel* Micro Cup) . .	190	9.0	28.0	4.0	25	650	7.0
beef vegetable (*Hormel* Micro Cup) . .	90	6.0	14.0	1.0	10	740	2.0
broccoli, cream of (*Knorr* Chef's), 2 tbsp.	60	2.0	9.0	1.5	0	660	2.0
broccoli-cheese:							
cheddar, creamy (*Fantastic* Cup)	130	6.0	23.0	1.5	5	480	2.0
creamy (*Cup-a-Soup*) . .	70	2.0	8.0	3.0	<5	550	1.0
w/ham (*Hormel* Micro Cup) . . .	170	4.0	10.0	13.0	60	700	1.0
and rice (*Uncle Ben's* Hearty) . .	160	7.0	26.0	3.0	5	870	1.0
chicken:							
(*Campbell's* Instant)	130	3.0	22.0	2.0	25	1290	1.0
cream of (*Cup-a-Soup*) . .	70	<1.0	12.0	2. 0	0	640	<1.0
hearty, supreme (*Cup-a-Soup*) . .	90	1.0	13.0	4.0	0	650	<1.0

Food and Measure	cal.	prot. (gms)	carbo. (gms)	fat (gms)	chol. (mgs)	sod. (mgs)	fiber (gms)
Soup mix, chicken *(cont.)*							
noodle *(Campbell's Soup/Recipe),* 3 tbsp.	100	2.0	18.0	1.5	10	790	1.0
noodle *(Cup-a-Soup)* . .	50	2.0	8.0	1.0	10	550	0
noodle, hearty *(Cup-a-Soup)* . .	60	3.0	10.0	1.0	15	590	0
noodle *(Hormel Micro Cup)* . . .	110	10.0	12.0	2.5	30	790	0
onion and rice *(Kettle Creations),* ¼ pkg.	120	4.0	24.0	1.0	<5	690	1.0
pasta and beans *(Kettle Creations),* ¼ pkg.	110	5.0	20.0	1.5	<5	690	3.0
rice *(Hormel* Micro Cup)	110	5.0	17.0	3.0	10	900	1.0
rice *(Mrs. Grass),* ¼ pkg.	80	2.0	15.0	1.0	0	1000	0
thyme *(Aunt Patsy's Pantry),* 2 tbsp.	100	4.0	20.0	.5	0	350	2.0
vegetable *(Smart Soup)*	130	6.0	24.0	1.5	25	590	1.0
chili:							
(Aunt Patsy's Pantry Cowgirl), 4 tbsp.	160	10.0	29.0	<1.0	0	490	4.0
black bean *(Aunt Patsy's Pantry),* 3 tbsp.	100	6.0	20.0	.5	0	350	3.0
chicken *(Aunt Patsy's Pantry),* 4 tbsp.	180	12.0	33.0	<1.0	0	490	3.0
chicken, white *(Buckeye),* ⅕ pkg.	260	18.0	49.0	1.0	0	590	4.0
hearty *(Fantastic Cha-Cha Cup)* . .	220	18.0	37.0	1.0	0	470	13.0
lentil *(Buckeye),* 4 tbsp.	170	14.0	29.0	1.0	0	540	6.0

Food and Measure	cal.	prot. (gms)	carbo. (gms)	fat (gms)	chol. (mgs)	sod. (mgs)	fiber (gms)
lentil (*Buckeye* Rip Roar'n), ⅛ pkg.	130	11.0	23.0	1.0	0	470	5.0
clam chowder, New England:							
(*Hormel* Micro Cup)	130	5.0	16.0	5.0	25	820	1.0
(*Knorr* Chef's), 3 tbsp.	90	4.0	12.0	3.0	10	970	0
corn chowder:							
(*Knorr* Cup)	140	3.0	26.0	3.0	5	700	2.0
(*Smart Soup*) . . .	100	4.0	23.0	1.0	0	300	1.0
and potato, creamy (*Fantastic* Cup)	170	7.0	34.0	1.0	0	580	2.0
w/tomatoes (*Health Valley*), ½ cup . .	90	4.0	20.0	0	0	360	3.0
couscous:							
(*Casbah* Moroccan Stew Cup)	180	5.0	38.0	0	0	460	2.0
w/lentil, hearty (*Fantastic* Cup)	230	12.0	44.0	1.0	0	480	7.0
gumbo, New Orleans (*Campbell's Soupsations*)	170	3.0	34.0	2.0	5	950	2.0
herb, 2 tbsp.:							
fine (*Knorr* Box) . .	100	3.0	13.0	5.0	<5	1010	0
golden, w/lemon (*Lipton Recipe Secrets*)	35	<1.0	7.0	.5	<5	510	0
Italian, w/tomato (*Lipton Recipe Secrets*)	40	1.0	9.0	.5	0	520	0
herb w/garlic, savory (*Lipton Recipe Secrets*), 1 tbsp. . .	35	1.0	6.0	.5	0	460	0
hot and sour (*Knorr* Box), 2 tbsp. . . .	45	<1.0	8.0	1.5	0	810	0
leek (*Knorr* Box), 2 tbsp.	70	2.0	9.0	3.0	<5	780	0

Food and Measure	cal.	prot. (gms)	carbo. (gms)	fat (gms)	chol. (mgs)	sod. (mgs)	fiber (gms)
Soup mix *(cont.)*							
lentil:							
(*Buckeye* Great Lean							
'n Lentils), 3 tbsp.	140	11.0	24.0	1.0	0	250	5.0
(*Smart Soup*) . . .	190	9.0	35.0	1.0	0	490	5.0
hearty (*Campbell's*							
Soup/Recipe) . .	240	2.0	42.0	2.5	<5	1320	7.0
hearty (*Campbell's*							
Soupsations) . .	240	2.0	42.0	15.0	<5	990	7.0
hearty (*Fantastic*							
Country Cup) . .	230	15.0	41.0	1.0	0	480	12.0
hearty (*Knorr* Cup)	220	13.0	42.0	.5	0	590	6.0
red (*Aunt Patsy's*							
Pantry), 2 tbsp.	80	5.0	15.0	.5	0	250	2.0
w/couscous (*Health*							
Valley), 1/3 cup . .	130	7.0	28.0	0	0	360	5.0
minestrone:							
(*Kettle Creations*),							
1/4 pkg.	110	4.0	22.0	1.5	0	750	4.0
(*Smart Soup*) . . .	120	4.0	24.0	.5	0	590	3.0
hearty (*Fantastic*							
Cup)	150	6.0	29.0	1.0	0	480	4.0
hearty (*Knorr* Cup)	120	4.0	28.0	1.0	<5	580	2.0
mushroom:							
beefy (*Lipton Recipe*							
Secrets), 2 tbsp.	35	<1.0	7.0	.5	0	650	0
cream of							
(*Cup-a-Soup*) . .	60	1.0	10.0	2.0	0	610	0
creamy (*Fantastic*							
Cup)	120	6.0	24.0	0	0	570	2.0
noodle:							
(*Nissin Top Ramen*							
Damae)	200	4.0	27.0	8.0	0	830	<1.0
(*Nissin Top Ramen*							
Oriental)	200	4.0	27.0	8.0	0	900	<1.0
(*Nissin Top Ramen*							
Low Fat Oriental)	150	3.0	31.0	1.0	0	1220	<1.0

Food and Measure	cal.	prot. (gms)	carbo. (gms)	fat (gms)	chol. (mgs)	sod. (mgs)	fiber (gms)
w/chicken broth (*Mrs. Grass*), ¼ pkg.	60	2.0	10.0	1.5	20	880	0
chicken free (*Fantastic* Cup)	140	8.0	26.0	.5	0	540	4.0
extra (*Lipton Soup Secrets*), 3 tbsp.	90	3.0	15.0	1.5	25	680	<1.0
homestyle (*Borden*), ¼ pkg.	70	3.0	11.0	1.5	15	730	0
onion and Oriental (*Sanwa* Ramen), ½ block	180	11.0	26.0	7.0	0	700	1.0
Oriental (*Campbell's* Ramen Low Fat)	220	2.0	45.0	1.5	0	1360	2.0
Oriental (*Campbell's* Ramen Low Fat), ½ block	140	2.0	29.0	1.0	0	740	1.0
Oriental (*Sanwa* Ramen), ½ block	180	11.0	26.0	7.0	0	850	1.0
ring noodle (*Cup-a-Soup*) . .	50	2.0	9.0	1.0	10	560	0
noodle, beef:							
(*Campbell's* Instant)	120	2.0	22.0	1.5	20	1260	1.0
(*Campbell's* Ramen Fried Cup)	280	17.0	40.0	11.0	<5	1240	3.0
(*Campbell's* Ramen Low Fat)	220	2.0	45.0	1.5	0	1370	2.0
(*Campbell's* Ramen Low Fat), ½ block	140	2.0	29.0	1.0	0	780	1.0
(*Campbell's/Sanwa* Ramen), ½ block	180	11.0	26.0	7.0	0	870	1.0
(*Nissin Cup Noodles*)	290	7.0	39.0	12.0	0	1540	2.0
(*Nissin Cup Noodles Twin*), 1.2 oz. . . .	160	4.0	20.0	7.0	0	870	<1.0
(*Nissin Top Ramen*)	200	4.0	27.0	8.0	0	1020	<1.0
(*Nissin Top Ramen Low Fat*)	150	3.0	31.0	1.0	0	1140	<1.0

Food and Measure	cal.	prot. (gms)	carbo. (gms)	fat (gms)	chol. (mgs)	sod. (mgs)	fiber (gms)
Soup mix, noodle, beef *(cont.)*							
onion (*Nissin Cup Noodles*)	280	6.0	40.0	11.0	0	1300	1.0
spicy (*Nissin Top Ramen*)	200	4.0	27.0	8.0	0	710	<1.0
noodle, chicken:							
(*Campbell's* Ramen)	280	17.0	40.0	11.0	0	1360	3.0
(*Campbell's* Ramen Low Fat)	210	2.0	45.0	1.0	0	1480	2.0
(*Campbell's* Ramen Low Fat), ½ block	140	2.0	29.0	1.0	0	790	1.0
(*Campbell's/Sanwa* Ramen)	310	20.0	41.0	13.0	0	1080	2.0
(*Knorr* Box), 2 tbsp.	90	3.0	17.0	1.0	15	800	0
(*Knorr* Cup)	110	4.0	19.0	2.0	20	800	0
(*Lipton Soup Secrets*), 3 tbsp.	80	3.0	12.0	2.5	15	650	0
(*Lipton Soup Secrets Giggle Noodle*), 2 tbsp.	80	3.0	11.0	2.0	15	730	0
(*Lipton Soup Secrets Ring-O-Noodle*), 2 tbsp.	70	2.0	10.0	2.0	10	710	0
(*Nissin Cup Noodles*)	300	6.0	39.0	12.0	<5	1220	2.0
(*Nissin Cup Noodles* Twin), 1.2 oz. . .	160	3.0	20.0	7.0	0	940	<1.0
(*Nissin Top Ramen*)	200	4.0	27.0	8.0	0	930	<1.0
(*Nissin Top Ramen* Low Fat)	150	3.0	31.0	1.0	0	1120	<1.0
(*Sanwa* Ramen Pride), ½ block	180	11.0	26.0	7.0	0	810	1.0
broth (*Campbell's* Instant)	130	3.0	23.0	2.0	20	1320	1.0
broth (*Campbell's* Soup/Recipe), ½ cup	190	4.0	35.0	2.5	35	820	1.0

Food and Measure	cal.	prot. (gms)	carbo. (gms)	fat (gms)	chol. (mgs)	sod. (mgs)	fiber (gms)
broth (*Lipton Soup Secrets*), 2 tbsp.	60	2.0	9.0	2.0	15	710	0
broth (*Mrs. Grass*), ¼ pkg.	60	2.0	10.0	1.5	20	880	0
curry (*Campbell's/ Sanwa* Ramen), ½ block	190	11.0	28.0	7.0	0	740	1.0
curry (*Sanwa* Ramen Pride) . .	310	22.0	40.0	14.0	0	1190	2.0
hearty (*Lipton Soup Secrets*), ¼ cup	80	4.0	14.0	2.0	20	670	0
mushroom (*Nissin Cup Noodles*) . .	300	6.0	39.0	13.0	0	1360	2.0
mushroom (*Nissin Top Ramen*) . . .	200	4.0	27.0	8.0	0	720	1.0
sesame (*Nissin Top Ramen*)	200	4.0	27.0	8.0	0	770	<1.0
spicy (*Campbell's Ramen Low Fat*), ½ block	140	2.0	29.0	1.0	0	910	1.0
spicy (*Nissin Cup Noodles*)	300	7.0	38.0	13.0	<5	1120	2.0
spicy (*Nissin Cup Noodles* Twin), 1.2 oz.	160	4.0	20.0	7.0	0	900	<1.0
w/vegetables (*Health Valley*), ⅓ cup . .	80	3.0	18.0	0	0	360	2.0
noodle, crab (*Nissin Cup Noodles*) . . .	290	6.0	39.0	12.0	0	1310	1.0
noodle, lobster (*Nissin Cup Noodles*) . . .	300	6.0	40.0	7.0	0	1300	2.0
noodle, pork: (*Campbell's* Ramen Low Fat)	220	2.0	45.0	1.5	5	1110	2.0
(*Campbell's* Ramen Low Fat), ½ block	140	2.0	29.0	1.0	0	850	1.0
(*Campbell's/Sanwa* Oriental), ½ block	180	11.0	26.0	7.0	0	760	1.0

Food and Measure	cal.	prot. (gms)	carbo. (gms)	fat (gms)	chol. (mgs)	sod. (mgs)	fiber (gms)
Soup mix, noodle, pork *(cont.)*							
(*Nissin Cup Noodles*)	290	7.0	39.0	12.0	0	1510	1.0
(*Nissin Top Ramen*)	200	4.0	27.0	8.0	0	820	<1.0
noodle, shrimp:							
(*Campbell's* Ramen)	310	22.0	40.0	14.0	0	1020	2.0
(*Campbell's* Ramen Low Fat)	220	2.0	46.0	1.0	10	1140	2.0
(*Campbell's* Ramen Low Fat), ½ block	140	2.0	29.0	1.0	0	720	1.0
(*Nissin Cup Noodles*)	290	7.0	39.0	12.0	15	1550	1.0
(*Nissin Cup Noodles* Twin), 1.2 oz. . .	150	4.0	20.0	6.0	0	900	<1.0
(*Nissin Top Ramen*)	200	4.0	27.0	8.0	0	1070	<1.0
(*Sanwa* Ramen Pride)	310	22.0	40.0	14.0	0	1020	2.0
picante (*Nissin Cup Noodles*)	290	6.0	40.0	12.0	5	1290	1.0
Thai (*Sanwa* Ramen), ½ block	190	11.0	28.0	7.0	0	730	1.0
Thai (*Sanwa* Ramen Pride)	310	20.0	40.0	13.0	10	1540	2.0
noodle, vegetable:							
beef (*Mrs. Grass*), ¼ pkg.	70	3.0	11.0	1.0	0	1030	0
beef (*Sanwa* Ramen Pride)	300	20.0	40.0	13.0	0	1410	2.0
curry (*Fantastic* Cup)	140	6.0	28.0	1.0	0	490	3.0
egg, in broth (*Campbell's* Soupsations)	150	3.0	27.0	2.0	20	980	2.0
garden (*Nissin Cup Noodles*)	290	6.0	40.0	12.0	0	1310	1.0
hearty (*Campbell's* Instant)	150	3.0	28.0	2.0	20	1050	1.0
hearty (*Lipton Soup Secrets*), 3 tbsp.	70	2.0	11.0	2.0	10	710	<1.0

Food and Measure	cal.	prot. (gms)	carbo. (gms)	fat (gms)	chol. (mgs)	sod. (mgs)	fiber (gms)
miso (*Fantastic* Cup)	130	5.0	25.0	1.0	0	540	2.0
tomato (*Campbell's/ Sanwa* Ramen Pride)	310	22.0	40.0	14.0	0	860	2.0
tomato (*Fantastic* Cup)	150	5.0	31.0	1.0	0	490	3.0
onion:							
(*Campbell's* Soup/ Recipe), 1 tbsp.	25	0	5.0	0	0	660	0
(*Campbell's* Soup/ Recipe), 2 tbsp.	50	2.0	10.0	1.0	0	760	1.0
(*Knorr* Box), 2 tbsp.	45	1.0	8.0	1.0	<5	980	0
(*Lipton Recipe Secrets*), 1 tbsp.	20	0	4.0	0	0	610	<1.0
(*Mrs. Grass* Soup/ Recipe), ¼ pkg.	35	1.0	6.0	.5	0	980	0
(*Mrs. Grass* Low Sodium), ¼ pkg.	35	1.0	7.0	0	0	490	0
beefy (*Lipton Recipe Secrets*), 1 tbsp.	25	<1.0	5.0	.5	0	610	0
golden (*Lipton Recipe Secrets*), 2 tbsp.	60	1.0	10.0	1.5	0	650	0
onion-mushroom:							
(*Lipton Recipe Secrets*), 2 tbsp.	35	1.0	6.0	1.0	0	620	0
(*Mrs. Grass* Soup/ Recipe), ⅓ pkg.	60	2.0	10.0	1.0	0	1080	0
orzo thyme (*Buckeye*), ¼ pkg.	210	7.0	41.0	1.0	0	270	2.0
oxtail (*Knorr* Box), 2 tbsp.	60	2.0	9.0	2.5	<5	910	0
pasta:							
(*Buckeye* Many Mac), ¹⁄₁₀ pkg. . . .	160	6.0	32.0	1.0	0	480	1.0
(*Buckeye* Starry), ¹⁄₁₀ pkg.	80	3.0	16.0	0	0	490	1.0

Food and Measure	cal.	prot. (gms)	carbo. (gms)	fat (gms)	chol. (mgs)	sod. (mgs)	fiber (gms)
Soup mix, pasta *(cont.)*							
Italiano (*Health Valley* Fat Free),							
½ cup	140	5.0	31.0	0	0	360	3.0
marinara, Parmesan, or Mediterranean (*Health Valley* Pasta Cup Fat Free), ½ cup . .	100	5.0	20.0	0	0	190	1.0
ruffle (*Lipton Soup Secrets*), 2 tbsp.	60	2.0	10.0	1.0	0	670	0
pasta and bean:							
(*Casbah Pasta Fasul*)	160	11.0	12.0	0	0	470	2.0
(*Kettle Creations*), ¼ pkg.	130	6.0	23.0	1.5	<5	690	4.0
(*Bean Cuisine* Ultima), 1 serving	117	7.0	22.0	<1.0	0	8	4.0
white bean (*Uncle Ben's* Hearty), ⅕ oz.	160	7.0	27.0	2.0	0	820	7.0
pea:							
green (*Cup-a-Soup*)	110	3.0	17.0	3.5	0	620	3.0
snow, cream of (*Knorr* Chef's), 3 tbsp.	70	2.0	10.0	2.0	0	700	0
pea, split:							
(*Aunt Patsy's Pantry*), 3 tbsp. . . .	160	12.0	28.0	.5	0	580	3.0
(*Bean Cuisine* Thick as Fog), 1 serving	116	8.0	21.0	<1.0	0	13	1.0
(*Buckeye* Country Pea Patchwork), ⅛ pkg.	160	12.0	29.0	1.0	0	340	3.0
(*Knorr* Cup)	150	8.0	29.0	.5	0	690	4.0
(*Smart Soup*) . . .	150	8.0	28.0	.5	0	460	7.0
hearty (*Fantastic* Cup)	190	12.0	35.0	1.0	0	470	8.0

Food and Measure	cal.	prot. (gms)	carbo. (gms)	fat (gms)	chol. (mgs)	sod. (mgs)	fiber (gms)
w/carrots (*Health Valley*), ½ cup . .	130	8.0	25.0	0	0	360	2.0
potato, w/broccoli (*Health Valley*), ⅓ cup	70	4.0	15.0	0	0	360	2.0
potato cheese, w/ham (*Hormel* Micro Cup)	190	4.0	16.0	13.0	60	730	1.0
potato leek:							
(*Knorr* Cup)	120	4.0	24.0	0	0	970	1.0
(*Smart Soup*) . . .	120	6.0	23.0	1.0	5	590	1.0
rice (*Casbah Thai Yum*)	160	4.0	30.0	0	0	470	2.0
rice and beans:							
(*Casbah* La Fiesta)	170	6.0	34.0	1.0	0	400	4.0
black (*Uncle Ben's* Hearty)	150	7.0	28.0	1.5	0	430	6.0
Cajun (*Casbah* Jambalaya) . . .	128	4.0	27.0	0	0	490	2.0
Cajun (*Fantastic* Cup)	240	10.0	47.0	1.5	0	480	6.0
Caribbean (*Fantastic* Cup)	230	10.0	44.0	1.5	0	480	6.0
curry, Bombay (*Fantastic* Cup)	260	12.0	46.0	3.0	0	470	8.0
Mexican (*Campbell's* Soupsations) . .	210	2.0	41.0	1.5	<5	930	6.0
Northern Italian (*Fantastic* Cup)	240	8.0	49.0	1.5	0	460	4.0
red (*Smart Soup*)	180	8.0	35.0	1.0	0	460	7.0
Szechuan (*Fantastic* Cup)	210	7.0	41.0	2.0	0	480	3.0
Tex-Mex (*Fantastic* Cup)	270	10.0	53.0	2.0	0	540	8.0
spinach, cream of (*Knorr* Box), 2 tbsp.	70	2.0	9.0	2.5	0	600	0
tomato:							
(*Cup-a-Soup*) . . .	90	2.0	20.0	1.0	0	510	<1.0
basil (*Knorr* Box), 2 tbsp.	80	2.0	14.0	2.0	0	970	0

Food and Measure	cal.	prot. (gms)	carbo. (gms)	fat (gms)	chol. (mgs)	sod. (mgs)	fiber (gms)
Soup mix, tomato *(cont.)*							
basil (*Uncle Ben's* Hearty)	110	3.0	18.0	2.5	10	680	2.0
rice Parmesano (*Fantastic* Cup)	200	6.0	41.0	2.0	0	550	2.0
vegetable (*Campbell's Soupsations*)	130	3.0	25.0	2.0	15	900	2.0
vegetable:							
(*Campbell's* Soup/ Recipe), 2 tbsp.	35	0	7.0	0	0	650	0
(*Knorr* Box), 2 tbsp.	30	1.0	6.0	0	0	730	1.0
(*Lipton Recipe Secrets*), 2 tbsp.	30	<1.0	7.0	0	0	580	1.0
(*Mrs. Grass* Soup/ Recipe), 1/4 pkg.	35	1.0	7.0	0	0	900	1.0
barley, hearty (*Fantastic* Cup)	150	6.0	29.0	.5	0	470	6.0
beef (*Mrs. Grass*), 1/4 pkg.	70	3.0	11.0	1.0	0	1030	0
chicken flavor (*Cup-a-Soup*) . .	50	1.0	10.0	1.0	10	520	0
chicken flavor (*Knorr* Cup) . . .	100	3.0	19.0	1.0	<5	770	0
chicken flavor, creamy (*Cup-a-Soup*) . .	90	2.0	10.0	4.0	0	590	<1.0
w/rice and pasta (*Ronco* Natural), 1/8 pkg.	90	5.0	16.0	.5	0	5	4.0
spring (*Cup-a-Soup*)	45	2.0	8.0	1.0	10	500	<1.0
spring (*Knorr*), 2 tbsp.	25	1.0	5.0	0	0	550	1.0
Soup base, bottled:							
(*Goya* Recaito), 1 tsp.	3	<1	0	0	0	35	0
(*Goya* Sofrito), 1 tsp.	5	0	1.0	0	0	45	0

Food and Measure	cal.	prot. (gms)	carbo. (gms)	fat (gms)	chol. (mgs)	sod. (mgs)	fiber (gms)
Soup base, mix, ⅛ pkg., except as noted:							
beef, ground, vegetable (*Soup Starter*)	80	3.0	17.0	.5	0	990	2.0
beef, ground, vegetable (*Soup Starter Quick Cook*), ¼ pkg.	80	3.0	17.0	.5	0	1020	2.0
beef barley vegetable (*Soup Starter*) . . .	100	3.0	20.0	.5	0	960	3.0
beef stew, hearty (*Soup Starter*), ⅟₇ pkg.	80	2.0	17.0	0	0	850	2.0
beef vegetable (*Soup Starter*)	90	3.0	19.0	.5	0	990	2.0
chicken noodle (*Soup Starter*)	80	2.0	17.0	.5	5	960	1.0
chicken noodle (*Soup Starter Quick Cook*), ¼ pkg.	80	2.0	16.0	1.0	0	1060	1.0
chicken and rice (*Soup Starter*) . . .	70	2.0	14.0	.5	0	780	1.0
chicken and rice (*Soup Starter Quick Cook*), ¼ pkg. . . .	50	1.0	12.0	0	0	900	<1.0
chicken vegetable (*Soup Starter*), ⅟₇ pkg.	70	2.0	16.0	0	0	850	2.0
chicken w/white and wild rice (*Soup Starter*)	70	2.0	15.0	0	0	790	1.0
Sour cream, see "Cream, sour"							
Sour cream dip mix (*Durkee*), 2 tsp. . . .	25	1.0	4.0	.5	0	200	0
Soursop, ½ cup . . .	75	1.1	18.9	.3	0	16	3.7
Soy beverage, 8 fl. oz.:							
(*EdenSoy*)	130	10.0	13.0	4.0	0	105	0

Food and Measure	cal.	prot. (gms)	carbo. (gms)	fat (gms)	chol. (mgs)	sod. (mgs)	fiber (gms)
Soy beverage *(cont.)*							
(*EdenSoy* Extra) . . .	130	9.0	12.0	5.0	0	100	0
(*Soy Moo* Fat Free)	110	6.0	22.0	0	0	60	1.0
carob (*EdenSoy*) . . .	150	6.0	23.0	4.0	0	105	0
milk	79	6.6	4.3	4.6	0	30	3.1
vanilla:							
(*EdenSoy*)	150	6.0	23.0	3.0	0	90	0
(*EdenSoy* Extra) . .	140	6.0	23.0	3.0	0	90	0
Soy beverage mix,							
dry, ¼ cup:							
(*Loma Linda Soyagen*							
No Sucrose)	130	6.0	12.0	6.0	0	160	3.0
all purpose (*Loma*							
Linda Soyagen) . .	130	6.0	12.0	6.0	0	150	3.0
carob (*Loma Linda*							
Soyagen)	130	6.0	13.0	6.0	0	170	2.0
Soy flour:							
(*Arrowhead Mills*),							
½ cup	200	16.0	16.0	9.0	0	0	8.0
stirred, 1 cup:							
full fat, raw	371	29.4	29.9	17.6	0	11	8.2
full fat, roasted . .	375	29.6	28.6	18.6	0	11	n.a.
defatted	329	47.0	38.4	1.2	0	20	17.5
lowfat	287	40.9	33.4	2.4	0	16	9.0
Soy meal, defatted,							
raw, 1 cup	414	54.8	49.0	2.9	0	3	14.0
Soy milk, see "Soy							
beverage"							
Soy protein, concen-							
trate, 1 oz.:							
w/alcohol	94	16.5	8.8	.1	0	1	<2.0
acid/water wash . . .	94	16.5	8.8	.1	0	255	<2.0
Soy sauce, 1 tbsp.,							
except as noted:							
(*House of Tsang*),							
.5-oz. pkt.	5	0	<1.0	0	0	770	0
(*House of Tsang*							
Light)	5	0	0	0	0	900	0

Food and Measure	cal.	prot. (gms)	carbo. (gms)	fat (gms)	chol. (mgs)	sod. (mgs)	fiber (gms)
(*House of Tsang* Low Sodium)	5	0	0	0	0	280	0
(*Kikkoman*)	10	2.0	0	0	0	920	0
(*Kikkoman* Light) . .	10	1.0	1.0	0	0	605	0
(*La Choy*)	10	1.5	1.0	0	0	1225	0
(*La Choy* Lite)	15	2.0	2.0	0	0	540	0
dark (*House of Tsang*)	10	0	1.0	0	0	860	0
ginger flavor (*House of Tsang*)	20	1.0	4.0	0	0	730	0
ginger or mushroom flavor (*House of Tsang* Low Sodium)	10	0	2.0	0	0	280	0
hot (*Try Me Dragon Sauce*), 1 tsp. . . .	5	<1.0	<1.0	0	0	260	0
tamari:							
(*Eden* Domestic) . .	15	2.0	2.0	0	0	970	0
(*Eden* Imported) . .	10	2.0	2.0	0	0	1130	0
shoyu:							
(*Eden* Imported) . .	15	2.0	2.0	0	0	1040	0
(*Eden* Traditional)	15	2.0	2.0	0	0	1010	0
Soybean, ½ cup:							
green:							
raw, shelled	188	16.6	14.1	8.7	0	n.a.	5.4
boiled, drained . . .	127	11.1	10.0	5.8	0	n.a.	3.8
dried:							
raw (*Arrowhead Mills*), ¼ cup . .	170	15.0	14.0	8.0	0	0	10.0
boiled	149	14.3	8.5	7.7	0	1	5.2
dry-roasted	387	34.0	28.1	18.6	0	2	7.0
roasted	405	30.3	28.9	21.8	0	140	7.0
Soybean cake or curd, see "Tofu"							
Soybean kernels, roasted, toasted:							
1 oz. or 95 kernels	129	10.5	8.7	6.8	0	1	1.0
whole, 1 cup	490	40.0	33.0	25.9	0	4	3.9
salted, whole, 1 cup	490	40.0	33.0	25.9	0	176	3.9

Food and Measure	cal.	prot. (gms)	carbo. (gms)	fat (gms)	chol. (mgs)	sod. (mgs)	fiber (gms)
Soybean sprouts (*Jonathan's*), 1 cup, 3 oz.	100	11.0	8.0	6.0	0	10	2.0
Spaghetti, see "Pasta"							
Spaghetti dinner, and meatballs, frozen (*Swanson*), 1 pkg.	300	18.0	36.0	12.0	20	1050	5.0
Spaghetti dishes, mix:							
w/meat sauce (*Kraft* Dinner), 5.5 oz. . .	330	12.0	46.0	11.0	15	830	3.0
mild (*Kraft* American Dinner), 2 oz. . . .	200	8.0	40.0	1.5	<5	520	1.0
tangy (*Kraft* Italian Dinner), 2 oz. . . .	200	9.0	38.0	2.0	<5	610	1.0
Spaghetti entree, canned, 1 cup, except as noted:							
(*Franco-American Garfield* Pizzos)	190	3.0	36.0	2.0	5	990	2.0
w/beef (*Franco-American Garfield* Pizzos)	260	17.0	31.0	11.0	20	1150	5.0
w/franks:							
(*Franco-American* SpaghettiO's) . .	250	17.0	32.0	11.0	25	1210	4.0
(*Van Camp's Weenee*), 1 can	230	7.0	34.0	8.0	20	670	1.0
rings (*Kid's Kitchen*), 7½ oz.	230	9.0	36.0	6.0	15	880	3.0
w/meatballs:							
(*Campbell's Superiore/Franco-American*)	270	15.0	35.0	10.0	30	1060	4.0
(*Franco-American* SpaghettiO's) . .	260	17.0	31.0	11.0	20	1150	5.0
(*Hormel* Micro Cup), 7½ oz.	210	10.0	28.0	7.0	20	940	2.0

Food and Measure	cal.	prot. (gms)	carbo. (gms)	fat (gms)	chol. (mgs)	sod. (mgs)	fiber (gms)
(*Libby's Diner*),							
7¾ oz.	190	2.0	27.0	5.0	20	940	2.0
(*Top Shelf*), 10 oz.	300	16.0	35.0	11.0	35	1650	3.0
mini meatballs							
(*Kid's Kitchen*),							
7½ oz.	220	11.0	28.0	8.0	25	940	2.0
rings (*Kid's*							
Kitchen), 7½ oz.	250	11.0	35.0	7.0	20	1200	3.0
rings (*Kid's Kitchen*),							
7½ oz.	190	8.0	34.0	2.0	10	920	2.0
tomato-cheese sauce:							
(*Franco-American*)	210	3.0	41.0	2.0	5	1020	3.0
(*Franco-American*							
SpaghettiO's) . .	190	3.0	36.0	2.0	5	990	2.0
Spaghetti entree,							
freeze-dried, w/							
meat, sauce (*Moun-*							
tain House), 1 cup	200	12.0	27.0	5.0	15	910	3.0
Spaghetti entree, fro-							
zen, 1 pkg.:							
Bolognese:							
(*Banquet*)	370	14.0	40.0	16.0	35	1040	6.0
(*Healthy Choice*) . .	260	14.0	43.0	3.0	15	470	5.0
marinara (*Marie Cal-*							
lender's)	270	10.0	35.0	10.0	10	540	3.0
w/meat sauce:							
(*The Budget Gour-*							
met Light &							
Healthy)	320	15.0	49.0	7.0	5	470	4.0
(*Lean Cuisine*) . . .	290	14.0	45.0	6.0	20	550	4.0
(*Morton*)	170	6.0	30.0	3.0	<5	600	4.0
(*Stouffer's Lunch*							
Express)	320	15.0	43.0	10.0	30	580	5.0
(*Weight Watchers*)	290	14.0	45.0	6.0	15	560	5.0
w/meatballs:							
(*Lean Cuisine*) . . .	290	17.0	40.0	7.0	30	520	4.0
(*Stouffer's*)	420	19.0	51.0	15.0	45	680	5.0
Spaghetti sauce, see							
"Pasta sauce"							

Food and Measure	cal.	prot. (gms)	carbo. (gms)	fat (gms)	chol. (mgs)	sod. (mgs)	fiber (gms)
Spaghetti squash,							
baked or boiled,							
drained, ½ cup . .	23	.5	5.0	.2	0	14	1.1
Spareribs, see "Pork"							
Spearmint, dried							
(*McCormick*),							
¼ tsp.	1	0	.1	0	0	1	0
Spelt flakes (*Arrow-*							
head Mills), 1 cup	100	5.0	22.0	1.0	0	60	3.0
Spelt flour (*Arrow-*							
head Mills), ¼ cup	100	4.0	24.0	.5	0	0	5.0
Spinach:							
fresh, ½ cup:							
raw, chopped . . .	6	.8	1.0	.1	0	22	.8
boiled, drained . . .	21	2.7	3.4	.2	0	63	2.2
canned, ½ cup:							
(*Allens Popeye*) . .	45	2.0	7.0	1.0	0	310	4.0
(*Allens Popeye* Low							
Sodium)	35	2.0	4.0	1.0	0	35	3.0
(*Del Monte*)	30	2.0	4.0	0	0	360	2.0
(*Del Monte* No Salt)	30	2.0	4.0	0	0	85	2.0
(*S&W*)	30	3.0	4.0	0	0	440	2.0
chopped (*Allens*							
Popeye/Sunshine)	40	2.0	6.0	1.0	0	310	4.0
frozen (see also							
"Spinach dishes"):							
(*Green Giant*),							
½ cup	25	3.0	3.0	0	0	65	3.0
(*Green Giant Har-*							
vest Fresh),							
½ cup	25	3.0	3.0	0	0	240	2.0
leaf (*Seabrook*),							
1 cup	20	2.0	2.0	0	0	110	2.0
chopped (*Seabrook*),							
⅓ cup	20	2.0	2.0	0	0	115	2.0
in butter sauce, cut							
(*Green Giant*),							
½ cup	40	2.0	5.0	1.5	<5	280	4.0

Food and Measure	cal.	prot. (gms)	carbo. (gms)	fat (gms)	chol. (mgs)	sod. (mgs)	fiber (gms)
Spinach, New Zealand, chopped:							
raw, 1 oz. or ½ cup	4	.4	.7	.1	0	37	n.a.
boiled, drained, ½ cup	11	1.2	2.0	.2	0	97	n.a.
Spinach dip (*Marie's*),							
2 tbsp.	140	2.0	3.0	14.0	10	200	0
Spinach dishes, frozen:							
au gratin (*The Budget Gourmet* Side Dish),							
5.5 oz.	150	6.0	9.0	11.0	30	730	1.0
creamed:							
(*Green Giant*),							
½ cup	80	4.0	10.0	3.0	0	520	2.0
(*Seabrook*), ½ cup	120	4.0	10.0	6.0	15	450	3.0
(*Stouffer's* Side Dish), ½ of							
9-oz. pkg.	160	4.0	8.0	12.0	15	380	2.0
(*Tabatchnick*),							
7.5 oz.	60	2.0	8.0	2.0	5	270	2.0
feta pocket (*Amy's*),							
1 pc.	200	9.0	27.0	7.0	15	420	2.0
Indian (*Deep* Palak Paneer), 5 oz. . . .	230	8.0	7.0	19.0	25	690	4.0
souffle (*Stouffer's* Side Dish), 4 oz.	150	6.0	9.0	10.0	120	480	9.0
Spinach salad, see "Salad blend mix"							
Spiny lobster, meat only:							
raw, 4 oz.	127	23.4	2.8	1.7	80	201	0
boiled or steamed, 2-lb. lobster w/shell	233	43.1	5.1	3.2	146	370	0
boiled or steamed, 4 oz.	138	29.9	3.5	2.2	102	257	0
Split peas, dried:							
(*Goya*), ¼ cup	110	11.0	27.0	0	0	25	11.0
boiled, ½ cup	116	8.2	20.7	.4	0	2	8.1

Food and Measure	cal.	prot. (gms)	carbo. (gms)	fat (gms)	chol. (mgs)	sod. (mgs)	fiber (gms)
Split peas *(cont.)*							
green, (*Arrowhead*							
Mills), ¼ cup . . .	170	12.0	31.0	.5	0	20	7.0
yellow (*Goya*), ¼ cup	110	10.0	28.0	0	0	20	12.0
Sports drink, 8 fl. oz.,							
except as noted:							
all flavors:							
(*Body Works*),							
12 fl. oz.	90	0	23.0	0	0	145	0
except orange							
(*Recharge*) . . .	70	0	18.0	0	0	25	0
fruit punch (*All Sport*)	80	0	22.0	0	0	55	0
grape (*All Sport*) . .	80	0	20.0	0	0	55	0
lemon-lime or orange							
(*All Sport*)	70	0	20.0	0	0	55	0
orange (*Recharge*) . .	70	4.0	18.0	0	0	25	0
Spot, meat only:							
raw, 4 oz.	140	21.0	0	5.6	n.a.	33	0
baked, broiled, or mi-							
crowaved, 4 oz. . .	179	26.9	0	7.1	n.a.	42	0
Sprouts (see also							
specific listings):							
bean:							
(*Frieda's*), 1 oz. . .	10	1.1	1.9	.1	0	1	n.a.
canned (*La Choy*),							
1 cup	10	1.0	2.0	0	0	20	1.0
hot and spicy (*Jona-*							
than's), 1 cup, 4 oz.	25	3.0	4.0	0	0	15	2.0
mixed:							
(*Jonathan's* Gour-							
met), 1 cup, 3 oz.	20	3.0	3.0	0	0	10	2.0
(*Shaw's*), 2 oz. . .	9	2.0	0	<1.0	0	40	2.0
lentil, adzuki, pea							
(*Jonathan's*),							
3 oz.	100	7.0	21.0	0	0	10	4.0
Squab, fresh, raw:							
meat w/skin, 4 oz. . . .	333	20.9	0	27.0	n.a.	n.a.	0
breast meat only,							
4 oz.	161	19.8	0	8.5	n.a.	n.a.	0

Food and Measure	cal.	prot. (gms)	carbo. (gms)	fat (gms)	chol. (mgs)	sod. (mgs)	fiber (gms)
Squash (see also specific squash listings):							
canned (*Stokely*), ½ cup	50	1.0	10.0	0	0	0	4.0
frozen (*Stilwell*), ½ cup	15	<1.0	2.0	0	0	15	1.0
Squid, meat only, raw, 4 oz.	104	17.7	3.5	1.6	265	50	0
Squid, canned:							
(*Goya*), ⅕ can	45	10.0	1.0	0	50	280	0
in juice (*Goya*), ¼ cup	120	8.0	2.0	9.0	15	350	0
Star fruit, see "Carambola"							
Steak, see "Beef"							
Steak sandwich, see "Beef sandwich"							
Steak sauce, 1 tbsp.:							
(*A.1.*)	15	0	3.0	0	0	250	0
(*A.1.* Bold)	20	0	5.0	0	0	190	0
(*A.1.* Thick and Hearty)	25	0	6.0	0	0	280	0
(*Alanna* Irish)	15	0	4.0	0	0	230	0
(*Heinz 57*)	15	0	4.0	0	0	220	0
(*HP*)	15	0	3.0	0	0	150	0
(*Hunt's*)	10	0	2.0	0	0	250	<1.0
(*Maull's*)	20	0	5.0	0	0	250	0
(*Texas Best*)	15	0	4.0	0	0	220	0
(*Trappey's* Great American)	16	0	4.0	0	0	150	0
and burger (*Try Me Bullfighter*)	15	0	4.0	0	0	220	0
Caribbean style (*Tabasco*)	15	0	4.0	0	0	130	0
garlic peppercorn (*Lea & Perrins*)	25	0	6.0	0	0	110	0
New Orleans style:							
(*Tabasco*)	10	0	2.0	0	0	90	0

Food and Measure	cal.	prot. (gms)	carbo. (gms)	fat (gms)	chol. (mgs)	sod. (mgs)	fiber (gms)
Steak sauce, New Orleans style *(cont.)*							
(*Trappey's Chef-Magic*)	10	0	2.0	0	0	70	<1.0
sweet:							
mild (*Maull's*) . . .	20	0	4.0	0	0	190	0
spicy (*Lea & Perrins*)	25	0	6.0	0	0	140	0
Stir-fry entree, frozen:							
lo-mein:							
(*Green Giant Create A Meal!*), 2⅓ cup[1]	160	7.0	32.0	.5	0	1070	5.0
(*Green Giant Create A Meal!*), 1¼ cup[2]	320	32.0	32.0	7.0	65	1140	5.0
sweet and sour:							
(*Green Giant Create A Meal!*), 2¾ cup[1]	130	3.0	29.0	0	0	390	5.0
(*Green Giant Create A Meal!*), 1¼ cup[2]	290	27.0	29.0	7.0	20	460	5.0
Szechuan:							
(*Green Giant Create A Meal!*), 2¾ cup[1]	150	6.0	21.0	5.0	0	1220	5.0
(*Green Giant Create A Meal!*), 1¼ cup[2]	320	27.0	21.0	14.0	20	1280	5.0
teriyaki:							
(*Green Giant Create A Meal!*), 2¾ cup[1]	100	5.0	19.0	0	0	870	4.0
(*Green Giant Create A Meal!*), 1¼ cup[2]	240	27.0	19.0	6.0	55	930	4.0
(*Lean Cuisine Lunch Express*), 9 oz.	260	15.0	39.0	5.0	30	550	4.0
vegetable almond:							
(*Green Giant Create A Meal!*), 2¾ cup[1]	150	6.0	22.0	4.5	0	1110	6.0
(*Green Giant Create A Meal!*), 1⅓ cup[2]	320	32.0	22.0	11.0	65	1190	6.0

[1] As packaged
[2] Mixture prepared as per package directions, with meat and oil.

Food and Measure	cal.	prot. (gms)	carbo. (gms)	fat (gms)	chol. (mgs)	sod. (mgs)	fiber (gms)
Stir-fry sauce (see also "Marinade," and specific listings), 1 tbsp., except as noted:							
(*House of Tsang* Classic)	25	0	4.0	1.0	0	570	0
(*House of Tsang Saigon Sizzle*)	40	0	8.0	1.0	0	350	0
(*House of Tsang Szechuan Spicy*) . .	20	0	4.0	.5	0	490	0
(*Ka-Me*)	10	1.0	1.0	0	0	570	0
(*Ken's Steak House*)	20	0	5.0	0	0	330	0
(*Kikkoman*)	15	<1.0	3.0	0	0	530	0
(*Lawry's*)	25	<1.0	4.0	.5	0	330	0
(*S&W* Oriental) . . .	20	1.0	5.0	0	0	390	0
honey (*Ken's Steak House*)	20	0	5.0	0	0	280	0
mandarin soy (*La Choy*), ½ cup . . .	70	2.0	16.0	0	0	850	1.0
and marinade (*Mary Rose* Halu)	25	0	6.0	0	0	340	0
and rib, garlic (*Mi-Kee*)	30	0	10	0	0	550	0
spicy (*La Choy* Szechuan), ½ cup	85	3.0	18.0	0	0	625	0
sweet and sour:							
(*House of Tsang*)	35	0	8.0	0	0	50	0
spicy (*La Choy*), ½ cup	140	2.0	36.0	0	0	750	3.0
teriyaki (*La Choy*), ½ cup	95	3.0	22.0	0	0	1155	2.0
Stomach, pork, raw, 1 oz.	44	4.7	0	2.7	55	15	0
Strawberry:							
fresh:							
1 pint	97	2.0	22.5	1.2	0	4	7.4
½ cup	23	.5	5.2	.3	0	1	1.7

Food and Measure	cal.	prot. (gms)	carbo. (gms)	fat (gms)	chol. (mgs)	sod. (mgs)	fiber (gms)
Strawberry *(cont.)*							
canned in heavy							
syrup, ½ cup . . .	117	.7	29.9	.3	0	5	2.2
frozen:							
unsweetened, ½ cup	26	.3	6.8	.1	0	1	1.6
(*Big Valley*), ⅔ cup	50	<1.0	12.0	0	0	0	2.0
(*Stilwell*), ⅔ cup	50	<1.0	13.0	1.0	0	5	2.0
Strawberry drink:							
(*Capri Sun* Cooler),							
6.75 fl. oz.	100	0	26.0	0	0	20	0
(*Farmer's Market*),							
8 fl. oz.	120	0	30.0	0	0	0	0
nectar:							
(*Kern's*), 8 fl. oz.	150	0	36.0	0	0	5	0
(*Libby's/Kern's*),							
11.5 fl. oz.	210	0	52.0	0	0	10	0
Strawberry drink							
blends, 8 fl. oz.:							
banana:							
(*R.W. Knudsen*) . .	120	0	30.0	0	0	25	0
cactus (*R.W. Knud-*							
sen)	120	0	29.0	0	0	10	0
nectar (*Kern's*) . . .	150	0	36.0	0	0	5	0
guava:							
(*R.W. Knudsen*) . .	110	0	27.0	0	0	25	0
(*Santa Cruz*)	100	0	24.0	0	0	25	0
kiwi (*R.W. Knudsen*)	120	0	30.0	0	0	25	0
melon (*Veryfine*							
Shivering Chillers)	120	0	29.0	0	0	5	0
orange banana (*Tree*							
Top)	120	0	29.0	0	0	25	0
Strawberry drink							
mix*, 8 fl. oz.:							
(*Kool-Aid*)	100	0	25.0	0	0	25	0
(*Kool-Aid* w/Sugar)	60	0	16.0	0	0	0	0
Strawberry juice,							
8 fl. oz.:							
(*Veryfine* Juice-Ups)	140	0	36.0	0	0	15	0

Food and Measure	cal.	prot. (gms)	carbo. (gms)	fat (gms)	chol. (mgs)	sod. (mgs)	fiber (gms)
nectar (*R.W. Knud-sen*)	120	0	30.0	0	0	25	0
Strawberry milk:							
(*Nestlé Quik*), 1 cup	230	7.0	31.0	9.0	30	100	0
lowfat:							
(*Nestlé Quik*), 1 cup	200	8.0	32.0	5.0	20	120	0
(*Nestlé Quik*), 8-fl.-oz. cont. . .	210	8.0	35.0	5.0	20	100	0
banana (*Nestlé Quik*), 8 fl. oz. . .	200	7.0	31.0	5.0	20	110	0
shake:							
(*Nestlé Killer*), 14 oz.	420	12.0	62.0	14.0	55	250	5.0
(*Nestlé Quik*), 9 oz.	270	8.0	40.0	9.0	35	160	3.0
Strawberry milk drink:							
canned, 10 fl. oz.:							
(*Sego*)	240	12.0	37.0	5.0	5	280	0
(*Sego* Lite)	150	11.0	18.0	4.0	0	400	0
creme (*Carnation Instant Breakfast*)	220	12.0	35.0	2.5	5	230	0
mix, powder:							
(*Nestlé Quik*), 2 tbsp.	90	0	22.0	0	0	0	0
creme (*Carnation Instant Breakfast*), 1 pkt.	130	4.0	28.0	0	<5	160	0
creme (*Carnation Instant Breakfast* No Sugar), 1 pkt. . .	70	4.0	12.0	0	<5	90	0
Strawberry syrup:							
(*Fox's No Cal*), 2 tbsp.	0	0	0	0	0	40	0
(*Hershey's*), 2 tbsp.	100	0	26.0	0	0	10	0
(*Knott's Berry Farm*), 2 tbsp.	120	0	30.0	0	0	0	0
(*R.W. Knudsen*), ¼ cup	150	0	38.0	0	0	0	0

Food and Measure	cal.	prot. (gms)	carbo. (gms)	fat (gms)	chol. (mgs)	sod. (mgs)	fiber (gms)
Strawberry syrup *(cont.)*							
(*S&W* Reduced Calorie), ¼ cup	60	0	15.0	0	0	105	0
Strawberry topping, 2 tbsp.:							
(*Kraft*)	110	0	29.0	0	0	15	0
(*Smucker's*)	100	0	26.0	0	0	0	0
Melba (*Dickinson's*)	90	0	23.0	0	0	0	0
String beans, see "Green beans"							
Stroganoff gravy (*Pepperidge Farm*), ¼ cup	30	2.0	4.0	1.0	<5	240	0
Stroganoff mix (see also "Tofu dishes, mix"), vegetarian (*Natural Touch*), 4 tbsp.	90	5.0	10.0	3.5	10	610	3.0
Stroganoff sauce, beef (*Lawry's*), 1 tbsp.	20	0	5.0	0	0	500	0
Stroganoff seasoning mix (*Durkee*), ⅛ pkg.	10	.5	3.0	0	0	350	0
Strudel, apple (*Entenmann's*), ¼ strudel	310	3.0	44.0	14.0	0	230	2.0
Stuffing (see also "Stuffing mix"):							
(*Arnold* Unspiced), 2 cups	250	9.0	50.0	3.0	0	460	2.0
apple and raisin (*Pepperidge Farm*), ½ cup	140	4.0	27.0	1.5	0	520	2.0
Cajun rice (*Good Harvest*), ½ cup . . .	130	3.0	24.0	2.0	0	390	1.0
chicken, classic (*Pepperidge Farm*), ½ cup	130	5.0	24.0	1.5	0	490	3.0

Food and Measure	cal.	prot. (gms)	carbo. (gms)	fat (gms)	chol. (mgs)	sod. (mgs)	fiber (gms)
corn bread:							
(*Arnold*), 2 cups . .	250	9.0	49.0	4.0	0	800	2.0
(*Brownberry*),							
2 cups	250	8.0	51.0	3.5	0	800	2.0
(*Pepperidge Farm*),							
¾ cup	170	4.0	33.0	2.0	0	480	2.0
honey pecan (*Pep-							
peridge Farm*),							
½ cup	140	3.0	23.0	5.0	0	400	<1.0
country style (*Pepper-							
idge Farm*), ¾ cup	140	5.0	27.0	1.5	0	380	2.0
cube:							
(*Pepperidge Farm*),							
¾ cup	140	4.0	28.0	1.5	0	530	2.0
bread, unseasoned							
(*Brownberry*),							
2 cups	240	8.0	51.0	3.0	0	500	3.0
garden and herb,							
country (*Pepperidge							
Farm*), ½ cup . . .	150	4.0	22.0	5.0	0	360	2.0
herb seasoned:							
(*Arnold*), 2 cups . .	240	9.0	48.0	3.0	0	740	4.0
(*Brownberry*), 1 cup	200	7.0	41.0	2.5	0	630	3.0
(*Pepperidge Farm*),							
¾ cup	170	5.0	33.0	1.5	0	600	3.0
sage and onion,							
2 cups:							
(*Arnold*)	240	9.0	48.0	3.0	0	960	4.0
(*Brownberry* 7 oz.)	240	9.0	49.0	3.5	0	980	3.0
(*Brownberry* 14 oz.)	240	9.0	49.0	3.0	0	980	3.0
sage and onion (*Pep-							
peridge Farm*),							
½ cup	150	5.0	28.0	1.5	0	520	2.0
Santa Fe (*Good Har-							
vest*), ½ cup . . .	110	3.0	21.0	1.5	0	330	.5
seasoned (*Arnold*),							
2 cups	250	9.0	49.0	3.0	0	820	2.0

Food and Measure	cal.	prot. (gms)	carbo. (gms)	fat (gms)	chol. (mgs)	sod. (mgs)	fiber (gms)
Stuffing *(cont.)*							
sourdough, San Francisco (*Good Harvest*), ½ cup . . .	110	3.0	19.0	2.0	0	480	.5
vegetable, harvest, and almond (*Pepperidge Farm*), ½ cup	140	5.0	23.0	3.0	0	300	2.0
wild rice and mushroom (*Pepperidge Farm*), ⅔ cup . . .	170	5.0	22.0	6.0	0	410	2.0
wild rice trio (*Good Harvest*), ½ cup . .	140	3.0	27.0	2.5	0	470	.5
Stuffing mix, ⅙ box dry, except as noted:							
(*Kellogg's Crouettes*), 1 cup	120	5.0	25.0	0	0	460	0
for beef (*Stove Top*)	110	4.0	22.0	1.0	0	520	1.0
chicken flavor:							
(*Stove Top*)	110	4.0	20.0	1.0	0	440	<1.0
(*Stove Top* Lower Sodium)	110	4.0	21.0	1.0	0	270	<1.0
(*Stove Top* Microwave)	130	4.0	20.0	3.5	0	450	<1.0
w/rice (*Rice-A-Roni*), 1 cup*	170	4.0	20.0	9.0	0	510	1.0
corn bread:							
(*Stove Top*)	110	3.0	21.0	1.0	0	510	1.0
homestyle (*Stove Top* Microwave)	120	3.0	20.0	3.5	0	450	1.0
w/rice (*Rice-A-Roni*), 1 cup*	170	3.0	21.0	8.0	0	650	0
herb (*Stove Top* Flexible Serve), 1 oz. . .	120	3.0	19.0	3.0	0	440	<1.0
herb and butter (*Rice-A-Roni*), 1 cup*	170	4.0	20.0	9.0	0	490	1.0

Food and Measure	cal.	prot. (gms)	carbo. (gms)	fat (gms)	chol. (mgs)	sod. (mgs)	fiber (gms)
herbs, savory (*Stove Top*)	110	4.0	20.0	1.0	0	510	<1.0
long grain/wild rice (*Stove Top*)	110	4.0	22.0	1.0	0	490	<1.0
mushroom/onion (*Stove Top*)	110	4.0	20.0	1.5	0	410	<1.0
for pork (*Stove Top*)	110	4.0	20.0	1.0	0	500	1.0
San Francisco style (*Stove Top*)	110	4.0	20.0	1.0	0	510	1.0
for turkey (*Stove Top*)	110	3.0	20.0	1.0	0	490	<1.0
w/wild rice (*Rice-A-Roni*), 1 cup*	170	4.0	20.0	9.0	0	570	1.0
Sturgeon, meat only:							
raw, 4 oz.	120	18.3	0	4.6	n.a.	n.a.	0
baked, broiled, or microwaved, 4 oz. . .	153	23.5	0	5.9	n.a.	n.a.	0
smoked, 4 oz.	196	35.4	0	5.0	n.a.	n.a.	0
Subway, 1 serving, except as noted:							
sandwiches:							
bologna, jumbo . .	446	n.a.	n.a.	27.0	57	1374	n.a.
bologna, junior . .	270	n.a.	n.a.	11.0	19	706	n.a.
ham, jumbo	259	n.a.	n.a.	5.0	36	1519	n.a.
ham, junior	208	n.a.	n.a.	4.0	12	754	n.a.
roast beef, jumbo	348	n.a.	n.a.	9.0	84	993	n.a.
roast beef, junior	232	n.a.	n.a.	5.0	27	574	n.a.
Subway Seafood & Crab:							
jumbo	472	n.a.	n.a.	27.0	52	772	n.a.
jumbo, w/lite mayo	348	n.a.	n.a.	13	48	808	n.a.
junior	279	n.a.	n.a.	11.0	17	505	n.a.
junior, w/lite mayo	238	n.a.	n.a.	6.0	16	517	n.a.
tuna:							
jumbo	632	n.a.	n.a.	47.0	52	818	n.a.
jumbo, w/lite mayo	406	n.a.	n.a.	22.0	47	898	n.a.
junior	332	n.a.	n.a.	18.0	17	521	n.a.

Food and Measure	cal.	prot. (gms)	carbo. (gms)	fat (gms)	chol. (mgs)	sod. (mgs)	fiber (gms)
Subway, sandwiches *(cont.)*							
junior, w/lite							
mayo	257	n.a.	n.a.	9.0	16	547	n.a.
turkey breast:							
jumbo	290	n.a.	n.a.	6.0	40	1926	n.a.
junior	218	n.a.	n.a.	4.0	13	877	n.a.
submarines, cold, 6″:							
Classic Italian							
B.M.T.	434	n.a.	n.a.	21.0	54	1586	n.a.
ham	273	n.a.	n.a.	4.0	24	1291	n.a.
mixed cold cuts . .	347	n.a.	n.a.	12.0	56	1222	n.a.
roast beef	299	n.a.	n.a.	6.0	42	837	n.a.
Subway Club	300	n.a.	n.a.	6.0	37	1261	n.a.
Subway Seafood &							
Crab	415	n.a.	n.a.	19.0	34	793	n.a.
Subway Seafood &							
Crab w/lite mayo	333	n.a.	n.a.	10.0	32	817	n.a.
tuna	522	n.a.	n.a.	33.0	35	824	n.a.
tuna w/lite mayo . .	372	n.a.	n.a.	15.0	31	877	n.a.
turkey breast	276	n.a.	n.a.	4.0	20	1303	n.a.
turkey breast & ham	275	n.a.	n.a.	4.0	22	1297	n.a.
Veggie Delite	223	n.a.	n.a.	3.0	0	526	n.a.
submarines, hot, 6″:							
chicken breast,							
roasted	321	n.a.	n.a.	5.0	49	1065	n.a.
meatball	411	n.a.	n.a.	15.0	34	1014	n.a.
steak & cheese . .	363	n.a.	n.a.	10.0	22	1079	n.a.
Subway Melt	361	n.a.	n.a.	12.0	40	1680	n.a.
salads:							
bread bowl	290	n.a.	n.a.	4.0	0	650	n.a.
chicken breast fillet,							
roasted	143	n.a.	n.a.	3.0	49	845	n.a.
Subway Club	123	n.a.	n.a.	3.0	37	1041	n.a.
Subway Seafood &							
Crab	238	n.a.	n.a.	17.0	34	573	n.a.
Subway Seafood &							
Crab w/lite mayo	155	n.a.	n.a.	8.0	32	597	n.a.
tuna	345	n.a.	n.a.	31.0	35	604	n.a.
tuna w/lite mayo . .	194	n.a.	n.a.	13.0	31	657	n.a.

Food and Measure	cal.	prot. (gms)	carbo. (gms)	fat (gms)	chol. (mgs)	sod. (mgs)	fiber (gms)
turkey breast	99	n.a.	n.a.	2.0	20	1083	n.a.
Veggie Delite	45	n.a.	n.a.	1.0	0	306	n.a.
salad dressings, 1 tbsp.:							
French	65	n.a.	n.a.	5.0	0	100	n.a.
French, fat free . .	15	n.a.	n.a.	0	0	85	n.a.
Italian, creamy . . .	65	n.a.	n.a.	6.0	4	132	n.a.
Italian, fat free . . .	5	n.a.	n.a.	0	0	152	n.a.
ranch	87	n.a.	n.a.	9.0	1	117	n.a.
ranch, fat free . . .	12	n.a.	n.a.	0	0	177	n.a.
Thousand Island . .	65	n.a.	n.a.	6.0	7	107	n.a.
condiments:							
bacon, 2 slices . .	45	n.a.	n.a.	4.0	8	182	n.a.
cheese, 2 triangles	41	n.a.	n.a.	3.0	10	201	n.a.
mayonnaise dressing, 1 tsp.	37	n.a.	n.a.	4.0	3	27	n.a.
mayonnaise dressing, lite, 1 tsp.	18	n.a.	n.a.	2.0	2	33	n.a.
mustard, 2 tsp. . .	8	n.a.	n.a.	0	0	0	n.a.
olive oil blend, 1 tsp.	45	n.a.	n.a.	5.0	0	0	n.a.
vinegar, 1 tsp. . . .	1	n.a.	n.a.	0	0	0	n.a.
cookies, 1.3-oz. piece:							
chocolate:							
double w/Brazil nut	200	n.a.	n.a.	11.0	10	75	n.a.
white w/macadamias . . .	174	n.a.	n.a.	10.0	17	118	n.a.
chocolate chip:							
regular	161	n.a.	n.a.	8.0	12	113	n.a.
M & M	162	n.a.	n.a.	8.0	12	113	n.a.
walnut	165	n.a.	n.a.	9.0	9	106	n.a.
white	166	n.a.	n.a.	8.0	10	189	n.a.
chocolate chunk . .	160	n.a.	n.a.	7.0	10	140	n.a.
oatmeal raisin . . .	147	n.a.	n.a.	6.0	10	114	n.a.
peanut butter . . .	169	n.a.	n.a.	9.0	0	151	n.a.
sugar	178	n.a.	n.a.	9.0	27	173	n.a.
toffee crunch . . .	153	n.a.	n.a.	8.0	9	114	n.a.

Food and Measure	cal.	prot. (gms)	carbo. (gms)	fat (gms)	chol. (mgs)	sod. (mgs)	fiber (gms)
Succotash, ½ cup, except as noted:							
fresh, boiled, drained	111	4.9	23.4	.8	0	16	n.a.
canned:							
cream-style corn . .	102	3.5	23.4	.7	0	325	n.a.
kernel (*S&W*) . . .	100	3.0	19.0	1.0	0	340	2.0
kernel (*Stokely*) . .	100	3.0	14.0	1.0	0	340	2.0
frozen, boiled, drained	79	3.7	17.0	.8	0	38	4.6
Sucker, white, meat only:							
raw, 4 oz.	105	19.0	0	2.6	47	45	0
baked, broiled, or mi-crowaved, 4 oz. . .	135	24.4	0	3.4	60	58	0
Sugar, beet or cane:							
brown:							
1 oz.	107	0	27.6	0	0	11	0
1 cup, not packed	546	0	141.0	0	0	57	0
1 cup, packed . . .	828	0	214.0	0	0	86	0
granulated:							
1 oz.	110	0	28.3	0	0	<1	0
1 cup	773	0	199.8	0	0	<1	0
1 tbsp.	46	0	12.0	0	0	<1	0
1 tsp.	15	0	4.0	0	0	<1	0
powdered or confec-tioner's:							
1 cup, sifted	389	0	99.5	0	0	1	0
1 tbsp., unsifted . .	31	0	8.0	0	0	<1	0
Sugar, maple, 1 oz.	99	0	25.5	0	0	4	0
Sugar, substitute:							
(*Equal*), 1 pkt.	4	0	<1.0	0	0	0	0
(*NutraSweet*), 1 tsp.	2	0	<1.0	0	0	0	0
(*Sweet 'n Low*), 1 pkt.	4	0	1.0	0	0	0	0
Sugar apple:							
1 medium, 9.9 oz. . .	146	3.2	36.6	.5	0	15	6.8
½ cup	118	2.6	29.6	.4	0	12	5.5
Sugar snap peas, see "Peas, edible-pod-ded"							

Food and Measure	cal.	prot. (gms)	carbo. (gms)	fat (gms)	chol. (mgs)	sod. (mgs)	fiber (gms)
Summer sausage:							
(*Old Smokehouse*),							
1 oz.	110	4.0	1.0	10.0	30	400	0
(*Oscar Mayer*),							
2 slices, 1.6 oz. . .	140	7.0	0	13.0	40	650	0
beef (*Oscar Mayer*),							
2 slices, 1.6 oz. . .	140	7.0	1.0	12.0	35	640	0
Sunburst squash, raw							
(*Frieda's*), 1 oz. . .	4	.3	.9	<.1	0	<1	n.a.
Sunfish, pumpkin-							
seed, meat only:							
raw, 4 oz.	101	22.0	0	.8	76	91	0
baked, broiled, or mi-							
crowaved, 4 oz. . .	129	28.2	0	1.0	98	117	0
Sunflower seed,							
1 oz., except as							
noted:							
dried, in shell (*Arrow-*							
head Mills), 1 cup,							
1.3 oz. edible . . .	180	8.0	6.0	15.0	0	10	2.0
dry-roasted, in shell:							
(*Planters*),							
3-oz. bag, 1.5 oz.							
edible	240	9.0	8.0	23.0	0	135	3.0
(*Planters*), ¾ cup,							
1 oz. edible . . .	160	6.0	5.0	15.0	0	90	2.0
(*Planters* Original),							
¾ cup, 1 oz. edi-							
ble	160	6.0	5.0	15.0	0	35	2.0
(*Planters Munch 'N*							
Go), .75 oz. edible	120	4.0	4.0	11.0	0	70	1.0
dry-roasted, kernels:							
salted	165	5.5	6.8	14.1	0	221	2.6
(*Planters*), ¼ cup	190	7.0	6.0	17.0	0	230	4.0
honey-roasted, kernels							
(*Planters*), 1.7 oz.	280	10.0	15.0	22.0	0	105	6.0
oil-roasted, kernels:							
(*Planters*), 1.7 oz.	290	11.0	9.0	25.0	0	260	7.0
(*Planters*), 2 oz. . .	340	13.0	11.0	29.0	0	310	8.0

Food and Measure	cal.	prot. (gms)	carbo. (gms)	fat (gms)	chol. (mgs)	sod. (mgs)	fiber (gms)
Sunflower seed, oil-roasted, kernels *(cont.)*							
(*Planters Munch 'N Go*), ¼ cup . . .	200	8.0	6.0	17.0	0	180	4.0
barbecued kernels:							
(*Planters*), 1.7 oz.	290	11.0	10.0	25.0	0	180	6.0
(*Planters Munch 'N Go*), 3 tbsp. . . .	150	6.0	6.0	13.0	0	100	3.0
salted kernels (*Planters*)	170	7.0	5.0	14.0	0	140	4.0
tamari-roasted (*Eden*)	170	8.0	9.0	11.0	0	50	3.0
Sunflower seed butter:							
1 tbsp.	93	3.2	4.4	7.6	0	1	.8
(*Roaster Fresh*), 1 oz.	160	6.0	5.0	14.0	0	1	0
Sunflower seed flour, partially defatted, 1 cup	261	38.5	28.7	1.3	0	2	4.2
Sunflower sprouts (*Jonathan's*), 1 cup	45.	2.0	2.0	4.0	0	0	1.0
Surimi, pollock, 4 oz.	112	17.2	7.8	1.0	34	162	0
Swamp cabbage:							
raw, .6-oz. shoot . .	2	.3	.4	<.1	0	15	.3
boiled, drained, chopped, ½ cup . .	10	1.0	1.8	.1	0	60	.9
Sweet peas, see "Peas, green"							
Sweet potato:							
raw, 5″ × 2″ potato	136	2.1	31.6	.4	0	17	3.9
baked in skin:							
5″ × 2″ potato . . .	118	2.0	27.7	.1	0	12	3.4
mashed, ½ cup . .	103	1.7	24.3	.1	0	10	3.0
boiled w/out skin:							
4 oz.	119	1.9	27.5	.3	0	15	2.8
mashed, ½ cup . .	172	2.7	39.8	.5	0	21	4.1
Sweet potato, canned, ½ cup, except as noted:							
in syrup, w/liquid . .	101	1.1	23.9	.2	0	50	2.1
in syrup, drained . .	106	1.3	24.9	.3	0	38	1.8

Food and Measure	cal.	prot. (gms)	carbo. (gms)	fat (gms)	chol. (mgs)	sod. (mgs)	fiber (gms)
whole (*Royal Prince/ Trappey's*), 4 pcs.	200	1.0	48.0	.5	0	40	4.0
halves (*Royal Prince*), 5.7 oz., 3 pcs. . . .	190	1.0	46.0	.5	0	40	4.0
cut or pieces (*Allens/ Sugary Sam/ Princella* Yams), ⅔ cup	160	0	40.0	.5	0	35	3.0
mashed (*Princella/ Sugary Sam*), ⅔ cup	120	1.0	28.0	.5	0	30	3.0
candied:							
(*Royal Prince*) . . .	210	1.0	50.0	.5	0	30	2.0
(*S&W*)	170	2.0	46.0	0	0	360	4.0
orange-pineapple (*Royal Prince*) . . .	210	1.0	43.0	.5	0	30	3.0
Sweet potato, frozen:							
baked, cubed, ½ cup	88	1.5	20.6	.1	0	7	2.6
candied:							
(*Mrs. Paul's*), 5 fl. oz.	300	2.0	73.0	1.0	0	130	3.0
(*Mrs. Paul's Sweets'n Apples*), 1 cup	270	0	66.0	0	0	90	3.0
(*Ore-Ida*), 5 pcs. . .	170	2.0	40.0	0	0	75	3.0
Sweet potato chips, 1 oz.:							
(*Terra* Chips)	140	1.0	18.0	7.0	0	10	2.0
cinnamon (*Terra* Chips)	140	1.0	17.0	7.0	0	70	2.0
Sweet potato leaf:							
raw, chopped, ½ cup	6	.7	1.1	.1	0	2	<1.0
steamed, ½ cup . . .	11	.7	2.3	.1	0	4	.6
Sweet and sour drink mixer (*Holland House/Mr. & Mrs. "T"/Rose's*), 4 fl. oz.	100	0	23.0	0	0	50	0

Food and Measure	cal.	prot. (gms)	carbo. (gms)	fat (gms)	chol. (mgs)	sod. (mgs)	fiber (gms)
Sweet and sour din- ner mix (*La Choy*), ¼ pkg.	90	1.0	22.0	0	0	840	2.0
Sweet and sour sauce, 2 tbsp., ex- cept as noted:							
(*Contadina*)	40	0	8.0	1.0	0	110	0
(*House of Tsang*) . .	30	0	7.0	0	0	45	0
(*House of Tsang*) .5-oz. pkt.	20	0	4.0	0	0	25	0
(*Kikkoman*)	35	0	9.0	0	0	190	0
(*Kraft*)	80	0	19.0	.5	0	180	0
(*La Choy*)	60	0	14.0	0	0	120	0
(*Sauceworks*)	60	0	14.0	0	0	125	0
(*Woody's*)	70	0	17.0	0	0	610	<1.0
concentrate (*House of Tsang*), 1 tsp. . . .	10	0	3.0	0	0	15	0
chicken (*Gold's Dip'n Joy*), 1 tbsp.	30	0	7.0	0	0	125	0
duck sauce:							
(*Ka-Me*)	80	0	20.0	0	0	480	0
(*La Choy*)	60	0	15.0	0	0	130	0
all varieties (*Gold's*)	60	0	14.0	0	0	250	0
Sweetbreads, see "Pancreas" and "Thymus"							
Swiss chard, ½ cup:							
raw, chopped	3	.3	.7	<.1	0	38	.3
boiled, drained, chopped	18	1.7	3.6	.1	0	158	1.8
Swiss steak gravy mix (*Durkee*), ¼ cup*	15	0	4.0	0	0	370	0
Swiss steak season- ing mix (*Durkee/ French's* Roasting Bag), ⅑ pkg. . . .	10	0	3.0	0	0	310	0

Food and Measure	cal.	prot. (gms)	carbo. (gms)	fat (gms)	chol. (mgs)	sod. (mgs)	fiber (gms)
Swordfish, fresh, meat only:							
raw, 4 oz.	137	22.5	0	4.6	45	102	0
baked, broiled, or microwaved, 4 oz. . .	176	28.8	0	5.8	57	130	0
Swordfish, frozen, steaks (*Peter Pan*), 4 oz.	160	29.0	0	5.0	55	65	0
Syrup, see specific listings							
Szechuan sauce (see also "Stir-fry sauce"):							
(*Ka-Me*), 1 tbsp. . . .	20	1.0	2.0	1.0	0	410	2.0
cooking (*Kylin* Chili & Tomato), ¼ cup . .	50	1.0	11.0	1.0	0	810	0

T

Food and Measure	cal.	prot. (gms)	carbo. (gms)	fat (gms)	chol. (mgs)	sod. (mgs)	fiber (gms)
Tabouli (*Frieda's*),							
½ cup	152	3.0	17.0	9.0	0	265	5.0
Tabouli mix:							
(*Casbah*), 1 oz. . . .	90	3.0	20.0	<1.0	0	350	1.0
(*Fantastic*), ¼ cup . .	120	4.0	26.0	.5	0	450	6.0
(*Near East*), ⅔ cup*	120	3.0	23.0	3.0	0	340	3.0
Taco Bell, 1 serving:							
burritos:							
bean	391	13.0	n.a.	12.0	5	1138	n.a.
beef	432	22.0	n.a.	19.0	57	1303	n.a.
Burrito Supreme:							
regular	443	18.0	n.a.	19.0	47	1184	n.a.
big beef	525	25.0	n.a.	25.0	72	1418	n.a.
chicken	520	27.0	n.a.	23.0	125	1130	n.a.
steak	500	26.0	n.a.	23.0	75	1350	n.a.
chicken	345	17.0	n.a.	13.0	57	854	n.a.
chili cheese	391	17.0	n.a.	18.0	47	980	n.a.
combo	412	17.0	n.a.	16.0	32	1221	n.a.
7 layer	485	15.0	n.a.	21.0	28	1115	n.a.
tacos/tostadas:							
soft taco	223	12.0	n.a.	11.0	32	539	n.a.
soft taco, chicken	223	14.0	n.a.	10.0	53	553	n.a.
soft taco, steak . .	217	12.0	n.a.	9.0	31	569	n.a.
soft *Taco Supreme*	268	13.0	n.a.	15.0	47	551	n.a.
taco	180	10.0	n.a.	11.0	32	276	n.a.
Taco Supreme . . .	225	11.0	n.a.	15.0	47	287	n.a.
tostada	242	9.0	n.a.	11.0	14	593	n.a.
specialty items:							
beef *MexiMelt* . . .	262	13.0	n.a.	14.0	38	711	n.a.
cinnamon twists . .	139	1.0	n.a.	6.0	0	189	n.a.
Mexican pizza . . .	574	19.0	n.a.	38.0	50	1003	n.a.

Food and Measure	cal.	prot. (gms)	carbo. (gms)	fat (gms)	chol. (mgs)	sod. (mgs)	fiber (gms)
nachos	345	7.0	n.a.	18.0	9	398	n.a.
nachos *BellGrande*	633	22.0	n.a.	34.0	49	952	n.a.
nachos supreme . .	364	12.0	n.a.	18.0	17	470	n.a.
pintos 'n cheese . .	190	9.0	n.a.	9.0	14	640	n.a.
taco salad	838	31.0	n.a.	55.0	79	1132	n.a.
sides/condiments:							
green sauce	4	0	n.a.	0	0	136	0
guacamole	36	0	n.a.	3.0	0	132	n.a.
nacho cheese sauce	51	2.0	n.a.	4.0	4	196	0
picante sauce . . .	3	0	n.a.	0	0	132	0
pico de gallo	6	0	n.a.	0	0	65	0
ranch dressing . . .	136	1.0	n.a.	14.0	20	330	0
red sauce	10	0	n.a.	0	0	261	0
salsa	27	1.0	n.a.	0	0	709	0
seasoned rice . . .	110	2.0	n.a.	3.0	5	230	n.a.
sour cream	44	1.0	n.a.	4.0	15	11	0
taco sauce, hot . .	2	0	n.a.	0	0	91	0
taco sauce, mild . .	0	0	n.a.	0	0	6	0
Taco entree, frozen mini, w/cheese sauce (*Swanson Fun Feast*), 1 pkg.	380	23.0	50.0	15.0	35	760	4.0
Taco John's, 1 serving:							
burritos:							
bean	340	14.8	45.2	11.1	15	654	n.a.
beef	415	22.4	39.4	18.9	43	703	n.a.
combination	378	18.1	46.1	13.4	30	659	n.a.
smothered, platter	972	38.1	123.0	37.5	61	2181	n.a.
super	424	19.6	45.0	18.8	35	736	n.a.
chimichanga platter	922	32.4	119.0	35.2	50	2347	n.a.
enchilada platter, double	901	41.8	103.0	36.5	73	2100	n.a.
fajitas, chicken:							
burrito	360	20.4	41.4	11.9	49	1201	n.a.
salad, no dressing	561	21.9	40.4	34.6	55	1507	n.a.
softshell	216	13.2	20.3	8.3	33	1083	n.a.
Mexi Rolls:							
w/guacamole	839	29.7	78.3	45.6	46	1054	n.a.

Food and Measure	cal.	prot. (gms)	carbo. (gms)	fat (gms)	chol. (mgs)	sod. (mgs)	fiber (gms)
Taco John's *(cont.)*							
w/nacho cheese . .	813	29.7	77.3	43.0	46	1201	n.a.
w/salsa	754	28.5	76.5	37.1	46	1388	n.a.
w/sour cream . . .	854	29.7	74.3	47.0	46	852	n.a.
Mexican pizza	636	25.8	53.1	35.9	55	1334	n.a.
nachos, super	848	18.8	76.9	49.9	50	1232	n.a.
Sampler platter . . .	1276	57.7	149.0	51.0	97	2737	n.a.
Sierra Chicken Fillet							
Sandwich	500	31.0	46.0	21.0	41	1493	n.a.
tacos:							
crispy	178	9.0	12.5	10.3	22	256	n.a.
kid's meal:							
w/crispy taco . . .	575	12.5	54.7	33.3	31	773	n.a.
w/soft shell taco . .	623	15.0	65.7	32.7	32	1021	n.a.
w/taco burger . . .	668	17.7	70.3	34.1	35	1081	n.a.
salad, w/out dress-							
ing	469	11.2	39.7	30.5	22	647	n.a.
soft shell	278	13.5	32.0	11.3	22	556	n.a.
Taco Bravo	332	14.7	37.7	13.6	23	654	n.a.
taco burger	275	14.5	28.9	11.2	26	566	n.a.
sides and condiments:							
beans, refried . . .	301	17.4	39.3	7.8	8	955	n.a.
chili, Texas style,							
w/2 crackers . . .	297	22.6	26.6	14.3	47	1425	n.a.
Mexican rice	567	7.9	93.9	17.7	0	1293	n.a.
nachos	294	1.8	30.9	16.8	6	447	n.a.
nacho cheese . . .	80	n.a.	5.0	6.0	n.a.	380	n.a.
Potato Oles	442	3.3	45.4	27.5	n.a.	385	n.a.
Potato Oles, w/							
nacho cheese . .	523	n.a.	49.8	33.7	6	832	n.a.
salad dressing,							
house	114	.3	2.9	11.4	<1	623	n.a.
sour cream	60	1.0	1.0	5.0	n.a.	15	n.a.
desserts:							
choco taco	320	3.0	38.0	17.0	20	100	n.a.
churro	147	2.0	17.4	7.8	4	160	n.a.
flauta, apple	84	1.0	18.8	1.1	0	72	n.a.
flauta, cherry . . .	143	2.1	26.7	3.6	0	110	n.a.
flauta, cream cheese	181	2.5	26.5	7.9	10	135	n.a.

Food and Measure.	cal.	prot. (gms)	carbo. (gms)	fat (gms)	chol. (mgs)	sod. (mgs)	fiber (gms)
Taco mix, dinner:							
(*Lawry's*), ⅕ pkg. . .	150	2.0	19.0	7.0	0	550	1.0
(*Old El Paso*),							
2 tacos*	270	2.0	21.0	13.0	60	910	4.0
(*Pancho Villa*),							
2 tacos*	270	2.0	20.0	13.0	60	840	4.0
soft (*Old El Paso*) . .	380	n.a.	45.0	10.0	63	1340	3.0
vegetarian (*Natural*							
Touch), 3 tbsp. . .	60	8.0	5.0	1.0	0	590	3.0
Taco sauce, 1 tbsp.,							
except as noted:							
(*Chi-Chi's* Thick &							
Chunky)	10	0	1.0	0	0	75	0
(*Hunt's Manwich*),							
¼ cup	30	1.0	7.0	0	0	590	1.0
(*Lawry's* Chunky),							
2 tbsp.	10	0	2.0	0	0	250	0
(*Lawry's* Sauce'n Sea-							
soner), 2 tbsp. . . .	15	<1.0	3.0	0	0	320	<1.0
(*Pancho Villa*), 2 tbsp.	15	0	3.0	0	0	170	0
green (*La Victoria*)	0	0	<1.0	0	0	95	0
hot (*Old El Paso*) . .	5	0	1.0	0	0	90	0
medium (*Old El Paso*)	5	0	1.0	0	0	70	0
mild (*Old El Paso*) . .	5	0	1.0	0	0	85	0
mild or medium (*Old*							
El Paso Chunky) . .	5	0	1.0	0	0	80	0
red (*La Victoria*) . . .	5	0	1.0	0	0	105	0
Taco seasoning							
(*Tone's*), 2 tsp. . .	20	1.0	4.0	0	0	440	1.0
Taco seasoning mix:							
(*Durkee* Pouch),							
⅛ pkg.	15	0	2.0	0	0	350	0
(*Durkee* Pouch Fam-							
ily), 1/16 pkg.	10	0	2.0	0	0	280	0
(*Lawry's*), 1 tbsp. . .	25	<1.0	5.0	0	0	360	0
(*McCormick*), 2 tsp.	20	0	3.0	0	0	430	<1.0
(*Old El Paso*), 2 tsp.	20	0	5.0	0	0	550	0
(*Old El Paso* Less							
Salt), 2 tsp.	20	0	4.0	0	0	330	0

Food and Measure	cal.	prot. (gms)	carbo. (gms)	fat (gms)	chol. (mgs)	sod. (mgs)	fiber (gms)
Taco seasoning mix *(cont.)*							
(*Pancho Villa*), 2 tsp.	20	0	5.0	0	0	550	0
chicken (*Lawry's*),							
2 tsp.	20	<1.0	5.0	0	0	450	0
mild (*Durkee* Pouch),							
⅛ pkg.	15	.5	3.0	0	0	320	0
salad:							
(*Durkee* Pouch),							
⅙ pkg.	20	.5	4.0	0	0	320	0
(*Lawry's*), 1 tsp. . . .	15	0	3.0	0	0	210	0
Taco shell:							
(*Gebhardt*), 3 shells	155	2.0	19.0	8.5	0	10	4.5
(*Lawry's*), 2 shells . .	120	2.0	13.0	6.0	0	110	1.0
(*Lawry's* Super Size),							
2 shells	180	2.0	22.0	10.0	0	180	1.0
(*Old El Paso*), 3 shells	170	2.0	18.0	10.0	0	130	2.0
(*Old El Paso* Super),							
2 shells	190	3.0	21.0	12.0	0	150	2.0
(*Pancho Villa*),							
3 shells	190	2.0	19.0	11.0	0	0	3.0
(*Rosarita*), 3 shells	155	2.0	19.0	8.5	0	10	4.5
mini (*Old El Paso*),							
7 shells	160	2.0	18.0	10.0	0	130	2.0
soft, see "Tortilla"							
tostada:							
(*Lawry's*), 2 shells	110	1.0	13.0	6.0	0	110	1.0
(*Old El Paso*),							
3 shells	160	2.0	19.0	10.0	0	220	2.0
(*Rosarita*), 2 shells	125	2.0	17.0	5.0	0	20	0
tostaco (*Old El Paso*),							
1 shell	130	2.0	14.0	7.0	0	10	1.0
white corn:							
(*Chi-Chi's*), 2 shells	170	3.0	22.0	8.0	0	0	2.0
(*Old El Paso*),							
3 shells	170	2.0	18.0	10.0	0	30	2.0
Tagliatelle, refriger-							
ated, spinach (*Con-*							
tadina), 1¼ cup . .	270	12.0	46.0	4.0	105	110	4.0

Food and Measure	cal.	prot. (gms)	carbo. (gms)	fat (gms)	chol. (mgs)	sod. (mgs)	fiber (gms)
Tahini:							
(*Arrowhead Mills*),							
1 oz.	170	6.0	4.0	17.0	0	<1	2.6
(*Joyva*), 2 tbsp. . . .	200	5.0	3.0	18.0	0	75	1.0
(*Krinos*), 2 tbsp. . . .	260	9.0	5.0	23.0	0	0	3.0
Tahini sauce mix							
(*Casbah*), 1 oz. . .	160	4.0	10.0	13.0	0	160	<1.0
Tamale, canned:							
(*Gebhardt*), 2 pcs. . .	270	5.0	19.0	20.0	30	770	2.5
(*Gebhardt* Jumbo),							
2 pcs.	330	5.5	24.0	25.0	35	930	3.0
(*Just Rite*), 3 pcs. . .	255	7.5	21.0	17.5	25	1035	4.0
(*Nalley*), 3 pcs. . . .	290	8.0	25.0	17.0	30	1000	1.0
(*Old El Paso*), 3 pcs.	330	7.0	31.0	19.0	30	590	5.0
(*Van Camp's*), 2 pcs.	210	6.0	20.0	13.0	20	610	3.0
beef:							
(*Hormel*), 7½-oz.							
can	290	5.0	20.0	21.0	35	1030	3.0
hot-spicy or regular							
(*Hormel*), 3 pcs.	280	15.0	20.0	21.0	35	1010	3.0
jumbo (*Hormel*),							
2 pcs.	270	10.0	18.0	20.0	35	940	3.0
chicken (*Hormel*),							
3 pcs.	210	7.0	23.0	10.0	60	1040	2.0
Tamale, frozen							
(*Goya*), 1 pc. . . .	300	6.0	28.0	18.0	35	450	2.0
Tamale pie, Mexican,							
frozen (*Amy's*),							
8 oz.	220	10.0	41.0	3.0	0	480	11.0
Tamari, see "Soy							
sauce"							
Tamarind:							
1 fruit, 3" × 1"	5	.1	1.3	<.1	0	1	.1
pulp, ½ cup	144	1.7	37.5	.4	0	17	3.1
pulp (*Frieda's*							
Tamarindo), 3.5 oz.	239	2.8	62.5	.6	0	51	n.a.
frozen, chunks							
(*Goya*), ⅓ pkg. . .	70	1.0	15.0	0	0	15	3.0

Food and Measure	cal.	prot. (gms)	carbo. (gms)	fat (gms)	chol. (mgs)	sod. (mgs)	fiber (gms)
Tamarind nectar							
canned (*Goya*),							
12 fl. oz.	240	1.0	59.0	0	0	20	1.0
Tandoori paste, mild							
(*Patak's*), 2 tbsp.	30	<1.0	3.0	1.0	0	1440	2.0
Tangerine:							
fresh:							
1 medium, 2⅜" . .	37	.5	9.4	.2	0	1	1.9
sections w/out mem-							
brane, ½ cup . .	43	.6	10.9	.2	0	2	2.2
canned:							
in juice, ½ cup . .	46	.8	11.9	<.1	0	7	.9
in juice (*S&W* Man-							
darin), ⅔ cup . .	70	1.0	16.0	0	0	0	0
in light syrup,							
½ cup	76	.6	20.4	.1	0	8	.9
in light syrup (*Del*							
Monte), ½ cup	80	0	19.0	0	0	10	<1.0
in light syrup (*S&W*							
Mandarin), ⅔ cup	100	1.0	23.0	0	0	15	1.0
Tangerine juice:							
fresh, 6 fl. oz.	80	.9	18.7	.4	0	2	.4
frozen* (*Minute Maid*							
Beverage), 8 fl. oz.	120	0	30.0	0	0	5	0
blend (*Dole* Manda-							
rin), 8 fl. oz.	140	1.0	35.0	0	0	30	0
Tapenade, see "To-							
mato tapenade"							
Tapioca, dry (*Minute*),							
1½ tsp.	20	0	5.0	0	0	5	0
Tapioca pudding, see							
"Pudding"							
Tarama, see "Caviar"							
Taramosalata, see							
"Caviar spread"							
Taro:							
raw, sliced, ½ cup	56	.8	13.8	.1	0	6	2.1
cooked:							
sliced, ½ cup . . .	94	.3	22.8	.1	0	10	3.4

Food and Measure	cal.	prot. (gms)	carbo. (gms)	fat (gms)	chol. (mgs)	sod. (mgs)	fiber (gms)
(*Frieda's*), 5 oz. . . .	150	1.0	36.0	n.a.	0	10	4.0
Taro chips:							
1 oz.	141	.7	19.3	7.1	0	97	n.a.
½ cup	57	.3	8.1	3.1	0	44	n.a.
spiced (*Terra*), 1 oz.	130	1.0	20.0	5.0	0	170	2.0
Taro leaf, ½ cup:							
raw	6	.7	.9	.1	0	1	.5
steamed	18	2.0	3.0	.3	0	2	n.a.
Taro root, cooked							
(*Frieda's*), 5 oz. . . .	150	1.0	36.0	n.a.	0	10	4.0
Taro shoots, ½ cup:							
raw, sliced	5	.4	1.0	<.1	0	<1	n.a.
cooked, sliced	10	.5	2.2	.1	0	1	n.a.
Taro, Tahitian:							
raw, sliced, ½ cup	25	1.7	4.3	.6	0	31	n.a.
cooked, sliced, ½ cup	30	2.8	4.7	.5	0	37	n.a.
Tarragon, dried:							
(*McCormick*), ¼ tsp.	1	0	.1	0	0	0	0
ground, 1 tsp.	5	.4	.8	.1	0	1	.1
Tart shell, see "Pastry shell"							
Tartar sauce, 2 tbsp.:							
(*Bookbinder's*)	120	0	4.0	11.0	0	210	0
(*Hellmann's/Best Foods*)	140	0	1.0	16.0	10	260	0
(*Hellmann's/Best Foods* Low Fat) . .	40	0	7.0	1.5	0	360	0
(*Nalley*)	190	0	1.0	20.0	15	250	0
(*Sauceworks*)	100	0	4.0	10.0	10	180	0
lemon herb flavor (*Sauceworks*) . . .	150	0	<1.0	16.0	15	170	0
TCBY, ½ cup, except as noted:							
nonfat yogurt:							
apple pie alamode	120	3.0	27.0	0	0	60	1.0
banana split	110	3.0	25.0	0	0	55	<1.0
cappuccino	120	4.0	26.0	0	0	60	1.0
chocolate:							
brown/white . .	120	4.0	26.0	0	0	60	1.0

Food and Measure	cal.	prot. (gms)	carbo. (gms)	fat (gms)	chol. (mgs)	sod. (mgs)	fiber (gms)
TCBY, nonfat yogurt *(cont.)*							
sundae, chewy	120	3.0	28.0	0	0	60	2.0
peach cobbler . . .	110	3.0	25.0	0	0	60	1.0
raspberry cheese-							
cake	120	3.0	27.0	0	0	65	<1.0
strawberry short-							
cake	120	3.0	26.0	0	0	85	1.0
vanilla caramel cus-							
tard	120	3.0	29.0	0	0	80	1.0
soft serve yogurt, all							
flavors:							
regular	130	4.0	23.0	3.0	15	60	0
nonfat	110	4.0	23.0	0	<5	60	0
nonfat, no sugar . .	80	4.0	20.0	0	<5	35	0
sorbet, all flavors . .	100	0	24.0	0	0	30	0
Yog•A•Bar, 1 bar:							
orange or raspberry							
swirl	80	2.0	18.0	.5	<5	30	0
vanilla:							
chocolate dipped	120	3.0	13.0	8.0	5	25	0
w/toasted al-							
monds	190	3.0	19.0	11.0	<5	30	0
w/*Heath* toffee	190	2.0	22.0	11.0	5	45	0
Tea (see also "Tea, iced"), 1 bag or tsp.:							
plain, regular or in-							
stant, all varieties	0	0	0	0	0	0	0
flavored, lemon, in-							
stant (*Lipton*),							
1 tsp.	0	0	1.0	0	0	0	0
Tea, iced, 8 fl. oz., except as noted:							
(*Schweppes*)	90	0	22.0	0	0	60	0
(*Snapple*)	70	0	18.0	0	0	10	0
(*Veryfine* Chillers) . .	80	0	19.0	0	0	5	0
all fruit flavors:							
(*Apple & Eve*) . . .	100	0	25.0	0	0	5	0
(*Lipton* Chilled) . .	80	0	20.0	0	0	15	0

Food and Measure	cal.	prot. (gms)	carbo. (gms)	fat (gms)	chol. (mgs)	sod. (mgs)	fiber (gms)
herbal (*R.W. Knudsen* Coolers) . . .	90	0	23.0	0	0	40	0
lemon:							
(*Snapple*)	100	0	25.0	0	0	10	0
(*Tropicana*)	100	0	25.0	0	0	25	0
(*Veryfine* Chillers)	90	0	23.0	0	0	10	0
mango or passion							
fruit (*Snapple*) . . .	110	0	27.0	0	0	10	0
mint (*Snapple*)	120	0	29.0	0	0	10	0
peach, 11.5 fl. oz.:							
(*Snapple*)	150	0	36.0	0	0	15	0
(*Tropicana*)	160	0	41.0	0	0	20	0
peach, raspberry, or							
strawberry (*Snapple*)	100	0	26.0	0	0	10	0
peach-kiwi (*Veryfine*							
Chillers)	80	0	18.0	0	0	5	0
raspberry:							
(*Snapple*),							
11.5 fl. oz.	150	0	37.0	0	0	15	0
(*Tropicana*),							
11.5 fl. oz.	160	0	41.0	0	0	15	0
(*Veryfine* Chillers)	100	0	24.0	0	0	5	0
Tea, iced, mix, 1⅔ tbsp.:							
lemon flavor (*Lipton*)	90	0	22.0	0	0	0	0
w/out lemon (*Lipton*)	80	0	19.0	0	0	0	0
Teff seed or flour (*Arrowhead Mills*),							
2 oz.	200	7.0	41.0	1.0	0	6	7.7
Tempeh:							
1 oz.	56	5.4	4.8	2.2	0	2	n.a.
½ cup	165	15.7	14.1	6.4	0	5	n.a.
Teriyaki sauce, 1 tbsp.:							
(*House of Tsang Korean Teriyaki*) . . .	30	0	6.0	.5	0	430	0
(*La Choy*)	20	1.0	3.0	0	0	920	0
(*La Choy* Lite)	20	1.0	3.5	0	0	440	0

Food and Measure	cal.	prot. (gms)	carbo. (gms)	fat (gms)	chol. (mgs)	sod. (mgs)	fiber (gms)
Teriyaki sauce *(cont.)*							
barbecue (*Mary Rose* Sumi)	30	0	7.0	0	0	420	0
baste and glaze:							
(*Kikkoman*)	50	1.0	11.0	0	0	810	0
w/honey and pineapple (*Kikkoman*)	80	1.0	18.0	0	0	770	0
cooking and marinade:							
(*S&W*)	25	1.0	5.0	0	0	480	0
(*S&W* Lite)	25	1.0	5.0	0	0	220	0
hot (*La Choy* Chun King)	20	2.0	3.0	0	0	995	0
marinade (*Lawry's*)	20	0	5.0	0	0	810	0
marinade and:							
(*Kikkoman*)	15	1.0	2.0	0	0	610	0
(*Lea & Perrins*) . .	15	0	4.0	0	0	210	0
light (*Kikkoman*) . .	15	<1.0	3.0	0	0	320	0
Teriyaki seasoning mix beef (*Durkee*), 1 tbsp.	30	1.0	6.0	1.0	0	700	0
Thai sauce (*World Harbors* Nong Khai), 1 tbsp.	20	0	5.0	0	0	200	0
Thyme, dried:							
(*McCormick*), ¼ tsp.	4	0	.2	0	0	<1	.1
ground, 1 tsp.	4	.1	.9	.1	0	1	.3
Thymus, 4 oz.:							
beef, braised	362	24.8	0	28.3	333	132	0
veal, braised	197	35.8	0	4.9	532	75	0
Tikka sauce, see "Curry sauce"							
Tilefish, meat only:							
raw, 4 oz.	108	19.9	0	2.6	n.a.	60	0
baked, broiled, or microwaved, 4 oz. . .	167	27.8	0	5.3	n.a.	67	0

Food and Measure	cal.	prot. (gms)	carbo. (gms)	fat (gms)	chol. (mgs)	sod. (mgs)	fiber (gms)
Toaster muffins and pastries, 1 pc., except as noted:							
apple:							
(*Toaster Strudel*)	180	3.0	27.0	7.0	5	190	<1.0
cinnamon (*Pop-Tarts*)	210	2.0	38.0	5.0	0	170	1.0
cinnamon (*Thomas' Toast-r-Cakes*) . .	100	1.0	18.0	3.0	<5	220	1.0
banana nut (*Thomas' Toast-r-Cakes*) . . .	110	2.0	16.0	5.0	<5	170	<1.0
blueberry:							
(*Pop-Tarts*)	210	2.0	36.0	7.0	0	210	1.0
(*Thomas' Toast-r-Cakes*)	100	1.0	17.0	3.0	<5	160	<1.0
(*Toaster Strudel*)	180	3.0	26.0	7.0	5	200	<1.0
frosted (*Pop-Tarts*)	200	2.0	37.0	5.0	0	210	1.0
frosted (*Toastettes*)	190	2.0	35.0	5.0	0	190	1.0
brown sugar-cinnamon:							
(*Pop-Tarts*)	220	3.0	32.0	9.0	0	210	1.0
frosted (*Pop-Tarts*)	210	3.0	34.0	7.0	0	180	1.0
frosted (*Toastettes*)	190	2.0	35.0	5.0	0	180	1.0
cherry:							
(*Pop-Tarts*)	200	2.0	37.0	5.0	0	220	1.0
(*Toaster Strudel*)	180	3.0	27.0	7.0	5	200	<1.0
frosted (*Pop-Tarts*)	200	2.0	37.0	5.0	0	220	1.0
frosted (*Toastettes*)	190	2.0	35.0	5.0	0	190	1.0
chocolate:							
(*Pop-Tarts Minis*), 1 pkt.	170	2.0	30.0	4.0	0	200	1.0
fudge, frosted (*Pop-Tarts*)	200	3.0	37.0	5.0	0	220	1.0
graham (*Pop-Tarts*)	210	3.0	36.0	6.0	0	220	1.0
chocolate-vanilla creme, frosted (*Pop-Tarts*)	200	3.0	37.0	5.0	0	230	1.0
cinnamon (*Toaster Strudel*)	190	3.0	26.0	8.0	5	200	<1.0

Food and Measure	cal.	prot. (gms)	carbo. (gms)	fat (gms)	chol. (mgs)	sod. (mgs)	fiber (gms)
Toaster muffins and pastries *(cont.)*							
corn (*Thomas'*							
Toast-r-Cakes) . . .	110	2.0	19.0	4.0	<5	180	<1.0
cream cheese:							
(*Toaster Strudel*)	190	3.0	23.0	10.0	15	230	0
blueberry or straw-							
berry (*Toaster*							
Strudel)	190	3.0	24.0	9.0	10	220	<1.0
French toast style							
(*Toaster Strudel*)	190	3.0	28.0	7.0	5	200	<1.0
fudge, frosted (*Toas-*							
tettes)	190	2.0	34.0	5.0	0	280	1.0
grape, frosted:							
(*Pop-Tarts*)	200	2.0	38.0	5.0	0	200	1.0
(*Pop-Tarts Minis*),							
1 pkt.	170	2.0	32.0	4.0	0	180	0
raisin bran (*Thomas'*							
Toast-r-Cakes) . . .	90	2.0	17.0	3.0	<5	170	1.0
raspberry:							
(*Toaster Strudel*)	180	3.0	26.0	7.0	5	200	<1.0
frosted (*Pop-Tarts*)	210	2.0	37.0	6.0	0	210	1.0
S'mores (*Pop Tarts*)	200	3.0	37.0	5.0	0	200	1.0
strawberry:							
(*Pop-Tarts*)	200	2.0	37.0	5.0	0	180	1.0
(*Pop-Tarts Minis*),							
1 pkt.	170	2.0	32.0	4.0	0	180	0
(*Thomas'*							
Toast-r-Cakes) . .	110	2.0	18.0	4.0	<5	160	<1.0
(*Toaster Strudel*)	180	3.0	26.0	7.0	5	200	<1.0
(*Toastettes*)	190	2.0	35.0	5.0	0	200	1.0
frosted (*Pop-Tarts*)	200	2.0	38.0	5.0	0	170	1.0
frosted (*Toastettes*)	190	2.0	35.0	5.0	0	190	1.0
Tofu:							
fresh:							
1 oz.	22	2.3	.5	1.4	0	2	.3
½ cup	94	10.0	2.3	5.9	0	9	1.5
extra firm (*Nasoya*),							
⅕ of 1-lb. block	90	11.0	1.0	5.0	0	10	0
firm, 1 oz.	41	4.5	1.2	2.5	0	4	.7

Food and Measure	cal.	prot. (gms)	carbo. (gms)	fat (gms)	chol. (mgs)	sod. (mgs)	fiber (gms)
firm, ½ cup	183	19.9	5.4	11.0	0	17	2.9
firm (*Nasoya*), ⅕ of 1-lb. block	80	9.0	2.0	4.0	0	10	0
pasteurized (*Frieda's*), 4.2 oz.	86	9.6	2.9	n.a.	0	8	0
silken (*Nasoya*), ⅕ of 1-lb. block	50	5.0	2.0	2.0	0	10	0
soft (*Nasoya*), ⅙ of 1-lb. block	60	7.0	2.0	3.0	0	5	0
flavored, ¼ block:							
5-spice (*Nasoya*)	70	8.0	0	4.0	0	70	0
French (*Nasoya*) . .	70	8.0	0	4.0	0	130	0
salted and fermented (fuyu), 1 oz.	33	2.3	1.5	2.3	0	814	<1.0
Tofu dishes, mix, dry:							
burger (*Fantastic*), ⅛ cup	70	3.0	12.0	1.5	0	320	2.0
chow mein, mandarin (*Fantastic*), ⅝ cup	170	6.0	33.0	1.5	0	720	3.0
shells 'n curry (*Fantastic*), ½ cup . . .	200	8.0	40.0	1.5	0	500	5.0
Stroganoff, creamy (*Fantastic*), ½ cup	190	10.0	35.0	5.0	5	660	3.0
Tofu seasoning mix, ¼ pkg.:							
breakfast scramble:							
(*Fantastic* Classics)	60	3.0	12.0	.5	0	480	3.0
(*TofuMate*)	15	0	3.0	0	0	340	0
eggless salad (*TofuMate*)	15	0	4.0	0	0	310	0
mandarin stir-fry (*TofuMate*)	30	1.0	6.0	0	0	310	0
Mediterranean herb (*TofuMate*)	15	1.0	3.0	0	0	310	0
Szechwan stir-fry (*TofuMate*)	25	1.0	4.0	0	0	290	0
Texas taco (*TofuMate*)	15	1.0	3.0	0	0	380	0

Food and Measure	cal.	prot. (gms)	carbo. (gms)	fat (gms)	chol. (mgs)	sod. (mgs)	fiber (gms)
Tom collins mixer (see also "Soft drinks"), bottled (*Holland House*), 3 fl. oz.	160	0	37.0	0	0	85	0
Tomatillo:							
1 medium, 1⅝″ diam.	11	.3	2.0	.4	0•	tr.	.6
chopped, ½ cup . . .	21	.6	3.8	.7	0	1	1.3
in jars:							
(*La Victoria* Entero), 5 pcs.	40	1.0	7.0	1.0	0	410	5.0
crushed (*La Victoria*), 4½ oz. . . .	45	2.0	8.0	.5	0	400	7.0
Tomato:							
raw:							
2⅗″ tomato	26	1.0	5.7	.4	0	11	1.4
chopped, ½ cup . .	19	.8	4.2	.3	0	8	1.0
boiled, ½ cup	32	1.3	7.0	.5	0	13	1.2
dried, see "Tomato, dried"							
Tomato, canned, (see also "Tomato sauce"), ½ cup, except as noted:							
(*Contadina* Pasta Ready)	40	1.0	5.0	2.0	0	620	1.0
(*Contadina* Recipe Ready)	25	1.0	5.0	0	0	200	1.0
(*Hunt's*)	30	1.0	7.0	0	0	30	1.5
whole:							
(*Del Monte*)	25	1.0	6.0	0	0	160	2.0
(*Hunt's*), 2 pcs. . . .	20	2.0	4.0	0	0	400	1.0
(*Hunt's* No Salt), 2 pcs.	20	1.0	4.5	0	0	5	1.0
Italian pear (*Contadina*)	25	1.0	4.0	0	0	220	1.0
Italian pear, w/basil (*S&W*)	25	1.0	4.0	0	0	220	1.0
pear (*Hunt's*) . . .	20	1.0	4.0	0	0	360	1.0

Food and Measure	cal.	prot. (gms)	carbo. (gms)	fat (gms)	chol. (mgs)	sod. (mgs)	fiber (gms)
peeled (*Contadina*)	25	1.0	4.0	0	0	20	1.0
peeled (*Progresso*)	25	1.0	4.0	0	0	220	1.0
peeled (*S&W*) . . .	25	1.0	4.0	0	0	220	1.0
peeled (*S&W* No-Salt)	20	2.0	4.0	0	0	90	1.0
w/basil (*Progresso*)	25	1.0	4.0	0	0	220	1.0
w/basil (*Progresso* Imported)	25	1.0	4.0	0	0	200	1.0
w/green chilies (*Ro*Tel*)	20	<1.0	4.0	0	0	370	1.0
aspic (*S&W*)	50	1.0	14.0	0	0	570	2.0
w/cheeses, three (*Contadina* Pasta Ready)	70	1.0	8.0	4.0	<5	650	<1.0
chunky:							
chili (*Del Monte*)	30	1.0	8.0	0	0	670	2.0
pasta (*Del Monte*)	45	1.0	11.0	0	0	560	2.0
salsa (*Del Monte*)	35	1.0	8.0	0	0	560	2.0
crushed:							
(*Contadina*), ¼ cup	20	<1.0	4.0	0	0	150	1.0
(*Eden*)	20	1.0	3.0	0	0	0	1.0
(*Hunt's*)	30	1.0	7.0	0	0	285	1.5
(*Hunt's* Angela Mia)	30	1.0	6.0	0	0	380	2.0
(*Progresso*)	20	1.0	4.0	0	0	95	1.0
(*S&W*), ¼ cup . .	20	1.0	4.0	0	0	95	1.0
cut:							
(*Hunt's* Choice Cut)	20	1.0	5.0	0	0	325	1.0
in juice (*S&W* Ready-Cut) . . .	25	1.0	4.0	0	0	190	1.0
in juice (*S&W* Ready-Cut No-Salt)	25	1.0	4.0	0	0	30	1.0
in juice, Italian style (*S&W* Ready-Cut)	25	1.0	4.0	0	0	190	1.0
in puree (*S&W* Ready-Cut) . . .	30	2.0	6.0	0	0	410	2.0
diced:							
(*Del Monte*)	25	1.0	6.0	0	0	25	2.0

Food and Measure	cal.	prot. (gms)	carbo. (gms)	fat (gms)	chol. (mgs)	sod. (mgs)	fiber (gms)
Tomato, canned, diced *(cont.)*							
w/basil (*Master Choice*)	40	1.0	9.0	0	0	330	n.a.
w/basil, garlic, oregano (*Del Monte*)	50	2.0	11.0	0	0	650	<1.0
w/green chiles (*Hunt's* Choice Cut), 2 tbsp. . . .	0	0	0	0	0	25	0
w/onion, garlic (*Del Monte*)	35	2.0	7.0	0	0	440	<1.0
w/roasted garlic (*Hunt's* Choice Cut)	25	1.0	5.0	0	0	505	<1.0
Italian herb (*Hunt's* Choice Cut) . . .	25	1.0	5.0	0	0	600	<1.0
w/green chilies:							
whole or diced (*Ro*Tel*)	20	<1.0	4.0	0	0	370	1.0
(*Old El Paso*), ¼ cup	100	0	2.0	0	0	310	2.0
diced (*Chi-Chi's*), ¼ cup	20	0	4.0	0	0	340	0
w/jalapeños (*Old El Paso*), ¼ cup . . .	15	1.0	3.0	0	0	290	3.0
w/mushrooms (*Contadina* Pasta Ready)	50	1.0	9.0	1.5	0	640	1.0
w/olives (*Contadina* Pasta Ready) . . .	60	1.0	8.0	3.0	0	640	1.0
paste, see "Tomato paste"							
primavera (*Contadina* Pasta Ready) . . .	50	1.0	8.0	1.5	0	600	1.0
puree, see "Tomato puree"							
w/red pepper, crushed (*Contadina* Pasta Ready)	60	1.0	8.0	3.0	0	690	1.0
stewed:							
½ cup	34	1.2	8.3	.2	0	325	.9

Food and Measure	cal.	prot. (gms)	carbo. (gms)	fat (gms)	chol. (mgs)	sod. (mgs)	fiber (gms)
(*Contadina*)	40	1.0	9.0	0	0	250	1.0
(*Del Monte*)	35	1.0	9.0	0	0	360	2.0
(*Del Monte* No Salt)	35	1.0	9.0	0	0	50	2.0
(*Green Giant* Classic)	35	1.0	7.0	0	0	360	2.0
(*Hunt's*)	35	1.0	7.0	0	0	360	2.0
(*S&W*)	35	1.0	7.0	0	0	270	2.0
(*S&W* No-Salt) . .	35	1.0	7.0	0	0	15	2.0
Cajun (*Del Monte*)	35	1.0	9.0	0	0	460	2.0
Italian (*Contadina*)	40	1.0	8.0	0	0	260	1.0
Italian (*Del Monte*)	30	1.0	8.0	0	0	420	2.0
Italian (*Green Giant*)	30	1.0	7.0	0	0	360	2.0
Italian (*S&W*) . . .	35	1.0	7.0	0	0	270	2.0
Mexican (*Contadina*)	40	1.0	9.0	0	0	220	1.0
Mexican (*Del Monte*)	35	1.0	9.0	0	0	400	2.0
Mexican (*Green Giant*)	35	1.0	7.0	0	0	400	2.0
wedges (*Del Monte*)	35	1.0	9.0	0	0	380	2.0
Tomato, dried:							
1 oz.	73	4.0	15.8	.8	0	594	3.5
1 pc. (32 per cup) . .	5	.3	1.1	.1	0	42	.3
½ cup	70	3.8	15.1	.8	0	566	3.3
(*Frieda's* No Salt), 1 oz.	86	3.7	21.2	.1	0	38	n.a.
bits (*Sonoma*), 2–3 tsp.	15	1.0	3.0	0	0	5	1.0
flakes (*Christopher Ranch*), 3 tbsp. . .	80	4.0	15.0	0	0	35	4.0
halves (*Sonoma*), 2–3 pcs.	15	1.0	3.0	0	0	5	1.0
julienne (*Sonoma*), 7–9 strips	15	1.0	3.0	0	0	5	1.0
in oil, drained (*Sonoma* Spice Medley), 1 tbsp.	50	1.0	3.0	4.0	0	200	1.0
pasta toss (*Sonoma*), ½ cup	70	4.0	13.0	0	0	75	3.0

Food and Measure	cal.	prot. (gms)	carbo. (gms)	fat (gms)	chol. (mgs)	sod. (mgs)	fiber (gms)
Tomato, dried *(cont.)*							
seasoning (*Sonoma*							
Season It), 2–3 tsp.	20	1.0	3.0	0	0	25	1.0
Tomato, green, 2³/₅"							
tomato	30	1.5	6.3	.3	0	16	1.8
Tomato, pickled,							
1 oz.:							
(*Claussen*)	5	0	1.0	0	0	320	<1.0
(*Hebrew National/*							
Shorr's), 1 oz. . . .	4	0	1.0	0	0	280	n.a.
half sour (*Rosoff*) . .	5	0	1.0	0	0	290	n.a.
Tomato, sun-dried,							
see "Tomato, dried"							
Tomato dip, sun-dried							
(*Marie's*), 2 tbsp.	140	2.0	2.0	14.0	15	135	<1.0
Tomato chutney, see							
"Chutney"							
Tomato juice,							
8 fl. oz.:							
(*Campbell's*)	50	1.0	9.0	0	0	860	1.0
(*Campbell's* Enhanced							
Flavor Low Sodium)	50	1.0	10.0	0	0	140	1.0
(*Del Monte*)	50	2.0	10.0	0	0	760	1.0
(*Del Monte* Not from							
Concentrate)	40	3.0	7.0	0	0	550	0
(*Hunt's*)	35	1.5	7.5	0	0	690	2.0
(*Hunt's* No Salt) . . .	35	1.5	7.5	0	0	10	2.0
(*R.W. Knudsen*) . . .	60	2.0	14.0	0	0	390	0
(*Sacramento*)	35	3.0	8.0	0	0	550	3.0
(*S&W*)	40	3.0	7.0	0	0	550	0
garlic (*R.W. Knudsen*)	60	2.0	13.0	0	0	32	0
Tomato paste,							
2 tbsp.:							
(*Contadina*)	30	2.0	6.0	0	0	20	1.0
(*Del Monte*)	30	1.0	7.0	0	0	25	2.0
(*Goya*)	30	2.0	6.0	0	0	20	1.0
(*Hunt's*)	30	1.0	6.0	0	0	90	2.0
(*Hunt's* No Salt) . . .	30	1.0	6.0	0	0	<10	2.0
(*Progresso*)	30	2.0	6.0	0	0	20	1.0

Food and Measure	cal.	prot. (gms)	carbo. (gms)	fat (gms)	chol. (mgs)	sod. (mgs)	fiber (gms)
(S&W)	30	2.0	6.0	0	0	20	1.0
w/garlic (Hunt's) . . .	30	1.0	6.0	0	0	280	2.0
Italian (Contadina) . .	40	1.0	7.0	1.0	0	320	1.0
Italian (Hunt's)	30	1.0	6.0	0	0	260	2.0
Tomato pesto, see "Pesto sauce"							
Tomato powder (AlpineAire), 2 oz. . . .	104	5.0	22.0	1.0	0	14	n.a.
Tomato puree, ¼ cup:							
(Contadina)	20	<1.0	4.0	0	0	15	<1.0
(Hunt's)	25	1.0	4.0	0	0	100	1.0
(Progresso)	25	1.0	5.0	0	0	15	1.0
thick (Progresso) . .	30	1.0	5.0	0	0	15	1.0
Tomato sauce, **canned** (see also "Pasta sauce" and "Tomato, canned"), ¼ cup, except as noted:							
(Contadina)	20	<1.0	4.0	0	0	280	<1.0
(Contadina Thick & Zesty)	20	1.0	3.0	0	0	340	1.0
(Del Monte)	20	<1.0	4.0	0	0	340	<1.0
(Del Monte No Salt)	20	<1.0	4.0	0	0	20	<1.0
(Goya)	20	1.0	4.0	0	0	280	1.0
(Hunt's)	15	1.0	3.0	0	0	360	1.0
(Hunt's No Salt) . . .	15	1.0	3.0	0	0	10	1.0
(Progresso)	20	1.0	4.0	0	0	260	1.0
(S&W)	20	1.0	4.0	0	0	300	1.0
chili, chunky (Hunt's Ready Sauce) . . .	20	1.0	3.0	0	0	320	1.0
chunky:							
(Hunt's Ready Sauce)	15	1.0	3.0	0	0	400	1.0
(Hunt's Ready Sauce Special)	20	1.0	4.0	<1.0	0	145	1.0
garden:							
(S&W Original) . .	20	0	4.0	0	0	200	1.0

Food and Measure	cal.	prot. (gms)	carbo. (gms)	fat (gms)	chol. (mgs)	sod. (mgs)	fiber (gms)
Tomato sauce, canned, garden *(cont.)*							
Italian herb (*S&W*),							
½ cup	35	2.0	9.0	0	0	470	2.0
mild Mexican							
(*S&W*)	20	1.0	4.0	0	0	190	1.0
garlic:							
(*Hunt's Ready*							
Sauce)	30	1.0	4.0	1.0	0	270	2.0
and herb (*Hunt's*							
Ready Sauce) . .	25	1.0	3.0	0	0	360	1.0
herb:							
(*Hunt's*)	30	1.0	5.0	1.0	0	270	1.0
country (*Hunt's*							
Ready Sauce) . .	35	1.0	5.0	1.0	0	255	1.0
and garlic (*S&W*							
Cooking Sauce),							
1 tbsp.	15	0	0	1.0	0	150	0
Italian:							
(*Contadina*)	15	<1.0	4.0	0	0	320	<1.0
(*Hunt's*)	30	1.0	5.0	1.0	0	210	1.0
(*Hunt's Ready*							
Sauce)	30	1.0	4.0	1.0	0	180	1.5
chunky (*Hunt's*							
Ready Sauce) . .	25	1.0	5.0	0	0	250	1.5
meatloaf (*Hunt's*							
Ready Sauce							
Meatloaf Fixin's) . .	20	1.0	4.0	0	0	600	1.0
Mexican, chunky							
(*Hunt's Ready*							
Sauce)	20	1.0	4.0	0	0	390	1.0
salsa (*Hunt's Ready*							
Sauce)	20	1.0	3.0	0	0	360	1.0
seasoned, lightly							
(*Eden*)	25	1.0	5.0	0	0	45	1.0
Tomato tapenade,							
dried (*Sonoma*),							
1 tbsp.	70	1.0	4.0	6.0	0	5	1.0

Food and Measure	cal.	prot. (gms)	carbo. (gms)	fat (gms)	chol. (mgs)	sod. (mgs)	fiber (gms)
Tomato-beef cocktail							
(*Beefamato*),							
8 fl. oz.	80	1.0	20.0	0	0	780	1.0
Tomato-chili cocktail							
(*Snap-E-Tom*):							
6 fl. oz.	40	2.0	8.0	0	0	500	1.0
10 fl. oz.	60	3.0	13.0	0	0	840	2.0
Tomato-clam cock-							
tail, 8 fl. oz.:							
(*Clamato*)	100	1.0	24.0	0	0	720	0
Caesar (*Clamato*) . .	100	0	24.0	0	0	780	0
Tongue, braised:							
beef, 4 oz.	321	25.1	.4	23.5	121	68	0
lamb, 4 oz.	312	24.5	0	23.0	214	76	0
pork, 4 oz.	307	27.3	0	21.1	166	124	0
veal (calf), 4 oz. . . .	229	29.3	0	11.5	n.a.	73	0
Tongue lunch meat,							
beef, corned (*He-*							
brew National),							
2 oz.	120	10.0	0	9.0	50	330	0
Tortellini, frozen or							
refrigerated:							
cheese, three, ¾ cup:							
(*Contadina*)	260	11.0	41.0	6.0	35	290	1.0
spinach (*Contadina*)	260	13.0	39.0	6.0	55	390	3.0
mushroom (*Con-*							
tadina), 1 cup . . .	310	11.0	49.0	8.0	45	250	2.0
spinach (*Putney*),							
1 cup	290	17.0	49.0	3.0	55	460	1.0
tofu:							
(*Soy-Boy*), ⅞ cup	190	8.0	32.0	3.0	0	140	1.0
(*Tofutti*), 1 cup . .	320	15.0	54.0	5.0	0	440	2.0
Tortellini dishes							
cheese, frozen (*The*							
Budget Gourmet							
Side Dish), 6.25 oz.	190	6.0	24.0	8.0	10	800	3.0

Food and Measure	cal.	prot. (gms)	carbo. (gms)	fat (gms)	chol. (mgs)	sod. (mgs)	fiber (gms)
Tortellini entree, canned:							
cheese, 1 cup:							
(*Chef Boyardee*) . .	230	9.0	46.0	1.0	15	770	5.0
(*Franco-American*)	240	6.0	44.0	4.0	25	1140	2.0
meat, 1 cup:							
(*Chef Boyardee*) . .	260	10.0	48.0	3.0	20	810	6.0
(*Franco-American*)	260	14.0	36.0	9.0	30	1 140	2.0
ground beef (*Chef Boyardee*), 7½ oz.	220	8.0	39.0	2.5	15	680	4.0
Tortilla:							
corn (*Tyson*), 3 pcs.	140	3.0	31.0	1.0	0	0	1.0
corn, white (*Goya*), 2 pcs.	120	2.0	26.0	1.5	0	0	3.0
flour, 1 pc.:							
(*Goya*)	110	3.0	18.0	2.5	0	290	3.0
(*Mesa 6″*)	80	2.0	15.0	1.5	0	210	<1.0
(*Old El Paso*) . . .	150	4.0	27.0	3.0	0	340	0
(*Tyson*), 1.4 oz. . .	120	3.0	21.0	3.0	0	290	1.0
(*Tyson*), 1.9 oz. . .	170	4.0	30.0	4.0	0	410	2.0
small (*Goya*)	80	3.0	14.0	2.0	0	220	2.0
flour, heat pressed (*Tyson*), 2 pcs. . .	180	4.0	30.0	4.5	0	420	2.0
soft taco (*Old El Paso*), 2 pcs. . . .	180	5.0	33.0	3.5	0	410	0
Tortilla chips, see "Corn chips, puffs, and similar snacks"							
Tostaco or tostada shell, see "Taco shell"							
Tostone, see "Plantain"							
Trail mix:							
(*Eden* Fruit & Nuts), 1 oz.	160	7.0	10.0	10.0	0	0	3:0
(*Sonoma*), ¼ cup . .	160	3.0	24.0	7.0	0	5	2.0
California:							
(*Dole*), 1.2 oz. . . .	130	5.0	23.0	2.5	0	0	3.0

Food and Measure	cal.	prot. (gms)	carbo. (gms)	fat (gms)	chol. (mgs)	sod. (mgs)	fiber (gms)
(*Dole*), 2 oz.	220	9.0	38.0	4.0	0	0	4.0
(*Eden* Harvest),							
1 oz.	130	4.0	14.0	7.0	0	0	3.0
Hawaiian:							
(*Dole*), 1.2 oz. . . .	150	2.0	26.0	4.0	0	20	3.0
(*Dole*), 2 oz.	250	4.0	44.0	6.0	0	35	4.0
Sierra:							
(*Del Monte*), .9 oz.	110	3.0	15.0	6.0	0	45	2.0
(*Del Monte*), 1 oz.	120	3.0	16.0	6.0	0	50	2.0
(*Del Monte*), ¼ cup	150	4.0	20.0	8.0	0	65	3.0
Tree fern, cooked,							
chopped, ½ cup . .	28	.2	7.8	.1	0	3	2.6
Triticale, whole grain,							
1 cup	646	25.1	138.5	4.0	0	10	34.8
Triticale flour, whole							
grain, 1 cup	440	17.1	95.1	2.4	0	3	19.0
Tropical punch, see							
"Fruit drink blends"							
and "Fruit juice							
blends"							
Trout, meat only:							
mixed species:							
raw, 4 oz.	168	23.6	0	7.5	66	59	0
baked, broiled, or							
microwaved, 4 oz.	215	30.2	0	9.6	84	76	0
rainbow, farmed:							
raw, 4 oz.	156	23.7	0	6.1	67	40	0
baked, broiled, or							
microwaved, 4 oz.	192	27.5	0	8.2	77	48	0
rainbow, wild:							
raw, 4 oz.	135	23.2	0	3.9	67	35	0
baked, broiled, or							
microwaved, 4 oz.	170	26.0	0	6.6	78	64	0
sea, see "Sea trout"							
smoked, peppered,							
rainbow (*Spence &*							
Co.), 2 oz.	100	14.0	0	5.0	30	430	0

Food and Measure	cal.	prot. (gms)	carbo. (gms)	fat (gms)	chol. (mgs)	sod. (mgs)	fiber (gms)
Tuna, meat only:							
bluefin:							
raw, 4 oz.	163	26.5	0	5.6	43	44	0
baked, broiled, or							
microwaved, 4 oz.	209	33.9	0	7.1	56	57	0
skipjack:							
raw, 4 oz.	117	25.0	0	1.2	53	42	0
baked, broiled, or							
microwaved, 4 oz.	150	32.0	0	1.5	68	53	0
yellowfin:							
raw, 4 oz.	123	26.5	0	1.1	51	42	0
baked, broiled, or							
microwaved, 4 oz.	158	34.0	0	1.4	66	53	0
Tuna, canned,							
drained, 2 oz. or							
¼ cup:							
chunk light, oil:							
(*Bumble Bee*) . . .	110	13.0	0	6.0	30	250	0
(*Chicken of the Sea*)	110	13.0	0	6.0	30	250	0
(*S&W*)	110	14.0	0	6.0	30	230	0
(*Star-Kist*)	110	13.0	0	6.0	30	250	0
chunk light, water:							
(*Bumble Bee*) . . .	60	13.0	0	.5	30	250	0
(*S&W*)	70	15.0	0	.5	35	230	0
solid, olive oil							
(*Progresso*)	160	13.0	0	12.0	30	250	0
solid light, water							
(*Star-Kist/Star-Kist*							
Prime Catch)	60	13.0	0	1.0	30	250	0
solid white, oil:							
(*Bumble Bee*) . . .	90	14.0	0	3.0	25	250	0
(*Chicken of the Sea*)	90	14.0	0	3.0	25	250	0
(*S&W*)	80	17.0	0	1.5	20	230	0
(*Star-Kist*)	90	15.0	0	3.0	25	250	0
solid white, water							
(*Bumble Bee*) . . .	70	15.0	0	1.0	25	250	0
Tuna, frozen, yellow-							
tail (*Peter Pan*),							
4 oz.	110	26.0	0	.5	35	35	0

Food and Measure	cal.	prot. (gms)	carbo. (gms)	fat (gms)	chol. (mgs)	sod. (mgs)	fiber (gms)
"Tuna," vegetarian, frozen (*Worthington Tuno*), drained, ½ cup	80	6.0	2.0	6.0	0	290	1.0
Tuna casserole, frozen, noodle, 1 pkg.:							
(*Stouffer's*)	320	20.0	37.0	10.0	40	1130	0
(*Swanson*)	320	17.0	38.0	11.0	25	800	1.0
(*Weight Watchers*) . .	270	13.0	39.0	7.0	35	590	4.0
Tuna entree mix, dry: broccoli, creamy (*Tuna Helper*), ⅔ cup	190	6.0	33.0	4.5	5	700	1.0
cheddar, garden (*Tuna Helper*), ⅔ cup . .	190	6.0	33.0	4.0	<5	850	1.0
pasta, ¾ cup: cheesy (*Tuna Helper*)	170	5.0	29.0	3.0	<5	710	<1.0
creamy (*Tuna Helper*)	190	5.0	29.0	6.0	<5	730	1.0
pot pie (*Tuna Helper*), ½ cup	340	5.0	35.0	20.0	0	920	1.0
Tuna salad spread (*Libby's Spreadables*), ⅓ cup . . .	130	7.0	6.0	8.0	15	370	3.0
Turbot, European, meat only: raw, 4 oz.	108	18.2	0	3.4	n.a.	170	0
baked, broiled, or microwaved, 4 oz. . .	138	23.3	0	4.3	n.a.	218	0
Turkey (see also "Turkey, frozen or refrigerated"), fresh, all classes, roasted: meat w/skin, 4 oz. . .	236	31.9	0	11.0	93	77	0
meat only: 4 oz.	193	3.2	0	5.6	86	79	0
diced, 1 cup	238	41.0	0	7.0	107	99	0
skin only, 1 oz. . . .	125	5.6	0	11.2	32	15	0

Food and Measure	cal.	prot. (gms)	carbo. (gms)	fat (gms)	chol. (mgs)	sod. (mgs)	fiber (gms)
Turkey *(cont.)*							
dark meat:							
w/skin, 4 oz.	251	31.2	0	13.1	101	86	0
meat only, 4 oz. . . .	212	32.4	0	8.2	96	90	0
meat only, diced,							
1 cup	262	40.0	0	10.1	119	110	0
light meat:							
w/skin, 4 oz.	223	32.4	0	9.4	86	71	0
meat only, 4 oz. . . .	178	33.9	0	3.7	78	73	0
meat only, diced,							
1 cup	219	41.9	0	4.5	97	89	0
breast, meat w/skin:							
½ breast, 1.9 lb.,							
(4.2 lbs. raw w/							
bone)	1637	248.1	0	64.1	643	541	0
4 oz.	214	32.6	0	8.4	84	71	0
ground, see "Turkey,							
ground"							
leg, meat w/skin:							
1.2 lb. (1.5 lbs. raw							
w/bone)	1133	152.2	0	53.6	466	420	0
4 oz.	236	31.6	0	11.1	96	87	0
wing, meat w/skin:							
6.6 oz. (9.9 oz. raw							
w/bone)	426	50.9	0	23.1	150	114	0
4 oz.	260	31.0	0	14.1	92	69	0
Turkey, canned,							
chunk, 2 oz.,							
¼ cup:							
(Hormel)	70	11.0	0	3.0	35	340	0
(Swanson Premium)	100	6.0	2.0	4.0	50	230	0
white:							
(Hormel)	60	13.0	0	1.0	25	320	0
(Swanson Premium)	90	3.0	4.0	2.0	35	220	1.0
Turkey, dried, diced							
(AlpineAire), ⅓ cup	80	13.0	n.a.	1.0	n.a.	n.a.	n.a.

Food and Measure	cal.	prot. (gms)	carbo. (gms)	fat (gms)	chol. (mgs)	sod. (mgs)	fiber (gms)
Turkey, frozen or re- **frigerated,** 4 oz., except as noted:							
whole, raw, young:							
(*Norbest* Family Tra- dition, 8–16 lbs.)	190	23.0	0	10.0	70	70	0
(*Norbest* Family Tra- dition, 16–24 lbs.)	170	23.0	0	8.5	80	80	0
basted (*Norbest,* 8–16 lbs.)	180	21.0	0	9.5	65	180	0
basted (*Norbest,* 16–24 lbs.) . . .	165	22.0	0	8.0	75	190	0
whole, cooked, 3 oz.:							
dark meat (*Perdue*)	200	19.0	0	14.0	95	55	0
white meat (*Perdue*)	170	22.0	0	9.0	70	35	0
barbecued (*Empire* Kosher), 5 oz. . .	250	35.0	0	12.0	100	320	0
breast, raw:							
basted (*Norbest*)	170	22.0	0	8.5	60	270	0
boneless (*Perdue*)	130	28.0	0	1.5	65	60	0
cutlets, thin sliced (*Perdue*), 3½ oz.	100	23.0	0	1.5	60	40	0
fillets (*Perdue*) . . .	120	27.0	0	1.0	65	60	0
roast, boneless (*Norbest*)	135	20.0	0	6.0	60	490	0
tenderloins (*Perdue*)	120	27.0	0	1.0	65	60	0
breast, cooked:							
(*Perdue* Whole), 3 oz.	170	23.0	0	2.5	65	30	0
(*Perdue* Half), 3 oz.	170	24.0	0	8.0	65	35	0
boneless or tender- loins (*Perdue*), 3 oz.	110	26.0	0	1.0	55	35	0
cutlets, thin sliced (*Perdue*), 2.5 oz.	90	21.0	0	1.0	50	25	0
fillets (*Perdue*), 3 oz.	110	26.0	0	1.0	55	50	0

Food and Measure	cal.	prot. (gms)	carbo. (gms)	fat (gms)	chol. (mgs)	sod. (mgs)	fiber (gms)
Turkey, frozen or refrigerated, breast, cooked *(cont.)*							
honey roasted							
(*Louis Rich*),							
2.8-oz. slice . . .	80	16.0	3.0	1.0	35	940	0
breast, oven roasted:							
(*Louis Rich*), 2.8 oz.	70	16.0	1.0	1.0	35	890	0
(*Hebrew National*),							
2 oz.	60	13.0	0	1.0	25	350	0
skinless (*Hebrew*							
National), 2 oz.	50	11.0	0	.5	25	450	0
breast, smoked:							
(*Hebrew National*),							
2 oz.	60	12.0	0	.5	25	330	0
(*Hormel Light &*							
Lean 97), 3 oz.	80	17.0	1.0	1.0	35	780	0
(*Louis Rich* Hick-							
ory), 2.8-oz. slice	80	16.0	2.0	1.0	35	1050	0
(*Perdue*), 3 oz. . .	150	22.0	0	7.0	100	70	0
ground, see "Turkey,							
ground"							
maple glaze (*Boar's*							
Head Honey Coat),							
3 oz.	100	21.0	3.0	1.0	45	660	0
roast, boneless							
(*Norbest*)	135	18.0	0	7.0	65	490	0
smoked, hickory							
(*Norbest* Young),							
3 oz.	145	16.0	0	9.0	50	720	0
steak, cubed, raw							
(*Perdue*)	110	23.0	0	2.0	90	95	0
thigh, cooked (*Per-*							
due), 3 oz.	180	20.0	0	11.0	100	55	0
wing, cooked:							
(*Perdue* Tom), 3 oz.	160	23.0	0	8.0	90	60	0
portion (*Perdue*),							
3 oz.	170	21.0	0	10.0	95	60	0
roasted (*Perdue*),							
3-oz. wing	180	22.0	0	10.0	95	60	0

Food and Measure	cal.	prot. (gms)	carbo. (gms)	fat (gms)	chol. (mgs)	sod. (mgs)	fiber (gms)
roasted (*Perdue* Drummettes), 3½-oz. pc.	180	24.0	0	9.0	100	65	0
Turkey, ground:							
raw, 4 oz.:							
(*Louis Rich*)	190	20.0	0	12.0	90	140	0
(*Norbest*)	170	16.0	0	10.0	75	75	0
(*Perdue*)	160	22.0	0	8.0	110	85	0
(*Shady Brook Farms*)	170	2.0	0	9.0	90	105	0
breast (*Perdue*) . .	120	27.0	0	1.5	65	70	0
breast (*Shady Brook Farms*)	120	28.0	0	1.0	70	55	0
cooked, 3 oz.:							
breast (*Perdue*) . .	110	24.0	0	1.5	55	40	0
regular or burger (*Perdue*)	170	21.0	0	9.0	110	65	0
"Turkey," vegetarian:							
canned (*Worthington Turkee*), 3 slices . .	130	13.0	3.0	14.0	0	580	2.0
frozen, smoked:							
roll (*Worthington*), ⅜″ slice	140	10.0	3.0	10.0	0	600	2.0
sliced (*Worthington*), 3 slices . .	140	10.0	3.0	10.0	0	620	2.0
Turkey bacon (*Louis Rich*), .5-oz. slice	30	2.0	0	2.5	10	190	0
Turkey bologna:							
(*Empire*), 3 slices . .	90	8.0	3.0	5.5	30	430	0
(*Louis Rich*), 1-oz. slice	50	3.0	1.0	3.5	20	270	0
(*Norbest*), 2 oz. . . .	130	7.0	0	11.0	45	640	0
Turkey dinner, frozen, 1 pkg.:							
breast:							
(*Healthy Choice*) . .	280	22.0	40.0	3.0	45	460	7.0
w/pasta (*Swanson*)	270	11.0	31.0	7.0	35	720	6.0

Food and Measure	cal.	prot. (gms)	carbo. (gms)	fat (gms)	chol. (mgs)	sod. (mgs)	fiber (gms)
Turkey dinner, breast *(cont.)*							
stuffed (*The Budget Gourmet* Light & Healthy)	260	23.0	29.0	6.0	35	660	7.0
mostly white meat:							
(*Swanson*)	300	9.0	42.0	6.0	35	1130	4.0
(*Swanson Hungry Man*)	510	23.0	59.0	15.0	45	1660	9.0
and gravy, w/dress-ing:							
(*Banquet*)	560	32.0	63.0	20.0	75	1910	7.0
(*Marie Callender's*)	530	33.0	51.0	17.0	85	230	2.0
Turkey entree, canned:							
gravy and dressing:							
(*Dinty Moore American Classics*), 10 oz.	290	22.0	32.0	8.0	45	1120	3.0
(*Libby's Diner*), 7 oz.	180	11.0	17.0	7.0	35	830	2.0
stew:							
(*Dinty Moore*), 1 cup	150	10.0	20.0	3.0	25	1080	3.0
(*Dinty Moore* Cup), 7.5 oz.	130	9.0	17.0	2.5	10	960	2.0
Turkey entree, freeze-dried, tetraz-zini (*Mountain House*), 1 cup . . .	210	14.0	20.0	8.0	45	1060	1.0
Turkey entree, fro-zen, 1 pkg., except as noted:							
(*Lean Cuisine* Home-style)	230	18.0	26.0	6.0	50	590	3.0
breast, stuffed (*Weight Watchers*)	230	17.0	28.0	5.0	15	680	6.0
fettuccine alla crema (*Healthy Choice*) . .	350	28.0	50.0	4.0	30	370	5.0

Food and Measure	cal.	prot. (gms)	carbo. (gms)	fat (gms)	chol. (mgs)	sod. (mgs)	fiber (gms)
glazed:							
(*The Budget Gour-*							
met Light &							
Healthy)	250	15.0	38.0	4.0	30	730	2.0
(*Lean Cuisine* Cafe							
Classics)	250	14.0	36.0	6.0	30	590	5.0
and gravy, w/dress-							
ing: (*Banquet*							
Homestyle)	270	15.0	31.0	10.0	45	1100	3.0
(*Swanson*)	230	8.0	30.0	5.0	30	1040	3.0
gravy and:							
(*Banquet* Family),							
2 slices	120	8.0	5.0	8.0	35	670	1.0
(*Banquet* Toppers),							
5-oz. bag	90	8.0	7.0	4.0	30	670	0
w/dressing (*Morton*)	230	14.0	27.0	8.0	35	1090	5.0
medallions (*Smart*							
Ones)	190	10.0	34.0	2.0	20	530	4.0
pie or pot pie:							
(*Banquet*)	370	10.0	38.0	20	45	850	3.0
(*Empire* Kosher) . .	470	21.0	46.0	23.0	25	820	11.0
(*Lean Cuisine*) . . .	300	20.0	34.0	9.0	50	590	3.0
(*Marie Callender's*)	710	17.0	57.0	46.0	20	770	4.0
(*Stouffer's*)	530	21.0	36.0	33.0	65	1040	3.0
(*Swanson*)	440	37.0	44.0	24.0	20	750	2.0
(*Swanson Hungry*							
Man)	650	52.0	65.0	34.0	45	1450	5.0
(*Tyson*)	550	15.0	49.0	33.0	20	780	4.0
open face, w/potato							
(*The Budget Gour-*							
met)	330	16.0	32.0	15.0	40	1010	3.0
roast:							
(*Healthy Choice*							
Country Inn) . . .	250	26.0	29.0	4.0	30	530	6.0
breast, and stuffing							
(*Lean Cuisine*) . .	290	16.0	48.0	4.0	25	530	3.0
w/mushrooms							
(*Healthy Choice*							
Country)	220	19.0	28.0	4.0	25	440	3.0

Food and Measure	cal.	prot. (gms)	carbo. (gms)	fat (gms)	chol. (mgs)	sod. (mgs)	fiber (gms)
Turkey entree, frozen, roast *(cont.)*							
and stuffing (*Stouffer's* Home-style)	280	19.0	25.0	11.0	40	950	1.0
tetrazzini (*Stouffer's*)	360	19.0	33.0	23.0	55	1060	1.0
Turkey fat, 1 tbsp.	115	0	0	12.8	13	0	0
Turkey frankfurter, 1 link:							
(*Empire* Kosher) . . .	90	9.0	<1.0	6.0	35	410	0
and beef (*Oscar Mayer* Hot Dogs)	40	7.0	2.0	0	15	460	0
and chicken:							
(*Louis Rich* 8/12 oz.), 1.5 oz.	80	6.0	1.0	6.0	40	480	0
(*Louis Rich* 10/16 oz.), 1.6 oz.	80	5.0	1.0	6.0	40	500	0
(*Louis Rich* Bun-Length)	110	7.0	3.0	8.0	50	630	0
cheese (*Louis Rich*)	90	5.0	2.0	7.0	40	420	0
Turkey giblets:							
simmered, 4 oz. . . .	189	30.1	2.4	5.8	474	67	0
simmered, diced, 1 cup	243	38.5	3.0	7.4	606	85	0
Turkey gravy, ¼ cup:							
(*Franco-American*) . .	25	2.0	3.0	1.0	<5	290	0
roasted (*Heinz*) . . .	25	1.0	3.0	1.0	0	360	0
seasoned, w/turkey (*Pepperidge Farm*)	30	2.0	4.0	1.0	<5	330	0
mix*:							
(*Durkee/French's*)	20	1.0	4.0	0	0	270	0
(*McCormick*)	20	<1.0	4.0	0	0	350	0
roasted (*Knorr*) . .	25	2.0	4.0	.5	<5	290	0
Turkey ham, 2 oz., except as noted:							
(*Healthy Deli*)	70	10.0	2.0	2.5	30	470	0
(*Louis Rich*)	70	11.0	1.0	2.5	40	620	0
(*Louis Rich* Round), 1-oz. slice	35	5.0	0	1.0	20	300	0

Food and Measure	cal.	prot. (gms)	carbo. (gms)	fat (gms)	chol. (mgs)	sod. (mgs)	fiber (gms)
(*Louis Rich* Square), 3 slices, 2.2 oz. . . .	70	11.0	1.0	2.5	45	710	0
(*Louis Rich Deli-Thin*), 4 slices, 2 oz.	60	10.0	0	1.5	35	580	0
(*Norbest* Tavern Ham) canned (*Hormel*)	70	9.0	0	4.0	40	600	0
chopped (*Louis Rich*), 1-oz. slice	40	5.0	0	2.5	20	290	0
honey cured (*Louis Rich*), 3 slices . . .	70	11.0	2.0	2.0	45	660	0
Turkey hash, roast (*Mary Kitchen*), 1 cup	210	23.0	23.0	3.0	60	950	2.0
Turkey lunch meat (see also "Turkey ham," etc.), 2 oz. breast, except as noted:							
(*Boar's Head* Premium Lower Sodium)	60	11.0	<1.0	2.0	25	310	0
(*Boar's Head* Premium Lower Sodium Skinless) . . .	60	12.0	<1.0	.5	25	340	0
(*Boar's Head Ovengold*)	60	12.0	1.0	1.5	35	360	0
(*Boar's Head Ovengold* Skinless)	60	13.0	0	1.0	20	350	0
(*Boar's Head Salsalito*)	60	13.0	1.0	.5	25	460	0
(*Hormel* Deli No Salt)	60	15.0	0	.5	30	35	0
(*Hormel* Deli Premium)	50	11.0	0	1.0	25	460	0
(*Hormel Light & Lean 97*)	50	10.0	1.0	.5	20	420	0
(*Hormel Light & Lean 97*), 1-oz. slice . .	30	5.0	0	.5	15	370	0
(*Hormel Sandwich Maker*)	45	8.0	2.0	.5	15	390	0

Food and Measure	cal.	prot. (gms)	carbo. (gms)	fat (gms)	chol. (mgs)	sod. (mgs)	fiber (gms)
Turkey lunch meat *(cont.)*							
(*Norbest* Bronze Label)	60	7.0	2.0	2.0	20	560	0
(*Norbest* Gold Label)	55	10.0	0	1.5	25	500	0
(*Norbest* Gold Label Golden Browned)	60	10.0	0	1.5	30	500	0
(*Norbest* Silver Label)	55	7.0	2.0	2.0	25	500	0
barbecued (*Louis Rich*)	60	2.0	2.0	1.0	25	630	0
Black Forest (*Healthy Deli*)	60	11.0	1.0	.5	20	480	0
cured (*Norbest* Gourmet)	70	7.0	0	4.5	35	620	0
honey roasted:							
(*Healthy Deli*) . . .	60	10.0	3.0	.5	20	480	0
(*Hormel Light & Lean 97*)	50	11.0	1.0	.5	20	530	0
(*Louis Rich*)	60	11.0	2.0	.5	25	660	0
lemon garlic (*Hebrew National*), 5 thin slices	50	0	11.0	.5	20	400	0
maple honey (*Boar's Head*)	70	14.0	2.0	.5	30	440	0
oven roasted:							
(*Alpine Lace*) . . .	50	12.0	0	0	25	290	0
(*Boar's Head Golden*)	60	11.0	0	2.0	25	340	0
(*Boar's Head* Golden Skinless)	60	13.0	<1.0	.5	25	350	0
(*Empire*), 3 slices	50	10.0	1.0	.5	15	200	0
(*Healthy Deli* Gourmet)	60	11.0	1.0	.5	20	440	0
(*Healthy Deli* Gourmet Brick Oven)	60	11.0	1.0	.5	20	470	0
(*Healthy Deli* Less Sodium)	60	10.0	1.0	.5	20	310	0
(*Healthy Deli* Natural Shape)	60	11.0	1.0	.5	20	480	0

Food and Measure	cal.	prot. (gms)	carbo. (gms)	fat (gms)	chol. (mgs)	sod. (mgs)	fiber (gms)
(*Hebrew National*), 5 thin slices . . .	50	11.0	0	.5	20	420	0
(*Hillshire Farm* Deli Select)							
(*Louis Rich*)	50	11.0	1.0	.5	25	620	0
(*Louis Rich* Fat Free), 1-oz. slice	25	4.0	1.0	0	10	310	0
(*Louis Rich Carving Board* Thin), 6 slices	60	12.0	0	.5	25	710	0
(*Louis Rich Carving Board* Traditional), 2 slices	40	9.0	0	.5	20	540	0
(*Louis Rich Deli-Thin* Fat Free), 4 slices	40	8.0	2.0	0	15	610	0
(*Oscar Mayer*), 1-oz. slice	25	5.0	1.0	.5	10	310	0
(*Oscar Mayer* Fat Free), 4 slices . .	40	8.0	2.0	0	15	610	0
glazed (*Healthy Deli Gourmet*)	60	11.0	1.0	.5	20	440	0
Italian (*Healthy Deli*)	70	10.0	4.0	.5	20	480	0
white (*Oscar Mayer*), 1-oz. slice	30	4.0	1.0	1.0	10	330	0
and white (*Louis Rich*)	60	9.0	2.0	1.0	20	630	0
and white (*Louis Rich*), 1-oz. slice	30	5.0	1.0	.5	10	310	0
and white (*Oscar Mayer Deli-Thin*), 4 slices	50	9.0	2.0	1.0	20	610	0
roast (*Oscar Mayer Deli-Thin*), 4 slices	50	9.0	2.0	1.0	20	580	0
skinless:							
(*Hormel*)	50	10.0	1.0	.5	20	420	0
(*Hormel* Deli) . . .	50	11.0	0	.5	20	480	0

Food and Measure	cal.	prot. (gms)	carbo. (gms)	fat (gms)	chol. (mgs)	sod. (mgs)	fiber (gms)
Turkey lunch meat *(cont.)*							
smoked:							
(*Boar's Head* Hickory)	70	12.0	<1.0	2.0	25	340	0
(*Boar's Head* Cracked Pepper Mill)	60	13.0	0	.5	30	460	0
(*Empire*), 3 slices	40	8.0	0	0	15	350	0
(*Healthy Deli* Mesquite)	60	11.0	1.0	.5	20	480	0
(*Hebrew National*), 5 thin slices . . .	60	0	11.0	.5	25	310	0
(*Hebrew National* Hickory)	60	0	11.0	.5	25	310	0
(*Hormel* Mesquite)	60	11.0	1.0	1.0	25	600	0
(*Hormel Light & Lean* 97 Mesquite), 1 oz. . . .	30	5.0	0	.5	15	370	0
(*Louis Rich* Hickory)	60	11.0	1.0	.5	25	740	0
(*Louis Rich* Hickory), 1-oz. slice	25	5.0	0	.5	10	260	0
(*Louis Rich* Fat Free Hickory), 1-oz. slice	25	4.0	1.0	0	10	300	0
(*Louis Rich* Carving Board), 2 slices	40	9.0	0	.5	20	540	0
(*Louis Rich* Deli-Thin Hickory), 4 slices	50	9.0	1.0	1.0	20	490	0
(*Norbest* Gold Label)	60	10.0	0	1.5	30	510	0
(*Oscar Mayer* Fat Free), 4 slices, 1.8 oz.	40	8.0	2.0	0	15	550	0
honey roasted (*Oscar Mayer* Deli-Thin), 4 slices, 1.8 oz.	60	10.0	2.0	1.0	20	520	0

Food and Measure	cal.	prot. (gms)	carbo. (gms)	fat (gms)	chol. (mgs)	sod. (mgs)	fiber (gms)
white (*Louis Rich*),							
1-oz. slice	30	5.0	0	1.0	15	280	0
Turkey nuggets,							
breaded (*Louis*							
Rich), 4 pcs.,							
3.25 oz.	260	13.0	15.0	16.0	35	640	0
Turkey pastrami,							
2 oz., except as							
noted:							
(*Boar's Head*)	60	14.0	0	.5	30	390	0
(*Empire*), 3 slices . .	60	9.0	0	2.0	30	270	1.0
(*Louis Rich*)	70	11.0	1.0	2.0	40	590	0
(*Louis Rich* Square),							
2 slices.	45	8.0	0	1.5	30	520	0
(*Healthy Deli*)	70	10.0	2.0	2.5	30	480	0
(*Hebrew National*) . .	60	10.0	0	2.5	45	560	0
(*Norbest*)	70	10.0	0	3.0	30	570	0
Turkey patty, breaded:							
(*Empire* Kosher),							
1 pc.	200	13.0	14.0	10.0	5	280	1.0
(*Louis Rich*), 1 pc.	220	12.0	13.0	13.0	35	550	0
Turkey pie, see "Tur-							
key entree"							
Turkey salad spread							
(*Libby's Spread-*							
ables), ⅓ cup . . .	150	7.0	6.0	10.0	25	310	2.0
Turkey salami:							
(*Empire*), 3 slices . .	70	9.0	1.0	3.5	35	350	0
(*Louis Rich*), 2 oz.	120	8.0	1.0	9.0	50	500	0
(*Louis Rich*),							
1-oz. slice	45	5.0	0	2.5	20	290	0
(*Norbest*), 2 oz. . . .	85	9.0	2.0	5.0	30	510	0
cooked, 1 oz.	56	4.6	.2	3.9	23	285	0
cotto (*Louis Rich*),							
1-oz. slice	40	5.0	0	2.5	25	290	0

Food and Measure	cal.	prot. (gms)	carbo. (gms)	fat (gms)	chol. (mgs)	sod. (mgs)	fiber (gms)
Turkey sandwich, frozen, 1 pc.:							
w/broccoli:							
(*Mrs. Paterson's* *Aussie Pie*) . . .	470	16.0	42.0	26.0	95	770	2.0
and cheese (*Lean* *Pockets*)	260	12.0	35.0	8.0	35	710	4.0
and ham w/cheddar:							
(*Hot Pockets*) . . .	320	14.0	38.0	13.0	35	680	1.0
(*Lean Pockets*) . .	260	15.0	35.0	7.0	35	810	4.0
Turkey sausage, raw, except as noted:							
(*Louis Rich* Links) 2 links, 2 oz. . . .	90	11.0	0	6.0	45	470	0
(*Shady Brook Farms* Old World), 4 oz.	190	20.0	3.0	11.0	65	850	0
breakfast:							
(*Perdue*), 2 links . .	100	9.0	0	6.0	45	450	0
(*Shady Brook* *Farms*), 4 oz. . .	160	20.0	1.0	9.0	70	950	0
breakfast, cooked (*Perdue*), 2 links . .	100	9.0	0	6.0	45	430	0
Italian, hot (*Shady* *Brook Farms*), 4 oz.	170	20.0	1.0	9.0	70	800	0
Italian, hot or sweet:							
(*Louis Rich*), 2.5 oz.	120	12.0	1.0	8.0	55	430	0
raw or cooked (*Perdue*), 1 link . . .	110	13.0	1.0	6.0	60	500	0
Italian, sweet (*Shady* *Brook Farms*), 4 oz.	170	20.0	2.0	9.0	70	730	0
smoked:							
(*Louis Rich*), 2 oz.	80	9.0	2.0	5.0	35	500	0
(*Louis Rich* Polska), 2 oz.	80	9.0	1.0	4.5	35	500	0
w/cheese (*Louis* *Rich*), 2 oz. . . .	90	9.0	2.0	5.0	35	540	0

Food and Measure	cal.	prot. (gms)	carbo. (gms)	fat (gms)	chol. (mgs)	sod. (mgs)	fiber (gms)
Turkey seasoning, w/ gravy (*McCormick Bag 'n Season*), 1 tsp.	15	<1.0	2.0	0	0	220	0
Turkey sticks, breaded (*Louis Rich*), 3 pcs.	230	12.0	12.0	15.0	35	580	0
Turmeric, dried:							
(*McCormick*), ¼ tsp.	2	.1	.4	0	0	<1	.1
ground, 1 tsp.	8	.2	1.4	.2	0	1	.5
Turnip, ½ cup, except as noted:							
fresh or stored:							
raw, cubed	18	.6	4.1	.1	0	44	1.2
boiled, cubed . . .	14	.6	3.8	.1	0	39	1.6
boiled, mashed . .	21	.8	5.6	.1	0	58	2.3
frozen, boiled, drained, 4 oz. . . .	26	1.7	4.9	.3	0	41	n.a.
Turnip greens, ½ cup, except as noted:							
fresh:							
raw, untrimmed, 1 lb.	85	4.8	18.2	1.0	0	126	7.6
raw, chopped . . .	7	.4	1.6	.1	0	11	.7
boiled, chopped . .	15	.8	3.1	.2	0	21	2.2
canned:							
w/liquid	17	1.6	2.8	.4	0	325	1.5
(*Allens/Sunshine*)	25	2.0	3.0	.5	0	15	2.0
chopped, w/diced turnip (*Allens/ Sunshine*)	30	1.0	5.0	.5	0	20	3.0
frozen:							
boiled, drained, w/turnips, 4 oz.	19	2.4	3.3	.2	0	17	3.5
w/diced turnips (*Seabrook*) . . .	30	2.0	2.0	0	0	20	2.0

Food and Measure	cal.	prot. (gms)	carbo. (gms)	fat (gms)	chol. (mgs)	sod. (mgs)	fiber (gms)
Turnover, frozen or refrigerated, 1 pc., except as noted:							
apple:							
(*Pepperidge Farm*)	330	4.0	48.0	14.0	0	180	6.0
(*Pillsbury*), 2 pcs.	350	4.0	45.0	17.0	0	660	1.0
iced (*Pepperidge Farm*)	360	4.0	53.0	14.0	0	190	2.0
mini (*Pepperidge Farm*)	140	2.0	15.0	8.0	0	80	1.0
blueberry (*Pepperidge Farm*)	340	4.0	45.0	16.0	0	200	6.0
cherry:							
(*Pepperidge Farm*)	320	4.0	46.0	13.0	0	190	6.0
(*Pillsbury*), 2 pcs.	360	4.0	48.0	17.0	0	650	<1.0
iced (*Pepperidge Farm*)	340	4.0	51.0	13.0	0	200	3.0
mini (*Pepperidge Farm*)	140	2.0	16.0	8.0	0	70	1.0
peach:							
(*Pepperidge Farm*)	340	4.0	47.0	15.0	0	180	6.0
cobbler, mini (*Pepperidge Farm*) . .	160	2.0	21.0	8.0	0	45	<1.0
raspberry:							
(*Pepperidge Farm*)	330	4.0	47.0	14.0	0	190	6.0
iced (*Pepperidge Farm*)	360	4.0	53.0	14.0	0	190	3.0
strawberry, mini (*Pepperidge Farm*) . . .	140	2.0	18.0	7.0	0	100	<1.0
Tzatziki (*Western Creamy*), 2 tbsp.	60	3.0	1.0	5.0	5	115	0

V

Food and Measure	cal.	prot. (gms)	carbo. (gms)	fat (gms)	chol. (mgs)	sod. (mgs)	fiber (gms)
Vanilla flavor drink:							
canned, 10 fl. oz.:							
(*Sego*)	240	12.0	37.0	5.0	5	280	0
(*Sego* Lite)	150	11.0	18.0	4.0	0	400	0
creme (*Sweet Success*)	200	12.0	38.0	3.0	5	220	6.0
French (*Sego* Lite)	150	11.0	18.0	4.0	0	380	0
mix, 1 pkt.:							
creamy (*Sweet Success*)	90	7.0	20.0	.5	<5	180	6.0
French (*Carnation Instant Breakfast*)	130	4.0	27.0	0	<5	110	0
French (*Carnation Instant Breakfast No Sugar*)	70	4.0	12.0	0	<5	90	0
Vanilla shake:							
(*Nestlé Killer*), 14 oz.	430	13.0	65.0	14.0	55	330	4.0
(*Nestlé Quik*), 9 oz.	280	8.0	42.0	9.0	35	210	3.0
Veal, meat only, 4 oz.:							
cubed, lean only, braised or stewed	213	39.6	0	4.9	164	105	0
ground, broiled . . .	195	27.6	0	8.6	117	94	0
leg:							
braised, lean w/fat	239	41.0	0	7.2	152	76	0
braised, lean only	230	41.6	0	5.8	159	76	0
roasted, lean w/fat	181	31.4	0	5.3	117	77	0
roasted, lean only	170	31.8	0	3.8	117	77	0
loin:							
braised, lean w/fat	322	34.2	0	19.5	134	91	0
braised, lean only	256	38.1	0	10.4	142	95	0

Food and Measure	cal.	prot. (gms)	carbo. (gms)	fat (gms)	chol. (mgs)	sod. (mgs)	fiber (gms)
Veal, loin *(cont.)*							
roasted, lean w/fat	246	28.1	0	14.0	117	105	0
roasted, lean only	198	29.8	0	7.9	120	109	0
rib:							
braised, lean w/fat	285	36.8	0	14.2	158	108	0
braised, lean only	247	39.1	0	8.9	163	112	0
roasted, lean w/fat	259	27.2	0	15.8	125	104	0
roasted, lean only	201	29.2	0	8.4	130	110	0
shoulder, whole:							
braised, lean w/fat	259	36.4	0	11.5	143	108	0
braised, lean only	226	38.2	0	6.9	147	110	0
roasted, lean w/fat	209	28.7	0	9.5	128	109	0
roasted, lean only	193	29.3	0	7.5	129	110	0
shoulder, arm:							
braised, lean w/fat	268	38.1	0	11.6	168	99	0
braised, lean only	228	40.5	0	6.0	176	102	0
roasted, lean w/fat	208	28.9	0	9.4	122	102	0
roasted, lean only	186	29.6	0	6.6	124	103	0
shoulder, blade:							
braised, lean w/fat	255	35.4	0	11.4	174	111	0
braised, lean only	224	37.0	0	7.3	179	115	0
roasted, lean w/fat	211	28.5	0	9.8	133	113	0
roasted, lean only	194	29.1	0	7.8	135	116	0
sirloin:							
braised, lean w/fat	286	35.4	0	14.9	122	90	0
braised, lean only	231	38.5	0	7.4	128	92	0
roasted, lean w/fat	229	28.5	0	11.9	116	94	0
roasted, lean only	191	29.8	0	7.1	118	96	0
"Veal," vegetarian, frozen (*Worthington Veelets*), 1 patty . .	180	14.0	10.0	9.0	0	390	5.0
Veal dinner, parmigiana, frozen, 1 pkg.:							
(*Swanson*)	400	28.0	40.0	18.0	85	1060	5.0
(*Swanson Hungry Man*)	640	35.0	74.0	23.0	75	2070	7.0

Food and Measure	cal.	prot. (gms)	carbo. (gms)	fat (gms)	chol. (mgs)	sod. (mgs)	fiber (gms)
Veal entree, parmigiana, frozen:							
(*Banquet*), 9 oz.	320	13.0	35.0	14.0	25	960	7.0
(*Morton*), 8.75 oz. . . .	280	8.0	30.0	13.0	20	950	4.0
(*Swanson*), 1 pkg. . . .	310	18.0	33.0	12.0	60	970	4.0
w/spaghetti (*Stouffer's* Homestyle),							
11⅞ oz.	420	20.0	43.0	19.0	75	1200	6.0
patties (*Banquet* Family), 1 patty	230	9.0	19.0	14.0	20	740	2.0
Vegetable antipasto,							
(*Paesana*), 3¾ oz.	260	2.0	3.0	12.0	0	250	.5
Vegetable burger, see " 'Hamburger,' vegetarian"							
Vegetable chips (*Eden*), 50 chips,							
1.1 oz.	130	<1.0	24.0	4.0	0	260	0
Vegetable dinner, frozen, 1 pkg.:							
(*Amy's* Country) . . .	380	11.0	60.0	12.0	15	570	9.0
loaf (*Amy's*)	260	8.0	47.0	5.0	0	690	7.0
Vegetable dishes, frozen (see also, "Vegetable entree, frozen" and specific listings):							
mandarin (*The Budget Gourmet* Side Dish),							
5.5 oz.	180	3.0	14.0	13.0	10	520	3.0
New England (*The Budget Gourmet* Side Dish), 5.5 oz.	240	6.0	22.0	16.0	33	490	2.0
samosa (*Deep* Indian Cuisine), 2 pcs. . .	130	3.0	15.0	7.0	0	370	1.0
spring, in cheese sauce (*The Budget Gourmet* Side Dish),							
5.5 oz.	150	6.0	10.0	10.0	25	450	2.0

Food and Measure	cal.	prot. (gms)	carbo. (gms)	fat (gms)	chol. (mgs)	sod. (mgs)	fiber (gms)
Vegetable entree, canned or in jars:							
Chinese, mixed (*La Choy*), ⅔ cup . . .	15	<1.0	3.0	0	0	30	1.0
chop suey (*La Choy*), ⅔ cup	15	1.0	3.0	0	0	320	1.0
curry (*Patak's*), ½ cup	180	6.0	18.0	10.0	10	580	3.0
Vegetable entree, frozen, 1 pkg., except as noted:							
Chinese, and chicken (*The Budget Gourmet* Light & Healthy)	290	1.0	42.0	9.0	15	720	4.0
country, and beef (*Lean Cuisine*) . . .	220	13.0	32.0	4.0	30	570	4.0
Italian, and chicken (*The Budget Gourmet* Light & Healthy)	280	10.0	44.0	7.0	25	660	3.0
pilaf, Indian (*Deep*), 1 cup	230	6.0	45.0	2.5	0	600	3.0
pot pie:							
(*Amy's*)	360	7.0	44.0	18.0	45	490	4.0
(*Amy's* Nondairy)	320	9.0	50.0	9.0	0	590	4.0
w/beef (*Morton*) . .	310	7.0	34.0	17.0	15	1380	2.0
w/cheese (*Banquet*)	390	8.0	49.0	18.0	15	1000	3.0
w/chicken (*Morton*)	320	8.0	32.0	18.0	25	1020	3.0
w/turkey (*Morton*)	300	8.0	29.0	18.0	25	1060	2.0
Shepherd's pie, nondairy (*Amy's*)	160	5.0	27.0	4.0	0	490	5.0
Vegetable entree mix, stew (*Knorr*), 1 pkg.	160	4.0	32.0	2.0	0	760	2.0
Vegetable juice, 8 fl. oz.:							
(*V-8* 100%)	50	1.0	10.0	0	0	620	1.0

Food and Measure	cal.	prot. (gms)	carbo. (gms)	fat (gms)	chol. (mgs)	sod. (mgs)	fiber (gms)
low sodium:							
(*R.W. Knudsen Very Veggie*)	50	3.0	10.0	1.0	0	32	n.a.
(*V-8*)	60	1.0	11.0	0	0	140	2.0
original, organic, or spicy (*R.W. Knudsen Very Veggie*)	50	3.0	10.0	1.0	0	32	n.a.
picante (*V-8*)	50	1.0	10.0	0	0	680	1.0
spicy hot (*V-8* 100%)	50	1.0	10.0	0	0	780	1.0
tangy (*V-8* 100%) . .	60	1.0	11.0	0	0	340	1.0
Vegetable oyster, see "Salsify"							
Vegetable pie, see "Vegetable entree"							
Vegetable pocket (see also specific listings), frozen, 1 pc.:							
Bar-B-Q (*Ken & Robert's Veggie Pockets*)	290	10.0	45.0	8.0	0	490	5.0
Greek (*Ken & Robert's Veggie Pockets*)	250	10.0	37.0	8.0	0	490	4.0
Indian (*Ken & Robert's Veggie Pockets*)	260	8.0	40.0	8.0	0	490	5.0
Oriental (*Ken & Robert's Veggie Pockets*)	250	8.0	40.0	8.0	0	490	5.0
pot pie:							
(*Amy's*)	230	7.0	37.0	6.0	0	420	2.0
(*Ken & Robert's Veggie Pockets*)	250	6.0	38.0	9.0	0	410	2.0
Santa Fe (*Ken & Robert's Veggie Pockets*)	250	8.0	39.0	8.0	0	550	5.0
Tex-Mex (*Ken & Robert's Veggie Pockets*)	280	9.0	46.0	8.0	0	490	6.0

Food and Measure	cal.	prot. (gms)	carbo. (gms)	fat (gms)	chol. (mgs)	sod. (mgs)	fiber (gms)
Vegetables, see specific listings							
Vegetables, mixed, fresh, 3 oz.:							
California style (*Dole*)	30	1.0	5.0	1.0	0	190	2.0
garden style (*Dole*)	30	2.0	4.0	.5	0	40	2.0
Italian style (*Dole*) . .	25	2.0	3.0	.5	0	280	3.0
New England (*Dole*)	50	2.0	9.0	.5	0	30	2.0
Oriental style (*Dole*)	30	2.0	4.0	.5	0	45	2.0
Vegetables, mixed, canned, ½ cup, except as noted:							
(*Del Monte*)	40	2.0	8.0	0	0	360	2.0
(*Del Monte* No Salt)	40	2.0	8.0	0	0	25	2.0
(*Goya*)	35	1.0	7.0	0	0	300	2.0
(*Green Giant*)	60	2.0	12.0	0	0	460	2.0
(*Green Giant Garden Medley*)	40	1.0	9.0	0	0	360	2.0
(*S&W*)	35	1.0	7.0	0	0	370	2.0
(*Stokely*)	35	1.0	7.0	0	0	320	2.0
(*Stokely* No Salt) . .	35	1.0	7.0	0	0	25	2.0
Chinese (*La Choy*), ⅔ cup	10	1.0	1.0	0	0	30	1.0
chop suey (*La Choy*)	15	1.0	3.0	0	0	325	1.0
and sauce:							
(*House of Tsang* Cantonese Classic)	70	1.0	14.0	1.0	0	960	1.0
hot and spicy (*House of Tsang* Szechuan)	70	1.0	14.0	1.0	0	1130	1.0
sweet and sour (*House of Tsang* Hong King) . . .	160	0	40.0	0	0	580	0
teriyaki (*House of Tsang* Tokyo) . .	100	1.0	23.0	0	0	1240	1.0
stew (*Stokely*)	45	1.0	10.0	0	0	320	2.0

Food and Measure	cal.	prot. (gms)	carbo. (gms)	fat (gms)	chol. (mgs)	sod. (mgs)	fiber (gms)
Vegetables, mixed, frozen:							
(*Goya*), ⅔ cup	60	3.0	11.0	0	0	50	2.0
(*Green Giant*), ¾ cup	50	2.0	11.0	0	0	35	3.0
(*Green Giant Harvest Fresh*), ⅔ cup . . .	50	2.0	10.0	0	0	125	3.0
(*Stilwell*), ½ cup . .	60	3.0	11.0	0	0	50	2.0
butter sauce (*Green Giant*), ¾ cup . . .	70	2.0	11.0	2.0	<5	240	3.0
California:							
(*Green Giant*), ¾ cup	25	1.0	2.0	0	0	15	2.0
(*Stilwell*), ½ cup	25	2.0	4.0	0	0	25	2.0
Capri (*Stilwell*), ½ cup	25	.5	4.0	0	0	20	1.0
English, cheddar (*Green Giant*), 4 oz.	120	4.0	15.0	5.0	5	390	3.0
French, garlic-Dijon (*Green Giant*), 4 oz.	60	2.0	6.0	3.0	10	380	2.0
Heartland (*Green Giant*), 1 cup	30	2.0	2.0	0	0	35	3.0
Italian, Parmesan (*Green Giant*), 4 oz.	70	4.0	8.0	2.5	5	250	3.0
Japanese, teriyaki (*Green Giant*), 4 oz.	50	3.0	9.0	0	0	400	2.0
Manhattan (*Green Giant*), 1 cup	25	2.0	1.0	0	0	15	2.0
New England (*Green Giant*), ⅔ cup . . .	70	2.0	13.0	1.5	0	70	3.0
Normandy, mushroom (*Green Giant*), 4 oz.	80	2.0	11.0	.5	10	270	2.0
San Francisco (*Green Giant*), ¾ cup . . .	30	1.0	6.0	0	0	20	2.0
Santa Fe (*Green Giant*), ¾ cup	60	2.0	4.0	0	0	10	2.0
Seattle (*Green Giant*), ¾ cup	25	1.0	2.0	0	0	15	2.0
stew (*Ore-Ida*), ⅔ cup	50	1.0	11.0	0	0	45	1.0

Food and Measure	cal.	prot. (gms)	carbo. (gms)	fat (gms)	chol. (mgs)	sod. (mgs)	fiber (gms)
Vegetables, mixed, frozen *(cont.)*							
tropical:							
(*Goya* Pasteles de Masa), 1 pouch	280	8.0	21.0	19.0	30	770	3.0
(*Goya* Viando Sancocho), 3 oz.	100	1.0	23.0	0	0	10	2.0
(*Goya* Yautia Malanga), ⅛ pkg.	130	2.0	30.0	0	0	40	2.0
Western (*Green Giant*), ¾ cup	50	1.0	9.0	1.5	0	10	2.0
Vegetables, mixed, freeze-dried, ½ cup:							
(*AlpineAire*)	71	3.0	16.0	.4	0	65	n.a.
garden (*AlpineAire*)	79	4.0	17.0	.5	0	20	n.a.
Vegetables, mixed, pickled (Gardiniera):							
(*Krinos*), 3 oz.	0	0	0	0	0	900	2.0
(*Perfecta*), 5.3 oz. . . .	0	0	0	0	0	900	0
(*Zorba*), ½ cup . . .	20	<1.0	2.0	1.0	0	850	n.a.
Vegetarian burger, see " 'Hamburger,' vegetarian"							
Vegetarian entree (see also specific listings):							
canned:							
(*Loma Linda Swiss Stake*), 1 pc. . .	120	9.0	8.0	6.0	0	430	4.0
(*Worthington Numete*), ⅜" slice	130	6.0	5.0	10.0	0	270	3.0
(*Worthington Protose*), ⅜" slice	130	13.0	5.0	7.0	0	280	3.0
choplet (*Worthington*), 2 pcs. . . .	90	17.0	3.0	1.5	0	500	2.0
cuts, dinner (*Loma Linda*), 2 pcs. . .	90	17.0	3.0	1.5	0	500	2.0
canned, cutlet:							
(*Worthington*), 1 pc.	70	11.0	3.0	1.0	0	340	2.0

Food and Measure	cal.	prot. (gms)	carbo. (gms)	fat (gms)	chol. (mgs)	sod. (mgs)	fiber (gms)
multigrain (*Worthington* 20 oz), 2 pcs.	100	15.0	5.0	2.0	0	390	4.0
multigrain (*Worthington* 50 oz.), 1 pc.	80	12.0	4.0	1.5	0	300	3.0
frozen:							
(*Worthington* FriPats), 1 patty	130	14.0	4.0	6.0	0	320	3.0
(*Worthington* Stakelets), 1 pc.	140	12.0	6.0	8.0	0	480	2.0
croquettes (*Worthington* Golden), 4 pcs.	210	14.0	14.0	10.0	0	600	6.0
dinner entree (*Natural Touch*), 3-oz. patty	220	19.0	2.0	15.0	0	380	2.0
nuggets, w/rice (*Hain* Hawaiian), 10 oz.	310	13.0	55.0	5.0	0	495	6.0
roast, dinner (*Worthington*), ¾" slice	180	12.0	5.0	12.0	<5	580	3.0
mix, dry, ⅓ cup:							
loaf, dinner (*Loma Linda*), ⅓ cup . .	90	14.0	7.0	1.5	0	560	5.0
patty (*Loma Linda*)	90	14.0	7.0	1.0	0	480	5.0
Vegetarian foods, see specific listings							
Venison, meat only, roasted, 4 oz. . . .	179	34.3	0	3.6	127	61	0
Vienna sausage, canned:							
(*Goya*), 4 links	170	7.0	1.0	15.0	70	430	0
(*Hormel*), 2 oz. . . .	140	6.0	1.0	13.0	45	420	0
(*Libby's*), 3 links . .	130	5.0	1.0	120	50	300	0
w/barbecue sauce (*Libby's* BBQ), 3 links	130	5.0	1.0	12.0	50	330	0

Food and Measure	cal.	prot. (gms)	carbo. (gms)	fat (gms)	chol. (mgs)	sod. (mgs)	fiber (gms)
Vienna sausage *(cont.)*							
w/hot sauce (*Goya*),							
3 links	130	5.0	1.0	12.0	50	320	0
chicken:							
(*Hormel*), 2 oz. . . .	110	6.0	1.0	10.0	55	420	0
(*Libby's*), 3 links	100	6.0	0	8.0	50	300	0
Vindaloo sauce, see							
"Curry sauce"							
Vine spinach, raw,							
untrimmed, 1 lb.	86	8.2	15.4	1.4	0	n.a.	4.0
Vinegar, 1 tbsp., ex-							
cept as noted:							
all varieties:							
(*Progresso*)	0	0	0	0	0	0	0
(*Regina*)	0	0	0	0	0	0	0
(*S&W*)	0	0	0	0	0	0	0
balsamic (*Pastorelli*							
Italian Chef)	5	0	2.0	0	0	0	0
red wine (*Pastorelli*							
Italian Chef)	2	0	0	0	0	0	0
Vodka sour mixer, in-							
stant (*Bar-Tenders*),							
2 pouches, 1.1 oz.	110	0	26.0	0	0	105	0

W

Food and Measure	cal.	prot. (gms)	carbo. (gms)	fat (gms)	chol. (mgs)	sod. (mgs)	fiber (gms)
Waffle, frozen, 2 pcs., except as noted:							
(*Downyflake* Butter & Syrup)	150	3.0	30.0	4.0	0	470	2.0
(*Downyflake* Crisp & Healthy)	170	4.0	34.0	2.0	0	340	2.0
(*Downyflake* Home-style), 4 pcs. . . .	230	4.0	29.0	4.0	0	620	2.0
(*Downyflake* Home-style Jumbo)	170	4.0	29.0	4.0	0	450	1.0
(*Downyflake* Hot 'n Buttery)	180	3.0	28.0	6.0	<5	490	2.0
(*Eggo* Homestyle) . .	220	5.0	30.0	8.0	25	470	0
(*Eggo Minis* Home-style), 3 sets	240	6.0	34.0	8.0	25	520	0
(*Nutri-Grain*)	190	5.0	30.0	6.0	0	430	4.0
(*Special K*)	140	6.0	29.0	0	0	250	0
apple cinnamon:							
(*Downyflake* Crisp & Healthy)	180	4.0	36.0	2.0	0	360	2.0
apple cinnamon (*Eggo*)	220	5.0	33.0	8.0	20	450	0
blueberry:							
(*Aunt Jemima*) . . .	190	4.0	38.0	7.0	10	530	1.0
(*Downyflake*)	180	3.0	31.0	4.0	0	480	1.0
(*Eggo*)	220	5.0	33.0	8.0	20	450	0
(*Eggo Minis*), 3 sets	240	6.0	37.0	8.0	25	510	0
buttermilk:							
(*Aunt Jemima*) . . .	170	4.0	27.0	6.0	10	410	1.0
(*Downyflake*)	160	4.0	28.0	4.0	<5	480	1.0
(*Eggo*)	220	5.0	30.0	8.0	25	480	0

Food and Measure	cal.	prot. (gms)	carbo. (gms)	fat (gms)	chol. (mgs)	sod. (mgs)	fiber (gms)
Waffle *(cont.)*							
cinnamon:							
(*Aunt Jemima*) . . .	180	4.0	28.0	6.0	10	470	1.0
toast (*Eggo*), 3 sets	280	5.0	44.0	9.0	25	470	0
multibran (*Nutri-*							
Grain)	200	5.0	32.0	6.0	0	400	6.0
nut and honey (*Eggo*)	240	6.0	32.0	10.0	25	480	0
oat bran:							
(*Common Sense*)	200	6.0	27.0	7.0	0	350	3.0
w/fruit and nut							
(*Common Sense*)	220	6.0	32.0	8.0	0	340	4.0
oatmeal (*Aunt Je-*							
mima)	170	4.0	27.0	7.0	0	660	3.0
raisin and bran (*Nutri-*							
Grain)	210	5.0	36.0	6.0	0	390	5.0
strawberry (*Eggo*) . .	220	5.0	32.0	8.0	20	460	0
whole grain (*Aunt Je-*							
mima)	170	5.0	24.0	7.0	0	450	2.0
Waffle breakfast, fro-							
zen (*Swanson Kids*							
Breakfast Blast),							
1 pkg.	330	26.0	39.0	17.0	75	250	1.0
Waffle mix, see "Pan-							
cake mix"							
Walnut, dried:							
(*Paradise/Wild Swan*),							
¼ cup, 1 oz.	190	4.0	3.0	18.0	0	0	3.0
black:							
(*Planters*),							
2-oz. pkg.	340	14.0	8.0	31.0	0	0	3.0
shelled, 1 oz. . . .	172	6.9	3.4	16.1	0	<1	1.4
chopped, 1 cup . .	759	30.4	15.1	70.7	0	2	6.3
English or Persian:							
shelled, 1 oz. . . .	182	4.1	5.2	17.6	0	3	1.4
pcs., 1 cup	770	17.2	22.0	74.2	0	12	5.8
halves, 1 cup . . .	642	14.3	18.3	61.9	0	10	4.8
halves:							
(*Planters*), ⅓ cup	220	5.0	5.0	22.0	0	0	1.0

Food and Measure	cal.	prot. (gms)	carbo. (gms)	fat (gms)	chol. (mgs)	sod. (mgs)	fiber (gms)
(*Planters Gold Measure*), 2-oz. pkg.	380	8.0	8.0	38.0	0	0	2.0
pieces (*Planters*), ¼ cup	190	4.0	4.0	20.0	0	0	1.0
Walnut topping, syrup (*Smucker's*), 2 tbsp.	190	2.0	23.0	10.0	0	0	0
Waterchestnuts, Chinese:							
fresh:							
4 medium, 2″ . . .	38	.5	8.6	<.1	0	5	1.1
sliced, ½ cup . . .	66	.9	14.8	.1	0	9	1.9
(*Frieda's*), 1 oz. . .	22	.4	5.4	.1	0	6	n.a.
canned:							
4 medium or 1 oz.	14	.3	3.5	<.1	0	2	.7
w/liquid, sliced, ½ cup	35	.6	8.7	<.1	0	6	1.8
(*La Choy*), 2 pcs.	10	0	2.0	0	0	0	1.0
sliced (*La Choy*), 2 tbsp.	10	0	3.0	0	0	0	1.0
sliced (*Sun Luck*), ¼ cup	15	0	4.0	0	0	0	1.0
Watercress:							
10 sprigs, 11¼″ . . .	3	.6	.3	<.1	0	10	.6
chopped, ½ cup . . .	2	.4	.2	<.1	0	7	.4
Watermelon:							
1″ slice, 10″ diam.	152	3.0	34.6	2.0	0	10	2.4
diced, ½ cup	25	.5	5.7	.3	0	2	.4
seedless (*Frieda's*), 1 oz.	7	.1	1.8	.1	0	<1	n.a.
Watermelon drink (*R.W. Knudsen* Cooler), 8 fl. oz. . .	120	0	29.0	0	0	10	0
Watermelon juice (*After the-Fall*), 8 fl. oz.	90	1.0	22.0	0	0	15	0
Watermelon seed, dried, 1 oz.	158	8.1	4.4	13.5	0	28	n.a.

Food and Measure	cal.	prot. (gms)	carbo. (gms)	fat (gms)	chol. (mgs)	sod. (mgs)	fiber (gms)
Wax beans:							
fresh, see "Green beans"							
canned, cut, ½ cup:							
(*S&W*)	20	1.0	4.0	0	0	400	1.0
(*Stokely*)	20	1.0	4.0	0	0	370	1.0
(*Stokely* No Salt)	20	1.0	4.0	0	0	25	1.0
golden (*Del Monte*)	20	1.0	4.0	0	0	360	2.0
frozen (*Seabrook*),							
⅔ cup	25	1.0	4.0	0	0	10	2.0
Wax gourd, boiled,							
cubed, ½ cup . . .	11	.4	2.6	.2	0	93	.9
Welsh rarebit, frozen							
(*Stouffer's*), 2.2 oz.	120	5.0	5.0	9.0	20	280	0
Wendy's, 1 serving:							
sandwiches:							
bacon cheeseburger							
Jr.	410	22.0	34.0	21.0	60	910	2.0
Big Bacon Classic	610	36.0	45.0	33.0	105	1510	3.0
cheeseburger:							
Jr.	320	17.0	34.0	13.0	45	770	2.0
Jr, deluxe	360	18.0	36.0	16.0	45	840	3.0
Kid's Meal . . .	320	17.0	33.0	13.0	45	770	2.0
chicken, grilled . .	290	24.0	35.0	7.0	55	720	2.0
chicken, breaded	440	28.0	44.0	18.0	60	840	2.0
chicken, spicy . . .	440	23.0	45.0	20.0	50	1220	8.0
chicken club	500	32.0	44.0	23.0	70	1090	2.0
hamburger:							
single, plain . .	360	25.0	31.0	16.0	65	460	2.0
single, everything	420	26.0	37.0	20.0	70	810	3.0
Jr.	270	15.0	34.0	10.0	30	560	2.0
Kid's Meal . . .	270	15.0	33.0	10.0	30	560	2.0
sandwich compo-							
nents:							
American cheese	70	3.0	1.0	5.0	15	320	0
American cheese Jr.	45	2.0	0	4.0	10	220	0
bacon, 1 slice . . .	30	2.0	0	2.5	5	125	0
ketchup, 1 tsp. . .	10	0	2.0	0	0	80	0

Food and Measure	cal.	prot. (gms)	carbo. (gms)	fat (gms)	chol. (mgs)	sod. (mgs)	fiber (gms)
mayonnaise,							
1½ tsp.	30	0	1.0	3.0	5	60	0
mustard, ½ tsp. . . .	0	0	0	0	0	55	0
onion, 4 rings . . .	0	0	1.0	0	0	0	0
pickles, 4 slices . .	0	0	0	0	0	140	0
chicken nuggets,							
5 pcs.	230	11.0	10.0	16.0	40	500	0
nuggets sauce, 1 oz.:							
barbecue	50	1.0	11.0	0	0	100	0
honey	45	0	12.0	0	0	0	0
honey mustard . .	130	0	6.0	12.0	0	n.a.	0
spicy buffalo wing	30	0	4.0	2.0	0	n.a.	0
sweet and sour . .	50	0	12.0	0	0	n.a.	0
chili:							
small, 8 oz.	210	15.0	21.0	7.0	30	800	5.0
large, 12 oz.	310	23.0	32.0	10.0	45	1190	7.0
cheddar cheese,							
shredded, 2 tbsp.	70	4.0	1.0	6.0	15	110	0
saltine crackers, 2	25	0	4.0	.5	0	80	0
baked potato:							
plain	310	7.0	71.0	0	0	25	7.0
bacon and cheese	540	17.0	78.0	18.0	20	1430	7.0
broccoli and cheese	470	9.0	80.0	14.0	5	470	9.0
cheese	570	14.0	78.0	23.0	30	640	7.0
chili and cheese . .	620	20.0	83.0	24.0	40	780	9.0
sour cream w/chive	380	8.0	74.0	6.0	15	40	8.0
fries:							
small	260	3.0	33.0	13.0	0	85	3.0
medium	380	5.0	47.0	19.0	0	120	5.0
Biggie	460	6.0	58.0	23.0	0	150	6.0
salads-to-go, fresh,							
w/out dressing:							
deluxe garden . . .	110	7.0	10.0	6.0	0	320	4.0
grilled chicken . . .	200	25.0	10.0	8.0	50	690	4.0
side salad	60	4.0	5.0	3.0	0	160	2.0
side salad, Caesar	110	8.0	8.0	5.0	10	660	2.0
taco salad	510	29.0	53.0	30.0	65	1230	10.0
soft breadstick . . .	130	4.0	24.0	3.0	5	250	1.0

Food and Measure	cal.	prot. (gms)	carbo. (gms)	fat (gms)	chol. (mgs)	sod. (mgs)	fiber (gms)
Wendy's *(cont.)*							
dressing, 2 tbsp.:							
blue cheese	170	1.0	0	19.0	15	190	0
French	120	0	6.0	10.0	0	330	0
French, fat free . .	30	0	8.0	0	0	150	0
French, sweet red	130	0	9.0	10.0	0	230	0
Italian, reduced fat/							
calorie	40	0	2.0	3.0	0	340	0
Italian Caesar . . .	150	1.0	1.0	16.0	20	250	0
ranch, *Hidden Valley*	90	0	1.0	10.0	10	240	0
ranch, *Hidden Valley*, reduced fat/							
calorie	60	0	2.0	5.0	10	240	0
Thousand Island . .	130	0	3.0	13.0	10	170	0
desserts:							
chocolate chip							
cookie	270	4.0	38.0	11.0	15	150	3.0
Frosty, small	340	9.0	57.0	10.0	40	200	3.0
Frosty, medium . .	460	12.0	76.0	13.0	55	260	4.0
Frosty, large	570	15.0	95.0	17.0	70	330	5.0
Wheat, whole grain:							
durum, 1 cup	650	26.3	136.6	4.7	0	3	n.a.
hard red:							
spring, 1 cup . . .	631	29.6	130.6	3.7	0	4	24.2
winter, 1 cup . . .	628	24.2	136.7	3.0	0	4	24.2
winter (*Arrowhead Mills*), ¼ cup . .	160	6.0	34.0	1.0	0	0	7.0
soft red winter, 1 cup	556	17.4	124.7	2.6	0	4	n.a.
hard white, 1 cup . .	656	21.7	145.7	3.3	0	n.a.	n.a.
soft white, 1 cup . .	571	18.0	126.6	3.3	0	n.a.	n.a.
Wheat, parboiled, see "Bulgur"							
Wheat, sprouted, 1 cup	214	8.1	45.9	1.4	0	18	n.a.
Wheat bran (see also "Cereal"), ¼ cup, except as noted:							
(*Arrowhead Mills*) . .	30	3.0	7.0	.5	0	0	6.0
(*Shiloh Farms*)	30	3.0	7.0	0	0	0	6.0

Food and Measure	cal.	prot. (gms)	carbo. (gms)	fat (gms)	chol. (mgs)	sod. (mgs)	fiber (gms)
crude, 2 tbsp.	15	1.1	4.5	.3	0	<1	3.0
toasted (*Kretschmer*)	30	4.0	6.0	1.0	0	210	7.0
unprocessed (*Quaker*),							
⅓ cup	30	3.0	11.0	0	0	0	8.0
Wheat grass (*Pines*),							
3 servings	29	2.6	4.0	0	0	3	1.6
Wheat flakes (*Arrow-*							
head Mills), ⅓ cup	110	4.0	24.0	.5	0	0	5.0
Wheat flour, ¼ cup,							
except as noted:							
all-purpose, white:							
1 cup	455	12.9	95.4	1.2	0	2	3.4
(*Goya*)	100	3.0	23.0	0	0	0	1.0
bleached (*Pills-*							
bury's)	100	3.0	23.0	0	0	0	<1.0
unbleached (*Pills-*							
bury)	100	3.0	21.0	0	0	0	<1.0
unbleached (*Arrow-*							
head Mills),							
⅓ cup	160	5.0	33.0	.5	0	0	0
unbleached, whole							
grain (*Arrowhead*							
Mills)	110	4.0	24.0	.5	0	0	4.0
cake, white:							
1 cup	395	8.9	85.1	.9	0	2	1.8
(*Swan's Down*) . .	100	2.0	22.0	0	0	0	0
bread, white (*Pills-*							
bury's)	100	4.0	22.0	0	0	0	<1.0
gluten (*Arrowhead*							
Mills), 3 tbsp. . . .	35	5.0	15.0	0	0	0	0
pastry, soft:							
white, unbleached							
(*Arrowhead Mills*)	100	3.0	23.0	.5	0	0	4.0
whole grain (*Arrow-*							
head Mills),							
⅓ cup	100	4.0	22.0	.5	0	0	3.0
presifted, white (*Pills-*							
bury Shake &							
Blend)	100	3.0	23.0	0	0	0	<1.0

Food and Measure	cal.	prot. (gms)	carbo. (gms)	fat (gms)	chol. (mgs)	sod. (mgs)	fiber (gms)
Wheat flour *(cont.)*							
self-rising, white:							
1 cup	442	12.4	92.8	1.2	0	1587	4.0
bleached or un-							
bleached (*Pills-*							
bury's)	100	3.0	22.0	0	0	360	<1.0
tortilla mix	449	10.7	74.5	11.8	0	751	n.a.
whole grain:							
1 cup	407	16.4	87.1	2.2	0	1	15.1
stone ground (*Ar-*							
rowhead Mills),							
¼ cup	130	5.0	25.0	.5	0	0	4.0
whole wheat (*Pills-*							
bury)	120	5.0	1.0	0	0	0	<1.0
Wheat germ:							
(*Kretschmer*), 2 tbsp.	50	4.0	6.0	1.0	0	140	2.0
crude, 1 oz.	102	6.6	14.7	2.8	0	3	3.7
honey crunch (*Kret-*							
schmer), 1⅔ tbsp.	50	4.0	8.0	1.0	0	135	1.0
raw (*Arrowhead*							
Mills), 3 tbsp. . . .	50	3.0	10.0	.5	0	0	2.0
toasted, 1 oz.	108	8.3	14.1	3.0	0	1	3.7
Wheat nuts (*So-*							
noma), 2 tbsp. . . .	60	0	8.0	3.0	0	140	1.0
Wheat pilaf mix							
(*Near East*), 1 cup*	220	6.0	42.0	4.5	0	690	5.0
Whelk, meat only,							
raw, 4 oz.	156	27.0	8.8	.5	74	234	0
Whey, fluid:							
acid, 1 cup	59	1.9	12.6	.2	0	118	0
sweet, 1 cup	66	2.1	12.6	.9	5	132	0
Whipped topping, see							
"Cream topping"							
Whiskey, see							
"Liquor"							
Whiskey sour mixer:							
bottled, 4 fl. oz.:							
(*Holland House*) . .	150	0	34.0	0	0	115	0
(*Mr. & Mrs. "T"*)	100	0	23.0	0	0	50	0

Food and Measure	cal.	prot. (gms)	carbo. (gms)	fat (gms)	chol. (mgs)	sod. (mgs)	fiber (gms)
mix:							
(*Bar-Tenders*),							
2 pkts.	130	0	30.0	0	0	90	0
(*Bar-Tenders* Lite),							
3 pkts.	20	0	2.0	0	0	70	0
(*Bar-Tenders*							
Slightly Sour),							
2 pkts.	120	0	28.0	0	0	65	0
White bean, ½ cup:							
dried:							
boiled	125	8.6	22.6	.3	0	6	5.7
small, boiled	127	8.1	23.2	.6	0	2	3.7
canned:							
w/liquid	153	9.5	28.7	.4	0	595	6.3
(*Goya*)	80	6.0	18.0	.2	0	386	7.0
small (*S&W*) . . .	80	7.0	19.0	.5	0	440	6.0
in tomato sauce							
(*Goya* Guisados)	110	6.0	19.0	1.0	0	600	9.0
White sauce mix:							
1¾-oz. pkt.	230	5.4	25.1	13.2	tr.	1691	<1.0
(*Knorr*), ⅛ pkg. . . .	25	0	4.0	1.0	0	200	0
Whitefish, meat only:							
raw, 4 oz.	153	21.7	0	6.7	68	58	0
baked, broiled, or mi-							
crowaved, 4 oz. . .	195	27.7	0	8.5	87	74	0
smoked, 4 oz.	122	26.5	0	1.1	37	1156	0
Whiting, meat only:							
raw, 4 oz.	102	20.8	0	1.5	76	82	0
baked, broiled, or mi-							
crowaved, 4 oz. . .	130	26.6	0	1.9	95	150	0
Wiener, see "Frank-							
furter"							
Wild rice:							
raw, 1 oz.	101	4.2	21.2	.3	0	2	1.7
raw (*Fantastic Foods*),							
¼ cup	140	6.0	28.0	0	0	0	2.0
cooked, 1 cup	166	6.5	35.0	.6	0	6	1.5
blends, see "Rice"							

Food and Measure	cal.	prot. (gms)	carbo. (gms)	fat (gms)	chol. (mgs)	sod. (mgs)	fiber (gms)
Wild rice dishes, see "Rice dishes"							
Wine, 1 fl. oz.:							
dessert or apertif[1] . .	41	tr.	2.3	0	0	1	0
dry or table[2]	25	tr.	1.2	0	0	1	0
Wine, cooking, 2 tbsp.:							
(*La Vina* Gold)	2	0	0	0	0	210	0
Marsala (*Holland House*)	35	0	2.0	0	0	190	0
red (*Holland House*)	20	0	1.0	0	0	190	0
red (*La Vina*)	2	0	0	0	0	220	0
sherry (*Holland House*)	45	0	2.0	0	0	190	0
vermouth (*Holland House*)	20	0	0	0	0	190	0
white (*La Vina*) . . .	2	0	0	0	0	230	0
white, regular or lemon flavor (*Holland House*)	20	0	0	0	0	190	0
Wine cooler, pear (*Bartles & Jaymes*), 12-oz. bottle:							
berry	220	0	33.0	0	0	0	0
black cherry	210	0	31.0	0	0	0	0
Fuzzy Navel	250	0	41.0	0	0	0	0
iced tea, Long Island	250	0	42.0	0	0	15	0
Mai Tai	250	0	41.0	0	0	0	0
margarita	270	0	45.0	0	0	40	0
original	200	0	29.0	0	0	0	0
peach	220	0	34.0	0	0	0	0
piña colada	280	0	48.0	0	0	0	0
strawberry	220	0	32.0	0	0	0	0
strawberry daiquiri	230	0	36.0	0	0	0	0

[1] *Includes fortified wines containing more than 15% alcohol, such as port, sherry, vermouth, etc.*
[2] *Includes wines containing less than 15% alcohol, such as burgundy, Chablis, champagne, etc.*

Food and Measure	cal.	prot. (gms)	carbo. (gms)	fat (gms)	chol. (mgs)	sod. (mgs)	fiber (gms)
tropical	240	0	37.0	0	0	0	0
Winged bean, ½ cup:							
fresh:							
raw, sliced	11	1.5	1.0	.2	0	1	n.a.
boiled, drained . . .	12	1.6	1.0	.2	0	1	n.a.
dried:							
raw	372	27.0	38.0	14.9	0	35	14.1
boiled	126	9.1	12.8	5.0	0	11	n.a.
Winged bean leaves,							
trimmed, 1 oz. . . .	21	1.7	4.0	.3	0	n.a.	n.a.
Winged bean tuber,							
trimmed, 1 oz. . . .	45	3.3	8.0	.3	0	n.a.	n.a.
Wolf fish, Atlantic,							
meat only:							
raw, 4 oz.	109	19.9	0	2.7	52	97	0
baked, broiled, or mi-							
crowaved, 4 oz. . .	139	25.4	0	3.5	67	124	0
Wonton wrapper:							
(*Frieda's*), 1 pc. . . .	13	.4	4.4	0	0	26	0
(*Nasoya*), 5 pcs. . . .	90	3.0	18.0	0	5	230	0
Worcestershire							
sauce, 1 tsp.:							
(*Lea & Perrins*) . . .	5	0	1.0	0	0	65	0
(*French's*)	0	0	<1.0	0	0	55	0
white wine (*Lea &*							
Perrins)	0	0	0	0	0	50	0
wine and pepper (*Try*							
Me)	0	0	1.0	0	0	90	0

Y

Food and Measure	cal.	prot. (gms)	carbo. (gms)	fat (gms)	chol. (mgs)	sod. (mgs)	fiber (gms)
Yam, ½ cup:							
baked or boiled . . .	79	1.0	18.8	.1	0	6	2.7
canned or frozen, see "Sweet potato"							
Yam, mountain, Hawaiian, ½ cup:							
raw, cubed	46	.9	11.1	.1	0	9	n.a.
steamed, cubed . . .	59	1.2	14.4	.1	0	9	n.a.
Yam bean tuber:							
raw:							
sliced, ½ cup . . .	23	.4	5.3	.1	0	3	n.a.
(*Frieda's*), 3.5 oz.	45	1.2	10.2	.1	0	n.a.	n.a.
boiled, drained, 4 oz.	43	.8	10.0	.1	0	5	n.a.
Yard-long bean:							
fresh, sliced, ½ cup:							
raw	22	1.3	3.8	.2	0	2	n.a.
boiled, drained . . .	25	1.3	4.8	.1	0	2	n.a.
dried, ½ cup:							
raw	292	20.4	52.0	1.1	0	14	4.0
boiled	102	7.1	18.1	.4	0	4	1.4
Yeast, baker's, all varieties (*Fleischmann's*), ¼ tsp. . . .	0	0	0	0	0	0	0
Yellow beans, dried, boiled, ½ cup . . .	126	8.1	22.2	1.0	0	4	n.a.
Yellow squash:							
fresh or frozen, see "Crookneck squash"							
canned (*Allen/Sunshine*), ½ cup . . .	25	0	5.0	0	0	160	2.0

Food and Measure	cal.	prot. (gms)	carbo. (gms)	fat (gms)	chol. (mgs)	sod. (mgs)	fiber (gms)
Yellowtail, meat only:							
raw, 4 oz.	166	26.3	0	6.0	n.a.	44	0
baked, broiled, or microwaved, 4 oz. . . .	212	33.6	0	7.6	n.a.	57	0
Yogurt, 1 cup or 8 oz., except as noted:							
plain:							
(*Breyers*)	130	11.0	15.0	3.0	20	150	0
(*Colombo* Lowfat)	120	8.0	12.0	4.5	20	150	0
(*Colombo* Nonfat)	110	11.0	16.0	0	5	170	0
(*Dannon* Lowfat), 8 oz.	140	12.0	16.0	2.0	20	150	0
(*Dannon* Lowfat), 1 cup	150	13.0	17.0	2.5	20	170	0
(*Dannon* Nonfat), 8 oz.	110	12.0	16.0	0	5	150	0
(*Dannon* Nonfat), 1 cup	120	13.0	17.0	0	0	170	0
(*Ultimate 90*) . . .	90	8.0	14.0	0	5	150	0
all fruit flavors:							
(*Light n'Lively Free 50 Cal*), 4.4 oz.	50	5.0	8.0	0	<5	60	0
except banana (*Dannon Sprinkl'ins*), 4.1 oz.	140	5.0	24.0	2.5	10	95	0
apple cinnamon (*Dannon* Fruit on Bottom)	240	9.0	46.0	3.0	15	140	1.0
apple spice or apricot (*Colombo*)	190	8.0	39.0	0	5	130	0
banana:							
(*Dannon Sprinkl'ins*), 4.1 oz. . . .	140	5.0	24.0	2.5	10	85	0
(*Tropifruita*), 6 oz.	150	7.0	30.0	0	5	105	0
banana cream pie (*Dannon*)	100	9.0	17.0	0	<5	150	0

Food and Measure	cal.	prot. (gms)	carbo. (gms)	fat (gms)	chol. (mgs)	sod. (mgs)	fiber (gms)
Yogurt *(cont.)*							
banana creme straw- berry (*Dannon* *Double Delights*), 6 oz.	170	7.0	30.0	2.5	10	90	1.0
banana strawberry:							
(*Colombo* Lowfat)	210	6.0	39.0	3.5	15	110	0
(*Colombo* Nonfat)	200	8.0	42.0	0	5	130	0
Bavarian creme rasp- berry (*Dannon* *Double Delights*), 6 oz.	170	7.0	31.0	2.5	10	115	0
berry, mixed:							
(*Breyers*)	250	8.0	48.0	2.5	15	110	0
(*Dannon* Fruit on Bottom)	240	9.0	45.0	3.0	15	150	1.0
(*Knudsen Free*), 6 oz.	170	8.0	33.0	0	5	105	0
(*Light n' Lively* *Free*), 6 oz. . . .	170	8.0	34.0	0	5	105	0
blueberry:							
(*Breyers*)	250	8.0	48.0	2.5	15	110	0
(*Colombo* Lowfat)	200	6.0	36.0	3.5	15	110	0
(*Colombo* Nonfat)	190	8.0	39.0	0	5	130	0
(*Dannon Danimals*), 4.4 oz.	140	6.0	25.0	2.0	10	90	0
(*Dannon* Fruit on the Bottom) . . .	240	9.0	46.0	3.0	15	140	1.0
(*Dannon* Nonfat) . .	100	9.0	20.0	0	<5	140	0
(*Knudsen Cal 70*), 6 oz.	70	7.0	12.0	0	5	80	0
(*Light n' Lively* Multi), 4.4 oz. . . .	140	5.0	27.0	1.0	10	65	0
(*Light n' Lively* *Free*), 6 oz. . . .	190	8.0	38.0	0	5	105	0
(*Light n' Lively Free* 70 Cal), 6 oz. . .	70	7.0	11.0	0	<5	80	0
and creme (*Ultimate* *90*)	90	8.0	14.0	0	5	140	3.0

Food and Measure	cal.	prot. (gms)	carbo. (gms)	fat (gms)	chol. (mgs)	sod. (mgs)	fiber (gms)
boysenberry (*Dannon* Fruit on Bottom) . .	240	9.0	45.0	3.0	15	150	1.0
cappuccino:							
(*Colombo*)	180	9.0	35.0	0	<5	140	0
(*Dannon*)	100	9.0	17.0	0	<5	140	0
(*Ultimate 90*) . . .	90	8.0	14.0	0	5	140	0
w/chocolate (*Dannon Light'n Crunchy*)	150	9.0	27.0	0	<5	170	0
caramel apple (*Dannon Light'n Crunchy*)	150	9.0	28.0	0	<5	180	0
cheesecake, strawberry/cherry (*Dannon Double Delights*), 6 oz.	170	7.0	30.0	2.5	10	90	1.0
cherry:							
(*Colombo*)	190	8.0	39.0	0	5	135	0
(*Dannon* Fruit on Bottom)	240	9.0	46.0	3.0	15	135	1.0
cherry, black:							
(*Breyers*)	260	8.0	50.0	2.5	15	110	0
(*Colombo*)	200	6.0	36.0	3.5	15	115	0
(*Knudsen Cal 70*), 6 oz.	70	7.0	12.0	0	5	85	0
(*Light n' Lively Free 70 Cal*), 6 oz. . .	70	7.0	11.0	0	<5	85	0
cherry jubilee (*Ultimate 90*)	90	8.0	14.0	0	5	140	0
cherry vanilla:							
(*Dannon*), 8 oz. . .	100	9.0	17.0	0	<5	140	0
(*Dannon*), 1 cup . .	110	9.0	19.0	0	<5	160	0
chocolate, white, and raspberry (*Yoplait*), 6 oz.	180	7.0	33.0	1.5	10	125	0
coffee:							
(*Breyers*)	220	10.0	38.0	3.0	20	135	0
(*Dannon*), 8 oz. . .	210	10.0	36.0	3.0	15	160	0
(*Dannon*), 1 cup . .	230	11.0	39.0	3.5	20	170	0

Food and Measure	cal.	prot. (gms)	carbo. (gms)	fat (gms)	chol. (mgs)	sod. (mgs)	fiber (gms)
Yogurt *(cont.)*							
coconut cream pie							
(*Yoplait*), 6 oz. . .	200	7.0	35.0	3.0	10	125	0
cranberry raspberry:							
(*Dannon*)	210	10.0	36.0	3.0	15	160	0
(*Ultimate 90*) . . .	90	8.0	14.0	0	5	140	0
cranberry strawberry							
(*Colombo*)	200	8.0	43.0	0	5	120	0
creme caramel (*Dan-*							
non)	100	10.0	15.0	0	<5	125	0
French roast (*Co-*							
lombo)	180	9.0	35.0	0	<5	140	0
fruit cocktail (*Co-*							
lombo)	190	8.0	39.0	0	5	130	0
guava (*Tropifruita*),							
6 oz.	150	7.0	29.0	0	5	105	0
lemon:							
(*Colombo*)	170	10.0	33.0	0	<5	150	0
(*Dannon* Lowfat),							
8 oz.	210	10.0	36.0	3.0	15	160	0
(*Dannon* Lowfat),							
1 cup	230	11.0	39.0	3.5	20	170	0
(*Dannon* Nonfat) . .	100	9.0	17.0	0	<5	140	0
(*Knudsen Cal 70*),							
6 oz.	70	7.0	11.0	0	5	100	<1.0
(*Knudsen Free*),							
6 oz.	160	8.0	33.0	0	5	105	0
(*Light n' Lively*							
Free), 6 oz. . . .	170	8.0	35.0	0	5	105	0
(*Light n' Lively Free*							
70 Cal), 6 oz. . .	70	7.0	12.0	0	<5	120	0
creamy (*Breyers*)	220	10.0	38.0	3.0	20	140	0
ice (*Dannon*							
Danimals), 4.4 oz.	130	6.0	22.0	2.0	10	90	0
lemon chiffon:							
(*Dannon*), 6 oz. . .	150	7.0	31.0	0	<5	110	0
(*Ultimate 90*) . . .	90	8.0	14.0	0	5	140	1.0

Food and Measure	cal.	prot. (gms)	carbo. (gms)	fat (gms)	chol. (mgs)	sod. (mgs)	fiber (gms)
w/blueberry (*Dannon Light'n Crunchy*)	140	9.0	26.0	0	<5	150	0
mango (*Tropifruita*), 6 oz.	150	7.0	31.0	0	5	105	0
orange (*Dannon* Fruit on Bottom)	240	9.0	45.0	3.0	15	135	0
orange-banana (*Dannon Danimals*), 4.4 oz.	140	6.0	24.0	2.0	10	80	0
papaya-pineapple (*Tropifruita*), 6 oz.	150	7.0	30.0	0	5	105	0
peach:							
(*Breyers*)	250	8.0	48.0	2.5	15	110	0
(*Colombo*)	190	8.0	39.0	0	5	130	0
(*Dannon* Fruit on Bottom)	240	9.0	45.0	3.0	15	140	1.0
(*Dannon* Nonfat) . .	100	9.0	18.0	0	<5	140	0
(*Knudsen Cal 70*), 6 oz.	70	7.0	11.0	0	5	80	<1.0
(*Knudsen Free*), 6 oz.	170	8.0	33.0	0	5	105	0
(*Light n' Lively* Multi), 4.4 oz. . .	140	5.0	27.0	1.0	10	65	0
(*Light n' Lively* Free), 6 oz. . . .	170	8.0	35.0	0	5	105	0
(*Light n' Lively Free* 70 Cal), 6 oz. . .	70	6.0	12.0	0	<5	80	0
(*Ultimate 90*) . . .	90	8.0	14.0	0	5	140	0
(*Yoplait* Tropical), 6 oz.	180	7.0	33.0	1.5	10	125	0
Melba (*Colombo* Lowfat)	200	6.0	36.0	3.5	15	115	0
pear (*Dannon* Fruit on the Bottom)	240	9.0	45.0	3.0	15	135	0
piña colada (*Tropifruita*), 6 oz.	150	7.0	30.0	0	5	105	0
pineapple:							
(*Breyers*)	250	8.0	49.0	2.5	15	110	0

Food and Measure	cal.	prot. (gms)	carbo. (gms)	fat (gms)	chol. (mgs)	sod. (mgs)	fiber (gms)
Yogurt, pineapple *(cont.)*							
(*Knudsen Cal 70*),							
6 oz.	70	7.0	11.0	0	5	80	0
(*Light n' Lively*							
Multi), 4.4 oz. . . .	140	5.0	27.0	1.0	5	60	0
plum (*Dannon* Fruit							
on Bottom)	240	9.0	45.0	3.0	15	160	0
raspberry:							
(*Breyers*)	250	8.0	48.0	2.5	15	110	2.0
(*Colombo* Lowfat)	210	6.0	39.0	3.5	15	115	0
(*Colombo* Nonfat)	190	8.0	39.0	0	5	130	0
(*Dannon* Fruit on							
Bottom)	240	9.0	45.0	3.0	15	150	1.0
(*Dannon* Nonfat) . .	100	9.0	18.0	0	<5	150	0
(*Knudsen Cal 70*)							
6 oz.	70	7.0	11.0	0	5	75	0
(*Knudsen Free*),							
6 oz.	160	8.0	31.0	0	5	105	0
(*Light n' Lively*							
Multi), 4.4 oz. . . .	130	5.0	24.0	1.0	10	65	0
(*Light n' Lively*							
Free), 6 oz.	180	8.0	36.0	0	5	105	0
(*Light n' Lively Free*							
70 Cal), 6 oz. . . .	70	7.0	11.0	0	<5	80	0
creme (*Ultimate 90*)	90	8.0	14.0	0	5	140	0
w/granola (*Dannon*							
Light 'n Crunchy)	150	10.0	17.0	0	<5	135	0
wild (*Dannon*							
Danimals), 4.4 oz.	130	6.0	22.0	2.0	10	80	0
strawberry:							
(*Breyers*)	250	8.0	47.0	2.5	15	110	0
(*Colombo* Lowfat)	200	6.0	36.0	3.5	15	110	0
(*Colombo* Nonfat)	190	8.0	39.0	0	5	135	0
(*Dannon Danimals*),							
4.4 oz.	140	6.0	24.0	2.0	10	85	0
(*Dannon* Nonfat),							
8 oz.	100	9.0	18.0	0	<5	140	0
(*Dannon* Nonfat),							
1 cup	110	9.0	19.0	0	<5	160	0

Food and Measure	cal.	prot. (gms)	carbo. (gms)	fat (gms)	chol. (mgs)	sod. (mgs)	fiber (gms)
(*Knudsen Cal 70*),							
6 oz.	70	7.0	11.0	0	5	85	0
(*Knudsen Free*),							
6 oz.	160	8.0	32.0	0	5	105	0
(*Light n' Lively*							
Multi), 4.4 oz. . .	140	5.0	26.0	1.0	10	65	0
(*Light n' Lively*							
Free), 6 oz. . . .	180	8.0	36.0	0	5	105	0
(*Light n' Lively Free*							
70 Cal), 6 oz. . .	70	7.0	11.0	0	<5	85	0
(*Tropifruita*), 6 oz.	150	7.0	31.0	0	5	105	0
(*Ultimate 90*) . . .	90	8.0	14.0	0	5	140	2.0
(*Yoplait*), 6 oz. . .	180	7.0	33.0	1.5	10	125	0
fruit basket (*Knud-*							
sen Cal 70), 6 oz.	70	7.0	11.0	0	5	90	0
fruit cup (*Dannon*)	100	9.0	18.0	0	<5	140	0
fruit cup (*Light n'*							
Lively Free), 6 oz.	170	8.0	35.0	0	5	105	0
fruit cup (*Light n'*							
Lively Multi),							
4.4 oz.	140	5.0	27.0	1.0	10	60	0
fruit cup (*Light n'*							
Lively Free							
70 Cal), 6 oz. . .	70	7.0	11.0	0	<5	80	0
wild (*Light n' Lively*							
Kidpack), 4.4 oz.	140	5.0	28.0	1.0	10	65	0
strawberry-banana:							
(*Breyers*)	250	9.0	50.0	2.5	15	115	<1.0
(*Dannon* Fruit on							
Bottom)	240	9.0	43.0	3.0	15	140	1.0
(*Dannon* Nonfat) . .	100	9.0	18.0	0	<5	140	0
(*Knudsen 70*), 6 oz.	70	7.0	11.0	0	5	85	0
(*Light n' Lively*							
Multi), 4.4 oz. . .	140	5.0	28.0	1.0	10	60	0
(*Light n' Lively Free*							
70 Cal), 6 oz. . .	70	7.0	11.0	0	<5	85	0
(*Tropifruita*), 6 oz.	150	7.0	31.0	0	5	105	0
(*Ultimate 90*) . . .	90	8.0	14.0	0	5	140	2.0

Food and Measure	cal.	prot. (gms)	carbo. (gms)	fat (gms)	chol. (mgs)	sod. (mgs)	fiber (gms)
Yogurt, strawberry-banana *(cont.)*							
(*Yoplait*), 6 oz. . .	180	7.0	33.0	1.5	10	125	0
strawberry-kiwi, 6 oz.:							
(*Tropifruita*)	150	7.0	30.0	0	5	105	0
(*Yoplait*)	180	7.0	33.0	1.5	10	125	0
strawberry pineapple							
orange (*Colombo*)	190	8.0	38.0	0	5	125	0
tropical fruit (*Dannon*)	100	9.0	19.0	0	<5	140	0
tropical punch (*Dan-non Danimals*),							
4.4 oz.	140	6.0	25.0	2.0	10	85	0
vanilla:							
(*Breyers*)	220	10.0	38.0	3.0	20	135	0
(*Colombo*)	170	10.0	32.0	0	5	150	0
(*Dannon Danimals*),							
4.4 oz.	140	6.0	24.0	2.0	10	80	0
(*Dannon* Lowfat),							
8 oz.	210	10.0	36.0	3.0	15	160	0
(*Dannon* Lowfat),							
1 cup	230	11.0	39.0	3.5	20	170	0
(*Dannon* Nonfat),							
8 oz.	100	9.0	17.0	0	<5	140	0
(*Dannon* Nonfat),							
1 cup	110	10.0	18.0	0	<5	160	0
(*Knudsen Cal 70*),							
6 oz.	70	7.0	11.0	0	5	80	0
(*Knudsen Free*),							
6 oz.	170	8.0	32.0	0	5	100	0
(*Light n' Lively Free*), 6 oz. . . .	160	8.0	32.0	0	5	105	0
(*Ultimate 90*) . . .	90	8.0	14.0	0	5	140	0
French (*Colombo*)	180	7.0	29.0	2.5	20	130	0
French (*Dannon* Nonfat), 6 oz. . .	160	7.0	31.0	0	<5	100	0
w/chocolate (*Dan-non Light'n Crunchy*)	150	9.0	26.0	0	<5	170	0

Food and Measure	cal.	prot. (gms)	carbo. (gms)	fat (gms)	chol. (mgs)	sod. (mgs)	fiber (gms)
vanilla peach apricot or strawberry (*Dannon Double Delights*), 6 oz.	170	7.0	30.0	2.5	10	90	0
Yogurt, frozen, ½ cup:							
banana:							
cream pie (*Dannon Light'n Crunchy*)	110	4.0	24.0	1.0	0	65	0
pudding, homestyle (*TCBY*)	120	3.0	22.0	2.0	5	55	0
cappuccino:							
(*Ben & Jerry's* Nonfat)	150	5.0	30.0	0	0	80	0
(*Dannon Light*) . .	80	4.0	19.0	0	0	70	0
caramel praline crunch (*Edy's*) . . .	100	4.0	22.0	0	5	70	0
cherry vanilla:							
black, swirl (*Edy's*)	90	4.0	19.0	0	5	65	0
chocolate cherry (*Dannon Pure Indulgence*)	150	4.0	26.0	3.0	15	85	0
chocolate chip (*Ben & Jerry's Cherry Garcia*)	160	3.0	30.0	3.0	5	70	0
swirl (*Dannon Light*)	90	3.0	21.0	0	0	65	0
chocolate:							
(*Ben & Jerry's* Nonfat)	130	3.0	29.0	0	0	50	1.0
(*Dannon Light*) . .	80	4.0	21.0	0	0.	60	1.0
(*Edy's*)	100	3.0	17.0	2.5	10	30	0
(*Edy's* Nonfat) . . .	90	4.0	19.0	0	0	65	0
(*Häagen-Dazs*) . . .	160	8.0	26.0	2.5	30	60	<1.0
brownie chunk (*Edy's*)	110	3.0	18.0	4.0	10	35	0
chip cookie dough (*Ben & Jerry's*)	210	5.0	39.0	3.5	10	110	<1.0
Dutch (*TCBY*) . . .	100	2.0	20.0	1.5	5	40	0

Food and Measure	cal.	prot. (gms)	carbo. (gms)	fat (gms)	chol. (mgs)	sod. (mgs)	fiber (gms)
Yogurt, frozen, chocolate *(cont.)*							
nut, chunky *(Dannon Pure Indulgence)*	150	6.0	25.0	3.0	0	65	0
triple *(Dannon Light 'n Crunchy)* . . .	110	4.0	28.0	0	0	60	0
chocolate fudge:							
(Dannon Pure Indulgence Coco-Nut)	160	5.0	28.0	3.0	15	70	0
(Edy's)	100	3.0	21.0	0	5	75	0
brownie *(Ben & Jerry's)*	180	6.0	34.0	2.0	5	115	2.0
citrus heights *(Edy's)*	80	2.0	18.0	2.5	10	25	0
coffee *(Häagen-Dazs)*	160	8.0	26.0	2.5	45	55	0
coffee fudge:							
(Ben & Jerry's Nonfat)	140	4.0	31.0	0	0	55	<1.0
sundae *(Edy's)* . . .	100	3.0	21.0	0	5	75	0
cookies 'n cream:							
(Dannon Pure Indulgence)	150	5.0	24.0	3.0	0	105	0
(Edy's)	120	3.0	20.0	4.0	10	70	0
(TCBY)	120	3.0	23.0	2.5	5	80	0
cone crunch, crispy *(TCBY)*	130	3.0	22.0	3.0	5	55	0
espresso, crunchy *(Dannon Pure Indulgence)*	150	5.0	26.0	3.0	15	85	0
lemon chiffon *(Dannon Light)*	90	4.0	22.0	0	0	65	0
marble fudge:							
(Edy's)	110	3.0	19.0	3.0	10	35	0
(Edy's Nonfat) . . .	100	3.0	22.0	0	5	75	0
mocha chocolate chunk *(Dannon Light'n Crunchy)* . .	110	4.0	26.0	1.0	0	60	0
Orange Tango (Häagen-Dazs) . . .	130	4.0	26.0	1.0	20	25	0

Food and Measure	cal.	prot. (gms)	carbo. (gms)	fat (gms)	chol. (mgs)	sod. (mgs)	fiber (gms)
orange vanilla swirl							
(Edy's)	100	3.0	17.0	2.5	10	30	0
peach:							
(TCBY)	110	3.0	21.0	1.0	5	45	0
perfectly (Edy's) . .	100	2.0	17.0	2.5	10	25	0
raspberry Melba							
(Dannon Light)	90	4.0	21.0	0	0	65	0
peanut butter fudge							
sundae (TCBY) . .	110	3.0	23.0	1.5	<5	50	0
peanut chocolate							
(Dannon Light'n							
Crunchy)	110	4.0	29.0	0	0	65	0
pecan praline crisp							
(TCBY)	110	3.0	23.0	1.5	5	50	0
piña colada (Häagen-							
Dazs)	130	3.0	26.0	1.5	25	25	0
pine-orange paradise							
(Edy's)	90	4.0	18.0	0	5	60	0
raspberry:							
(Edy's)	100	2.0	17.0	2.5	10	25	0
(Edy's Nonfat) . . .	90	3.0	18.0	0	5	50	0
black (Ben & Jerry's							
Nonfat)	140	3.0	32.0	0	0	55	0
vanilla swirl (Edy's)	100	3.0	17.0	2.5	10	30	0
Raspberry							
Randezvous							
(Häagen-Dazs) . . .	130	4.0	26.0	1.5	20	25	1.0
(Starburst), 1 cup . .	80	2.0	14.0	1.5	5	35	0
strawberry:							
(Edy's)	100	2.0	17.0	2.5	10	25	0
(Edy's Nonfat) . . .	90	3.0	18.0	0	5	55	0
cheesecake (Dannon							
Light)	90	4.0	22.0	0	0	60	0
chocolate chip							
(Edy's)	120	3.0	19.0	4.0	10	25	0
summertime (TCBY)	100	3.0	20.0	1.0	5	40	0
Strawberry Duet							
(Häagen-Dazs) . . .	130	3.0	26.0	2.0	25	25	<1.0

Food and Measure	cal.	prot. (gms)	carbo. (gms)	fat (gms)	chol. (mgs)	sod. (mgs)	fiber (gms)
Yogurt, frozen *(cont.)*							
toffee crunch:							
(*Ben & Jerry's*							
Heath)	190	3.0	32.0	6.0	10	115	0
(*Dannon Pure Indul-*							
gence Heath) . .	150	5.0	25.0	3.0	5	105	0
(*Edy's Heath*) . . .	120	4.0	19.0	4.0	10	50	0
vanilla:							
(*Dannon Light*) . .	80	4.0	21.0	0	0	65	0
(*Edy's*)	100	3.0	17.0	2.5	10	30	0
(*Edy's* Nonfat) . . .	90	4.0	19.0	0	5	65	0
(*Häagen-Dazs*) . . .	160	8.0	26.0	2.5	45	55	0
classic (*TCBY*) . . .	110	3.0	21.0	1.5	5	50	0
vanilla blueberry swirl							
(*Dannon Light 'n*							
Crunchy)	110	4.0	26.0	1.0	0	65	0
vanilla chocolate swirl							
(*Edy's*)	90	4.0	18.0	0	5	65	0
vanilla fudge (*Ben &*							
Jerry's Nonfat) . . .	160	5.0	35.0	0	0	85	<1.0
vanilla raspberry truf-							
fle (*Dannon Pure In-*							
dulgence)	150	5.0	25.0	3.0	15	70	1.0
Yogurt bar, frozen,							
1 pc.:							
all flavors (*Starburst*)	70	2.0	13.0	1.0	<5	25	0
Brownie Nut Blast							
(*Häagen-Dazs Ex-*							
träas)	220	8.0	29.0	8.0	40	65	1.0
cherry chocolate:							
chip (*Ben & Jerry's*							
Cherry Garcia) . .	260	5.0	31.0	14.0	15	70	2.0
fudge (*Häagen-*							
Dazs)	240	5.0	26.0	13.0	35	45	1.0
chocolate almond							
(*Frozfruit*)	130	4.0	23.0	4.0	0	10	0
chocolate fudge							
(*Edy's*)	240	4.0	26.0	15.0	10	45	0

Food and Measure	cal.	prot. (gms)	carbo. (gms)	fat (gms)	chol. (mgs)	sod. (mgs)	fiber (gms)
peach:							
(*Frozfruit*)	100	3.0	22.0	0	0	95	0
(*Häagen-Dazs*) . . .	90	2.0	20.0	1.0	15	20	0
piña colada (*Häagen-Dazs*)	100	3.0	19.0	1.0	15	45	0
raspberry and vanilla (*Häagen-Dazs*) . . .	90	3.0	19.0	1.0	15	25	0
strawberry/strawberry banana (*Frozfruit*)	100	3.0	22.0	0	0	85	0
Strawberry Cheesecake Craze (*Häagen-Dazs Exträas*) . . .	220	7.0	31.0	8.0	65	140	0
strawberry daiquiri (*Häagen-Dazs*) . . .	90	2.0	18.0	1.0	15	20	0
toffee crunch (*Edy's*)	250	3.0	31.0	14.0	15	75	0
Tropical Orange Passion (*Häagen-Dazs*)	100	2.0	20.0	1.0	15	20	0
vanilla almond (*Edy's*)	230	4.0	24.0	15.0	10	40	0
Yuca:							
boiled, drained (*Frieda's*), 4 oz.	77	1.2	38.6	.2	0	2	n.a.
frozen (*Goya*), ½ cup	191	1.4	44.0	1.0	0	8	1.7

Z

Food and Measure	cal.	prot. (gms)	carbo. (gms)	fat (gms)	chol. (mgs)	sod. (mgs)	fiber (gms)
Ziti dishes, frozen, marinara sauce (*The Budget Gourmet Side Dish*), 6.25 oz.	220	9.0	25.0	10.0	15	720	2.0
Zucchini, ½ cup, except as noted:							
fresh, raw:							
sliced	9	.8	1.9	.1	0	2	.8
baby, 1 large, 3⅛″	3	.4	.5	.1	0	tr.	n.a.
fresh, boiled, drained:							
sliced	14	.6	3.5	.1	0	2	1.3
mashed	19	.8	4.7	.1	0	3	1.7
canned, Italian style:							
(*Del Monte*)	30	1.0	7.0	0	0	490	1.0
(*Progresso*)	40	2.0	7.0	2.0	0	400	2.0
w/tomato juice . . .	33	1.2	7.8	.1	0	424	1.0
frozen, sliced (*Stilwell*), ⅔ cup	15	<1.0	2.0	0	0	15	1.0
Zucchini, breaded, frozen (*Empire*), 1 pc.	100	5.0	18.0	0	0	280	1.0